Handbook of Medical Emergencies in the Dental Office

Handbook of
Medical Emergencies
in the
Dental Office

STANLEY F. MALAMED, D.D.S.

Associate Professor, Division of Surgical Sciences,
Section of Anesthesia and Medicine,
University of Southern California School of Dentistry,
Los Angeles, California

Chapter 4, Medical-Legal Considerations, by
KENNETH S. ROBBINS, B.A., LL.B.

Attorney in private practice; Honolulu, Hawaii

THIRD EDITION
with **194** illustrations

The C. V. Mosby Company

ST. LOUIS • WASHINGTON, D.C. • TORONTO   1987

MOSBY

A TRADITION OF PUBLISHING EXCELLENCE

Editor: Darlene Barela Cooke
Assistant editor: Donna Saya Sokolowski
Project editor: Suzanne Seeley
Manuscript editor: Kathy Corbett Hickman
Designer: Susan E. Lane
Production: Kathy Burmann

THIRD EDITION

The C.V. Mosby Company
11830 Westline Industrial Drive, St. Louis, Missouri 63146

Library of Congress Cataloging-in-Publication Data

Malamed, Stanley F., 1944-
    Handbook of medical emergencies in the dental office.

    Includes bibliographies and index.
    1. Medical emergencies—Handbooks, manuals, etc.
2. Dental emergencies—Handbooks, manuals, etc.
I. Robbins, Kenneth S. II. Title. [DNLM: 1. Dentistry.
2. Emergencies. WB 105 M236h]
RC86.8.M34 1987   616'.025'0246176   86-23763
ISBN 0-8016-3102-5

VT/VH/VH 9 8 7   03/A/305

To my
mother and **father,**
who made it all possible, and
to my wife **Beverly** and children, **Heather, Jennifer,** and **Jeremy,**
who make it all so worthwhile,

I dedicate this book.

Foreword

In the past 20 years, dental physicians have truly joined the ranks of health professionals by developing competence in internal medicine, psychosedation, physical evaluation, and emergency medicine. Although technical excellence must never be sacrificed, the role of dentistry is broadening to include adequate pain and anxiety control, significant health screening, and emergency preparedness.

Is there anything more noble than the saving of a life? It is just as noble to avoid mortality or serious morbidity by proper pretreatment physical evaluation and by appropriate modification of dental therapy. It is equally as noble to discover undiagnosed disease and to refer the patient for proper care, thus adding significantly to longevity.

In a time when the credibility and motives of health professionals are under constant scrutiny, dentistry has added immeasurably to its public and professional image by extending its treatment scope in the public interest. This book on medical emergencies will be a valued addition to the library of the dental physician who has extended his or her horizons to include the broad health picture and has made the transition from the oral cavity to the complete patient. It is an excellent contribution to our literature.

Frank M. McCarthy, M.D., D.D.S.

Note

The treatment modalities and the indications and dosages of all drugs in the *Handbook of Medical Emergencies in the Dental Office* have been recommended in the medical literature. Unless specifically indicated, drug dosages are those recommended for adult patients.

The package insert for each drug should be consulted for use and dosages as approved by the FDA. Because standards of usage change, it is advisable to keep abreast of revised recommendations, particularly those concerning new drugs.

Preface

In December of 1975 I began writing the manuscript for *Handbook of Medical Emergencies in the Dental Office.* The book was completed and published in April of 1978. As I mentioned in the preface to that first edition, my primary aim in writing the book was, and still is, to stimulate the members of the dental profession—the doctor, dental hygienist, dental assistant, and all other office personnel—to improve and maintain their skills in the prevention of medical emergencies and in the management of emergencies that inevitably occur.

However, it is acknowledged that with proper patient management virtually all medical emergency situations within the dental office can be prevented. What then is the need for a textbook on the management of medical emergencies? This thought has occurred to me on many occasions over the past few years. Do these situations really happen? The answer, unfortunately, is yes, they definitely do. I have received numerous letters and telephone calls and have met many doctors and other dental personnel who have had real-life experiences with life-threatening medical problems. Virtually all of these situations have occurred within the dental office, but a significant number happened outside: on family outings, driving in a car, or at home.

There is still a need for increasing the awareness of the dental profession in the area of emergency medicine. Although a growing number of states currently mandate continued certification in cardiopulmonary resuscitation (CPR) for dental relicensure, all too many states have not yet addressed this important issue. As an Affiliate Faculty in Basic Life Support and as CPR Chairman for the American Heart Association Greater Los Angeles Affiliate's Metropolitan Division, I see the immense value in training all adults in the simple procedures

collectively known as basic life support. Local and state dental societies should continue to present courses in basic life support or should initiate them posthaste.

Visible progress has been made. The awareness of our profession has been elevated, and laudable achievements continue. Yet because of the very nature of the problem, what we require in dentistry is a continued maintenance of our high level of skill in the prevention, recognition, and management of medical emergencies. To do so, we must all participate in ongoing programs devised by individual doctors to meet the needs of their offices. These programs should include attendance at continuing education courses in emergency medicine, constant access to information on this subject (through journals and texts), semiannual or annual recertification in basic life support or advanced cardiac life support, and in-office practice sessions in emergency procedures for the entire office staff. Such a program is discussed more fully in Chapter 3. The ultimate goal in preparation of a dental office for emergencies should be for you, the reader, to be able to put yourself in the position of a victim of a serious medical emergency in your dental office, and for you to be confident that your office staff would be able to react promptly and effectively in the management of your problem.

Emergency medicine is a constantly evolving medical specialty, and because of this many changes have occurred since publication of the first and second editions of this text. My goal now, as it was then, is to enable you to manage the given emergency situation in an effective yet uncomplicated manner. Alternative treatments and alternative drugs, which are also effective, are advocated by some authors. Our goal, as well as theirs, is simply to preserve the life of the victim.

Continual revision and updating of essential materials is evident in this third edition. Significant changes have occurred in the sections that relate to the implementation of techniques of basic life support (BLS). In June of 1985 the American Heart Association met in Dallas, Texas to discuss and revise the techniques of basic life support and advanced cardiac life support. The findings and recommendations of this meeting were published in the Journal of the American Medical Association in June of 1986 and are contained in this third edition. The first section of the book, Prevention, has been thoroughly revised, as well as "Unconsciousness: General Considerations" (Chapter 5); "Airway Obstruction" (Chapter 11); "Diabetes Mellitus: Hyperglycemia and Hypoglycemia" (Chapter 17); and "Cardiac Arrest and Cardiopulmonary Resuscitation" (Chapter 30).

The basic format of the text—based on clinical signs and symptoms rather than on a systems-oriented approach—remains quite well received and is therefore unchanged in this edition.

As with the first two editions of this text, I have again been quite fortunate in having the opportunity to work with a number of people who made the job of revision somewhat more tolerable and, to a degree, enjoyable. While it is impossible to mention everyone involved in the production of this book, I must mention specifically the following persons, without whose help this volume could not have been completed: Dr. Christine L. Quinn, Dr. Hyrum Hatch, Patricia Sroka, Karine Bolton, and Jerry Drucker—all of whom participated as photographic models. As always, the tolerance and patience of Beverly Malamed and the rest of the Malamed clan were necessary and appreciated. Last, but by no means least, I want to thank my guardian angels at The C.V. Mosby Company: Donna Sokolowski, Melba Steube, and Darlene Barela Cooke, without whose gentle urging this third edition might not have been completed.

Reader input concerning the prior editions of this text has proven to be a valuable means of evaluating the needs for future revision, additions, or deletions. I greatly appreciate and indeed want to solicit comment from my readers.

Stanley F. Malamed

Contents

Handbook of Medical Emergencies in the Dental Office

1 *Introduction*

Life-threatening emergencies can and do occur in the practice of dentistry. They may happen to anyone: the dental patient, the doctor, members of the dental office staff, even a person who is simply waiting to accompany a patient home from the dental office. Although life-threatening emergency situations do not occur frequently within the typical dental practice, a number of factors may increase the rate at which these incidents arise. These include (1) the increasing number of older persons seeking dental treatment, (2) recent therapeutic advances by the medical profession, (3) the trend toward longer dental appointments, and (4) the increasing utilization and administration of drugs in the practice of dentistry. On the other hand, there are a number of other factors that the dental profession has at its disposal that will minimize the possibility of life-threatening situations occurring. Included are (1) the pretreatment physical evaluation of the dental patient, consisting of the patient-completed medical history questionnaire, physical examination of the patient, and the dialogue history, and (2) possible modification in dental therapy to decrease medical risk to the patient. It has been estimated that through the effective use of these procedures, all but about 10% of life-threatening situations can be prevented.

MORBIDITY IN DENTAL PRACTICE

In spite of the most meticulous precautions designed to prevent these situations from arising, some will still occur. What is the nature of the life-threatening emergencies that develop in dental practice? It must be stated at the outset that there are no medical emergency situations unique to the practice of dentistry. Any acute medical situation may arise. Table 1-1 lists the life-threatening situations that occurred at the School of Dentistry of the University of Southern California from 1973 to 1985. Although most of these problems arose during dental therapy, with the patient seated in the dental chair, others occurred elsewhere in the dental school: one patient had an episode of orthostatic hypotension while in the restroom, several patients suffered convulsive seizures while in the patient waiting room, and another patient suffered a seizure just outside the entrance to the dental clinic. Dental patients were not the only victims of these emergencies: an adult who was accompanying a patient home developed an allergic skin reaction following ingestion of aspirin for a headache, and a dental student seated in a lecture hall suffered episodes of vasodepressor syncope, as did a dentist who was treating a patient. Therefore it is not just the dental patient who is at risk during dental treatment!

Although all forms of medical emergency may develop in dental practice, some are seen with greater frequency. These are situations produced entirely by stress or those that are acutely exacerbated when the patient is under stress. These situations include vasodepressor syncope, the hyperventilation syndrome, and acute cardiovascular emergencies. Effective management of stress in the dental office will be instrumental in minimizing the occurrence of these situations.

Other life-threatening situations that occur with greater frequency in dental practice are those reactions associated with the administration of drugs. The most frequently observed reactions are those associated with the administration of local anesthetics, the most commonly used drugs in dentistry. Drug administration may bring with it a variety of adverse reactions, most frequently psychogenic reactions, drug overdose, and drug allergy. The majority of these reactions are stress related (psycho-

Table 1-1. Summary of medical emergency situations occurring at the USC School of Dentistry (1973-1985)

Nature of situation	
Hyperventilation	34
Convulsive seizures	31
Hypoglycemia	20
Vasodepressor syncope	19
Angina pectoris	11
Postural hypotension	11
Allergic reactions	10
Acute asthmatic attacks	6
Acute myocardial infarction	1
Site of occurrence	
Patient (during treatment)	88
Patient (before or after treatment)	31
Dental personnel	18
Other persons in dental office	6

Table 1-2. Years of life expected at birth in the United States

Year	Total	White male	White female	Black male	Black female
1981	74.2	71.1	78.5	64.4	73.0
1980	73.7	70.7	78.1	63.7	72.3
1979	73.8	69.9	77.8	—	—
1978	73.3	69.5	77.2	—	—
1975	72.5	68.7	76.5	—	—
1970	70.8	67.1	74.6	60.0	68.3
1960	69.7	66.6	73.1	—	—
1950	68.2	66.6	71.1	—	—
1940	62.9	60.8	65.2	—	—
1930	59.7	58.1	61.6	—	—
1920	54.1	53.6	54.6	—	—
1910	47.3	46.3	48.2	—	—

Data from Division of Vital Statistics, National Center for Health Statistics, 1985.

genic); however, many reactions are produced by the drug itself. Although not all of these adverse drug responses are preventable, most are. Thorough knowledge of drugs and proper techniques of drug administration are essential in preventing adverse drug reactions.

DEATH AND DENTAL PRACTICE

Most of the emergency situations that arise in dental practice are life threatening—threats to the life of the victim. Fortunately, however, it is only rarely that a patient actually dies in the dental office. Although accurate statistics on dental morbidity and mortality are difficult to obtain, surveys of dental practice have been taken by various investigators and organizations, including the Southern California Society of Oral Surgeons (Lytle, 1974) and the American Dental Association (Moen, 1963). In the 1962 American Dental Association survey, which included almost 4000 dentists, 45 deaths in dental offices were reported. Seven of these deaths occurred in the waiting room before the patient had undergone dental treatment. In a survey of dentists in the state of Texas, Bell (1967) reported eight deaths occurring in dental offices. Six occurred in the offices of general practitioners and two in oral surgery practices. One death occurred in the waiting room before treatment. Only two deaths were associated with the administration of general anesthetics. More recently, a number of dental office deaths have been reported in Califor-

nia associated with the administration of local anesthetics and parenteral medications.

Any life-threatening situation could potentially lead to a fatality. Failure to recognize clinical signs and symptoms may rapidly change a relatively "innocuous" emergency into an office tragedy.

Adequate physical evaluation of the dental patient before treatment and the proper use of the many techniques of pain and anxiety control will prevent much of the morbidity and many of the mortalities. However, people will still die in dental offices, just as people will die while asleep in bed or watching a football game.

It is my firm conviction that prevention of all life-threatening situations is the goal that we must pursue. Chapter 2 is devoted to this goal, as are two excellent recently published textbooks. *Dental management of the medically compromised patient*, ed. 2, by Little and Falace (St. Louis, 1984, The C.V. Mosby Company) is a concise manual applicable for chairside use, and *Internal medicine for dentistry*, by Rose and Kaye (St. Louis, 1983, The C.V. Mosby Company) is a comprehensive review of medicine in dentistry.

However, as effective as certain steps may be in preventing most life-threatening situations, it is a fact that not all are preventable. Ten percent of all nonaccidental deaths that occur per year in the United States are of a sudden, unexpected nature, occurring in persons supposedly in good health. The usual cause of death in these cases is cardiac

Table 1-3. Leading causes of death by age in the United States

	5-14 yr	15-24 yr	25-44 yr	45-64 yr	65 yr and over
1.	Accidents	Accidents	Accidents	Heart disease	Heart disease
2.	Neoplasms	Neoplasms	Heart disease	Neoplasms	Neoplasms
3.	Congenital malformations	Homicide	Neoplasms	Cerebrovascular accidents	Cerebrovascular accidents
4.	Influenza and pneumonia	Suicide	Suicide	Accidents	Influenza and pneumonia
5.	Heart disease	Heart disease	Homicide	Cirrhosis of liver	Atherosclerosis

The World almanac and book of facts, 1977 edition. Copyright © Newspaper Enterprise Association, 1976. (Source: Division of Vital Statistics, National Center for Health Statistics, 1974 data.)

arrest, most frequently ventricular fibrillation. Preventive measures cannot as yet eliminate this from occurring; therefore, preparation is of extreme importance. All members of the dental office team must be well versed in the recognition and management of these life-threatening situations. The survey by the Southern California Society of Oral Surgeons (SCSOS) (Lytle, 1974) reported two patients with cardiac arrest who were successfully resuscitated. In both cases the necessary resuscitative equipment was available, and proper resuscitative measures were promptly carried out by the dental office team.

Not all dentistry-related deaths occur within the dental office. The stress of dental treatment may trigger events that result in the death of the patient within a few days after the appointment. In the SCSOS survey (Lytle, 1974), 10 such incidents were reported. Of particular interest are three deaths caused by myocardial infarction and one caused by cerebral vascular accident. Another death was reported to have been related to an allergic reaction to propoxyphene HCl prescribed for postoperative pain relief.

McCarthy (1973) estimates that one or two office-related deaths will occur over the practice lifetime of the typical dental practitioner. He further states that the number of office-related deaths would increase to five if dental patients were observed for 7 days following treatment.

FACTORS INCREASING THE INCIDENCE OF LIFE-THREATENING EMERGENCIES
Increased Number of Older Patients

The life expectancy of persons born in the United States has increased steadily during this century (Table 1-2). Greater numbers of older persons are therefore seeking dental care. Although many of these persons appear to be in good health, it is important to remember that significant disease of a subclinical nature may be present. Of primary concern will be the cardiovascular system. In the normal process of aging, cardiovascular function decreases in efficiency. In some instances, this decreased efficiency may become clinically evident (heart failure, angina pectoris); however, in many persons no overt clinical manifestations will appear. Yet under stress, demands on the cardiovascular system for increased supplies of oxygen and other nutrients may not be met, a condition leading to the development of acute cardiovascular complications. Disease of the cardiovascular system represents the leading cause of death in the United States today in persons over 45 years of age (Table 1-3). It is evident, then, that the older patient becomes more stress intolerant. Situations that might have proved innocuous to a person at a younger age may well prove to be harmful 20 years later. This relative inability of older persons to tolerate undue stress was demonstrated in a survey on the effects of age in fatally injured automobile drivers. Baker and Spitz (1970) found the proportion of drivers aged 60 years or older to be five times as high among those killed as among drivers who survived multivehicle crashes. Many of the fatally injured drivers aged 60 and over died following crashes that did not prove fatal to younger drivers. The association between age and length of survival suggests that whereas younger drivers are recovering from injuries, many older ones succumb to complications.

The aging process involves both physiologic and pathologic changes that may alter the patient's ability to respond to stress. Table 1-4 lists the many changes frequently encountered in the geriatric

Table 1-4. Physiologic and pathologic changes in geriatric patients

Central nervous system	***Respiratory system***
Decreased number of brain cells	Senile emphysema
Cerebral arteriosclerosis	Arthritic changes in thorax
CVA	Pulmonary problems related to pollutants
Decreased memory	Interstitial fibrosis
Emotional changes	
Parkinsonism	***Genitourinary system***
	Decreased renal blood flow
Cardiovascular system	Decreased number of functioning glomeruli
Coronary artery disease	Decreased tubular reabsorption
Angina pectoris	Benign prostatic hypertrophy
Myocardial infarction	
Arrythmias	***Endocrine system***
Decreased contractility	Decreased response to stress
High blood pressure	Maturity–type one adult–onset diabetes mellitus
Renovascular disease	
Cerebrovascular disease	
Cardiac disease	

Modified from Lichtiger, M., and Moya, F.: Curr. Rev. Nurse Anesth. **1**(1):1, 1978.

patient. Decrease in tissue elasticity is a major physiologic change that has significant effect on organs throughout the body. For example, when a person is 75 years of age, cerebral blood flow is 80% of what it was at the age of 30, cardiac output has declined to 65%, and renal blood flow has decreased to 45% of its earlier volume. The decrease in renal perfusion has potentially significant bearing on the actions of certain drugs, primarily those in which urinary excretion is a principal means of removing the drug and its metabolites from the body. Drugs such as penicillin, tetracycline, and digoxin exhibit a greatly increased beta half-life in geriatric patients.

Decreased tissue elasticity also affects the lungs; pulmonary compliance decreases with aging and in fact may progress to senile emphysema. Other pulmonary factors that tend to decrease respiratory function include the chronic exposure of the geriatric patient to smoke, dust, and pollutants, which may produce respiratory disorders. Pulmonary function in the geriatric patient is considerably diminished when compared to that in the younger patient (Table 1-5).

Because of these changes, the older patient is less able to tolerate stress than a younger patient and must be considered a greater medical risk during dental therapy even in the absence of clinically evident disease. In addition, steps must be taken to minimize this risk as much as possible (Stress Reduction Protocol).

Advances Made by the Medical Profession

With increasing age, the incidence of many diseases rises greatly. Diabetic patients and patients with cardiovascular disease (heart failure, arteriosclerosis) faced significantly shorter life expectancies a decade or two ago than they do today. This was also true for many other medical disorders, all of which commonly proved fatal at an early age. At best many of these patients lived confined to bed or a wheelchair, unable to work for a living and unlikely to seek dental care. Today, however, because of unprecedented advances in drug therapy and surgical technique, many of these patients live apparently normal lives. Radiation and chemotherapy enable many cancer victims to live longer lives; surgical procedures such as the coronary artery bypass and graft operation and heart valve replacement enable previously incapacitated patients to be virtually asymptomatic. Organ transplants are becoming commonplace. Drug therapy has been introduced for management of many disorders, such as high blood pressure, that were previously untreatable and were associated with a high mortality rate at a young age.

These medical advances are truly significant, yet they also mean that the dental practitioner is called on to manage the oral health needs of patients with a potential risk. It is necessary to keep in mind that most of these patients have not been cured of their illnesses; these chronic disorders are merely being kept under control, and the underlying disease is still present. McCarthy has termed these persons "the walking wounded" and "accidents looking for a place to happen."

Longer Dental Appointments

In recent years a significant number of doctors have increased the length of their dental appointments. Although appointments of less than 60 minutes are still commonplace, many doctors now schedule 1- to 3-hour treatment sessions. Dental therapy is stressful to the patient (and doctor and staff, too!), and longer appointments are more stressful than shorter ones. Medically compromised patients are more likely to react adversely under these conditions than are "healthy" individuals, yet even the so-called normal, healthy patient becomes stressed during longer procedures and is more likely to exhibit unwanted reactions. Stress reduction has become an important part of many dental procedures.

Increased Use of Drugs

Drugs are an integral part of the practice of dentistry. Drugs for the prevention of pain, the reduction of anxiety, and the treatment of infection are an important part of every doctor's armamentarium. Yet drug use carries with it an inherent risk. All drugs exert multiple actions, and no drug is totally safe. Knowledge of the pharmacologic actions of the drug and proper technique of administration will greatly decrease the occurrence of drug-related emergencies.

Drugs not prescribed by the doctor are yet another source of increased risk. Halpern (1975) found that 18% of his patient population was taking medication of one form or another. This incidence rose with age (41% of the patients over the age of 60 took medication regularly). Situations may arise in the dental office related either to the pharmacologic actions of these drugs or to complex drug interactions between commonly used dental drugs and other medications. An example of the former is orthostatic hypotension, which is associated with many drugs used to manage high

Table 1-5. Pulmonary changes in geriatric patients (age 65 and older)

Function	Percentage compared to capacity at age 30
Total lung capacity	100
Vital capacity	58
O$_2$ uptake during exercise	50
Maximum breathing capacity	55

From data in Lichtiger, M., and Moya, F.: Curr. Rev. Nurse Anesth. 1(1):1, 1978.

blood pressure. Potentially fatal interactions between the monoamine oxidase (MAO) inhibitors and narcotics (such as meperidine) exemplify the latter.

• • •

One of the aims of this textbook is to make the dental team more aware of possible high-risk patients so that appropriate modification may be incorporated into dental therapy to minimize the risk to the patient. A second aim relates to the prompt recognition and effective management of those situations that occur in spite of our efforts at prevention. Goldberger (1985) wrote in the preface to his textbook, *Treatment of Cardiac Emergencies,* "When you prepare for an emergency, the emergency ceases to exist." Adequate preparation before an emergency arises will greatly increase the probability of a successful outcome. The ultimate aim in the management of any emergency is the preservation of life. This primary goal is the thread that ties all sections of this textbook together.

CLASSIFICATION OF LIFE-THREATENING SITUATIONS

Several methods are available for the classification of medical emergencies. The approach traditionally employed has been the systems-oriented classification. In such a classification, major organ systems are listed, and life-threatening situations associated with that system are discussed. The following is an example of a systems-oriented classification:

Infectious diseases
Immune diseases
  Allergy
    Angioneurotic edema
    Contact dermatitis
    Anaphylaxis
Skin and appendages
Eye
Ear, nose, and throat
Respiratory tract
  Asthma
Cardiovascular system
  Arteriosclerotic heart disease
    Angina pectoris
    Myocardial infarction
    Heart failure
Blood
Gastrointestinal tract and liver
Obstetrics and gynecology
Nervous system
  Unconsciousness
  Syncope
    Hyperventilation syndrome
    Vasodepressor syncope
    Orthostatic hypotension
  Convulsive disorders
    Epilepsy
  Drug overdose reactions
  Cerebrovascular accident
Endocrine disorders
  Diabetes mellitus
    Hyperglycemia
    Hypoglycemia
  Thyroid gland
    Hyperthyroidism
    Hypothyroidism
  Adrenal gland
    Acute adrenal insufficiency

Although this approach is the approach of choice for educational purposes, it is faulty from a clinical standpoint.

A second method of classifying emergency situations is to divide them into several broad categories: cardiovascular and noncardiovascular; stress-related and non-stress-related. This system offers us a very general breakdown of life-threatening emergencies that may be of use in dentistry. Combining the two systems, we have four categories to work with:

Noncardiovascular emergencies
  Stress-related
  Non-stress-related
Cardiovascular emergencies
  Stress-related
  Non-stress-related

This system can assist the doctor in preparing a workable treatment plan for the prevention of such situations. The risk of a stress-related emergency occurring may be reduced through the employment of several stress-reducing modifications in dental therapy. Such factors will include psychosedative techniques, effective pain control, and limitations on the length of the dental appointment. A complete description of these factors may be found in Chapter 2. Classification by this system follows:

Noncardiovascular emergencies
  Stress-related
    Vasodepressor syncope
    Hyperventilation syndrome
    Hypoglycemic reactions
    Epilepsy
    Acute adrenal insufficiency
    Thyroid crisis
    Asthma
  Non-stress-related
    Orthostatic hypotension
    Overdose reaction
    Hyperglycemia
    Allergy
Cardiovascular emergencies
  Stress-related
    Angina pectoris
    Acute myocardial infarction
    Heart failure
    Cerebral ischemia and infarction
  Non-stress-related
    Acute myocardial infarction

As effective as this system will be in the *prevention* of emergencies, we also need a system that will be of use in the *clinical recognition* and *management* of these situations. For this to be effective we must abandon classifications based on organ systems, because in most clinical situations the underlying pathologic condition is not immediately clear.

The doctor is forced to recognize and initiate management of a situation with only obvious clinical signs and symptoms as a guide. For this reason, a classification of emergency situations based on clinically apparent signs and symptoms appears useful, and indeed has proven to be so. Initial management of emergency situations will necessarily be based on these clinical clues until a more definitive diagnosis can be determined. Commonly seen signs and symptoms include unconsciousness, respiratory difficulty, altered consciousness, seizures, drug-related emergencies, and chest pain. In all

2 *Prevention*

Through the use of a complete system of physical evaluation for all prospective dental patients, approximately 90% of life-threatening situations can be prevented. The remaining 10% will occur in spite of all efforts at prevention. "When you prepare for an emergency, the emergency ceases to exist" is accurate to the degree that preparation for an emergency will diminish the danger or possibility of death and morbidity. Prior knowledge of a patient's physical status will enable the doctor to incorporate modifications into the planned dental therapy. Prior knowledge is important: "To be forewarned is to be forearmed." Stated in another way: "Never treat a stranger."

This chapter* will present a detailed discussion of the most important components of physical evaluation, which, when properly employed, will lead to a significant reduction in the occurrence of acute medical emergencies. Continual reference to this chapter will be made throughout this text as the prevention of specific emergencies is discussed.

GOALS OF PHYSICAL AND PSYCHOLOGIC EVALUATION

In the following discussion a comprehensive but easy-to-employ program of physical evaluation will be described. Its use, as recommended, will enable the doctor to accurately assess the potential risk presented by a patient before the start of treatment. The following are goals that are sought in the use of this system:

---

*Portions of this chapter have appeared in a slightly different form in *Sedation: a guide to patient management* (Malamed, St. Louis, 1985, The C.V. Mosby Co.).

1. To determine the patient's ability to physically tolerate the stresses involved in dental treatment
2. To determine the patient's ability to psychologically tolerate the stresses involved in dental treatment
3. To determine whether treatment modifications are required to enable the patient to better tolerate the stresses of dental treatment
4. To determine whether the use of psychosedation is indicated
5. To determine which technique of sedation is most appropriate for the patient
6. To determine whether contraindications exist to any of the medications to be employed

The first two goals involve the patient's ability to tolerate the stress involved in dental treatment. Stress may be of a physiologic or psychologic nature. Patients with underlying medical problems will be less able to tolerate the usual levels of stress associated with various forms of dental therapy. These patients will be more likely to develop an acute exacerbation of their medical problems during these periods of stress. Examples of such disease processes include angina pectoris, epilepsy, asthma, and sickle cell disease. Although most of these patients will be able to safely receive dental therapy, it is the obligation of the doctor and staff to determine (1) whether this problem does exist and (2) the level of severity of the problem.

Excessive stress can also be detrimental to the patient who is not medically compromised; fear and anxiety produce acute changes in the normal homeostasis of the body. Many patients experience fear-related emergencies, including hyperventilation and vasodepressor syncope (fainting).

The third goal is to determine whether or not the usual treatment regimen for a patient will require modification so that the patient can better tolerate the stress of treatment. In many instances a healthy patient will be unable to psychologically tolerate the planned treatment. Treatment may be modified to minimize the stress faced by this patient. The medically compromised patient will also benefit from treatment modification aimed at minimizing stress. The Stress Reduction Protocols will be introduced later in this chapter; they are designed to aid the doctor in minimizing treatment-related stress in both the healthy and medically compromised patient.

In those instances in which it is believed that the patient will require some assistance in coping with dental treatment, the use of psychosedation will be considered. The last three goals involve the determination of the need for use of these techniques, selection of the most appropriate technique, and selection of the most appropriate medication(s) for the patient.

PHYSICAL EVALUATION

The term *physical evaluation* will be employed to discuss the steps involved in fulfilling the goals mentioned above. Physical evaluation in dentistry consists of the following three components:

1. Medical history questionnaire
2. Physical examination
3. Dialogue history

With the information collected from these three steps the doctor will be better able to (1) determine the physical and psychologic status of the patient (establish a risk factor classification for the patient), (2) seek medical consultation if indicated, and (3) institute appropriate modifications in dental therapy if indicated. Each of the three steps in the evaluation process will now be discussed.

Medical History Questionnaire

The use of a written, patient-completed medical history questionnaire is a moral and legal necessity in the practice of both medicine and dentistry. In addition, a questionnaire provides the doctor with valuable information about the physical, and in some cases the psychologic, condition of the prospective patient.

Many forms of medical history questionnaires are available. However, most are simply modifications of two basic types: the *short form* and the *long form*. The short form medical history questionnaire provides basic information concerning a patient's medical history and is ideally suited for the doctor with considerable clinical experience in physical evaluation. When employing the short form history, the doctor must have a firm grasp of the appropriate dialogue history required to aid in determination of the relative risk presented and must also be experienced in the use and interpretation of the techniques of physical evaluation. Unfortunately, most doctors will employ the short form or a modification of it in their office primarily as a convenience to the patient. The long form medical history questionnaire provides a more detailed data base concerning the physical condition of the prospective patient. It is used most often in teaching situations and represents an ideal instrument for teaching physical evaluation.

Either form of medical history questionnaire may be used to accurately determine the physical status of the patient. Either form of medical history questionnaire can also prove to be entirely worthless. The ultimate value of the medical history questionnaire will rest on the ability of the doctor to interpret its meaning and to then elicit additional information through the physical examination and dialogue history. The adult and pediatric medical history questionnaires used at the University of Southern California (USC) School of Dentistry (Figs. 2-1 and 2-2, respectively) have combined the best of both short and long forms.

Although both the long and short forms of medical history questionnaires are valuable in the determination of a patient's physical risk during treatment, a decided failing of most available health history questionnaires is their lack of questions relating to the patient's attitudes toward dentistry. It is recommended therefore that one or more questions be added to the questionnaire that relate to this all-important subject. The following questions are included in the USC School of Dentistry adult health history questionnaire:

Do you feel very nervous about having dentistry treatment?

Have you ever had a bad experience in the dental office?

It has been my experience that many adult patients will be reluctant to verbalize their fears about the proposed treatment to the doctor, hygienist, or assistant for fear of being labeled a "baby." This is especially true of young men, usually in their early twenties. These persons, rather than expressing their fears, will attempt to "take it like a man" or

MEDICAL HISTORY

CIRCLE

1. Are you having pain or discomfort at this time? . . . . YES NO
2. Do you feel very nervous about having dentistry treatment? . . . . YES NO
3. Have you ever had a bad experience in the dentistry office? . . . . YES NO
4. Have you been a patient in the hospital during the past two years? . . . . YES NO
5. Have you been under the care of a medical doctor during the past two years? . . . . YES NO
6. Have you taken any medicine or drugs during the past two years? . . . . YES NO
7. Are you allergic to (i.e., itching, rash, swelling of hands, feet or eyes) or made sick by
   penicillin, aspirin, codeine, or any drugs or medications? . . . . YES NO
8. Have you ever had any excessive bleeding requiring special treatment? . . . . YES NO
9. Circle any of the following which you have had or have at present:

Heart Failure	Emphysema	AIDS
Heart Disease or Attack	Cough	Hepatitis A (infectious)
Angina Pectoris	Tuberculosis (TB)	Hepatitis B (serum)
High Blood Pressure	Asthma	Liver Disease
Heart Murmur	Hay Fever	Yellow Jaundice
Rheumatic Fever	Sinus Trouble	Blood Transfusion
Congenital Heart Lesions	Allergies or Hives	Drug Addiction
Scarlet Fever	Diabetes	Hemophilia
Artificial Heart Valve	Thyroid Disease	Venereal Disease (Syphilis, Gonorrhea)
Heart Pacemaker	X-ray or Cobalt Treatment	Cold Sores
Heart Surgery	Chemotherapy (Cancer, Leukemia)	Genital Herpes
Artificial Joint	Arthritis	Epilepsy or Seizures
Anemia	Rheumatism	Fainting or Dizzy Spells
Stroke	Cortisone Medicine	Nervousness
Kidney Trouble	Glaucoma	Psychiatric Treatment
Ulcers	Pain in Jaw Joints	Sickle Cell Disease
		Bruise Easily

10. When you walk up stairs or take a walk, do you ever have to stop because of pain in your chest,
    or shortness of breath, or because you are very tired? . . . . YES NO
11. Do your ankles swell during the day? . . . . YES NO
12. Do you use more than 2 pillows to sleep? . . . . YES NO
13. Have you lost or gained more than 10 pounds in the past year? . . . . YES NO
14. Do you ever wake up from sleep short of breath? . . . . YES NO
15. Are you on a special diet? . . . . YES NO
16. Has your medical doctor ever said you have a cancer or tumor? . . . . YES NO
17. Do you have any disease, condition, or problem not listed? . . . . YES NO
18. WOMEN: Are you pregnant now? . . . . YES NO
    Are you practicing birth control? . . . . YES NO
    Do you anticipate becoming pregnant? . . . . YES NO

To the best of my knowledge, all of the preceding answers are true and correct. If I ever have any change in my health, or if my medicines change, I will inform the doctor of dentistry at the next appointment without fail.

_____   _____   _____
Date   *Faculty Signature*   *Signature of Patient, Parent or Guardian*

. . . .

MEDICAL HISTORY / PHYSICAL EVALUATION UPDATE

Date   *Addition*   *Student/Faculty Signatures*

_____   _____   _____   _____

_____   _____   _____   _____

_____   _____   _____   _____

Fig. 2-1. Medical history questionnaire. Room is provided for periodic updates on USC medical history questionnaire. (From Malamed, S.F.: Sedation, St. Louis, 1985, The C.V. Mosby Co.)

Child's Name: _____ Date of Birth: _____ Age _____ Date: _____

Address: _____ Telephone: (_____) _____

Physician's name (Medical Doctor): _____ Telephone: (_____) _____

Please circle the appropriate answer

1. Does your child have a health problem? .... YES NO
2. Was your child a patient in a hospital? .... YES NO
3. Date of last physical exam: _____
4. Is your child now under medical care? .... YES NO
5. Is your child taking medication now? .... YES NO
   If so, for what? _____
6. Has your child ever had a serious illness or operation? ...... YES NO
7. If so, explain: _____
8. Does your child have (or ever had) any of the following diseases?
   a. Rheumatic fever or rheumatic heart disease .... YES NO
   b. Congenital heart disease .... YES NO
   c. Cardiovascular disease (heart trouble, heart attack, coronary insufficiency, coronary occlusion, high blood pressure, arteriosclerosis, stroke) .... YES NO
   d. Allergy?   Food □,   Medicine □,   Other □ .... YES NO
   e. Asthma □ Hay Fever □ .... YES NO
   f. Hives or a skin rash .... YES NO
   g. Fainting spells or seizures .... YES NO
   h. Hepatitis, jaundice or liver disease .... YES NO
   i. Diabetes .... YES NO
   j. Inflammatory rheumatism (painful or swollen joints) .... YES NO
   k. Arthritis .... YES NO
   l. Stomach ulcers .... YES NO
   m. Kidney trouble .... YES NO
   n. Tuberculosis (TB) .... YES NO
   o. Persistent cough or cough up blood .... YES NO
   p. Veneral disease .... YES NO
   q. Epilepsy .... YES NO
   r. Sickle Cell disease .... YES NO
   s. Thyroid disease .... YES NO
   t. AIDS .... YES NO
   u. Emphysema .... YES NO
   v. Psychiatric treatment .... YES NO
   w. Cleft lip / palate .... YES NO
   x. Cerebral palsy .... YES NO
   y. Mental retardation .... YES NO
   z. Hearing disability .... YES NO
   aa. Developmental disability .... YES NO
       If yes, explain: _____
   bb. Was your child premature? .... YES NO
       If yes, how many weeks _____
   cc. Other: _____
9. Does your child have to urinate (pass water) more than six times a day? .... YES NO
10. Is your child thirsty much of the time? .... YES NO
11. Has your child had abnormal bleeding associated with previous surgery, extractions or accidents? .... YES NO

12. Does he/she bruise easily? .... YES NO
13. Has he/she ever required a blood transfusion? .... YES NO
14. Does he/she have any blood disorders such as anemia, etc? .... YES NO
15. Has he/she ever had surgery, x-ray or chemotherapy for a tumor, growth, or other condition? .... YES NO
16. Does your child have a disability that prevents treatment in a dental office? .... YES NO
17. Is he/she taking any of the following?
    a. Antibiotics or sulfa drugs .... YES NO
    b. Anticoagulants (blood thinners) .... YES NO
    c. Medicine for high blood pressure .... YES NO
    d. Cortisone or steroids .... YES NO
    e. Tranquilizers .... YES NO
    f. Aspirin .... YES NO
    g. Dilantin or other anticonvulsant .... YES NO
    h. Insulin, tolbutamide, Orinase, or similar drug .... YES NO
    i. Any other? _____
18. Is he/she allergic to, or has he/she ever reacted adversely to, any of the following?
    a. Local anesthetics .... YES NO
    b. Penicillin or other antibiotics .... YES NO
    c. Sulfa drugs .... YES NO
    d. Barbituates, sedatives, or sleeping pills .... YES NO
    e. Aspirin .... YES NO
    f. Any other? _____
19. Has he/she any serious trouble associated with any previous dental treatment? .... YES NO
    If so, please explain: _____
21. Has your child been in any situation which could expose him/her to x-rays or other ionizing radiators? .... YES NO
22. Last date of dental examination: _____
23. Has he/she ever had orthodontic treatment (worn braces)? .... YES NO
24. Has he/she ever been treated for any gum diseases (gingivitis, periodontitis, trenchmouth, pyorrhea)? ..... YES NO
25. Does his/her gums bleed when brushing teeth? .... YES NO
26. Does he/she grind or clench teeth? .... YES NO
27. Has he/she often had toothaches? .... YES NO
28. Has he/she had frequent sores in his/her mouth? .... YES NO
29. Has he/she had any injuries to his/her mouth or jaws? ...... YES NO
    If yes, explain: _____
30. Does he/she have any sores or swellings of his/her mouth or jaws? .... YES NO
31. Have you been satisfied with your child's previous dental care? .... YES NO

ADOLESCENT WOMEN:

32. Are you pregnant now, or think you may be? .... YES NO
33. Do you anticipate becoming pregnant? .... YES NO
34. Are you taking the Pill? .... YES NO

To the best of my knowledge, all of the preceding answers are true and correct. If my child ever has a change in his/her health or his/her medicines change, I will inform the doctor at the next appointment without fail.

Parent's Signature: _____ Date _____

....

MEDICAL HISTORY / PHYSICAL EXAMINATION REVIEW

Date	Addition	Student/Faculty Signatures
_____	_____	_____ _____
_____	_____	_____ _____
_____	_____	_____ _____

Fig. 2-2. USC pediatric medical history questionnaire.

"grin and bear it." Unfortunately, all too often the outcome of such "macho" behavior is an episode of syncope. Whereas an open admission of their fears before the episode usually is nonexistent, my experience has demonstrated that these same patients will volunteer this information in writing if questions are included in the medical history questionnaire. Other means of identifying anxiety will be discussed later in this chapter.

The USC adult questionnaire will be reviewed, providing the basic significance of each of the questions.

QUESTION 1. Are you having pain or discomfort at this time?

COMMENT. The primary thrust of this question is related to dentistry. The question is asked to try to determine what it was that actually brought the patient to seek dental treatment at this time. Should pain or discomfort be present, it may be necessary for the doctor to institute treatment at this first visit; in a more normal situation, treatment would not begin until future visits.

QUESTION 2. Do you feel very nervous about having dentistry treatment?

QUESTION 3. Have you ever had a bad experience in the dentistry office?

COMMENT. The inclusion of questions relating to a patient's attitudes toward dentistry is a significant addition to the medical history questionnaire. Most questionnaires, unfortunately, ignore questioning along this important line. It has been my experience that many adult patients, who would never verbally admit to being fearful, will indicate their fears or prior negative experiences on the written questionnaire.

QUESTION 4. Have you been a patient in the hospital during the past 2 years?

COMMENT. Knowledge of the reasons for hospitalization of the patient will greatly increase the doctor's ability to adequately evaluate the patient's ability to tolerate the stresses involved in dental treatment.

QUESTION 5. Have you been under the care of a medical doctor during the past 2 years?

COMMENT. As with the previous question, knowledge of any medical problems for which the patient required medical intervention can greatly increase the ability to fully evaluate the patient prior to the start of treatment.

QUESTION 6. Have you taken any medicine or drugs during the past 2 years?

COMMENT. Knowledge of the medications taken by a patient for the control or treatment of a medical disorder is vitally important. Frequently patients take medications but are unaware of the condition for which they are being taken; in addition, many patients do not even know the names of medications they are taking. For these two reasons it is essential that the doctor have available one or more means of identifying these medications, which the patient may carry with them. Several sources are available, including the *Physicians' Desk Reference* (*PDR*) and *Clinical Management of Prescription Drugs* (Long, 1984). The *PDR*, although primarily a compilation of drug package inserts, is a valuable reference. It contains a section that permits the visual identification of a medication should the patient be unaware of its name.

Knowledge of the drugs and medications being taken by a patient is essential because (1) it permits identification of the medical disorder being treated, (2) there are potential side effects to most medications, some of which may be of significance in dentistry (such as postural hypotension), and (3) drug interactions can develop between a patient's medication and the drugs administered during dental treatment. The box on pp. 14-15 lists interactions of drugs that might be used in dentistry.

QUESTION 7. Are you allergic to (i.e., itching, rash, swelling of hands, feet, or eyes) or made sick by penicillin, aspirin, codeine, or any drugs or medications?

COMMENT. Question 7 attempts to determine whether the patient has experienced any adverse drug reactions (ADRs). ADRs are not uncommon; the most frequently reported reactions are labeled "allergy." However, true allergic drug reactions are relatively uncommon, in spite of the great frequency with which they are reported. The doctor must evaluate all ADRs quite thoroughly, especially in those situations in which closely related medications are to be administered to or prescribed for the patient. Evaluation of alleged allergy and other adverse drug reactions is discussed in Section VI.

QUESTION 8. Have you ever had any excessive bleeding requiring special treatment?

COMMENT. Bleeding disorders, such as hemophilia, can lead to modification in certain forms of dental therapy (for example, surgery, local anesthetic administration) and must therefore be made known to the doctor prior to the start of treatment.

DENTAL DRUG INTERACTIONS

Dental drug	Interacting agents	Resulting effect
Anesthetics, general	Antidepressants	Hypotension
	Antihypertensives	Hypotension
Antihistamines	Alcohol	CNS depression
	Phenothiazines (Compazine, Thorazine)	Increased sedation
Anticholinergics (atropine)	Antihistamines	Increased anticholinergic effect
	Levodopa	Increased anticholinergic effect
	Phenothiazines	Increased anticholinergic effect
	Antidepressants, tricyclic (Vivactil, Surmontil, Tofranil)	Increased anticholinergic effect
Barbiturates	Alcohol	Enhanced sedation, increased respiratory depression
	Anticoagulants, oral	Decreased anticoagulant effect
	Antidepressants, tricyclic (Vivactil, Surmontil, Tofranil)	Decreased antidepressant effect
	Beta-adrenergic blockers (Lopressor, Inderal)	Decreased beta-blocker effect
	Corticosteroids	Decreased steroid effect
	Digitoxin (digitalis)	Decreased digitoxin effect
	Doxycycline	Decreased doxycycline effect
	Griseofulvin (Fulvicin, Grisactin, Grifulvin II)	Decreased griseofulvin effect
	Phenothiazines	Decreased phenothiazines effect
	Quinidine	Decreased quinidine effect
	Rifampin	Decreased barbiturate effect
	Valproic acid	Increased phenobarbital effect
Benzodiazepines (Librium, Serax, Valium)	Alcohol	Enhanced sedation
	Barbiturates	Enhanced sedation and increased respiratory depression
Carbamazepine	Anticoagulants, oral	Decreased anticoagulant effect
	doxycycline,	Decreased doxycycline effect
	propoxyphene	Increased carbamazepine effect
Cephalosporin antibiotics	Aminoglycoside antibiotics	Increased nephrotoxicity
	Ethacrynic acid	Increased nephrotoxicity
	Furosemide	Increased nephrotoxicity
Clindamycin	Curariform drugs	Neuromuscular blockade
	Lomotil	Increased diarrhea, colitis
Corticosteroids	Barbiturates	Decreased corticosteroid effect
	Ephedrine	Decreased dexamethasone effect
	Phenytoin	Decreased corticosteroid effect
	Rifampin	Decreased corticosteroid effect
Erythromycin	Lincomycin	Decreased antimicrobial effect
Fluoride	Aluminum hydroxide	Decreased fluoride absorption

Modified from Council on Dental Therapeutics, J. Am. Dent. Assoc. **107**:885, 1983.

Dental drug	Interacting agents	Resulting effect
Lincomycin	Curariform drugs	Neuromuscular blockade
	Kaolin-pectin	Decreased lincomycin effect
	Diphenoxylate-atropine and similar products (Lomotil)	Increased diarrhea, colitis
Meperidine	Barbiturates	Increased CNS depression
	Curariform drugs	Increased respiratory depression
	MAO inhibitors (Marplan, Nardil, Parnate)	Hypertension
Phenothiazines	Alcohol	Increased sedation
(Promethazine)	Guanthidine	Decreased phenothiazine effect
	Levodopa	Decreased levodopa effect
	Lithium	Decreased phenothiazine effect
Propoxyphene	Alcohol	Increased respiratory depression
	Carbamazepine	Increased carbamazepine effect
	Curariform drugs	Increased respiratory depression
Salicylates (aspirin)	Acetazolamide	Increased salicylate CNS toxicity
	Antacids	Decreased salicylate levels
	Anticoagulants, oral	Increased bleeding risk
	Dipyridamole	Increased effect on platelet function
	Hypoglycemics	Increased hypoglycemia
	Methotrexate	Increased methotrexate toxicity
	Probenecid	Decreased uricosuric effect
Sympathomimetic	Antidepressants, tricyclic (Vivactil, Surmontil, Tofranil)	Hypertension, hypertensive crisis
amines	Antihypertensive drugs	Decreased hypertensive effect
(epinephrine,	Beta-adrenergic blockers (Lopressor, Inderal)	Hypertension with epinephrine
phenylephrine,	Halogenated anesthetics	Cardiac arrhythmias
nordefrin)	Digitalis drugs	Tendency to cardiac arrhythmias
	Indomethacin	Severe hypertension
	MAO inhibitors (Marplan, Nardil, Parnate)	Hypertensive crisis
Tetracyclines	Antacids	Decreased tetracycline effect
	Barbiturates	Decreased doxycycline effect
	Bismuth subsalicylate	Decreased tetracycline effect
	Carbamazepine	Decreased doxycycline effect
	Iron, oral	Decreased tetracycline effect
	Methoxyflurane	Increased nephrotoxicity
	Milk and dairy products	Decreased tetracycline effect
	Phenytoin	Decreased doxycycline effect
	Zinc sulfate	Decreased tetracycline effect

Table 2-1. Guidelines for blood pressure (adult)

Blood pressure (mm Hg, or torr)	ASA classification	Dental therapy considerations
<140 and <90	I	1. Routine dental management 2. Recheck in 6 months
140 to 160 and/or 90 to 95	II	1. Recheck blood pressure prior to dental treatment for 3 consecutive appointments; if all exceed these guidelines, medical consultation is indicated 2. Routine dental management 3. Stress Reduction Protocol as indicated
160 to 200 and/or 95 to 115	III	1. Recheck blood pressure in 5 minutes 2. If still elevated, medical consultation before dental therapy 3. Routine dental therapy 4. Stress Reduction Protocol
>200 and/or >115	IV	1. Recheck blood pressure in 5 minutes 2. Immediate medical consultation if still elevated 3. No dental therapy, routine or emergency,* until elevated blood pressure is corrected 4. Emergency dental therapy with drugs (analgesics, antibiotics) 5. Refer to hospital if immediate dental therapy indicated

*When the blood pressure of the patient is slightly above the cut-off for category IV, and where anxiety is present, the use of inhalation sedation may be employed in an effort to diminish the blood pressure (via the elimination of stress) below the 200/115 level. The patient should be advised that if the N_2O-O_2 succeeds in decreasing the blood pressure below this level, the planned treatment will proceed. However, should the blood pressure remain elevated, the planned procedure will be postponed until the elevated blood pressure has been lowered to a more acceptable range.

QUESTION 9. Circle any of the following which you have had or have at present:

COMMENT. This question presents a list of the more common illnesses and disorders afflicting the adult population in the United States.

Heart failure

COMMENT. The degree of heart failure must be assessed through the dialogue history. In the presence of more serious congestive heart failure (CHF) (such as dyspnea at rest) the patient will require strict modification in therapy and possibly the administration of supplemental oxygen throughout treatment.

Heart disease or attack

COMMENT. Heart attack is the lay term for myocardial infarction (MI). Knowledge of its severity, residual damage, and time that has elapsed since its occurrence is essential because therapy modifications may be warranted for this patient. Dental treatment should be postponed for 6 months following the MI.

Angina pectoris

COMMENT. A history of angina usually indicates the presence of a significant degree of coronary artery atherosclerosis. The risk factor for the typical anginal patient is an ASA III. Stress reduction is strongly recommended in these patients.

High blood pressure

COMMENT. Elevated blood pressure measurements are not uncommon in the dental environment, primarily because of the added stresses associated with dental treatment. Whenever patients report a history of high blood pressure, the doctor should determine the side effects and potential drug interactions of the medications they are taking to manage their blood pressure. Guidelines for clinical evaluation of risk based on adult blood pressure determinations are presented in Table 2-1.

Heart murmur

COMMENT. Heart murmurs are not uncommon; however, not all murmurs are clinically significant.

The doctor should seek to determine if a murmur is functional (nonpathologic) or if clinical signs and symptoms of either valvular stenosis or regurgitation are present and antibiotic prophylaxis is warranted. A major clinical symptom of a significant murmur is undue fatigue.

Rheumatic fever

COMMENT. A history of rheumatic fever should lead the doctor to an in-depth dialogue history seeking the presence of rheumatic heart disease (RHD). If RHD is present, antibiotic prophylaxis is indicated to minimize the risk of subacute bacterial endocarditis (SBE). Additional therapy modification may be desirable to further minimize risk to the patient, depending on the degree of cardiac involvement. The box on p. 18 presents the recently revised (May 1985) guidelines for antibiotic prophylaxis of the American Heart Association, which are included in a clinical implications bulletin of the University of Southern California School of Dentistry.

Congenital heart lesions

COMMENT. An in-depth dialogue history is required to determine the nature of the lesion and, of greater significance, the degree of disability produced by it. Medical consultation may be required, especially for the pediatric patient. Prophylactic antibiotics may be required before dental treatment.

Scarlet fever

COMMENT. Produced by group A beta-hemolytic streptococci, scarlet fever rarely produces cardiovascular sequelae such as valvular damage.

Artificial heart valve

COMMENT. Patients with artificial heart valves are no longer uncommon. The primary concern of the doctor is to determine which antibiotic regimen is appropriate for the patient during dental treatment. Medical consultation before the start of therapy is recommended in these patients.

Heart pacemaker

COMMENT. Pacemakers are implanted beneath the skin of the upper chest or the abdomen, with pacing wires extending into the myocardium. The most frequent indication for the use of a pacemaker is the presence of a clinically significant arrhythmia. Fixed-rate pacemakers provide the heart with a regular, continuous rate of firing regardless of the inherent rhythm of the heart, whereas the more commonly employed demand pacemakers remain inactive while the rhythm of the heart is normal but take over pacing of the heart when the inherent rhythm of the heart becomes abnormal. Although there is little indication for the administration of antibiotics in these patients, medical consultation is recommended before the start of the initial treatment to obtain the specific recommendations of the patient's physician.

Heart surgery

COMMENT. This is a very general term that may include any procedure, from the implantation of a pacemaker to a valve replacement to coronary artery bypass surgery to a heart transplant. A *yes* response to this question should elicit a vigorous dialogue history from the doctor.

Artificial joint

COMMENT. The replacement of hips, knees, and elbows with prosthetic devices is becoming more and more common. However, it is unknown at this time whether bacteremia produced in many dental procedures significantly increases the risk of joint infection. For this reason it is recommended that consultation with the patient's surgeon be obtained before the start of any dental procedure.

Anemia

COMMENT. Anemia is relatively common in the adult population, especially among younger women. The concern with anemic patients is the decreased ability of their blood to carry oxygen. This may be of special significance during procedures in which hypoxia is more likely to develop. Although this should never occur during dental treatment, the use of deeper levels of intramuscular (IM) or intravenous (IV) sedation without supplemental oxygen administration is more likely to produce hypoxia, which would be of greater consequence in these patients.

Sickle cell anemia will be seen in some black patients. A differentiation between sickle cell disease and sickle cell trait must be made.

The presence of congenital or idiopathic methemoglobinemia represents a relative contraindication to the administration of the local anesthetics articaine and prilocaine.

GUIDELINES FOR ANTIBIOTIC PROPHYLAXIS
University of Southern California—School of Dentistry
May 1, 1985

Rationale

Antibiotic chemoprophylaxis is medicolegally desirable in certain medically compromised patients to prevent bacterial metastasis from oral invasive procedures even though such procedures have not been proven medically or scientifically effective nor any patient risk/benefit ratio ever determined.

Prevention of infective endocarditis (IE) & other vascular infections

The medically compromised patients at risk from bacteremias are placed in the Very High, High, and Intermediate Risk categories.[1-5] Patients in the Low Risk category do not require antimicrobial prophylaxis.[1-5]

Dental procedures for which prophylaxis is indicated

All dental procedures likely to induce gingival bleeding (not simple adjustment of orthodontic appliances or shedding of deciduous teeth)[5] or any invasive procedure such as local anesthetic injection or intravenous sedation.

RELATIVE RISK RATE FOR BACTEREMIA-INDUCED INFECTIONS OR IE

Very high risk*
Previous episode of IE
Heart valve prosthesis
Coarctation of the aorta
Indwelling vascular catheter (left side of heart)

High risk*
Rheumatic heart disease (or other acquired valvular heart disease)
Congenital heart disease
  Ventricular septal defect
  Patent ductus arteriosus
  Tetralogy of Fallot
  Aortic stenosis
  Complex cyanotic heart disease
  Systemic-pulmonary artery shunt
Idiopathic hypertrophic subaortic stenosis (HSS)
Mitral valve prolapse (MVP) with mitral insufficiency
Indwelling vascular catheter (right side of heart)
Renal dialysis with A-V shunt appliance
Mitral valve surgery
Ventriculoatrial shunts for hydrocephalus

Intermediate risk*
Tricuspid valve disease
Assymetric septal hypertrophy

Low risk*
Mitral valve prolapse (MVP) without mitral insufficiency
Congenital pulmonary stenosis
Indwelling transvenous cardiac pacemakers†
Uncomplicated secundum septal atrial defect
Coronary artery disease or coronary bypass
Atherosclerotic plaques
Six months or longer after surgery for:
  Ligated ductus arteriosus
  Vascular grafts (autogenous)
  Surgically closed atrial or septal defects (without Dacron patches)

*Very High, High, and Intermediate Risk patients must receive antibiotic prophylaxis; Low Risk patients do not require chemoprophylaxis.[1-5] (*Reprinted with permission of the Dental Drug Service Newsletter [1]*)
†ADA recommendations are equivocal: prophylactic antibiotics *may* (not *should*) be employed.[5]

Heart valve prosthesis

Both the American Heart Association (AHA)[5] and The Medical Letter[6] recommend parenteral antibiotic prophylaxis for these patients. However, the AHA[5,7] allows for oral antibiotic prophylaxis for routine dental procedures (not extensive procedures especially extractions or oral or gingival surgery) in patients ". . . in whom a high level of oral health is being maintained . . .".

Prevention of recurrent rheumatic fever

The current AHA Guidelines[8] state that "Patients who have had rheumatic fever but who do not have evidence of rheumatic heart disease do not need endocarditis prophylaxis" but also acknowledge that high recurrence rates occur in patients ". . . with an attack of rheumatic fever in the preceding 5 years . . .". Some experts suggest antibiotic prophylaxis during this 5 year High Risk period.[9,10] No studies have been performed to demonstrate a direct relationship between dentally induced bacteremias and recurrent rheumatic fever (RF). Due to a high incidence of penicillin-resistant streptococci, patients receiving continuous penicillin to prevent recurrent RF require antibiotic prophylaxis with erythromycin, a cephalosporin or a parenteral regimen.[8]

Metallic prosthetic joint replacement

There are no established guidelines for antibiotic prophylaxis in prosthetic joint replacement patients.[9,11,12] The risk for prosthesis infection from dentally induced bacteremias appears very low (0.05%).[9,11,12] Consultation with the orthopedic surgeon is mandatory and if prophylaxis is recommended, the drug of choice is cephalexin (Keflex) or cephradine (Velosef) in the same two-dose regimen and dosage as with penicillin for IE prophylaxis.

Immunocompromised patients

Dental patients with a suppressed leukocyte count (cancer chemotherapy, blood dyscrasias, graft recipients) may be at-risk from dentally induced bacteremias if the WBC is 3500/mm or below.[13] These patients should only be treated for non-elective (emergency) dental situations. The antibiotic prophylaxis schedule is penicillin V (or erythromycin or a cephalosporin in allergic patients) at a dosage of 500 mg every 6 hours beginning one day before the dental procedure and continuing for 7 days after[13] along with physician consultation.

ORAL ANTIBIOTIC PROPHYLAXIS REGIMENS*

Drug	Adult dosage	Pediatric dosage
Penicillin V	2 grams 1 hour before procedure and 1 gram 6 hours after the initial dose	>60 pounds (27 kg) = Adult dose <60 pounds = Half the adult dose 1 hour before procedure and 6 hours later
Erythromycin (penicillin allergy)	1 gram 1 hour before procedure and 500 mg 6 hours after the initial dose	20 mg/kg 1 hour before procedure and 10 mg/kg 6 hours later

*Parenteral regimens and the complete AHA[5] or Medical Letter[6] Prophylaxis Guidelines are available upon request at the Dental School Pharmacy.

Continued.

GUIDELINES FOR ANTIBIOTIC PROPHYLAXIS
University of Southern California—School of Dentistry
May 1, 1985—cont'd.

REFERENCES

1. Pallasch, T.J.: New antibiotic prophylaxis regimens. *Dent. Drug Serv. Newsletter* **5:**13, 1984.
2. Friedman, L.R.: *Infective Endocarditis and Other Intravascular Infections,* 1982, Plenum Medical Book Company, New York.
3. Durack, D.T.: Prophylaxis of infective endocarditis. In: *Principles and Practice of Infectious Diseases* (Mandell, G.L., Douglas, R.G. Jr., and Bennett, J.E., eds.), 1979, John Wiley & Sons, New York.
4. Land, M.A. and Bisno, A.L.: Antimicrobial prophylaxis of bacterial infections. In: *Clinical Manual of Infectious Diseases* (Rytel, M.W. and Mogabgab, W., eds.), 1984, Year Book Medical Publishers, Chicago.
5. Shulman, S.T. et al.: Prevention of Bacterial Endocarditis: A Statement for Health Professionals· by the Committee on Rheumatic Fever and Infectious Endocarditis of the Council on Cardiovascular Disease in the Young. *Circulation* **70:**1123-A, 1984.
6. Prevention of bacterial endocarditis. *The Medical Letter on Drugs and Therapeutics* **26:**3, 1984.
7. American Heart Association. Prevention of Bacterial Endocarditis. *Circulation* **56:**139-A, 1977.
8. Shulman, S.T. et al.: Prevention of Rheumatic Fever: A Statement for Health Professionals by the Committee on Rheumatic Fever and Infectious Endocarditis of the Council on Cardiovascular Disease in the Young. *Circulation* **70:**1118-A, 1984.
9. Pallasch, T.J.: Principles of antibiotic therapy XII. Prophylactic use of antibiotics. Part III. Prophylaxis for other cardiac and non-cardiac risk patients. *Dent. Drug Serv. Newsletter* **4:**5, 1983.
10. Calin, A.: Acute Rheumatic Fever. In: *Scientific American Medicine* (Rubinstein, E. and Federman, D.D., eds.), 1984, Scientific American, Inc., New York.
11. Little, J.W. and Falace, D.A.: Therapeutic considerations in special patients. *Dent. Clin. No. Amer.* **28:**455, 1984.
12. Little, J.W.: The need for antibiotic coverage for dental treatment of patients with joint replacement. *Oral Surg.* **55:**20, 1983.
13. Sonis, S.T., Fazio, R.C. and Fang, L.: *Principles and Practice of Oral Medicine,* 1984, W.B. Saunders Company, Philadelphia.

Stroke

COMMENT. Stroke or cerebrovascular accident (CVA) must be evaluated carefully, because patients with a history of CVA are also at greater risk when exposed to hypoxic levels of oxygen. If sedation is necessary, only lighter levels, such as those provided by inhalation sedation, are recommended. Transient cerebral ischemia (TCI) is a prodromal syndrome to CVA and must be evaluated carefully.

Kidney trouble

COMMENT. The nature of diseases of the kidney should be evaluated. Treatment modifications, including antibiotic prophylaxis (see box on opposite page), may be appropriate for several chronic forms of kidney disease.

Ulcers

COMMENT. The presence of stomach or intestinal ulcers may indicate acute or chronic anxiety and the possible use of medications such as tranquilizers and antacids. Knowledge of which drugs are being taken is important before additional medications are administered in the dental office.

Emphysema

COMMENT. Emphysema is a form of chronic obstructive pulmonary disease (COPD). The patient with emphysema has a decreased respiratory reserve to draw on in the event that the cells of his body require additional oxygen. Supplemental oxygen therapy during dental treatment is strongly recommended in more severe cases of emphysema.

Cough

COMMENT. The presence of a chronic cough may indicate active tuberculosis or other chronic respiratory disorders such as chronic bronchitis. The administration of CNS depressants, especially those with greater respiratory depressant properties, must be carefully evaluated in these patients with diminished respiratory reserve.

Tuberculosis

COMMENT. The status of the disease (active, arrested) should be determined before the start of dental therapy. Medical consultation is recommended if doubt persists, with possible modification of dental therapy. Inhalation sedation is not recommended for use in patients with active tuberculosis because of the likelihood of contamination of the rubber goods and the difficulty in sterilizing them. If the doctor treats many patients with tuberculosis, disposable rubber goods for inhalation sedation units are available.

Asthma

COMMENT. Asthma represents a partial obstruction of the lower airway. The doctor must seek to determine the nature of the asthma, its frequency of occurrence, the causative factors in its onset, the patient's method of management of the acute episode, and any drugs that the patient may be taking on a regular basis to minimize the risk of an acute episode developing. Stress is a common cause of acute asthmatic attacks.

Hay fever

COMMENT. Hay fever will indicate the presence of allergy to a foreign protein material (for example, pollen, cat dander, dust, dirt). Dental treatment should be avoided, if possible, during periods in which acute exacerbations of a patient's allergy are more frequent.

Sinus trouble

COMMENT. Sinus trouble may indicate the presence of allergy (to be pursued in the dialogue history) or of an upper respiratory infection (such as a cold). The patient may experience some respiratory distress when placed in more supine positions or if a rubber dam is used. Specific treatment modifications, such as postponement of treatment until the patient is better able to breathe, may be warranted.

Allergies or hives

COMMENT. Any allergy must be thoroughly evaluated before the start of dental treatment and drug administration.

Diabetes

COMMENT. A positive response requires further inquiry to determine the type, severity, and degree of control of the diabetes. The patient with diabetes does not usually represent a significant risk during dental therapy or during the administration of medications for the management of pain or anxiety. The greatest concerns about dental management of this patient relate to the possible effect of dental treatment on eating habits and to the development of hypoglycemia. Modification of insulin dosage

---

DENTAL REFERRAL LETTER

Dear Doctor:

The patient who bears this note is on long-term chronic hemodialysis treatment because of chronic kidney disease. In providing dental care to these patients, there are certain precautions to be observed:

1. Dental manipulations are most safely done one day *after* their last dialysis treatment, or at least eight (8) hours thereafter. Residual heparin may make hemostasis difficult. (Some patients are on long-term anticoagulant therapy.)

2. We are concerned about bacteremic seeding of the arteriovenous shunt devices and heart valves. We recommend prophylactic antibiotics pre- and post-dental manipulation. Antibiotic selection and dosage can be tricky in renal failure.

   a) We recommend Penicillin V 2 grams 1 hour before procedure and 1 gram 6 hours later.

   b) In penicillin allergy: Erythromycin, 1 gram 1 hour before procedure and 500 mg 6 hours later, is recommended.

Sincerely,

Courtesy Kaiser Permanente Medical Center, Los Angeles, Calif. Reprinted by permission.

may be required in situations in which the patient does not obtain a normal food intake.

Thyroid disease

COMMENT. The presence of either hyperthyroidism or hypothyroidism leads the doctor to be more cautious in the administration of certain drug groups to these patients. In most instances, however, the patient seen will have had a hyperthyroid or hypothyroid condition at one time, but at present will be functioning at a normal level of thyroid hormone activity (euthyroid) because of either surgical intervention or drug therapy.

X-ray or cobalt treatment
Chemotherapy (cancer, leukemia)

COMMENT. The presence or prior existence of cancer of the head or neck may require specific modification in dental therapy. Irradiated tissues may have a decreased resistance to infection and a diminished vascularity with reduced healing capacity. There is no specific contraindication to the administration of any medication for pain or anxiety control. Many patients with cancer may also be receiving long-term therapy with central nervous system (CNS) depressants such as antianxiety drugs, hypnotics, or narcotics. Consultation with the patient's physician may be in order before dental treatment is begun.

Arthritis
Rheumatism
Cortisone medicine

COMMENT. A history of arthritis may be associated with chronic use of salicylates (aspirin) or other nonsteroidal antiinflammatory agents (NSAIAs), some of which may alter blood clotting. Arthritic patients may also be receiving long-term corticosteroid therapy with the possible risk of acute adrenal insufficiency. Such patients will require modification in the dosage of corticosteroids during the period of dental therapy to enable them to respond appropriately to any additional stress associated with dental treatment. An additional concern is the possible difficulty the doctor may have in attempting to position the patient for dental treatment. Modification may be necessary to accommodate the patient's physical disability.

Glaucoma

COMMENT. For patients with glaucoma, administration of an agent to diminish salivary gland secretions will be of concern. Atropine, scopolamine, and glycopyrrolate are contraindicated in these patients as they increase intraocular pressure.

Pain in the jaw joints

COMMENT. Chronic temporomandibular joint (TMJ) pain is seen with increasing frequency today. Evaluation as to the cause(s) should be sought.

AIDS
Hepatitis A (infectious)
Hepatitis B (serum)
Liver disease
Yellow jaundice
Blood transfusion
Drug addiction

COMMENT. The preceding diseases or procedures are either highly transmissible (such as AIDS and hepatitis A and B) or are possible indicators of a state of hepatic dysfunction. When any of these disorders is encountered, the doctor should seek to determine the status of the disease process and of the patient by consulting with the patient's physician.

Most medications used in dentistry undergo biotransformation in the liver. The presence of liver dysfunction will lead to a decreased rate of drug inactivation and to an increased risk of overdosage and/or prolonged clinical duration of action.

In patients who have undergone blood transfusion or who admit present or past drug addiction, there is a higher-than-normal incidence of liver disease. In addition, drug addicts also have a significantly greater risk of valvular damage in the heart and may require antibiotic prophylaxis.

Hemophilia

COMMENT. Hemophilia and other bleeding disorders must be fully evaluated before the start of any procedure, especially one in which bleeding may occur. It is prudent to avoid (where possible) the administration of regional nerve blocks in which the risk of positive aspiration of blood is great. In most instances, alternative techniques of pain control are available.

Venereal disease (syphilis, gonorrhea)
Cold sores
Genital herpes

COMMENT. The possibility of infection of the dentist is increased with these patients. Where oral lesions are present, dental therapy should be postponed, if possible. The use of protective rubber gloves, eyeglasses, and a mask provides the operator with a degree of protection but not absolute protection.

Epilepsy or seizures

COMMENT. The type of seizure activity, its frequency of occurrence, and the drug(s) used to prevent its occurrence must be determined before the start of dental treatment. Stress reduction and other treatment modifications are frequently in order during treatment of these patients.

Fainting or dizzy spells

COMMENT. The presence of chronic postural (orthostatic) hypotension or of symptomatic hypotension or anemia may be detected if patients report these symptoms. Transient ischemic attacks (TIA), a form of "prestroke," may also be detected by this question. Further evaluation, including consultation with the patient's physician, is recommended.

Nervousness
Psychiatric treatment

COMMENT. The presence of undue nervousness (in general or specifically related to dentistry) and the need for psychiatric treatment should place the doctor on guard before the start of dental therapy. These patients may be receiving any number of drugs for the management of their disorders, drugs that in many instances may produce interactions with other medications used in dentistry for the control of pain and anxiety (see box on p. 14). Medical consultation is recommended in these cases.

Sickle cell disease

COMMENT. Sickle cell disease is seen exclusively in the black patient. A sickle cell crisis can be precipitated in periods of unusual stress or when the patient does not receive an adequate oxygen supply (becomes hypoxic). When sickle cell disease is present, supplemental oxygenation of the patient during treatment is strongly recommended.

Bruise easily

COMMENT. A positive response to this statement may indicate the presence of a bleeding disorder, which should be evaluated before the start of dental treatment.

QUESTION 10. When you walk up stairs or take a walk, do you ever have to stop because of pain in your chest, or shortness of breath, or because you are very tired?

COMMENT. Although the patient may have indicated above that she does not have angina, heart failure, or pulmonary emphysema, clinical signs and symptoms may be present. This question will help the doctor to defer dental treatment until the patient's physician can further evaluate the patient's status.

QUESTION 11. Do your ankles swell during the day?

COMMENT. Congestive heart failure (CHF) immediately comes to mind when one thinks of swelling of ankles (pitting edema or dependent edema); however, there are several other conditions in which ankle edema is observed. These include varicose veins, pregnancy, and renal dysfunction. In addition, healthy persons who spend a great deal of their time standing on their feet (for example, mail carriers) may also exhibit edematous ankles.

QUESTION 12. Do you use more than two pillows to sleep?

COMMENT. Persons with more severe CHF exhibit orthostatic hypotension, which is the inability to breathe comfortably when lying down. These patients may require additional pillows under their back, in effect propping them up in bed, so that they may breathe more comfortably.

QUESTION 13. Have you lost or gained more than 10 pounds in the past year?

COMMENT. The question refers primarily to an unexpected gain or loss of weight (as opposed to dieting). Such weight changes may be observed in patients with heart failure (increased weight) or with widespread carcinoma or uncontrolled diabetes mellitus (weight loss), among other disorders.

QUESTION 14. Do you ever wake up from sleep short of breath?

COMMENT. Paroxysmal nocturnal dyspnea is a clinical manifestation of more severe left-side heart failure.

QUESTION 15. Are you on a special diet?

COMMENT. This question will elicit dietary alterations resulting from certain medical disorders (diabetes, high blood pressure, heart failure) and also diets that the patient may be on (either through a physician's consultation or a personal dieting plan) in an attempt to lose weight.

QUESTION 16. Has your medical doctor ever said you have a cancer or tumor?

COMMENT. This question refers to the comments made previously concerning x-ray or cobalt treatment, as well as chemotherapy (see pp. 21-22).

QUESTION 17. Do you have any disease, condition, or problem not listed?

COMMENT. The patient is permitted to comment on specific matters that were not previously discussed. Examples of such disorders that might be mentioned at this time include porphyria, atypical plasma cholinesterase, and malignant hyperthermia.

QUESTION 18. Women: are you pregnant now? Are you practicing birth control? Do you anticipate becoming pregnant?

COMMENT. Pregnancy is a relative contraindication to extensive elective dental therapy, particularly during the first trimester. Consultation with the patient's physician is recommended. Although the use of local anesthetics is indicated, the use of sedative modalities should receive careful consideration, weighing the risks vs the benefits. Of the available techniques, inhalation sedation with N_2O-O_2 is the most highly recommended. Table 2-2 lists many commonly used drugs and their possible prenatal effects.

• • •

The final statement on the form, "To the best of my knowledge, all of the preceding answers are true and correct. If I ever have any change in my health, or if my medicines change, I will inform the doctor of dentistry at the next appointment without fail," is essential from a medical-legal standpoint. It must be accompanied by the date and signatures of the patient (or parent/guardian) and doctor. In effect, this is a contract obliging the patient (or parent/guardian) to report any changes in the patients' health or medications. Brady and Martinoff (1980) demonstrated that patients' analysis of their own personal health is frequently optimistic and that pertinent health matters are sometimes not immediately reported. For these reasons the questionnaire should be updated periodically—approximately every 6 months—or following a prolonged lapse in treatment. The entire form need not be redone; the following questions need only be asked.

1. Has there been any change in your general health in the past 6 months?
2. Are you now under the care of a medical doctor? If so, what is the condition being treated?
3. Are you taking any drug or medicine?

If a positive response is elicited, a detailed dialogue history with the patient should follow. The responses to these questions are recorded on the patient's chart (Fig. 2-1).

The complete medical history questionnaire should be repeated annually. It should be completed by the patient (or parent/guardian) IN INK. Any correction or deletion made subsequently by the doctor should be done by drawing a single line through the original, not obliterating it. The change is then added, with the doctor initialing the change.

All positive responses on the medical history questionnaire should be addressed by the doctor during the dialogue history, with an appropriate notation placed on the chart.

Physical Examination

The medical history questionnaire is quite important in the overall assessment of a patient's physical and psychologic status. However, there are limitations to the value of the questionnaire. For the questionnaire to be valuable the patient must (1) be aware of the presence of any medical condition and (2) be willing to share this information with the dentist.

Most patients will not knowingly deceive the dentist by omitting important information from the medical history questionnaire, although cases in which such deception has been attempted are on record. For example, a patient seeking treatment for an acutely inflamed tooth decided to withhold from the doctor the fact that he had had a myocardial infarction 2½ months earlier because he knew that to tell the doctor would mean that he would not receive treatment. Examples such as this are quite rare but have occurred.

The other factor, a patient's lack of knowledge of his physical status, is a more likely cause of misinformation on the questionnaire. Most healthy persons do not visit their physician regularly for routine checkups. In fact, recent information has suggested that annual visits be discontinued in the healthy patient under 40 years of age because the annual physical examination has not proved to be as valuable an aid in preventive medicine as was once thought. Be that as it may, most patients simply do not visit their physicians on a regular basis, doing so, instead, whenever they become ill. Therefore it stands to reason that the true state of the patient's physical condition may be unknown to the patient. Feeling well, although usually a reliable indicator of good health, does not guarantee good health. Many disease entities may be present for a considerable length of time in a subclinical state without exhibiting any overt signs or symptoms that warn the patient of their presence. When such signs and symptoms are present, they are often mistaken for other, more benign problems. Although they may be answering the questions in the medical history questionnaire to the best of their ability, patients cannot give a positive reply to a question un-

Table 2-2. Known prenatal effects of drugs

Drug	Effect
Amobarbital	No adverse effects reported
Anesthetics, local	No adverse effects in dentistry
Atropine	Sympathomimetic effects
Barbiturates	Concentration is greater in fetus than mother because fetal kidneys are unable to eliminate barbiturate
Bupivacaine	Does not cross placenta readily; no adverse effects in dentistry
Chlordiazepoxide	In initial 42 days of pregnancy, congenital abnormalities more frequent
Diazepam	In first trimester, cleft lip and palate increased fourfold
Epinephrine	No adverse effects reported for dental use
Halothane	May be hazardous to pregnant operating-room personnel
Hydroxyzine	Hypotonia reported
Lidocaine	No adverse effects reported in dentistry
Meperidine	Decreased neonatal respiration
Mepivacaine	No adverse effects reported in dentistry
Meprobamate	Possible increased congenital abnormalities during first 42 days of pregnancy
Morphine	With chronic usage, smaller newborns; withdrawal symptoms noted
N_2O	With few exposures, no adverse effects reported when a 30% oxygen level is maintained and employed as an anesthetic for dental procedures; evidence suggests an increase in spontaneous abortion among wives of heavily exposed (> 9 hours/week) dentists and among female chairside assistants; increase in congenital anomalies in offspring of heavily exposed (> 9 hours/week) dental chairside assistants
Pentazocine	Fetal addiction and withdrawal symptoms of hypertonia, tremors, hyperactivity, and inability to feed
Promethazine	Congenital hip dislocation
Prilocaine	No adverse effects reported in dentistry
Scopolamine	No adverse effects reported

Modified from Council on Dental Therapeutics: J. Am. Dent. Assoc. **107**:887, 1983.

less they are aware that they do, in fact, have the problem. The first few questions on most history forms relate to the length of time since the last physical examination of the patient. The value of the answers dealing with disease processes can be gauged from the patient's responses to these questions.

Because of these problems, which are inherent in the use of a patient-completed medical history questionnaire, the doctor must seek additional sources of information concerning the physical status of the patient.

Physical examination of the patient will provide much of this information. This consists of the following:
1. Monitoring of vital signs
2. Visual inspection of the patient
3. Function tests, as indicated
4. Auscultation of heart and lungs, and laboratory tests, as indicated

Minimal physical evaluation of all potential patients should consist of measurement of vital signs and visual inspection of the patient.

The primary value of the physical examination is that it provides the doctor with important information concerning the physical condition of the patient immediately before the start of treatment, as contrasted with the questionnaire, which provides historical information. The patient should undergo this minimal physical evaluation during an initial visit to the office, before the initiation of any form of treatment.

Vital signs

There are six vital signs:
1. Blood pressure
2. Heart rate (pulse) and rhythm
3. Respiratory rate
4. Temperature
5. Height
6. Weight

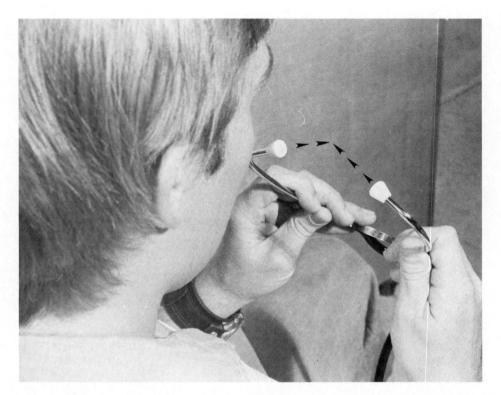

Fig. 2-3. Stethoscope ear pieces are inserted facing in an anterior direction.

The technique of recording vital signs, as well as guidelines for the interpretation of the measurements obtained, follow.

Blood pressure

Technique. The following technique is recommended for the accurate determination of blood pressure. A stethoscope (Fig. 2-3) and sphygmomanometer, or blood pressure cuff (Figs. 2-4 and 2-5) are the required equipment. The most accurate and reliable of these devices is the mercury-gravity manometer (Fig. 2-5). The aneroid manometer (Fig. 2-4), probably the most frequently employed, is calibrated to be read in millimeters of mercury (mm Hg, or torr) and is also quite accurate if well maintained. Rough handling of the aneroid manometer may lead to erroneous readings. The aneroid manometer should be recalibrated at least annually by checking it against a mercury manometer. In recent years many automatic blood pressure monitoring devices have been introduced on the market. The earliest of these devices left much to be desired in accuracy, sensitivity, and reliability. Some of the more recent automatic blood pressure devices appear to be considerably more reliable.

For the routine preoperative recording of blood pressure, the patient should be seated in an upright position. The patient's arm should be at the level of the heart—relaxed, slightly flexed, and supported on a firm surface. The patient should be permitted to sit for at least 5 minutes before the blood pressure is recorded. This will permit the patient to relax somewhat so that the blood pressure recorded will be closer to the patient's usual "baseline" reading. During this time other nonthreatening procedures may be carried out, such as review of the medical history questionnaire.

The blood pressure cuff should be deflated before its being placed on the arm. The cuff should be wrapped evenly and firmly around the arm, with the center of the inflatable portion over the brachial artery and the rubber tubing along the medial aspect of the arm. The lower margin of the cuff should be placed approximately 1 inch (2 to 3 cm) above the antecubital fossa. A cuff is too tight if two fingers cannot be placed under the lower edge of the cuff. Too tight a cuff will decrease venous return from the arm, leading to erroneous measurements. A cuff is too loose (a much more common

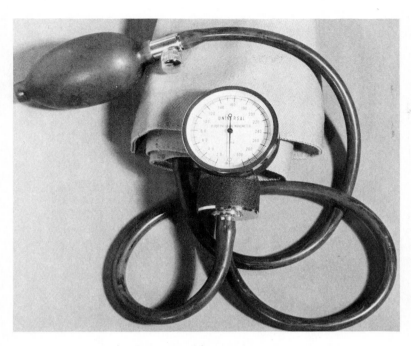

Fig. 2-4. Aneroid type manometer.

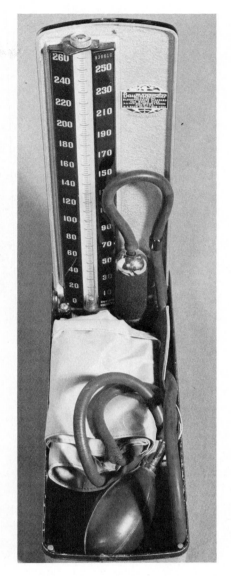

Fig. 2-5. Mercury type manometer.

problem) if it may be pulled off the arm with gentle tugging. A slight resistance should be present when a cuff is properly applied (Fig. 2-6).

The radial pulse must be palpated and then the pressure in the cuff increased rapidly to a point approximately 30 torr above the point at which the radial pulse disappears. The cuff should then be slowly deflated at a rate of 2 to 3 torr per second until the radial pulse reappears. This is termed the *palpatory systolic pressure.* Pressure in the cuff should then be released.

Determination of blood pressure by the more accurate auscultatory method requires palpation of the brachial artery, which is located on the medial aspect of the antecubital fossa (Fig. 2-7). The earpieces of the stethoscope should be placed, facing forward (Fig. 2-3), firmly in the recorder's ears. The diaphragm of the stethoscope must be placed firmly on the medial aspect of the antecubital fossa, over the brachial artery. To reduce extraneous noise, the stethoscope should not touch the blood pressure cuff or rubber tubing.

The blood pressure cuff should be rapidly inflated to a level 30 torr above the previously determined palpatory systolic pressure. Pressure in the cuff should be gradually released (2 to 3 torr per second) until the first sound is heard through the

stethoscope. This is referred to as *the systolic blood pressure.*

As the cuff deflates further, the sounds undergo changes in quality and intensity (Fig. 2-8). As the cuff pressure approaches the diastolic pressure, sounds become dull and muffled and then cease. The diastolic blood pressure is best indicated at the point of complete cessation of sounds. In some instances, however, complete cessation of sound does not occur. In these instances, the point at which the sounds became muffled will be the diastolic pressure. The cuff should be slowly deflated to a point

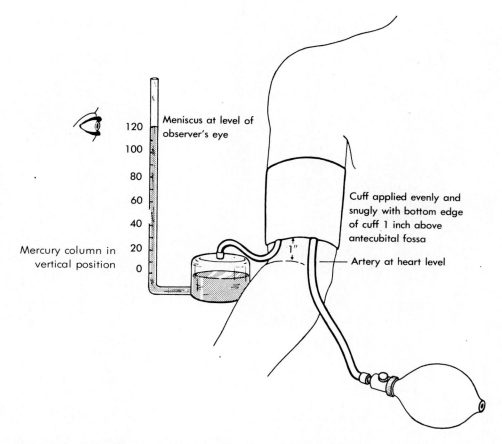

120   Meniscus at level of
100   observer's eye

80

60   Cuff applied evenly and
        snugly with bottom edge
40   of cuff 1 inch above
        antecubital fossa

Mercury column in   20
vertical position   0   Artery at heart level

Fig. 2-6. Proper placement of blood pressure cuff (sphygmomanometer). (From Burch, G.E., and DePasquale, N.P.: Primer of clinical measurement of blood pressure, St. Louis, 1962, The C.V. Mosby Co.)

10 torr beyond the point of disappearance and then totally deflated.

Should additional recordings be necessary, a wait of at least 15 seconds is required before reinflating the blood pressure cuff. This permits blood trapped in the arm to leave, providing more accurate readings.

Blood pressure is recorded on the patient's chart or sedation/anesthesia record as a fraction: *130/90 R* (right) or *L* (left), depending on the arm used to obtain the blood pressure reading.

Common errors in technique. There are some relatively common errors associated with the recording of blood pressure. Lack of awareness of these may lead to unnecessary medical consultation, adding financial burden to the patient, and a loss of faith in the doctor.

1. Applying the blood pressure cuff too loosely will give falsely elevated readings. This probably represents the most common error in recording blood pressure.

2. Use of the wrong cuff size can result in erroneous readings. A "normal adult" blood pressure cuff placed on an obese patient's arm will produce falsely elevated readings. This same cuff applied to the very thin arm of a child or adult will produce false-low readings. Sphygmomanometers are available in a variety of sizes. The width of the compression cuff should be approximately 20% greater than the diameter of the extremity on which the blood pressure is being recorded (Fig. 2-9).

3. An auscultatory gap may be present (Fig. 2-10). This gap represents a loss of sound between systolic and diastolic pressures, the sound reappearing at a lower level. For example, systolic sounds are noticed at 230 torr; however, the sound then disappears at 198 torr, reappearing at approximately 160 torr. All sound is lost at 90 torr. In

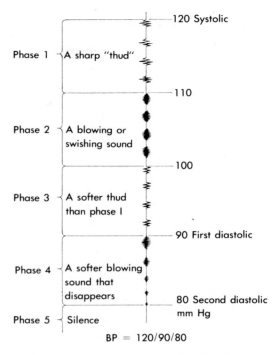

Phase 1 — A sharp "thud"

Phase 2 — A blowing or swishing sound

Phase 3 — A softer thud than phase I

Phase 4 — A softer blowing sound that disappears

Phase 5 — Silence

120 Systolic

110

100

90 First diastolic

80 Second diastolic mm Hg

BP = 120/90/80

Fig. 2-8. Korotkoff sounds. Systolic blood pressure is recorded at the first phase, and diastolic blood pressure is recorded at the point of disappearance of sound (fifth phase). (From Burch, G.E., and DePasquale, N.P.: Primer of clinical measurement of blood pressure, St. Louis, 1962, The C.V. Mosby Co.)

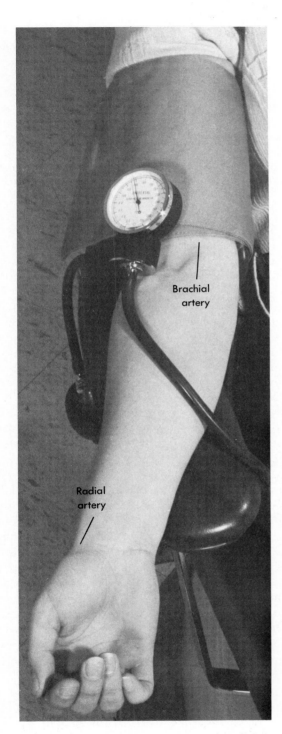

Fig. 2-7. Location of brachial artery and radial artery. Brachial artery is located in the medial half of the antecubital fossa; radial artery is located in the lateral volar aspect of the wrist.

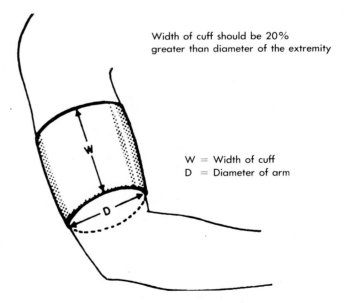

Width of cuff should be 20% greater than diameter of the extremity

W = Width of cuff
D = Diameter of arm

Fig. 2-9. Determination of proper size of blood pressure cuff. (From Burch, G.E., and DePasquale, N.P.: Primer of clinical measurement of blood pressure, St. Louis, 1962, The C.V. Mosby Co.)

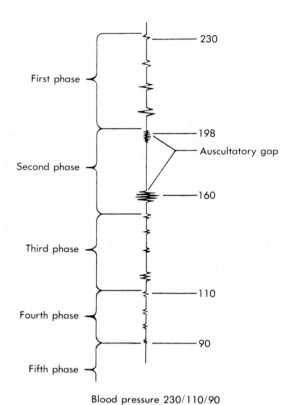

Blood pressure 230/110/90

Fig. 2-10. Korotkoff sounds, illustrating auscultatory gap. Sound is heard at 230 torr, disappears at 198 torr, and reappears at 160 torr. Sound disappears (fifth phase) at 90 torr. (From Burch, G.E., and DePasquale, N.P.: Primer of clinical measurement of blood pressure, St. Louis, 1962, The C.V. Mosby Co.)

this situation, if the person taking the blood pressure has not palpated (estimated) the systolic blood pressure before auscultation, the cuff might be inflated to some arbitrary pressure, such as 165 torr. At this level no sound would be heard because this lies within the auscultatory gap. Sounds would first be noticed at 160 torr, with disappearance at 90 torr, levels well within therapy limits for adults (see guidelines, Table 2-2). In reality, however, this patient has a blood pressure of 230/90, a significantly elevated pressure that represents a greater risk to the patient during dental therapy. Although the auscultatory gap occurs only infrequently, the possibility of error may be eliminated by first using the palpatory technique. The pulse will be present in the gap although the sound will disappear. Although there is no pathologic significance to its presence, the auscultatory gap is found most often in patients with high blood pressure.

4. The patient may be anxious. Sitting in the dental chair and having one's blood pressure recorded may produce anxiety, causing transient elevations in blood pressure, primarily the systolic. This is even more likely to be noted in the patient who is to receive sedation for management of dental anxieties. For this reason it is recommended that baseline measurements of vital signs be taken at a visit before the start of treatment, perhaps at the first office visit, when the patient will only be completing various forms. Measurements are more likely to be the norm for the particular patient at this time.

5. Blood pressure is based on the Korotkoff sounds (Fig. 2-8) produced by the passage of blood through obstructed, partially obstructed, or unobstructed arteries. Watching a mercury column or needle on an aneroid manometer for "pulsations" will lead to the recording of falsely elevated systolic pressures. These pulsations are observed approximately 10 to 15 torr before the first Korotkoff sounds are heard.

6. Use of the left or right arm will produce differences in recorded blood pressure. A difference of 5 to 10 torr exists between arms, the left arm being slightly higher.

Guidelines for clinical evaluation. The USC physical evaluation system is based on the American Society of Anesthesiologists ASA Physical Status Classification System (see p. 37). It provides four risk categories based on a patient's medical history and physical evaluation. These categories for blood pressure recordings are presented in Table 2-1.

For the adult patient with a blood pressure in the ASA I range (<140/<90 torr) it is suggested that the blood pressure be recorded every 6 months, unless specific forms of dental therapy demand more frequent monitoring. The administration of local anesthesia and the use of any parenteral or inhalation route of drug administration also require the more frequent recording of vital signs.

Patients falling into ASA II, III, or IV categories for blood pressure should be monitored at every appointment as outlined in the guidelines. Patients with known high blood pressure should also have their blood pressure monitored at each visit to determine if it is adequately controlled. The routine monitoring of blood pressure in all patients according to the treatment guidelines will effectively minimize the occurrence of acute complications of high blood pressure.

When parenteral or inhalation sedation tech-

Table 2-3. Normal blood pressure measurements for various ages*

Ages	Mean systolic ±2 S.D.	Mean diastolic ±2 S.D.
Newborn	80 ± 16	46 ± 16
6 mo-1 yr	89 ± 29	60 ± 10†
1 yr	96 ± 30	66 ± 25†
2 yr	99 ± 25	64 ± 25†
3 yr	100 ± 25	67 ± 23†
4 yr	99 ± 20	65 ± 20†
5- 6 yr	94 ± 14	55 ± 9
6- 7 yr	100 ± 15	56 ± 8
7- 8 yr	102 ± 15	56 ± 8
8- 9 yr	105 ± 16	57 ± 9
9-10 yr	107 ± 16	57 ± 9
10-11 yr	111 ± 17	58 ± 10
11-12 yr	113 ± 18	59 ± 10
12-13 yr	115 ± 19	59 ± 10
13-14 yr	118 ± 19	60 ± 10

From Nadas, A.S., and Fyler, D.C.: Pediatric cardiology, ed. 3, Philadelphia, 1972, W.B. Saunders Co.
*Adapted from data in the literature; figures have been rounded off to nearest decimal place.
†In this study the point of muffling was taken as the diastolic pressure.

niques or general anesthesia procedures are to be employed, there is a greater need for baseline vital signs. One of the factors employed to determine a patient's recovery from the effects of sedation and readiness to be discharged from the office will be a comparison of the posttreatment vital signs with baseline values.

Yet another reason for routine monitoring of blood pressure relates to the management of emergencies. After the basic steps of management in each emergency, certain specific steps are necessary for definitive treatment. Primary among these is the monitoring of vital signs, particularly blood pressure. Blood pressure recorded during an emergency situation is an important indicator of the status of the cardiovascular system. However, unless a baseline or nonemergency blood pressure had been recorded earlier, the measurement obtained during the emergency is less significant. A recording of 80/50 torr is less ominous in a patient with a preoperative reading of 110/70 than if the pretreatment recording were 190/110. The absence of blood pressure is an indication for cardiopulmonary resuscitation.

Normal blood pressures in younger patients will be somewhat lower than those presented above.

Table 2-3 presents a normal range of blood pressure measurements in infants and children.

Heart rate and rhythm

Techniques of measurement. Heart rate or pulse may be measured using any readily accessible artery. Most commonly employed for routine measurement are the brachial artery located on the medial aspect of the antecubital fossa and the radial artery on the radial and volar aspects of the wrist. Other arteries such as the carotid and femoral may be used; however, these are rarely used in routine situations because of their inaccessibility. In emergency situations it is recommended that the carotid artery be palpated in lieu of others, because the goal in managing life-threatening situations is the maintenance of life, and the carotid artery is the artery that carries oxygenated blood to the brain. Prompt and accurate location of this artery is essential in emergency situations. The technique of locating the carotid artery (in the neck) is reviewed in Chapter 5.

When palpating for a pulse, use the fleshy portions of the first two fingers, pressing gently enough to feel the pulsation but not so firmly that the artery is occluded and no pulsation felt. The thumb should not be used to monitor any pulse, because the thumb contains a fair-sized artery that pulsates. Situations have arisen in which the measured heart rate has been the rescuer's, not the victim's.

In the infant the precordium is no longer recommended as the site to determine the presence of an effective heartbeat. The brachial artery in the upper arm is recommended (Fig. 2-11).

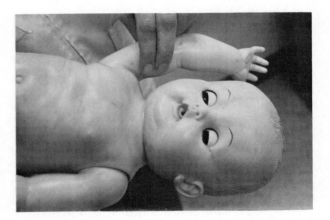

Fig. 2-11. Pulse determination in the infant is best accomplished in the brachial artery located on the medial side of the upper arm.

Table 2-4. Average pulse rates at different ages

Age	Lower limits of normal	Average	Upper limits of normal
Newborn	70	120	170
1-11 mo	80	120	160
2 yr	80	110	130
4 yr	80	100	120
6 yr	75	100	115
8 yr	70	90	110
10 yr	70	90	110

From Behrman, R.E., and Vaughn, V.C., III: Nelson textbook of pediatrics, ed. 12, Philadelphia, 1983, W.B. Saunders Co. Reprinted by permission.

Guidelines for clinical evaluation. Three factors should be evaluated while the pulse is monitored. These factors are as follows:

1. The heart rate (recorded as beats per minute)
2. The rhythm of the heart (regular or irregular)
3. The quality of the pulse (for example, thready, bounding, or weak)

The heart rate should be evaluated for a minimum of 30 seconds, and ideally for 1 minute. The normal resting heart rate for an adult ranges from 60 to 100 beats per minute. It is frequently lower in a well-conditioned athlete and elevated in the apprehensive individual. However, clinically significant pathologic conditions may also produce slow heart rates (bradycardia) or rapid heart rates (tachycardia). It is suggested that any adult heart rate under 60 or above 110 beats per minute be evaluated. When no obvious cause is located (endurance sports, anxiety), medical consultation should be considered.

The normal pulse maintains a relatively regular rhythm. Occasional premature ventricular contractions (PVCs) are so common that they are not necessarily considered abnormal. PVCs may be produced by smoking, fatigue, stress, various medications (such as epinephrine), and alcohol. If, however, PVCs are present at a rate of 5 or more per minute in a patient with other risk factors of coronary artery disease, medical consultation should be considered. Clinically PVCs are detected as breaks in a generally regular heart rate in which a longer-than-normal pause (skipped beat) is noted followed by resumption of normal rhythm. Unusually frequent PVCs (more than 5 per minute in the presence of other cardiovascular disease risk fac-

tors) indicate myocardial irritability and may presage ventricular fibrillation.

A second important disturbance in pulse is termed *pulsus alternans.* It is not truly an arrhythmia but is a regular heart rate characterized by a pulse in which strong and weak beats alternate. It is produced by the alternating contractile force of a diseased left ventricle. Pulsus alternans is observed frequently in left ventricular failure, severe arterial high blood pressure, and coronary artery disease. Medical consultation is indicated.

The quality of the pulse is commonly described as bounding, thready, or weak. These adjectives relate to the "feel" of the pulse and are used to describe situations such as "full bounding" pulse (as noted in severe arterial high blood pressure) or a "weak thready" pulse often noted in patients with hypotension and signs of shock.

As may be noted in Table 2-4, normal heart rates in pediatric patients are more rapid than those seen in adults.

Respiratory rate

Technique. Determination of the respiratory rate must be made surreptitiously. Patients aware that their breathing is being observed will not breathe normally. Therefore it is recommended that respiration be monitored immediately after the heart rate. The observer's fingers are left on the patient's radial or brachial pulse after the pulse rate has been determined; however, the doctor counts respirations instead (by observing the rise and fall of the chest) for a minimum of 30 seconds, ideally for 1 minute.

Guidelines for clinical evaluation. Normal respiratory rate for an adult is 16 to 18 breaths per minute. Bradypnea (abnormally slow rate) may be produced by narcotic administration, and tachypnea (abnormally rapid rate) is seen in fever and alkalosis. The most common change in ventilation in dental practice will be hyperventilation, an abnormal increase in rate and depth of respiration. Hyperventilation is also seen in diabetic acidosis. The most common cause of hyperventilation in dental settings is extreme psychologic stress.

Any significant variation in respiratory rate should be evaluated further before dental therapy. Absence of spontaneous ventilation is an indication to begin artificial ventilation.

Table 2-5 presents the normal range of respiratory rates at different ages.

• • •

Blood pressure, heart rate and rhythm, and respiratory rate are vital signs that provide information about the functioning of the cardiorespiratory system of the patient. It is recommended that they be recorded as a part of the routine physical evaluation for all potential patients. Recording of the remaining vital signs—temperature, height, and weight—is desirable but may be considered optional. However, in cases in which parenteral medications are to be administered, especially in lighter-weight, younger patients, recording of a patient's weight becomes considerably more important.

Temperature

Technique. Temperature should be monitored orally. The thermometer, sterilized and shaken down, is placed under the tongue of the patient, who has not eaten, smoked, or had anything to drink in the previous 10 minutes. The thermometer remains in the closed mouth for 2 minutes before removal. Disposable thermometers (Fig 2-12), as well as digital thermometers, are gaining acceptance today.

Guidelines for clinical evaluation. The "normal" oral temperature of 98.6° F is only an average. The true range of normal is considered to be from 97° F to 99.6° F. Temperatures vary (from 0.5° to 2.0°) throughout the day, being lowest in the early morning and highest in the late afternoon.

Fever represents an increase in temperature beyond 99.6° F. Temperatures in excess of 101° F usually indicate an active disease process. Full evaluation of the cause is necessary before treatment. When dental infection is considered a probable cause of elevated temperature, immediate treatment and antibiotic and antipyretic therapy are indicated. If the patient's temperature is 104° F or higher, immediate medical consultation is indicated. With elevated temperature, dental therapy is contraindicated and treatment should be limited to drug administration (antibiotics and antipyretics) because a person is less able than usual to withstand stress.

Height and weight

Technique. Patients should be asked to state their height and weight. The ranges of normal height and weight are quite variable and are indicated on charts developed by various insurance companies.

Guidelines for clinical evaluation. Gross obesity or underweight may be indicative of an active disease process. Obesity will be noted in various endocrine

Table 2-5. Respiratory rates by age

Age	Rate/minute
Neonate	40
1 wk	30
1 yr	24
3 yr	22
5 yr	20
8 yr	18
12 yr	16
21 yr	12

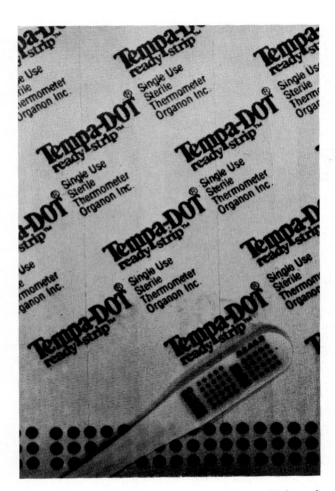

Fig. 2-12. Disposable thermometer. (From Malamed, S.F.: Sedation, St. Louis, 1985, The C.V. Mosby Co.)

disorders such as Cushing's syndrome, whereas extreme underweight may be noted in pulmonary tuberculosis, malignancy, and hyperthyroidism. In all instances of gross obesity or extreme underweight, medical consultation before the start of treatment is recommended. Excessively tall persons are referred to as giants, whereas persons who are decidedly shorter than normal are called dwarfs. In both instances endocrine gland dysfunction may be present. Medical consultation relative to dental treatment is usually not necessary for these patients.

Visual inspection of the patient

Visual observation of the patient may provide the doctor with valuable information concerning the medical status and the patient's level of apprehension toward dentistry. Observation of the patient's posture, body movements, speech, and skin can assist in a diagnosis of possibly significant disorders that may previously have gone undetected.

Patients with CHF and other chronic pulmonary disorders may be forced to sit in a more upright position in the chair because of orthopnea. The arthritic patient with a rigid neck may need to rotate his entire trunk when turning toward the doctor or to view an object from the side. Recognition of these factors will better enable the doctor to determine necessary treatment modifications.

Involuntary body movements occurring in conscious patients may indicate significant disorders. Tremor is noted in disorders such as fatigue, multiple sclerosis, parkinsonism, hyperthyroidism, and, of great importance to dentistry, hysteria and nervous tension.

The character of a patient's speech may also be significant. CVA may cause muscle paralysis leading to speech difficulties. Anxiety about impending dental treatment may also be noted by listening to a patient's speech. Rapid response to questions or a nervous quiver to the voice may indicate the presence of increased anxiety and the possible need for sedation during dental therapy.

Other possible disorders may be uncovered by the detection of odor on the patient's breath. A sweet, fruity odor of acetone is present in diabetic acidosis and ketosis. The smell of ammonia is noted in uremia. Probably the likeliest odor to be on the breath of a patient is that of alcohol. Detection of alcohol on a patient's breath should lead the doctor to consider the possibility of heightened anxiety toward dentistry.

The skin is an important source of information about the patient. It is my belief that the doctor should shake hands with patients on greeting them as a matter of routine. Much information can be gathered from the feel of a patient's skin. For example, the skin of a very apprehensive person will feel cold and wet, that of a patient with a hyperthyroid condition will be warm and wet, and that of a patient with diabetic acidosis will be warm but dry.

Looking at skin is also valuable. The color of the skin is significant. Pallor may indicate anemia or heightened anxiety. Cyanosis, indicating heart failure, chronic pulmonary disease, or polycythemia, will be most notable in the nail beds and mucous membranes (lips). Flushed skin may suggest apprehension, hyperthyroidism, or elevated temperature, and jaundice may indicate past or present hepatic disease.

Additional factors revealed through a visual examination of the patient include the presence of prominent jugular veins (in a patient seated upright), an indication of possible right-side heart failure; clubbing of the fingers (cardiopulmonary disease); swelling of the ankles (seen in right-side heart failure, varicose veins, renal disease, and occasionally in pregnancy); and exophthalmos (hyperthyroidism). Each of these findings will be discussed more fully in the section on prevention within each specific chapter.

For a more complete discussion of the art of observation and its importance in medical diagnosis, the reader is referred to *A Guide to Physical Evaluation* (Bates, 1979).

Additional evaluation procedures

After the completion of these three steps (written medical history questionnaire, recording of vital signs, and physical examination), a follow-up with additional evaluation for specific medical disorders may on occasion be necessary. This examination may include auscultation of the heart and lungs, testing for urinary and blood glucose levels, retinal examination, function tests for cardiorespiratory status (such as the breath-holding test), electrocardiographic examination, and blood chemistries. At present, many of these tests are used in dental offices but do not represent the standard of care in dentistry. Explanation and evaluation of many of the tests are beyond the scope of this text. Specific tests that may be used by the doctor in an effective and efficient manner will be referred to throughout this textbook. Examples are urinary and blood glucose testing and function tests for cardiopulmonary status.

Dialogue History

On completion of gathering all of the information (data base), the doctor must sit down with the patient and attempt to determine the severity of any disorder(s) and the potential risk represented by the patient during the planned treatment. The process of discussion with the patient is termed *the dialogue history,* and it forms an integral part of patient evaluation. The doctor must use all available knowledge of the disease to accurately assess the degree of risk to the patient. The dialogue history will be emphasized in the discussion on prevention of specific emergency situations.

In response to a positive reply to the question "Are you diabetic?" the dialogue history that follows should include these questions:

1. At what age did you develop diabetes? (adult or juvenile onset)
2. How do you control your diabetes? (insulin- or non-insulin-dependent)
3. How often do you check your urine or blood for sugar, and what are the measurements? (monitoring the degree of control of the disease)
4. Have you ever required hospitalization for your diabetic condition?

The following is a dialogue history to be initiated after a patient's affirmative reply to angina pectoris:

1. What precipitates your angina?
2. How frequently do you suffer anginal episodes?
3. How long do your anginal episodes last?
4. Describe a typical anginal episode.
5. How does nitroglycerin affect the anginal episode?

RECOGNITION OF ANXIETY

Thus far the primary thrust of our evaluation of the patient has been the prior medical history. Few if any questions have been directed at the patient's feelings toward the upcoming dental treatment. The typical (long-form) questionnaire has questions that ask, "Do you have fainting spells or seizures?" and "Have you had any serious trouble associated with any previous dental treatment?" The typical short-form history contains no questions that relate to this important area. Heightened anxiety and fear of dentistry are stresses that can lead

to the exacerbation of medical problems, such as angina, seizures, or asthma, or to other stress-related problems, such as hyperventilation or vasodepressor syncope. One of the goals of patient evaluation is to determine whether the patient is psychologically able to tolerate the stresses associated with dental therapy.

Three methods are available to recognize the presence of anxiety. First is the medical history questionnaire, second is the anxiety questionnaire, and third is the art of observation.

Earlier in this chapter it was recommended that one or more questions that relate to a patient's attitudes toward dentistry be added to the medical history questionnaire. It has been our experience at the USC School of Dentistry that patients who will

---

ANXIETY QUESTIONNAIRE

1. If you had to go to the dentist tomorrow, how would you feel about it?
   a. I would look forward to it as a reasonably enjoyable experience.
   b. I would not care one way or the other.
   c. I would be very uneasy about it.
   d. I would be afraid that it would be unpleasant and painful.
   e. I would be very frightened of what the dentist might do.
2. When you are waiting in the dentist's office for your turn in the chair, how do you feel?
   a. Relaxed.
   b. A little uneasy.
   c. Tense.
   d. Anxious.
   e. So anxious that I almost break out in a sweat or almost feel physically sick.
3. When you are in the dentist's chair waiting for him or her to get the drill ready and begin working on your teeth, how do you feel? (same choices as question 2)
4. You are in the dentist's chair to have your teeth cleaned. While you are waiting and the dentist is getting out the instruments with which to scrape your teeth around the gums, how do you feel? (same choices as question 2)
5. In general, do you feel uncomfortable or nervous about receiving dental treatment?
   a. Yes
   b. No

From Corah, N.: J. Dent. Res. **48**:596, 1969.

not verbally admit their fears to the doctor will in fact record on the chart that they are apprehensive. An affirmative response to any of these questions should alert the doctor to begin a more in-depth interview with the patient, seeking to determine the cause of the individual's fear of dentistry.

An additional aid in the recognition of anxiety is the anxiety questionnaire (see box on p. 35) devised by Corah (1969). Used since 1973 at the USC School of Dentistry, this questionnaire has proved to be a reliable aid in the recognition of anxiety. Answers to individual questions are scored 1 through 5 (a = 1, e = 5). Maximum score is 20. Scores of 8 or above indicate higher than usual levels of dental anxiety that should be addressed by the doctor.

In the absence of such questions or in the absence of an affirmative response to such questions, careful observation of the patient will enable the doctor and staff members to recognize the presence of unusual degrees of anxiety. Some patients will volunteer to the doctor and staff that they are quite apprehensive; however, the vast majority of apprehensive adult patients will do everything within their power to attempt to conceal their anxiety. The usual feeling of patients is that their fear is irrational and probably even a bit childish. They do not wish to tell the doctor of their fear because they are afraid of being labeled "childish." Because of this attitude in many adult patients, members of the dental staff must be trained to recognize clinical signs and symptoms of heightened anxiety.

While there are a number of levels into which anxiety may be subdivided, for the purposes of this discussion two will be discussed: moderate anxiety and severe (neurotic) anxiety.

Patients with *severe anxiety* will usually not attempt to hide this fact from the doctor. In fact, these patients will usually do anything within their power to avoid having to be dental patients. It is estimated that between 20 and 40 million adults in the United States avoid dental treatment because of their intense fears. These persons constitute the severe anxiety group. When in the dental office, they may be recognized by the following:

1. Increased blood pressure and heart rate
2. Trembling
3. Excessive sweating
4. Dilated pupils

Severely anxious patients will most commonly appear in the dental office when they have a serious toothache or infection. On questioning, they state that they have had this problem for quite some time, not just a few days, and have attempted every available means of home remedy (for example, toothache drops), which have apparently worked for some time. The reason that they are finally in the dental office is that within the past few nights they have been unable to sleep because of intense pain that none of their home remedies has been able to alleviate. Therefore these patients are driven by pain to the dental office, where they usually expect to have the tooth removed. These patients represent quite a management problem. Although they desire to have their problem treated, when it comes time for treatment to begin, their underlying fear of dentistry comes to the forefront and often makes it impossible for them to tolerate the procedure. In addition, the doctor is often faced with the unpleasant prospect of having either to extract an acutely inflamed tooth or to extirpate the pulp of an acutely sensitive tooth—two situations in which achieving clinically adequate pain control can be difficult in the best of circumstances.

Because of these factors, severely anxious patients will very often be candidates for the use of either IV sedation or general anesthesia. Other techniques, such as oral, IM, or inhalation sedation, used as suggested, will have little likelihood of success primarily because of their limited effectiveness or the constraints that are properly placed on their use.

Children with severe anxiety levels are frequently candidates for either IM or submucosal premedication or for general anesthesia.

Patients with more *moderate degrees of anxiety* will be much more frequently seen. Many of these patients will try to hide their fears from the doctor because they believe that, being adults, they should not admit to being afraid of the dentist. Children, on the other hand, being less inhibited than the typical adult, will immediately let the dental staff know of their feelings toward dentistry.

Assuming then that adult patients may attempt to hide their dental fears, the doctor and staff should remain observant both before and during the dental treatment.

The "front-office" people, such as the receptionist, will be able to overhear patients in the waiting room talking among themselves. Patients might ask important questions of the receptionist, such as "Is the doctor gentle?" or "Does the doctor use gas?" The receptionist should be trained to immediately inform the doctor whenever a patient makes statements that might indicate an increased degree of concern about the upcoming treatment. This is also true for chairside personnel.

Shaking hands with the patient may lead to a presumption of anxiety when the patient's palms are cold and sweaty, especially if the office is not especially cool.

Discussing a patient's prior dental experiences may give an indication of the dental anxiety status. The patient who has a history of emergency treatments only (for example, extractions or incision and drainage [I and D]) but who cancels or does not appear for subsequent appointments may be a fearful individual. A patient with a history of multiple cancelled appointments may also be a fearful patient. This history should be discussed with the patient in an attempt to determine the reasons behind this pattern of treatment (or nontreatment).

Once the patient is seated in the chair, he should be watched and listened to. Apprehensive patients remain alert and on guard at all times. They sit at the edge of the chair; their eyes roam all around the room, taking everything in. Their posture appears unnaturally stiff, and their arms and legs are tense. They may nervously fiddle with a handkerchief or tissue, occasionally being unaware that they are doing so. The "white-knuckle" syndrome may be observed, in which the patient clutches the armrest of the dental chair tightly enough that the knuckles turn white.

Profuse diaphoresis (sweating) of the palms or forehead may be noted, explained by the patient as "Gee, it's hot in here!"

The moderately apprehensive patient will be overly willing to aid the dentist. Actions are carried out quickly, usually without thinking. Questions to this patient are answered very quickly, usually too quickly.

Once anxiety has been recognized, be it through the questionnaire or observation, the patient must be confronted with it. The straightforward approach is surprisingly successful. The dentist might say, "Mr. Smith, I see from your medical history that you have had several unpleasant experiences in a dental office. Would you kindly describe these to me?" Or, when the anxiety is determined visually, "Mrs. Smith, you appear to be somewhat nervous today. Is something bothering you?" I have been truly astonished at how rapidly patients will drop all pretense at being calm once it is known that the doctor is aware of their fears. They usually will say, "Doctor, I didn't think you could tell." Once in the open, determination of the exact source of the patient's fears, such as injections or the drill, should be attempted. Once fears are known, steps may be instituted to minimize their occurrence.

The patient with moderate anxiety will usually prove to be treatable. In most cases, psychosedation will prove to be effective in management of the patient. This technique may involve the administration of a drug (pharmacosedation) or may be a nondrug form of sedation (iatrosedation). General anesthesia will only rarely be needed for the effective management of these patients.

• • •

With the information that has been gathered concerning the patient's past and present medical and dental histories, vital signs, and physical examination, the basic goals of evaluation can now be completed.

DETERMINATION OF MEDICAL RISK

Having completed all of the components of the physical evaluation and a thorough dental examination, the doctor must then gather all of this information and answer the following questions:

1. Is the patient capable, physiologically and psychologically, of tolerating in relative safety the stresses involved in the proposed dental therapy?
2. Does the patient represent a greater risk (of morbidity or mortality) than normal during dental therapy?
3. If the patient does represent an increased risk, what modifications will be necessary in the planned dental therapy to minimize this risk?
4. Is the risk too great for the patient to be managed safely in the dental office?

In an attempt to answer these questions, the USC School of Dentistry has developed a physical evaluation system that attempts to assist the doctor in categorizing patients from the standpoint of risk factor orientation. Its function is to place each patient in an appropriate risk category so that dental therapy can be provided in comfort and greater safety. The system is based on the ASA Physical Status Classification System, which will now be described.

PHYSICAL STATUS CLASSIFICATION SYSTEM

In 1962 the American Society of Anesthesiologists adopted what is now commonly referred to as the ASA Physical Status Classification System. It represents a method of estimating the medical risk presented by a patient undergoing a surgical procedure. The system was designed primarily for patients about to receive a general anesthetic, but since its introduction the classification system has been used for all surgical patients regardless of anesthetic technique (for example, general anesthesia, regional anesthesia, or sedation). The system has been in continuous use since 1962 virtually without change and has proved to be a valuable method of determining surgical and anesthetic risk before the actual procedure. The classification system follows:

ASA I: A patient without systemic disease; a normal, healthy patient

ASA II: A patient with mild systemic disease

ASA III: A patient with severe systemic disease that limits activity but is not incapacitating

ASA IV: A patient with incapacitating systemic disease that is a constant threat to life

ASA V: A moribund patient not expected to survive 24 hours with or without operation

ASA E: Emergency operation of any variety; E precedes the number, indicating the patient's physical status (for example, ASA E-III)

When this system was adopted for use in the typical outpatient dental setting, ASA V was eliminated, and an attempt has been made to correlate the remaining four classifications with possible treatment modifications for dental therapy. Fig. 2-13 illustrates the USC physical evaluation form on which a summary of the patient's physical and psychologic status is presented, along with treatment modifications.

Each of the classifications will be reviewed below, with specific examples listed.

ASA I

ASA I patients are considered to be normal and healthy. Review of these patients' medical histories, physical evaluations, and any other parameters that have been evaluated indicate no abnormalities. Physiologically these patients should be capable of tolerating the stresses involved in dental treatment with no added risk of serious complications. Psychologically these patients should represent little or no difficulty in handling the proposed treatment. Healthy patients with little or no anxiety are classified as ASA I patients. Therapy modifications

A

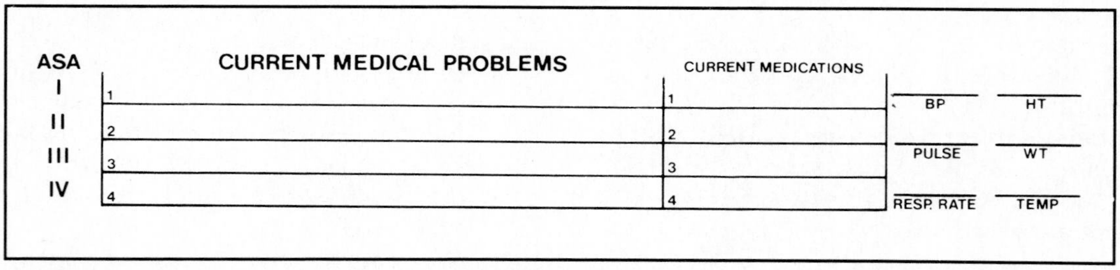
ASA
I
II
III
IV
CURRENT MEDICAL PROBLEMS
1
2
3
4
CURRENT MEDICATIONS
1
2
3
4
BP
HT
PULSE
WT
RESP. RATE
TEMP

B

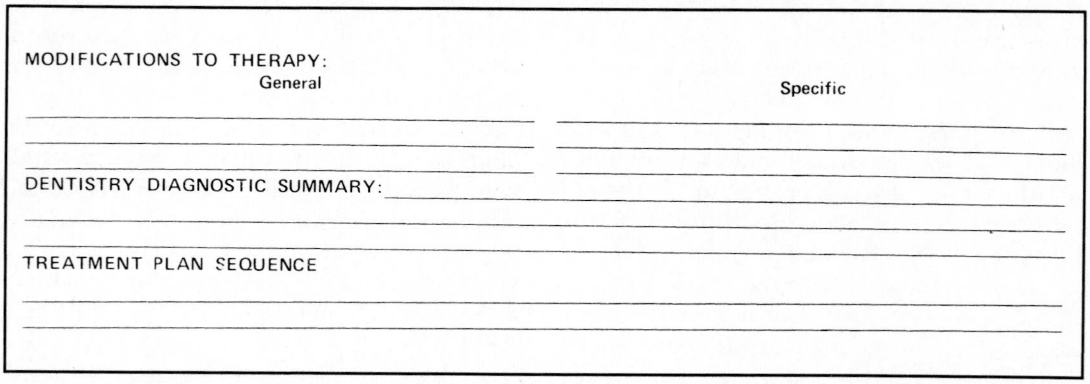
MODIFICATIONS TO THERAPY:
General
Specific
DENTISTRY DIAGNOSTIC SUMMARY:
TREATMENT PLAN SEQUENCE

Fig. 2-13. A, The physical evaluation section on the health history form provides room for summary of medical problems, vital signs, and ASA classification. **B,** Possible treatment modifications are listed on the patient's chart. (From Malamed, S.F.: Sedation, St. Louis, 1985, The C.V. Mosby Co.)

are usually not warranted for the patients in this group.

ASA II

ASA II patients have mild systemic disease or are healthy (ASA I) patients with more extreme anxiety and fear toward dentistry. ASA II patients are generally somewhat less stress tolerant than ASA I patients; however, they still represent a minimal risk during treatment. Routine treatment is in order with possible treatment modifications or special considerations as warranted by the particular condition. Examples of such modifications include the use of prophylactic antibiotics or sedative techniques, limiting the duration of treatment, and possible medical consultation.

Examples of ASA II patients include (1) patients with well-controlled, non-insulin-dependent diabetes, (2) patients with well-controlled epilepsy, (3) patients with well-controlled asthma, (4) patients with well-controlled hyperthyroid or hypothyroid conditions who are under care and presently have normal thyroid function, (5) ASA I patients with upper respiratory infection (URI), (6) healthy, pregnant women, (7) otherwise healthy patients with allergies, and (8) otherwise healthy patients with extreme dental fears. In general the ASA II patient will be able to perform normal activity* without experiencing such distress as undue fatigue, dyspnea, or precordial pain.

ASA III

ASA III patients have severe systemic disease that limits activity but is not incapacitating.

ASA III patients are even less stress tolerant than those classified ASA II. Dental treatment is still indicated; however, the need for stress reduction techniques and other treatment modifications is increased.

Examples of ASA III patients include (1) the typical patient with angina pectoris or a previous myocardial infarction, (2) patients who have had a CVA, (3) patients with insulin-dependent diabetes, (4) patients with CHF with orthopnea and ankle edema, and (5) patients with COPD, or chronic obstructive pulmonary disease (emphysema or chronic bronchitis and exercise-induced asthma). In general the ASA III patient will experience distress during normal activities.

---

*Normal activity is defined as the ability to climb a flight of stairs or walk two level city blocks.

ASA IV

ASA IV patients have an incapacitating disease that is a constant threat to life.

Patients in this category have a medical problem that is of greater importance than the planned dental treatment. Whenever possible, the planned treatment should be postponed until such time as the patient's medical condition has improved to at least ASA III. All elective dental therapy falls into this category. This patient represents a significant risk during treatment.

The management of dental emergencies, such as infection or pain, should be treated as conservatively as possible until the patient's condition improves. Where possible, treatment should consist of the prescription of medications such as analgesics for pain and antibiotics for infection. In situations in which it is believed that immediate intervention is required (I and D, extraction, pulpal extirpation), it is recommended that the patient receive such care within the confines of an acute care facility (that is, hospital). Although the risk to the patient is still significant, the chance of survival will be increased should an acute medical emergency arise.

Examples of ASA IV patients include patients with unstable angina pectoris (preinfarction angina), myocardial infarction within the past 6 months, blood pressure levels (for adults) greater than 200/115, severe CHF or COPD, CVA within the past 6 months, uncontrolled epilepsy, or uncontrolled insulin-dependent diabetes. In general, the ASA IV patient will experience distress while at rest.

• • •

This system is quite easy to employ when a patient has an isolated medical problem. However, many patients are initially seen with histories of several significant diseases. In these cases the doctor must weigh the significance of each disease and make a judgment as to the appropriate ASA category. The system is not meant to be inflexible; rather, it is meant to function as a relative value system based on the doctor's clinical judgment. When the doctor is unable to determine the clinical significance of one or more disease processes, consultation with the patient's physician or other medical or dental colleagues is recommended. In all cases, however, the ultimate decision either to treat or to postpone treatment must be made by the doctor. Liability rests solely in the hands of the doctor who treats or does not treat the patient.

MEDICAL CONSULTATION

Take patient's history
  Dental and medical
Perform physical examination
  Oral and general
Make initial evaluation
  Oral needs
  General systemic assessment (physical status category)
Consult the patient's physician when appropriate via telephone
  Physician's receptionist:
    Introduce yourself and give patient's name
  Physician:
    Introduce yourself
    Patient's name and reason for visit to you
    Relate *briefly* your summary of patient's general condition
    Ask for additional information
    Present your treatment plan *briefly,* including medications and degree of stress
    Discuss if necessary
Following consultation
  Write complete report of conversation for records

Modified with permission from W.H. Davis, D.D.S., Bellflower, CA.

Medical consultation

In the box above are the steps of a typical medical consultation. It is strongly suggested that the medical consultation not be made until the dental and physical evaluations have been completed. The dentist should be fully prepared to discuss the proposed dental therapy and any anticipated problems. One of the most important considerations in medical consultation is to determine the ability of the patient to tolerate the stress of dental therapy in relative safety. The physician's advice should be carefully considered, and the dentist must then institute steps to minimize the risk to the patient. The final responsibility for the dental treatment plan and the risks of treatment rests solely with the dentist. It cannot be shared with the physician. In most cases medical consultation leads to little or no basic alteration in planned dental therapy. Specific modifications, such as those offered on p. 41 in the Stress Reduction Protocol, represent potentially important steps in decreasing a patient's risk factor during dental therapy.

STRESS REDUCTION PROTOCOLS

At this point in our pretreatment evaluation of the patient, we have reviewed all of our history and physical evaluation data and have assigned a physical status classification. Most patients will be assigned an ASA I status, fewer will be ASA II, and fewer still will be categorized as ASA III or IV.

As discussed earlier, virtually every dental procedure is potentially stress inducing. Stress may be of a physiologic nature (pain, strenuous exercise) or of a psychologic nature (anxiety, fear). In either case, however, one of the responses of the body involves an increase in catecholamine release (epinephrine and norepinephrine) from the adrenal medulla into the cardiovascular system, which results in an increased cardiovascular workload (increased heart rate, increased strength of myocardial contraction, increased myocardial oxygen requirement). Although the ASA I patient may be quite able to tolerate such changes in cardiovascular activity, ASA II, III, and IV patients will be increasingly less able to safely tolerate these changes. The patient with angina may respond with an episode of chest discomfort, and various arrhythmias may develop. Patients with CHF may develop pulmonary edema. Patients with noncardiovascular disorders may also respond adversely when faced with increased levels of stress. For example, the patient with asthma may develop an acute episode of breathing difficulty, whereas the patient with epilepsy may have a seizure.

Unusual degrees of stress in the ASA I patient may be responsible for several psychogenically induced emergency situations, such as hyperventilation or vasodepressor syncope.

Interviews with apprehensive dental patients have demonstrated that many persons will begin to worry 1 or 2 days before their upcoming dental appointment. These persons may be unable to sleep well at night before the appointment, thus becoming fatigued and even more stress intolerant. The risk presented by these patients during dental treatment is increased even further.

The Stress Reduction Protocols are two series of procedures that, when used either individually or collectively, act to minimize stress during treatment and thereby decrease the risk presented by the patient. These protocols are predicated on the belief that the prevention or reduction of stress ought to begin before the start of treatment and continue throughout the treatment and, if indicated, the postoperative period.

Stress Reduction Protocol: Normal, Healthy, Anxious Patient (ASA I)

1. Recognition of anxiety
2. Premedication on night before dental appointment, as needed
3. Premedication immediately before dental appointment, as needed
4. Appointment scheduled in morning
5. Minimize waiting time
6. Psychosedation during therapy
7. Adequate pain control during therapy
8. Length of appointment variable
9. Postoperative pain/anxiety control
10. Telephone the highly anxious or fearful moderate-to-high-risk patient later on the same day that treatment was given.

Stress Reduction Protocol: Medical Risk Patient (ASA II, III, IV)

1. Recognition of medical risk
2. Medical consultation before dental therapy, as needed
3. Appointment scheduled in morning
4. Preoperative and postoperative vital signs monitored and recorded
5. Psychosedation during therapy, as needed
6. Adequate pain control during therapy
7. Length of appointment variable—not to exceed patient's limits of tolerance
8. Postoperative pain/anxiety control
9. Telephone the highly anxious or fearful moderate-to-high-risk patient later on the same day that treatment was given.
10. Arrange the appointment for the highly anxious or fearful moderate-to-high-risk patient during the first few days of the week when the office will be open for emergency care and when the treating doctor is available.

Recognition of Medical Risk and Anxiety

Recognition of these factors represents the starting point for the management of stress in the dental or surgical patient. Medical risk assessment will be accurately determined by strict adherence to the measures previously described in this chapter. The recognition of anxiety is often a more difficult task. As has been described previously, visual observa-

tion of the patient, as well as verbal communication, can provide the doctor with clues as to the presence of anxiety.

Medical Consultation

Medical consultation should be considered in those situations in which the doctor is uncertain as to the degree of risk represented by the patient. Medical consultation is neither required nor recommended for all patients with medical problems. In all cases it must be remembered that a consultation is a request for additional information concerning a specific patient or disease process. The doctor is seeking information that will aid in determining the degree of risk and therapy modifications that may be needed. The final responsibility for the care and safety of patients rests with the person who treats them.

Premedication

Many apprehensive patients state that their fear of dentistry is so great that they are unable to sleep well the night before their scheduled treatment. Fatigued the next day, these patients are less able to tolerate the additional stresses placed on them by dental treatment. Should the patient be medically compromised, the risk of an acute exacerbation of the patient's problem is greatly increased. In the ASA I patient, such additional stress may provoke a psychogenically induced response. Clinical manifestations of increased fatigue include a lowered pain reaction threshold. This patient is more likely to respond to a given stimulus as being painful than is a well-rested patient.

Restful sleep the night before a scheduled appointment is desirable. Therefore whenever it has been determined that heightened anxiety exists, it should also be determined if this anxiety interferes with sleep. Oral premedication is one method of achieving restful sleep. An antianxiety or sedative-hypnotic drug such as triazolam or flurazepam may be prescribed to be taken 1 hour before sleep.*

As the scheduled appointment approaches, the anxiety level of the patient will heighten. In many cases, the administration of an antianxiety or sedative-hypnotic agent approximately 1 hour prior to the scheduled appointment will decrease the patient's anxiety level to such a degree that the

---

*Appropriate dosages of these and other agents may be found in *Sedation: a guide to patient management* (Malamed, The C.V. Mosby Co., 1985).

thought of dental treatment is no longer as frightening. Oral medications should be administered approximately 1 hour before the scheduled start of treatment to permit a therapeutic blood level of the agent to develop. Oral agents may be taken by the patient while at home or in the confines of the dental office. Wherever an oral antianxiety drug has been prescribed to be taken by the patient at home, the doctor must advise the patient against driving a car or operating other potentially hazardous machinery.

The appropriate use of oral antianxiety or sedative-hypnotic agents is an excellent method of diminishing preoperative stress. Agents such as diazepam, oxazepam, hydroxyzine, promethazine, and chloral hydrate have been proven effective.

Appointment Scheduling

Apprehensive patients or medically compromised patients are best able to tolerate stress when they are well rested. In most cases, therefore, the ideal time to schedule these patients will be early in the day. This is also the case for the management of apprehensive or medically compromised children.

When the appointment is scheduled for the afternoon, the apprehensive patient must contend with the ominous specter of the dental appointment, which casts a pall over everything the patient does before it, allowing more time to think and to worry about it. The patient becomes more anxious, thereby increasing the likelihood of adverse psychogenic reactions. The morning appointment permits this patient to "get it over with" and to then continue with usual activities unburdened by anxiety.

For the medically compromised patient the situation is somewhat similar. As fatigue sets in, the patient becomes less and less able to manage increases in stress. A dental appointment scheduled later in the day may result in a medically compromised patient who has spent many hours at work, has driven through traffic, and possesses little or no ability to adequately handle additional stress. The earlier appointment provides the doctor and patient with a degree of flexibility in patient management.

The doctor should schedule the moderately to highly anxious medical-risk patient for treatment early in the week so that if postoperative complications arise, the patient is able to contact and be seen readily by the original treating doctor. In addition, the doctor should routinely contact the moderately to highly anxious, medically compromised patient later the same day following dental treatment to "see how they are doing." Such personal contact is greatly appreciated by the patient and serves as a means of preventing or at least minimizing any posttreatment complications.

Minimized Waiting Time

Once in the dental office setting, the apprehensive patient should not be required to sit in the waiting room or dental chair for extended periods of time before treatment commences. It is well known that anticipation of a procedure can induce more fear than the actual procedure. Sitting and waiting allows the patient to smell dental-office odors and hear dental-office sounds and to fantasize about the "horrible things" that are going to happen. Cases of serious morbidity and of death have occurred in the waiting room in dental offices. This factor is of greater significance in the apprehensive patient.

Vital Signs (Preoperative and Postoperative)

Before the start of dental therapy on the medically compromised patient the doctor should routinely measure and record the patient's vital signs. (Vital signs can be recorded by a trained auxiliary.) Those recorded should include blood pressure, pulse rate and rhythm, and respiratory rate. Comparison of these signs to the baseline values recorded at an earlier visit can serve as indicators of the patient's physical status on any given day. Although vital sign recordings are particularly relevant for patients with cardiovascular disease, it is recommended that they be taken on all medically compromised (all ASA III and appropriate ASA II) patients.

Postoperative vital signs should also be measured and recorded in these same patients on a routine basis.

Psychosedation During Therapy

Should additional stress reduction be considered necessary during dental treatment, any of the techniques of sedation or general anesthesia may be considered. Nondrug techniques include iatrosedation and hypnosis, whereas the more commonly used pharmacosedation procedures include oral, inhalation, IM, and IV sedation. The primary goal of all these techniques is the same: the decrease or elimination of stress in a conscious patient. When appropriate techniques are properly employed, this goal may be achieved without added risk to the patient.

Adequate Pain Control During Therapy

For stress reduction to be successful, it is essential that adequate pain control be present. The successful management of pain is probably of greater importance in the medically compromised patient than in the ASA I individual. The potentially adverse actions of endogenously released catecholamines on cardiovascular function in the patient with clinically significant heart or blood vessel disease warrants the inclusion of vasoconstrictors in the local anesthetic solution. Judicious use of these agents along with proper injection techniques must, of course, be effected. Without adequate control of pain, sedation and stress reduction are impossible to achieve.

Duration of Dental Appointment

The length of the treatment period is significant to both the medically compromised and apprehensive patient.

In the absence of any medical factors dictating the need for shorter appointments, the length of the appointment should be decided by the doctor after consideration of the patient's desires. In many instances, the apprehensive patient (ASA I) may prefer to have as few dental appointments as possible regardless of their length. Appointments 3 hours or longer may constitute preferred management for this otherwise healthy patient. However, attempting to satisfy the patient's desires for longer appointments is inadvisable when the doctor believes that there are appropriate reasons for shorter appointments. Cases of serious morbidity and of death have occurred when the doctor complied with parents' wishes to complete treatment of their child in one long appointment.

Unlike the anxious ASA I patient, the medically compromised patient should not be permitted to undergo longer appointments. In a dental chair 1 hour is stressful for many persons. Even an ASA I patient may have difficulty tolerating 2- or 3-hour procedures. To allow the higher risk patient to undergo extended treatment will unnecessarily increase risk. Dental appointments in the medically compromised patient should be of shorter duration, never exceeding the limit of the patient's tolerance. Signs that this limit has been reached include evidence of fatigue, restlessness, sweating, and evident discomfort. The most prudent way of managing the patient at this time is to terminate the procedure as expeditiously as possible and reschedule the treatment.

Postoperative Control of Pain and Anxiety

Of equal importance to preoperative and intraoperative pain and anxiety control is the management of pain and anxiety in the posttreatment period. This is especially relevant for the patient who has undergone a potentially traumatic procedure such as endodontics, periodontal or oral surgery, extensive oral reconstruction, or restorative procedures. The doctor must carefully consider the possible complications that might arise during the 24 hours immediately following dental therapy, discuss these with the patient, and then take steps to assist the patient in managing them. These steps include any or all of the following when indicated:

1. Availability of the doctor by telephone for 24 hours
2. Pain control: prescription for analgesic medication, as needed
3. Antibiotics if possibility of infection exists
4. Antianxiety agents, if in the doctor's opinion the patient may require them
5. Muscle relaxant agents after prolonged therapy or multiple injections into one area (such as inferior alveolar nerve block)

Availability of the doctor by telephone 24 hours a day has become a standard of care in dentistry. With answering services and telephone answering machines readily available, the patient should be able to contact the doctor whenever necessary.

Several studies have demonstrated that unexpected pain is rated as being more uncomfortable than expected pain. Should the possibility of discomfort exist following a procedure, the patient should be forewarned and an analgesic medication should be made available. When the possibility of posttreatment pain has not been discussed and it does develop, the patient will immediately think that something "has gone wrong." Such pain is recorded as being more intense and anxiety-provoking than expected pain. Should the posttreatment discomfort, which has been discussed, fail to materialize, the patient will be all the more relaxed and confident in the doctor's abilities.

• • •

In addition to the general modifications in patient management discussed in the preceding Stress Reduction Protocols, there are specific ther-

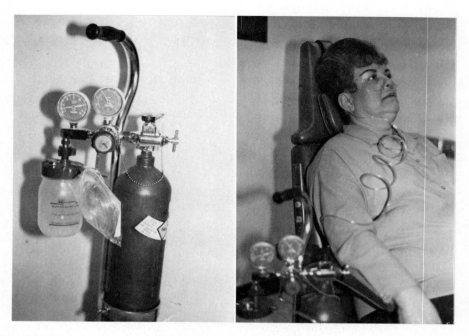

Fig. 2-14. Supplemental oxygen may be administered through a nasal cannula and humidifier.

apy modifications that will benefit certain groups of medically compromised patients. Both the general and specific therapy modifications indicated for a given patient should be entered on a patient's permanent record (Fig. 2-13) for future reference. Examples of specific therapy modification include:

1. Administration of intraoperative oxygen through a nasal cannula at a flow of 3 liters per minute; the oxygen should be humidified (Fig. 2-14)
2. Modification of patient positioning during treatment; the patient may be unable to tolerate the recommended supine or semisupine position and will require placement in a more upright position
3. The use of rubber dam—highly recommended for all dental procedures when its placement is possible—may be contraindicated in patients with certain cardiovascular or respiratory disorders; if a rubber dam cannot be used, the patient should be warned about the danger of swallowing or aspirating a foreign body, and a note to this effect should be entered on the patient's chart

Through the use of the steps included in the Stress Reduction Protocols and specific treatment modifications, patient management has been enlarged to include the preoperative and postoperative periods, as well as the intraoperative period. These protocols have made it possible to manage the dental health needs of a broad spectrum of anxious and medically compromised patients with a minimal complication rate.

BIBLIOGRAPHY

American Heart Association: Recommendations for human blood pressure determination by sphygmomanometry, Dallas, 1967, The Association.

American Society of Anesthesiologists: New classification of physical status, Anesthesiology **24:**111, 1963.

Bates, B.: A guide to physical examination, ed. 3, Philadelphia, 1984, J.B. Lippincott Co.

Brady, W.F., and Martinoff, J.T.: Validity of health history data collected from dental patients and patient perception of health status, J. Am. Dent. Assoc. **101:**642, 1980.

Bricker, S.L., and Langlais, R.P.: Principles of identification and management, Dent. Clin. North Am. **27:**221, 1983.

Burch, D.E., and DePasquale, N.P.: Primer of clinical measurement of blood pressure, St. Louis, 1962, The C.V. Mosby Co.

Corah, N.: Development of dental anxiety scale, J. Dent. Res. **48:**596, 1969.

Corah, N.L., Gale, E.N., and Illig, S.J.: Assessment of a dental anxiety scale, J. Am. Dent. Assoc. **97:**816, 1981.

Cottone, J.A., and Kafrawy, A.H.: Medications and health histories: a survey of 4365 dental patients, J. Am. Dent. Assoc. **98:**713, 1979.

DeGowen, E.L., and DeGowen, R.L.: Bedside diagnostic examination, ed. 3, New York, 1976, Macmillan Publishing Co., Inc.

deJulien, L.F.: Causes of severe morbidity/mortality cases, C.D.A.J. **11:**45, 1983.

Denborough, M.A., and Lovell, R.R.: Anesthetic deaths in a family, Lancet **2:**45, 1960.

DePaola, L.G., Kutcher, M.J., and Bowers, G.M.: The dentist's role in the detection of the undiagnosed diabetic patient, Compend. Contin. Educ. Dent. **3:**187, 1984.

Gier, R.E., and Janes, D.R.: Dental management of the pregnant patient, Dent. Clin. North Am. **27:**419, 1983.

Goebel, W.M.: Reliability of the medical history of identifying patients likely to place dentists at an increased hepatitis risk, J. Am. Dent. Assoc. **98:**907, 1979.

Goupil, M.T., and Roche, W.C.: Preoperative and operative considerations in malignant hyperthermia, J. Am. Dent. Assoc. **96:**1033, 1978.

Halpern, I.L.: Patient's medical status: a factor in dental treatment, Oral Surg. **39:**216, 1975.

Heard, E., Staples, A.F., and Czerwinski, A.W.: The dental patient with renal disease: precautions and guidelines, J. Am. Dent. Assoc. **96:**792, 1978.

Little, J.W., and Falace, F.A.: Dental management of the medically compromised patient, ed. 2, St. Louis, 1984, The C.V. Mosby Co.

Malamed, S.F.: The stress reduction protocols: a method of minimizing risk in dental practice, Paper presented at the fifth annual Continuing Education Seminar in Practical Considerations in IV and IM Dental Sedation, Mt. Sinai Medical Center, Miami, 1979.

Malamed, S.F.: Blood pressure evaluation and the prevention of medical emergencies in dental practice, J. Prev. Dent. **6:**183, 1980.

Malamed, S.F.: Sedation: a guide to patient management, St. Louis, 1985, The C.V. Mosby Co.

Marshall, J.R.: Preoperative evaluation and choice of anesthesia. In Lichtiger, M., and Moya, F., editors: Introduction to the practice of anesthesia, New York, 1979, Harper & Row Publishers, Inc.

McCarthy, F.M.: Vital signs: the six minute warning, J. Am. Dent. Assoc. **100:**682, 1980.

McCarthy, F.M.: Stress reduction and therapy modifications, C.D.A.J. **9:**41, 1981.

McCarthy, F.M.: Medical history: the best insurance, C.D.A.J. **11:**61, 1983.

McCarthy, F.M.: The medical revolution in dentistry, C.D.A.J. **12:**105, 1984.

McCarthy, F.M.: Safe treatment of the emphysema patient, J. Am. Dent. Assoc. **108:**761, 1984.

McCarthy, F.M.: A new, patient-administered medical history developed for dentistry, J. Am. Dent. Assoc. **111:**595, 1985.

McCarthy, F.M., and Malamed, S.F.: Physical evaluation manual, Los Angeles, 1975, University of Southern California School of Dentistry.

McCarthy, F.M., and Malamed, S.F.: Physical evaluation system to determine medical risk and indicated dental therapy modifications, J. Am. Dent. Assoc. **99:**181, 1979.

Oksas, R.M.: Epidemiologic study of potential adverse drug reactions in dentistry, Oral Surg. **45:**707, 1978.

Owens, W.D., Felts, J.A., and Spitznagel, E.L., Jr.: ASA physical status classifications: a study of consistency of ratings, Anesthesiology **49:**239, 1978.

Pearson, R.E.: Anxiety in the dental office. In Bennett, C.R., Conscious-sedation in dental practice, ed. 2, St. Louis, 1978, The C.V. Mosby Co.

Prior, J.A., Silberstein, J.S., and Stang, J.M.: Physical diagnosis, ed. 6, St. Louis, 1981, The C.V. Mosby Co.

Ramaprasad, R., and others: Dentists and blood pressure measurement: a survey of attitudes in practice, J. Am. Dent. Assoc. **108:**767, 1984.

Rose, L.F., and Kaye, D.: Internal medicine in dentistry, St. Louis, 1983, The C.V. Mosby Co.

Stout, F., and Doering, P.: The problematic drug history, Dent. Clin. North Am. **27:**387, 1983.

Streeten, D.H.P.: Corticosteroid therapy. I. Pharmacological properties and principles of corticosteroid use, JAMA **232:**944, 1975.

Streeten, D.H.P.: Corticosteroid therapy. II. Complications and therapeutic indications, JAMA **232:**1046, 1975.

Trieger, N., and Goldblatt, L.: The art of history taking, J. Oral Surg. **36:**118, 1978.

Westbrook, S.D.: Dental management of patients receiving hemodialysis and kidney transplants, J. Am. Dent. Assoc. **96:**464, 1978.

3 *Preparation*

In spite of our efforts to prevent life-threatening emergencies, these situations will arise on occasion. Prevention therefore is not enough. The dental office staff must also be fully prepared to assist in the recognition and management of any emergency situation that may develop. Unless all office personnel are capable of effectively managing those few serious emergencies that may develop during the practice lifetime of the doctor, those situations may well become office catastrophies.

What will constitute adequate preparation of a dental office and staff for the rapid and effective management of life-threatening situations? Of importance will be (1) training all members of the dental office staff in the recognition and management of life-threatening situations, (2) a team approach to managing emergencies, (3) emergency "fire drills" in the dental office, and (4) office preparation, including emergency telephone numbers and emergency drugs and equipment (Table 3-1).

GENERAL PREPARATION
Office Personnel
Training

Probably the most important factor in the preparation of a dental office for medical emergencies will be training all office personnel, including nonchairside personnel, in the recognition and management of these situations. Training should include an annual refresher course in emergency medicine that provides a general review of all aspects of the subject, such as seizures, chest pain, and respiratory difficulty, rather than just a review of basic life support (BLS). Such continuing education courses are listed in the *Journal of the American Dental Association*. Of equal if not greater importance is a clinical course in basic life support (cardiopulmonary resuscitation, or CPR). All office personnel should be required to receive certification at the

BLS-provider level (American Heart Association) at least once and preferably twice a year. The ability of the staff to perform basic life support effectively represents the single most important step in preparation of the dental office for medical emergencies. In all emergency situations, initial management always entails the application, as needed, of the steps of basic life support. The technique of basic life support is described in Chapters 5 and 30. Most emergency situations occurring in dental practice will prove to be readily manageable through the use of basic life support. Drug therapy will usually be relegated to a secondary role.

Training in advanced cardiac life support (ACLS) is being advocated more and more today. Such training involves the following subjects: adjuncts for airway control and ventilation (including intubation); monitoring and dysrhythmia recognition; defibrillation and synchronized cardioversion; cardiovascular pharmacology; acid-base balance; venipuncture; and resuscitation of infants, including the newborn. Although not essential for all dental practitioners, the knowledge of and ability to use these techniques in emergency situations is invaluable. Advanced cardiac life support programs are given by hospitals under the auspices of the American Heart Association. Enrollment is limited to physicians, dentists, and registered nurses. In some states, paramedical personnel are permitted to be trained in ACLS. ACLS training is especially valuable for doctors employing parenteral sedation or general anesthetic techniques in their offices. For information concerning ACLS training, contact your local American Heart Association affiliate.

Team management

With all office personnel trained in the recognition and management of life-threatening situations, it is possible for each person to maintain the life of a victim alone or as a member of a trained emergency team. Although management of most emergencies is possible with a single rescuer, the combined efforts of several trained persons are more efficient. Because most dental offices will have more than one staff person present during working hours (when most life-threatening emergencies would occur), a team approach to management is possible.

The emergency team consists of two or three members, each having a predefined role in the management of an emergency. The doctor will lead the team and is responsible for directing the actions of all other team members.

Team member 1 is the person, usually the doctor, who is with the victim or who first reaches the victim when the emergency situation is noticed. The primary task assigned to member 1 is the initiation of the steps of basic life support (*A*irway *B*reathing *C*irculation), as indicated by physical assessment of the victim. Member 1 should remain with the victim throughout the emergency unless relieved by another team member. If the initial person at the scene of the incident is not the doctor, the doctor will assume the role of team member 1 on arrival at the scene.

Member 2 will act as a "circulating nurse" or "circulating assistant." For example, a chairside assistant working alongside the doctor will serve in this capacity if the patient is the victim. In another situation, member 2 may be the next person to come to the aid of member 1. Primary assignments for member 2 are to assist member 1 with basic life support, as required; to monitor the vital signs of the victim (blood pressure, pulse, respirations); and to otherwise assist as needed, such as positioning the victim, loosening a collar or belt, or activating the EMS (emergency medical services) system by dialing the appropriate telephone number, 911.

The third team member will be responsible for gathering up the emergency kit and portable oxygen. This person is also assigned to regularly check the supply of emergency drugs and oxygen to make certain they will be readily available when needed (see discussion of emergency drugs and equipment on p. 70). When an emergency does occur, team member 3 will immediately bring this material to the site of the emergency. In the event that drug administration is required, team member 3 prepares the drug(s) for use by the doctor. In addition, member 3 is available to assist in basic life support, summon medical assistance, and keep a record of

Table 3-1. Summary of preparation

1. Personnel
   Semiannual certification as basic life support provider
   Annual review program in emergency medicine
2. Office
   Team approach to management
   Check drugs and equipment regularly
   Emergency telephone numbers:
     Paramedics
     Oral and maxillofacial surgeon
     Emergency ambulance service
     Physician
     Hospital with 24-hour, fully staffed emergency room
   Emergency practice drills
3. Emergency drugs and equipment
   Drugs, checked weekly
   Oxygen, checked daily

the proceedings. In the absence of a third team member, member 2 will fulfill these requirements, leaving the victim and member 1 if need be to gather the emergency equipment and/or summon additional medical assistance.

It is important that all office personnel be capable of joining the team. In addition, all team members should be able to carry out any of the functions of the entire team. Practice thus becomes a vitally important factor.

Emergency Practice Drills

If life-threatening situations occurred regularly in dental practice, there would be little need for emergency practice sessions. Team members would receive their training under actual emergency conditions. Fortunately, life-threatening situations do not occur with such frequency. Because of this fortunate infrequency, members of the dental office emergency team quickly become "rusty" from the lack of opportunity to use their knowledge and skills. For this reason, annual refresher courses are invaluable in maintaining the overall knowledge of the team. Of even greater importance, however, is the ability of the team to perform well in the office setting. In-office emergency drills are a means of maintaining an efficient emergency team in the absence of true emergency situations. On an irregular basis, the doctor may stage a simulated life-threatening situation. All members of the team should be able to respond exactly as they must under emergency conditions. Many doctors have even purchased mannequins for practicing cardiopulmonary resuscitation and hold frequent practice sessions for all staff members.

An example of an emergency situation and the team approach to its management follows: The doctor is preparing to administer a local anesthetic to a patient. As the syringe is inserted in the patient's mouth, the patient loses consciousness. The doctor (member 1) calls the other members of the team (with a code word or communication device, such as a light or buzzer). Member 2, the chairside assistant working with the doctor, remains with the doctor and victim, ready to assist as needed. Member 3 gets the portable oxygen and the emergency drug kit and brings them to the site of the emergency. Member 1, in this case the doctor in charge of the situation, initiates basic life support by positioning the victim and establishing a patent airway. Member 2 monitors the victim's vital signs, first recording the heart rate (carotid, brachial, or radial pulse). Member 3 prepares the oxygen for possible use and locates the aromatic ammonia vaporoles. If possible, and if needed, member 3 will chronologically record the management of this situation. Should the victim not regain consciousness in a reasonable period of time, member 2 or 3 will be sent to activate the emergency medical services system, meet the emergency personnel (extremely important in a large facility or office building), and escort them to the site of the emergency. Should emergency drug administration be considered necessary, it is the doctor who should, if at all possible, administer the drugs.

The remaining sections of this book will provide the dental staff with the proper knowledge to manage these situations. It is only through practice, however, that efficiency can be expected in these difficult circumstances.

Outside Medical Assistance

Although most dental office emergencies will be readily manageable by the emergency team, there may be occasion to call for outside medical assistance. Therefore emergency telephone numbers must be readily available and conspicuous at all telephones in the dental office (Fig. 3-1). Telephone numbers to be included are: local emergency medical services (EMS), a well-trained dental or medical professional, emergency ambulance service, and a hospital emergency room.

Many communities have instituted the universal emergency number 911 to expedite activation of

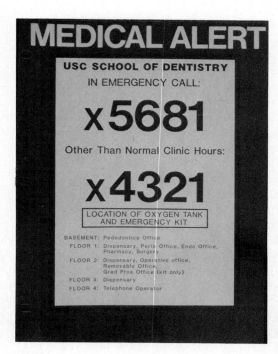

Fig. 3-1. Emergency telephone numbers should be prominently displayed.

the EMS. This number immediately connects the caller to the rescue service. When emergency medical care is required, the community EMS is the preferred source of immediate assistance. However, since not all areas have instituted the 911 system, proper emergency numbers must be posted.

When contacting the EMS operator, it is important for the caller to remain calm and to clearly give the operator any and all requested information. This may include the nature of the emergency in general terms (for example, consciousness, unconsciousness, chest pain, or seizures) and the location of the emergency (address). For this reason, the address of the dental office should be posted at every telephone in the office. Should the doctor's office be located in a large professional building, a member of the staff should be sent to wait in the lobby of the building to (1) hold an elevator for immediate use by emergency personnel and (2) escort them directly to the appropriate office.

A well-trained dental or medical professional can also serve as a source of emergency medical care. It is important, however, to discuss this arrangement before its actual need. Be absolutely certain that the person called in for aid is, in fact, well versed in emergency medicine and likely to be available during office hours. It has been my experience that the best-trained individuals in emergency medicine are emergency medicine physicians, anesthesiologists, surgeons (M.D.), and oral and maxillofacial surgeons (D.D.S.). Unfortunately, the first two groups are hospital based and are not readily available. However, a surgeon (M.D.) or oral and maxillofacial surgeon (D.D.S.) may be available. Prior arrangement with these persons will avoid potential misunderstandings and increase their usefulness in emergency situations in your office.

Many emergency ambulance services require that their personnel be trained as emergency medical technicians (EMTs). This can be an alternate source of assistance should the other sources be unavailable.

The location of the hospital closest to the dental office should be determined; it should have a 24-hour emergency room staffed with fully trained emergency personnel. It is also recommended that all staff members determine the nearest fully equipped hospital to their place of residence.

When should emergency medical personnel be summoned to aid in the management of the situation? Quite simply put, it is prudent to seek outside assistance when you (as team member 1) feel that the situation has gotten the upper hand—when, despite your efforts, the condition of the victim has not improved. Calling for outside assistance is justified in this situation. If, conversely, the patient appears to improve—that is, the skin or mucous membranes become more pink, blood pressure increases, wheezing or seizures cease, chest pain stops, or consciousness returns—then you may elect to continue management without seeking outside assistance. The question of when to seek outside assistance is a very personal one. The doctor's prior training, experience, and personality will dictate the need to summon assistance. Always remember that it is better to err on the side of caution—to seek help a little too soon rather than a little too late.

Emergency Drugs and Equipment

Emergency drugs and equipment must be available in the dental office. Although most emergency situations will not require drug administration, emergency drugs may prove to be life-saving on some occasions. In the acute systemic allergic response (anaphylaxis), the administration of epinephrine is essential. In most other situations, however, drug administration will play a secondary

role to the steps of basic life support in overall management.

Commercial versus homemade emergency kits

A number of emergency kits are available from commercial manufacturers for sale to dental and medical professionals (Fig. 3-2). Although some of these kits are rather well designed, many others are not and *contain drugs and equipment of little functional value in a dental office.* The Council on Dental Therapeutics of the American Dental Association issued a report on the subject of drug emergency kits in

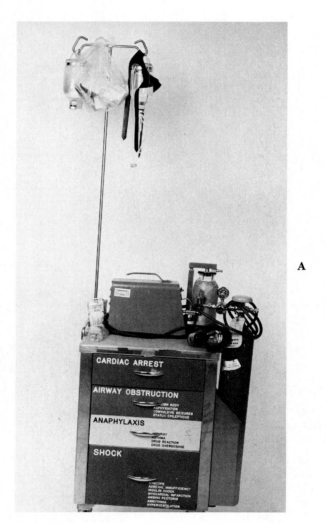

A

Fig. 3-2. A, Self-made emergency kit for office with personnel who are well trained in emergency medicine.

Continued.

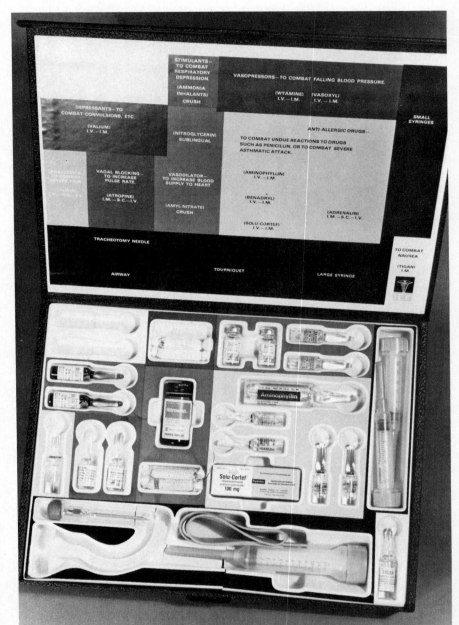

Fig. 3-2, cont'd. B, Commercial drug emergency kit. C, Basic self-made drug emergency kit for dental office.

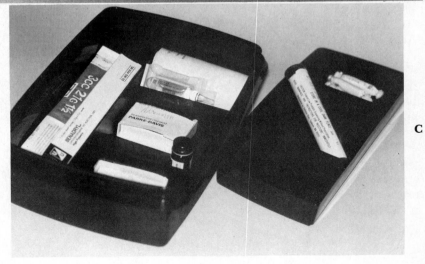

October, 1973. The following statement, equally true in 1986, is excerpted from this report:*

None of these kits is compatible with the needs of all practitioners, and their promotion is sometimes misleading. All dentists must be prepared to diagnose and treat expeditiously life-threatening emergencies that may arise in their practices. The best way to accomplish this objective is by taking continuing education courses on the subject of emergencies to remain informed on current practices recommended for handling emergencies in the office. A false sense of security may be engendered by the purchase of a kit if the purchaser presumes that it will fulfill all the needs of an emergency situation. The most important factors in the effective treatment of emergencies are the knowledge, judgment, and preparedness of the dentist. . . . Since emergency kits should be individualized to meet the special needs and capabilities of each clinician, no stereotyped kit can be approved by the Council on Dental Therapeutics. Practitioners are encouraged to assemble their own individual kit that will be safe and effective in their hands or to purchase a kit that contains drugs that they are fully trained to administer.

The most desirable approach to emergency drug kits for the dental office is for doctors to prepare a kit that is individualized to meet their requirements and capabilities. In my experience, commercially prepared emergency kits are quickly placed in a cabinet where they will not be touched until they are needed. The doctor and staff do not spend any time familiarizing themselves with the contents of the kit or the indications for the use of these agents, and the emergency kit quickly becomes a security blanket. It is there, ready for use, but in many instances it will prove useless when needed because the doctor and staff are unfamiliar with the kit. This is the primary reason I advocate homemade kits. By preparing an individualized kit, the doctor will of necessity become familiar with all of the drugs and equipment included in it. This intimate knowledge will prove to be of immense benefit when the doctor is called on to use the kit during an emergency situation.

EMERGENCY DRUG KITS

The dental office emergency kit need not—and indeed should not—be complicated. It ought to remain as simple as possible. Pallasch's statement

---

*Council on Dental Therapeutics: Emergency Kits, J. Am. Dent. Assoc. **87**:909, 1973. Copyright by the American Dental Association. Reprinted by permission.

> **REMEMBER**
>
> 1. Drugs are NOT necessary for the proper management of most emergencies.
> 2. Primary management of all emergency situations is *basic life support (BLS)*.
> 3. When in doubt, NEVER medicate.

(1976) that "complexity in a time of adversity breeds chaos" is all too true.

The emergency kit described in the following sections is a simply organized collection of drugs and equipment that has been found to be highly effective in managing those life-threatening situations that indicate the administration of drugs. However, it cannot be emphasized too much that in most emergency situations drugs are *not* necessary for proper management of the patient. First and foremost in the management of these situations will be the steps of basic life support. It is only after these steps have been taken that the doctor should consider the use of drugs. One exception to this will be the management of the acute allergic reaction, in which there is immediate respiratory embarrassment or circulatory collapse or both. In this situation, treatment of choice will be the administration of epinephrine as soon as possible following the institution of basic life support.

What should be included in the emergency kit? The following guidelines will be useful in the development of an office emergency kit. Categories of drugs will be listed, with suggestions of specific agents within each grouping and an explanation of the selection criteria for each drug mentioned. This approach will lead to the development of a useful and effective emergency kit.

All of the categories of drugs should be considered for inclusion in the emergency kit; however, the doctors should select only those drugs with which they are familiar and which they are able to employ. Suggested drugs are listed below, and alternatives have been given in many instances. It is my feeling that the doctor should carefully evaluate everything that goes into the emergency kit. If doubt remains concerning any of the categories, consult first with a physician (preferably an emergency room physician) or a hospital pharmacist, but above all determine their reasons for suggesting a

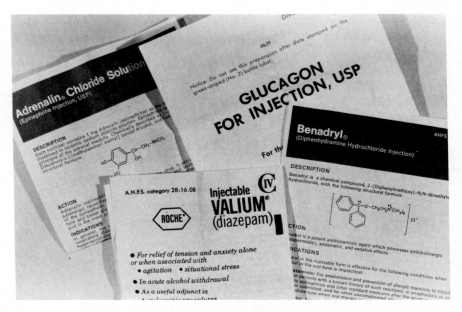

Fig. 3-3. Drug package inserts.

certain drug. Why is one drug more desirable than another drug?

All drugs come with a package insert (Fig. 3-3). Save this insert, read it, and make note of important information concerning the drug, such as indications, usual dose (both pediatric and adult), adverse reactions, and expiration date. Many doctors transfer this information to a 3- by 5-inch index card for quick reference.

Two categories of drugs will be described: (1) injectable drugs and (2) noninjectable drugs. The emergency equipment necessary is described beginning on p. 65. These drug categories will be further divided into two additional groups: (1) primary drugs (items that are considered to be essential) and (2) secondary drugs and equipment (items that can be included but are not absolutely essential). In reading the following material, always keep in mind that the types of drugs and equipment included in the emergency kit must be appropriate for the level of training of the office personnel who will be using the kit. *Simple but effective* is the goal to work toward in preparing this emergency kit. A complete description of the use of each item will be given in sections on management of specific emergencies.

What constitutes the minimum (bare bones) emergency kit? As always, basic life support training is the most significant asset. I also recommend that the following three items be included in all emergency kits: (1) epinephrine, (2) oxygen plus delivery system, and (3) nitroglycerin tablets, or spray.

• • •

The emergency kit to be described is designed for use in either the adult or pediatric patient. The primary distinction between these kits will be the therapeutic dose of the drug administered, pediatric doses usually being somewhat lower than adult doses. Specific dosages will not be discussed in this chapter—rather, they will be presented in the discussion of the management of each emergency situation. Dosage forms of most drugs—that is, the manner in which they are supplied for clinical use—rarely differ, there being no dosage form specific for pediatric use with another form for the adult. Naloxone, however, is an exception, being available in both adult and pediatric strengths.

Several items of emergency equipment should be available in both adult and pediatric sizes, especially in dental offices in which many children are treated. These items include the full-face mask and oropharyngeal and nasopharyngeal airways. Indeed, the pediatric dentist must have a wider range of equipment available—in both pediatric (for the patient-victim) and adult (for the doctor- or staff-victim) sizes—than the doctor who does not treat younger patients.

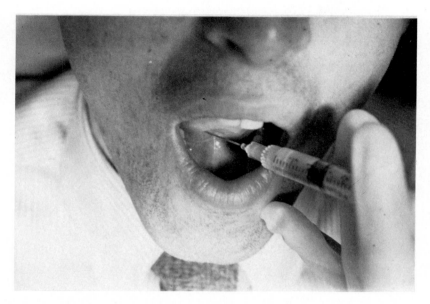

Fig. 3-4. Parenteral drug administration via sublingual injections intraorally or extraorally.

Injectable Drugs

Twelve drugs make up the list of injectable drugs that are considered for inclusion in the dental office emergency kit. The following categories of injectable drugs should be considered essential (primary) drugs:

1. Epinephrine (for management of acute allergic reactions)
2. Antihistamine
3. Anticonvulsant
4. Narcotic antagonist

Nonessential (secondary) drugs are:

5. Analgesic
6. Vasopressor
7. Corticosteroid
8. Antihypoglycemic

A third category of injectable drugs is included for those doctors who are trained in ACLS. The drugs in the ACLS category are:

9. Sodium bicarbonate
10. Calcium chloride
11. Lidocaine (cardiac)
12. Atropine

How and where are these injectable drugs to be administered to the victim? For the drug to exert a therapeutic action, a minimum therapeutic blood level must be achieved in the target organ (such as the brain or heart) or target system. In other words, enough of the drug has to get into the bloodstream and then be transported to the part of the body in which it is needed. With this in mind, then, the ideal technique of emergency drug administration will be the intravenous (IV) technique. Onset of action is rapid, and the drug effect is most reliable using this route of administration. Unfortunately, unless an IV has been started on this patient before the onset of the emergency, it often becomes quite difficult if not impossible to secure an IV during an emergency. Unless the doctor is quite adept at venipuncture, this route, although the most nearly ideal, ought not be used. Emergency medications may be administered intramuscularly (IM) into various sites, most often the anterolateral aspect of the thigh (vastus lateralis), the upper-outer quadrant of the gluteal region, and the mid-deltoid region. Of these three traditional IM sites, the mid-deltoid region provides the most rapid uptake of most medications (a result of greater tissue perfusion) and is therefore the site of choice.

However, one additional site provides a somewhat more effective and more rapid uptake than even the mid-deltoid region: the tongue. Emergency medications can be injected into the body of the tongue or into the sublingual region with every expectation of a somewhat more rapid uptake and onset of clinical action. The drug may be administered under the tongue, either intraorally (Fig. 3-4) or extraorally. Onset of action is approximately 5

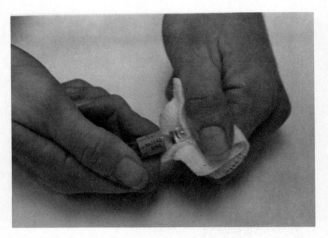

Fig. 3-5. Glass ampule is broken at pre-scored narrow neck. Gauze prevents injury.

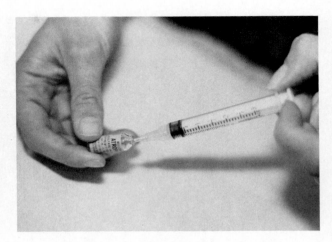

Fig. 3-6. Syringe is loaded with medication.

to 10 minutes if there is effective circulation. The steps of basic life support must be continued as needed while the emergency team awaits the onset of the drug's action.

Remember that in the absence of effective circulation neither intravenously nor intramuscularly administered drugs will be effective. In this situation, drugs ought not be the first consideration in treatment—the implementation of the ABCs of basic life support should take precedence.

To prepare an injectable emergency drug for administration, the rescuer breaks the unit dose ampule, covering the prescored neck with a gauze (Fig. 3-5), and then loads the syringe with the medication (Fig. 3-6).*

Some information about the injectable emergency drugs follows. First, all emergency drugs are available in the form known as a "unit dose" or "therapeutic dose." The one milliliter (1 ml) form of the drug is its adult (not pediatric) therapeutic dose. Remember that a milliliter is a unit of volume, not of a drug's strength. However, 1 ml (50 mg) of diphenhydramine is equipotent to 1 ml (10 mg) of chlorpheniramine. Administration of the 1-ml form of any emergency drug discussed below to an adult victim would be appropriate. One major exception to this basic statement is epinephrine. Although the 1-ml form of 1:1000 epinephrine is considered the adult therapeutic dose, a smaller dose—0.3 to 0.5 ml—is initially administered, with

*The technique of intramuscular drug administration is reviewed in depth in *Sedation: a guide to patient management* (Malamed, St. Louis, 1985, The C.V. Mosby Co.).

subsequent doses based on the patient's response. Pediatric doses are of necessity proportionately smaller, usually one quarter to one half the adult dose.

Second, all emergency drugs are available in preloaded syringes. I strongly recommend that these agents NOT be available in a preloaded form in the dental office. They become too easy to administer. In most situations, there is absolutely no urgent need to administer any substance other than oxygen. The only basic drug that should be available in a preloaded form is epinephrine—because in the acute allergic reaction, this drug needs to be administered as soon as possible. With only one drug available in a preloaded form there can be no confusion in drug selection in this time of near panic. ACLS drugs are available in preloaded form but are kept separate from basic emergency drugs.

Primary injectable drugs *(Fig. 3-7)*

Drug for acute allergic reaction
Drug of choice: Epinephrine
Alternative drug: None available
Drug class: Natural catecholamine

Epinephrine (Adrenalin) is the drug of choice for the management of the acute allergic reaction (signs and symptoms appearing within 1 hour of drug administration). Epinephrine will be of primary value in the management of the respiratory and cardiovascular manifestations of allergic reactions. Desirable properties of this agent include rapid onset of action; potent action as a bronchial smooth muscle dilator (beta properties); antihis-

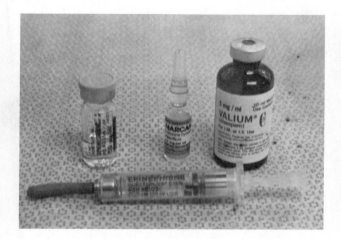

Fig. 3-7. Primary injectable drugs.

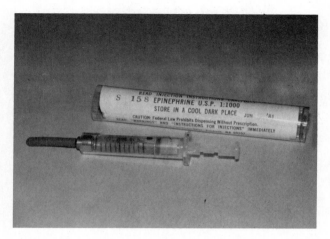

Fig. 3-8. Preloaded epinephrine syringe with rectangular plunger permits the administration of not more than 0.5 ml of solution at one time.

taminic properties; vasopressor properties; and its actions on the heart, which include increased heart rate (21%), increased systolic blood pressure (5%), decreased diastolic blood pressure (14%), increased cardiac output (51%), and increased coronary blood flow. Undesirable actions will include its tendency to predispose the heart to arrhythmias and its relatively short duration of action.

Therapeutic indications: Acute allergic reactions (within 1 hour—Chapter 24); acute asthmatic attacks (see also noninjectable drugs—Chapter 13); cardiac arrest (ACLS—Chapter 30).

Side effects, contraindications, and precautions: Tachyarrhythmias, both supraventricular and ventricular, may develop. Epinephrine should be used with caution in pregnancy because it decreases placental blood flow and may induce premature labor. When used, all vital signs should be frequently monitored.

Availability: Epinephrine for parenteral administration will be supplied in a 1:1000 concentration (1 g [1000 mg]/liter); thus each milliliter will contain 1 mg of the agent. Because of the potency of this drug, it is advisable to have it available in a 1 ml dosage form rather than in a multidose vial. Time is another factor relevant to the dosage forms of epinephrine. In the acute allergic reaction, it will be desirable to administer this agent as soon as possible after the onset of symptoms. For this reason it is recommended that a preloaded syringe be available, as well as 1 ml ampules. Because of the short duration of action of epinephrine, multiple administrations may be necessary during the acute

phase of treatment. Unit dose (1 ml) ampules are preferred over multidose vials because the unit dose form will prevent the rescuer from inadvertently administering an overdose. A little epinephrine may be life-saving, but a lot may be lethal.

Although the 1 ml ampule of 1:1000 epinephrine is considered to be the adult therapeutic dose, it is usual to start administration of epinephrine with 0.3 to 0.5 ml of solution, IM or subcutaneously (SC), with additional doses administered later as needed. Unfortunately, in what may be a near-panic situation (for example, anaphylaxis or cardiac arrest) the doctor may administer an overly large dose of this agent to the victim. A preloaded syringe is available (from Hollister-Stier Laboratories, Spokane, WA) that makes it impossible to administer a 1 ml dose (Fig. 3-8). The plunger on this 1 ml syringe is rectangular, as is its guide channel. However, at the 0.5 ml mark the rectangle shifts 90 degrees, making it impossible for the doctor to administer more than 0.5 ml at a time. To administer an additional dose, the plunger must be rotated. Such a syringe is highly recommended for inclusion in the dental emergency drug kit.

Suggested for emergency kit: One preloaded syringe (1 ml of 1:1000 [1 mg epinephrine]) and three to four ampules of 1:1000 epinephrine, also available as 1 mg diluted in 10 ml fluid for intravenous administration (1:10,000)

Antihistamine

Drug of choice: Chlorpheniramine (Chlor-Trimeton)

Alternative drug: Diphenhydramine HCl (Benadryl)

Antihistamines will be of value in the treatment of the delayed allergic response (onset of symptoms more than 1 hour after administration of the allergen) and in the definitive management of the acute allergic reaction (administered after epinephrine has terminated the acute life-threatening phase of the reaction). Antihistamines are competitive antagonists of histamine. They do not prevent the release of histamine from cells in response to injury, drugs, or antigens but do prevent access of histamine to its receptor site in the cell and thereby block the response of the effector cell to histamine. Thus antihistamines are more potent in *preventing* the actions of histamine than in reversing these actions once they develop. An interesting action of many antihistamines is that they are also potent local anesthetics, diphenhydramine and tripelennamine being particularly potent in this regard. The choice of an antihistamine for the emergency kit was made after considering that most dental patients are ambulatory and may leave the dental office unescorted (probably to drive a car). A potential side effect of many antihistamines is a degree of cortical depression (sedation) that will prevent the patient from leaving the dental office unescorted. Diphenhydramine HCl (Benadryl) causes sedation in nearly 50% of individuals. Chlorpheniramine (Chlor-Trimeton), on the other hand, produces less sedation (10%) than diphenhydramine for an equivalent antihistaminic action.

Therapeutic indications: Delayed allergy, definitive management of acute allergy; for local anesthesia, when history of alleged allergy is present (Chapter 24)

Side effects, contraindications, and precautions: Side effects of antihistamines include central nervous system (CNS) depression, decreased blood pressure, and a thickening of bronchial secretions resulting from the drug's drying action. Antihistamines are contraindicated in the management of acute asthmatic episodes.

Availability: Chlorpheniramine, 10 mg/ml (1 ml ampule), 10 mg/ml (2 ml ampule); diphenhydramine, 10 mg/ml (10 and 30 ml multidose vial), 50 mg/ml (1 ml ampule and 10 ml multidose vial)

Suggested for emergency kit: Chlorpheniramine, 10 mg/ml (three to four 1 ml ampules) or diphenhydramine, 50 mg/ml (three to four 1 ml ampules)

Anticonvulsant

Drug of choice: Diazepam

Alternative drug: Barbiturate

Seizure disorders may occur in the dental office in several circumstances: overdose reactions to local anesthetics, epileptic seizures, and febrile convulsions. Only rarely will an anticonvulsant medication be needed to terminate seizure activity. However, an anticonvulsant drug should be in the dental emergency kit so that it will be readily available if required. The choice of anticonvulsant has become somewhat simpler with the introduction of diazepam into clinical use. Until about 20 years ago, barbiturates were the drugs of choice in the management of seizure disorders. Diazepam has since become the preferred drug because seizure disorders are characterized by stimulation of the central nervous and cardiorespiratory systems followed by a period of depression of these same systems. When barbiturates are administered to terminate seizure activity, the degree of depression is accentuated and its duration prolonged because of the pharmacologic actions of the barbiturate. When seizure activity has been significant, the ensuing depression will be profound, leading to compromised respiration and a period of hypotension. When barbiturates are used to terminate seizures, the ensuing depression may be accentuated, leading to respiratory arrest and a profound cardiovascular depression or collapse. If the doctor is not capable of managing this situation, the patient may be in a more difficult situation after the seizure than during it. Diazepam, unlike barbiturates, will usually terminate seizure activity without the pronounced depression of the respiratory and cardiovascular systems.

Therapeutic indications: Termination of prolonged seizures (status epilepticus—Chapter 21), local anesthetic seizures (febrile convulsions—Chapter 23); hyperventilation syndrome (for sedation—Chapter 12); thyroid storm (for sedation—Chapter 18)

Side effects, contraindications, and precautions: The major side effect of diazepam is respiratory depression or arrest; however, with careful titration during administration this is unlikely to occur.

Availability: Diazepam (Valium), 5 mg/ml (2 ml preloaded syringe), 5 mg/ml (2 ml ampule), 5 mg/ml (10 ml vial); pentobarbital (Nembutal), 50 mg/ml (2 ml ampule), 50 mg/ml (5 ml ampule), 50 mg/ml (20 ml vial)

Suggested for emergency kit: One 10 ml vial of diazepam, 5 mg/ml

Narcotic antagonist

Drug of choice: Naloxone (Narcan)

Alternative drug: Nalbuphine (Nubain)

If a narcotic analgesic or pentazocine is included in the drug emergency kit or used for psychosedation techniques, a narcotic antagonist must be readily available. Narcotic antagonists are indicated for reversal of narcotic depression, including respiratory depression.

Therapeutic indications: Respiratory depression caused by narcotics or pentazocine (Chapter 23)

Side effects, contraindications, and precautions: Naloxone has been notably free of adverse side effects, although Pallasch (1981) has reported on several unexpected deaths following its administration. NOTE: The duration of naloxone is short—quite possibly shorter than that of the narcotic it is reversing. This situation may lead to a recurrence of respiratory depression following a period of apparent recovery. For this reason all patients receiving naloxone must be observed for at least 1 hour after its administration. A longer-acting narcotic antagonist, naltrexene, should be available in the near future.

Availability: Naloxone (Narcan), 0.4 mg/ml (1 ml ampule)

Suggested for emergency kit: Naloxone, 0.4 mg/ml (two to three 1 ml ampules)

Secondary injectable drugs *(Fig. 3-9)*

Secondary injectable drugs are agents that are deemed important but not absolutely essential to the successful management of emergency situations. Their inclusion in the kit is recommended only if the doctor has the background and ability to safely and effectively employ these agents clinically. Without this ability, these agents need not be present in the drug kit.

Analgesic drug

Drug of choice: Morphine sulfate

Alternative drug: Meperidine (Demerol)

Analgesic medications will be useful during emergency situations in which acute pain or anxiety is present. In most instances, the presence of pain or anxiety will cause an increase in the workload of the heart that may prove detrimental to the well-being of the patient. Two such circumstances are acute myocardial infarction and congestive heart failure. The choice of analgesic drugs includes the narcotic agonists morphine sulfate and meperidine (Demerol).

Therapeutic indications: Intense, prolonged pain and/or anxiety; acute myocardial infarction (Chapter 28); congestive heart failure (Chapter 14)

Side effects, contraindications, and precautions: Narcotic analgesics are potent CNS and respiratory depressants. Vigilant monitoring of vital signs is mandatory whenever these agents are used. Use of narcotics is contraindicated in victims of head injury and multiple trauma; they should be used with care in persons with compromised respiration.

The respiratory depressant actions of narcotic agonists may be reversed through administration of naloxone. Analgesic action is also reversed by naloxone.

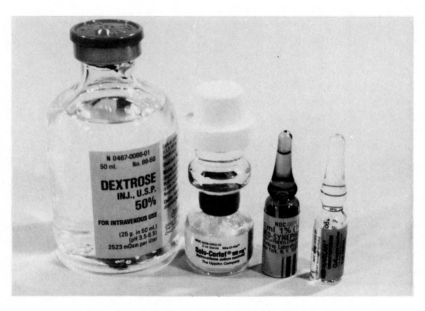

Fig. 3-9. Secondary injectable drugs.

Availability: Morphine sulfate, 10 mg/ml (in 1 ml ampules); meperidine (Demerol), 50 mg/ml (1 ml ampules and 10 and 30 ml vials), 100 mg/ml (1 ml ampules and 10 and 30 ml vials)

Suggested for emergency kit: Morphine sulfate, 10 mg/ml (two to three 1 ml ampules) or meperidine, 50 mg/ml (two to three 1 ml ampules)

NOTE. In recent years emergency medical services in many countries have employed mixtures of nitrous oxide (N_2O) and oxygen (O_2) in the management of pain associated with acute myocardial infarction in place of narcotic analgesics. Concentrations of N_2O have varied between 35% and 50%. At these levels, a mixture of 35% to 50% N_2O and 50% to 65% oxygen decreases pain, relaxes the victim somewhat, and provides the victim with 2½ to 3 times the ambient level of oxygen. Clinical use of nitrous oxide and oxygen in this situation is discussed in Chapter 28. When a dental office has N_2O-O_2 available, it may be used in place of the narcotic analgesics. In its absence, however, a narcotic analgesic should be available.

Vasopressors

Drug of choice: Methoxamine (Vasoxyl)

Alternative drug: Phenylephrine (Neo-Synephrine)

Although one potent vasopressor (epinephrine) has already been included in our kit, it is important that a second one be considered for inclusion. In most emergency situations in which a vasopressor is indicated in the dental office (see therapeutic uses below), an agent such as epinephrine will not be the drug of choice. Epinephrine will be used primarily in the management of acute allergic reactions and is rarely employed in cases of mild to moderate clinical hypotension. One of the major reasons for this is that epinephrine elicits an extreme antihypotensive response. In addition to an increase in blood pressure, epinephrine causes an increase in the workload of the heart through its effects on heart rate and cardiac contraction; it also increases the irritability of the myocardium (sensitizing it to arrhythmias). In most of the situations listed below, the blood pressure of the victim has fallen to a level of about 60 to 80 torr systolic and has not returned to its baseline level in an appropriate period of time. What is called for is an agent that will elevate the blood pressure approximately 30 to 40 torr for a sustained period of time and will allow the body to return to its normal functioning. Furthermore, in most instances the cardiovascular status of the patient will be unknown (unless electrocardiographic

monitoring is being carried out). For this reason, it seems desirable to utilize a vasopressor that will produce a moderate increase in blood pressure without stimulating the myocardium. Vasopressors such as methoxamine (Vasoxyl) and phenylephrine (Neo-Synephrine) are drugs that produce moderate blood pressure elevations through the mechanism of peripheral vasoconstriction. Methoxamine is a clinically useful vasopressor with sustained action and with little effect on the myocardium or central nervous system. Its vasopressor action is associated with a marked increase in the peripheral resistance and no increase in cardiac output. A compensatory bradycardia accompanies the rise in blood pressure. The onset of the pressor action is almost immediate following IV administration and may persist for up to 60 minutes. After IM injection the response occurs within 15 minutes and persists for 90 minutes. Phenylephrine acts in similar fashion, a 5 mg dose IM causing a 30 torr elevation of systolic blood pressure and a 20 torr elevation of diastolic blood pressure, with the response being noted for 50 minutes. As with methoxamine, a pronounced and persistent bradycardia will be noted (average decline in heart rate from 70 to 44 beats per minute).

Therapeutic indications: The vasopressors will be useful in the management of hypotension, in which the status of the heart is unknown and the intent is to raise the blood pressure without cardiac stimulation. Possible uses are in syncopal reactions (Section II), drug overdose reaction (Chapter 23), postseizure states (Chapter 21), acute adrenal insufficiency (Chapter 8), and allergy (Chapter 24).

Side effects, contraindications, and precautions: Parenteral administration of most vasopressors is contraindicated in patients with high blood pressure or ventricular tachycardia, and the drugs are to be used with extreme caution in patients with hyperthyroidism, bradycardia, partial heart block, myocardial disease, or severe atherosclerosis.

Availability: Methoxamine (Vasoxyl), 10 mg/ml and 20 mg/ml (1 ml ampules and 10 ml vials) or phenylephrine (Neo-Synephrine), 10 mg/ml (1 ml ampules)

Suggested for emergency kit: Methoxamine, 10 mg/ml (two to three 1 ml ampules) or phenylephrine, 10 mg/ml (two to three 1 ml ampules)

Corticosteroid

Drug of choice: Hydrocortisone sodium succinate (Solu-Cortef)

Alternative drug: Methylprednisolone sodium succinate (Solu-Medrol)

Corticosteroids will be employed in the management of the acute allergic reaction, but only after the acute phase has been brought under control through the use of epinephrine and the antihistamines. The primary value of the corticosteroids is in the prevention of recurrent episodes of anaphylaxis. Corticosteroids are also important in the management of acute adrenal insufficiency. Studies have demonstrated that corticosteroids have a slow onset of action even when administered intravenously. Because maximal effectiveness may not occur for up to 60 minutes after intravenous administration, many authorities question the effectiveness of these agents in the management of allergic reactions in patients with a normally functioning adrenal gland. It appears likely that the antiallergic effects of the corticosteroids are simply a manifestation of the nonspecific anti-inflammatory action of the adrenal glucocorticoids (hydrocortisone and cortisone). Dexamethasone (Decadron) and methylprednisolone sodium succinate (Solu-Medrol) are contraindicated for use in acute adrenal insufficiency. Therefore hydrocortisone sodium succinate is considered the drug of choice for our emergency kit.

Therapeutic indications: Definitive management of acute allergy (Chapter 24); acute adrenal insufficiency (Chapter 8)

Side effects, contraindications, and precautions: As used in the management of life-threatening medical emergencies, there are no contraindications to the corticosteroids. When administered for nonemergency treatment, there are many factors to be considered, such as presence of pre-existing infection, peptic ulcer, and hyperglycemia. (Consult a pharmacology textbook for more detailed information.)

Availability: Hydrocortisone sodium succinate (Solu-Cortef), 50 mg/ml (2-ml vial); methylprednisolone sodium succinate (Solu-Medrol), 40 mg/ml (1 ml vial)

Suggested for emergency kit: Hydrocortisone sodium succinate, 50 mg/ml (one 2 ml vial)

Antihypoglycemics

Drug of choice: 50% dextrose solution

Alternative drug: Glucagon

In the management of the hypoglycemic patient the mode of therapy will depend in large part on the patient's level of consciousness. Oral carbohydrate is much the preferred mode of therapy; however, if a patient is unconscious or severely obtunded, the oral route must *not* be employed. In this situation, 50 ml of a 50% dextrose solution may be administered intravenously. When the intravenous route is not available, glucagon may be administered intramuscularly. Glucagon is normally produced in the pancreas and acts to rapidly elevate the blood glucose level by mobilizing hepatic glycogen and converting it to glucose; thus glucagon will be effective only if hepatic glycogen is available. It will not be effective in starvation or chronic hypoglycemic states. Oral carbohydrate is administered as soon as the patient begins to respond (that is, regains consciousness).

Therapeutic indications: Hypoglycemia (Chapter 17); diagnostic tool in unconsciousness or seizures of unknown origin

Side effects, contraindications, and precautions: Fifty percent dextrose may produce tissue necrosis should infiltration occur. There are no specific contraindications to its use. If by chance a bolus of 50% dextrose is given to an already hyperglycemic patient, the blood sugar level will not be elevated significantly. Glucagon, either IM or IV, is contraindicated in starvation states and in chronic hypoglycemia.

Availability: Glucagon, 1 mg (1 unit) dry powder with 1 ml diluent; 10 mg dry powder with 10 ml diluent; 50% dextrose (50 mg bottle)

Suggested for emergency kit: Glucagon, 1 mg/ml (two or three 1 ml vials) or 50% dextrose solution (1 bottle) if IV route is available

Injectable drugs for advanced cardiac life support (ACLS)

The following drugs are classified as essential drugs in emergency cardiac care by the American Heart Association. Their use is limited to persons trained in advanced cardiac life support, including certain physicians, nurses, dental practitioners, and some emergency medical technicians. These drugs should be available in the drug emergency kit or in a separate kit in dental offices where the doctor is trained in advanced cardiac life support. Essential drugs in emergency cardiac care include the following, some of which have previously been discussed: oxygen, sodium bicarbonate, epinephrine, atropine, lidocaine, morphine, and calcium chloride (Fig. 3-10).

Sodium bicarbonate ($NaHCO_3$). During cardiopulmonary arrest, both metabolic and respiratory acidosis occur. Effective ventilation of the lungs is a major factor in management of the acidosis accompanying cardiac arrest, especially in the removal of

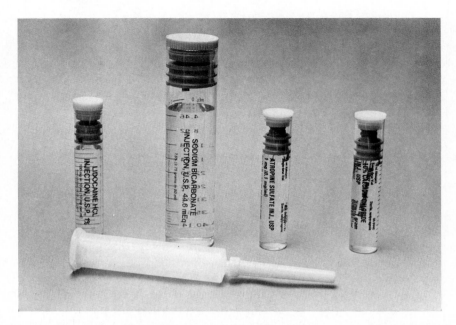

Fig. 3-10. ACLS injectables: lidocaine, sodium bicarbonate, atropine, and calcium chloride.

carbon dioxide that has been retained (hypercarbia) by ventilatory failure or insufficiency. Reversal of acidosis during cardiopulmonary arrest is important because it has been demonstrated clinically that ventricular fibrillation may be terminated by countershock more readily if $NaHCO_3$ is given prior to defibrillation. Acidosis also decreases ventricular contractile force and decreases myocardial responsiveness to catecholamines.

Sodium bicarbonate is effective in the management of metabolic acidosis. The HCO_3^- ion combines with the hydrogen (H^+) ion in the blood, thereby elevating the pH of the blood. Adequate ventilation is necessary whenever $NaHCO_3$ is administered because carbon dioxide is produced during the reaction:

$$HCO_3^- + H^+ \rightleftharpoons H_2CO_3 \rightleftharpoons CO_2 + H_2O$$

Therapeutic indications: Reversal of metabolic acidosis occurring during anaerobic metabolism in cardiopulmonary arrest (Chapter 30)

Side effects, contraindications, and precautions: Side effects from overadministration of sodium bicarbonate include metabolic alkalosis, with a possible consequent impairment of release of oxygen from hemoglobin to the tissues; and sodium and water overload, with hypernatremia and hyperosmolality

Availability: 1 mEq/ml (50 ml ampule)

Suggested for emergency kit: Four 50 ml ampules

Atropine sulfate. Atropine is a parasympatholytic drug that decreases vagal tone through its vagolytic action, thereby increasing the rate of discharge of the sinoatrial node.

Therapeutic indications: Management of severe sinus bradycardia when accompanied by symptomatic hypotension or hypotension that might impair coronary artery blood flow (Chapters 6 and 30)

Side effects, contraindications, and precautions: Acceleration of the heart rate in patients with acute myocardial infarction may prove deleterious. Increases in heart rate increase myocardial oxygen consumption. Atropine administration is therefore not recommended when bradycardia is not associated with hemodynamic compromise (hypotension).

Availability: Atropine, 0.5 mg (5 ml [0.1 mg/ml] preloaded syringe), 0.5 mg/ml (1 ml ampules)

Suggested for emergency kit: One preloaded syringe and two to three 1 ml ampules

Lidocaine. Lidocaine has been used extensively in the management of cardiac arrhythmias, especially those of ventricular origin that develop following acute myocardial infarction.

Therapeutic indications: Premature ventricular contractions (PVCs) occurring more than 5 times per minute, closely coupled PVCs, multifocal PVCs, and those occurring in bursts of two or more in succession. Lidocaine administration is also in-

Table 3-2. Injectable drugs for the emergency drug kit

Category	Drug of choice		Suggested for emergency kit	
	Generic	Proprietary	Quantity	Availability
Primary drugs				
Allergy	Epinephrine	Adrenalin	1 preloaded syringe and 3-4 1 ml ampules	1:1000
Antihistamine	Chlorpheniramine	Chlor-Trimeton Maleate	3-4 1 ml ampules	10 mg/ml
Anticonvulsant*	Diazepam	Valium	1 10 ml vial	5 mg/ml
Narcotic antagonist†	Naloxone	Narcan	2-3 1 ml ampules	0.4 mg/ml
Secondary drugs				
Analgesic	Morphine sulfate		2-3 1 ml ampules	10 mg/ml
Vasopressor	Methoxamine HCl	Vasoxyl	2-3 1 ml ampules	20 mg/ml
Corticosteroid	Hydrocortisone succinate	Solu-Cortef	1 2 ml Mix-o-vial	50 mg/ml
Antihypoglycemic	50% Dextrose	—	1 50 ml vial	500 mg/ml
	Glucagon	Glucagon	2-3 1 ml ampules	1 mg/ml
Advanced cardiac life support injectables				
	Sodium bicarbonate		1 preloaded syringe and 2-3 ampules	44.6 mEq
	Atropine sulfate		1 preloaded syringe and 2-3 ampules	0.5 mg
	Lidocaine	Xylocaine	1 ampule	20 mg/ml
	Calcium chloride		1 ampule	100 mg/ml

*Anticonvulsant is a primary drug only where the doctor is able to administer the drug intravenously.
†Narcotic antagonist is primary drug if any narcotic is employed in patient management. It need not be present if narcotics are never used.

dicated in ventricular tachycardia and ventricular fibrillation that is refractory to defibrillation (Chapter 30).

Side effects, contraindications, and precautions: Excessive doses of lidocaine produce myocardial, circulatory, and central nervous system depression. Clinical signs and symptoms of lidocaine overdose include drowsiness, paresthesias, and muscle twitching. More severe overdose may produce tonic-clonic seizure activity. Decreased hepatic function or hepatic blood flow slows the rate of lidocaine biotransformation, thus leading to prolonged elevated blood levels and a greater risk of lidocaine overdose. Impaired hepatic blood flow is frequently observed in the presence of acute reductions in cardiac output, as seen in myocardial infarction and congestive heart failure.

Availability: Lidocaine, 10 mg/ml (10 ml preloaded syringe), 20 mg/ml (5 ml ampules)

Suggested for emergency kit: One preloaded syringe or one 5 ml ampule

Calcium chloride ($CaCl_2$). Calcium has long been known to increase the force of myocardial contrac-

tion. In addition, calcium ions also enhance ventricular excitability. For this reason, calcium chloride is effective in profound cardiovascular collapse in which an orderly electrical rhythm is associated with an ineffective ejection of blood from the heart (electromechanical dissociation). $CaCl_2$ may also be useful in restoring an electrical rhythm in the presence of ventricular standstill (asystole).

Therapeutic indications: Cardiac arrest: electromechanical dissociation and ventricular asystole (Chapter 30)

Side effects, contraindications, and precautions: If the heart is beating, rapid administration of $CaCl_2$ can produce a severe sinus bradycardia or sinus arrest. Calcium cannot be administered along with sodium bicarbonate because the calcium will precipitate out.

Availability: Calcium chloride, 10% (100 mg/ml) (10 ml preloaded syringe or 10 ml ampule)

Suggested for emergency kit: One preloaded syringe or one ampule

Table 3-2 summarizes the injectable drugs recommended for the emergency kit.

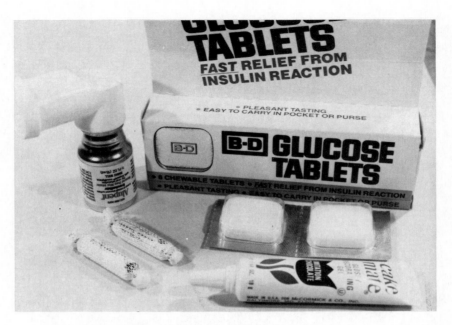

Fig. 3-11. Secondary noninjectable drugs.

Noninjectable Drugs

The five groups of noninjectable drugs are (1) oxygen, (2) vasodilating agents, (3) respiratory stimulants, (4) antihypoglycemic agents, and (5) bronchodilating agents. Primary drugs are oxygen and vasodilators. The others are listed as secondary (Fig. 3-11).

Primary noninjectable drugs

Oxygen

Alternative drugs: None

The most important drug in the entire emergency kit is oxygen. Oxygen is supplied in a variety of cylinder sizes but the minimal acceptable size is the E cylinder, which is quite portable. In emergency situations it has been shown that an E cylinder will provide oxygen for approximately 30 minutes. Larger cylinders (H cylinder) provide more oxygen but tend to be less portable; smaller cylinders (A through D) contain too little oxygen to be clinically effective for more than a short duration. Oxygen supplied in canisters through a chemical reaction is not adequate for the emergency kit and should not be considered. A portable E cylinder of oxygen should also be available in offices in which nitrous oxide-oxygen is available. Because emergencies occur in other parts of the dental office than the dental chair (Table 1-1), oxygen must be available anywhere within the office.

Therapeutic indications: Emergency situations in which respiratory difficulty is evident

Side effects, contraindications, and precautions: None to the emergency use of oxygen

Availability: Compressed gas cylinders in a variety of sizes

Suggested for emergency kit: Minimum for the emergency kit is one E cylinder (Fig. 3-12)

Vasodilator

Drug of choice: Nitroglycerin

Alternative drug: Amyl nitrite

Vasodilators are used in the immediate management of chest pain (such as occurs with angina pectoris and acute myocardial infarction). Two varieties of vasodilators are available: nitroglycerin (TNG) as a tablet and a spray, and an inhalant, amyl nitrite. The patient with a history of angina pectoris will usually carry a supply of nitroglycerin tablets. Prior to dental therapy the doctor should have the patient place the tablets on the bracket table so that if needed they will be readily available. Taken sublingually, nitroglycerin acts in 1 to 2 minutes. The patient's drug should be used if possible, but if it is not available or is ineffective, the 0.3 mg dosage form should be available in the emergency kit. The shelf life of TNG once exposed to air is quite short (about 6 weeks). Nitroglycerin tablets, when placed sublingually, usually taste bitter and sting. Suspect that the drug is outdated if the bitter taste is absent.

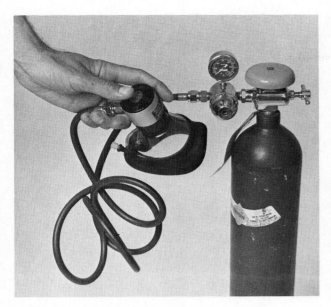

Fig. 3-12. E cylinder of oxygen with delivery system.

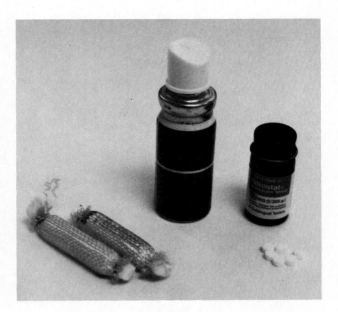

Fig. 3-13. Vasodilators.

Nitroglycerin spray has recently (January 1986) been introduced which has a significantly longer shelf life than the tablets. Amyl nitrite, another vasodilator, is available for use as an inhalant. It is supplied in a yellow vaporole, 0.3 ml, which when crushed and placed under the victim's nose will act in about 10 seconds to produce profound vasodilation. The duration of action of amyl nitrite is shorter than that of TNG; however, the shelf life of the vaporole is considerably longer.

Therapeutic indications: Immediate management of chest pain: angina pectoris (Chapter 27); acute myocardial infarction (Chapter 28)

Side effects, contraindications, and precautions: Side effects of nitroglycerin include transient pulsating headache, facial flushing, and hypotension. It is contraindicated in hypotensive patients. Because nitroglycerin, as a tablet, is a very unstable drug (short shelf life once opened), it must be replaced, usually within 6 weeks of its initial use. Side effects of amyl nitrite are more intense than those of nitroglycerin. These include flushing of the face, a pounding pulse, dizziness, intense headache, and hypotension.

Availability: Nitroglycerin tablets, 0.1, 0.3, 0.6 mg tablet; nitroglycerin spray (Nitrolingual, 0.4 mg/dose; amyl nitrite vaporoles (yellow), 0.3 ml

Suggested for emergency kit: One spray bottle of nitroglycerin (0.4 mg) (Fig. 3-13)

Secondary noningectable drugs (Fig. 3-11)

Respiratory stimulant

Drug of choice: Aromatic ammonia
Alternative drug: None

Aromatic ammonia is the agent of choice as a respiratory stimulant for the emergency kit. It is available in a silver-gray vaporole, which is crushed and placed under the victim's nose until respiratory stimulation is effected. Aromatic ammonia (a noxious odor) acts by irritating the mucous membrane of the upper respiratory tract, thereby stimulating the respiratory and vasomotor centers of the medulla; this in turn increases respiration and blood pressure.

Therapeutic indications: Respiratory depression not induced by narcotic analgesics; vasodepressor syncope (Chapter 6)

Side effects, contraindications, and precautions: Ammonia should be employed with caution in persons with chronic obstructive pulmonary disease (COPD) or asthma because it may precipitate bronchospasm resulting from its irritating effects on the mucous membranes of the upper respiratory tract.

Availability: Silver-gray vaporole (0.3 ml aromatic ammonia)

Suggested for emergency kit: Twelve vaporoles

COMMENT. Next to oxygen, aromatic ammonia will be the most commonly used drug in the emergency kit. I have found it convenient to tape one or

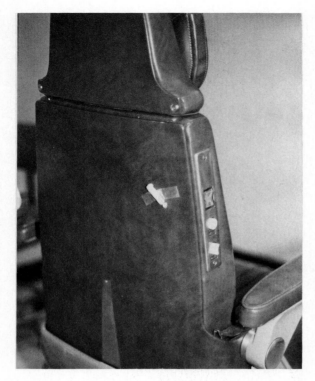

Fig. 3-14. Aromatic ammonia should be kept close at hand in all patient treatment areas. Ammonia is taped to back of dental chair.

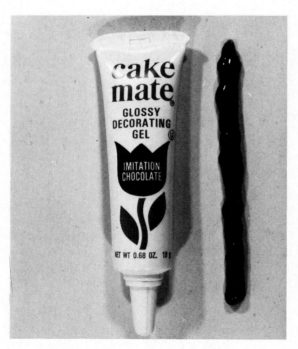

Fig. 3-15. Small tube of cake icing. Ribbon of icing is placed in maxillary and mandibular buccal folds.

two vaporoles close to every dental chair (for example, behind the back of the head rest) so that when it is required, time need not be spent looking for it (Fig. 3-14). The vaporoles should be located so that the operator can reach them without having to leave the patient (assume that there is no assistance at hand). In addition, several vaporoles ought to be kept in the emergency kit for use in other areas of the dental office.

Antihypoglycemic (oral)
Agent of choice: Carbohydrate

Antihypoglycemic agents will be useful in the management of hypoglycemic reactions occurring in patients with diabetes mellitus or in the nondiabetic patient with hypoglycemia. The diabetic patient will usually carry a ready source of carbohydrate such as a chocolate bar or hard candy. Such items should also be available in the dental office for use in the conscious patient with hypoglycemia. For management of the unconscious hypoglycemic patient, refer to the discussion of injectable drugs on p. 59.

Therapeutic indications: Hypoglycemic states secondary to diabetes mellitus or fasting hypoglycemia (in conscious patient) (Chapter 17)

Side effects, contraindications, and precautions: Oral carbohydrates should not be administered to patients who do not have an active gag reflex or who are unable to drink without assistance. Parenteral antihypoglycemics must be administered in these situations. There are no side effects when oral carbohydrates are administered as directed.

Small tubes of decorative icing are useful in the management of unconscious hypoglycemic individuals. These tubes contain a thickened paste of concentrated sugar that can be applied in the form of a ribbon to the buccal mucosa in the maxilla and mandible (Fig. 3-15). Because it is thick, this paste will not run and possibly obstruct the airway. Absorption into the cardiovascular system does not occur rapidly, requiring a minimum of 10 minutes. Basic life support is continued during this period.

Availability: Glucola, Gluco-Stat, Instaglucose, cola beverages, fruit juices, sugar, tubes of icing

Suggested for emergency kit: Any of the sources of carbohydrates listed above

Bronchodilating agent
Drug of choice: Metaproterenol
Alternative drug: Epinephrine, isoproterenol

Asthmatic patients and patients with allergic reactions manifested primarily by respiratory difficulty will require the use of bronchodilator drugs.

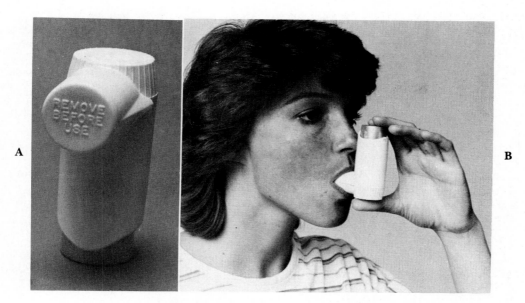

Fig. 3-16. A, Aerosol bronchodilator. **B,** Use of bronchodilator aerosol.

Although epinephrine still remains the drug of choice in the management of bronchospasm, its wide-ranging effects on systems other than the respiratory tract have resulted in the introduction of newer, more specific agents known as beta-2 sympathomimetics. These agents, of which metaproterenol is an example, have specific bronchial, smooth muscle–relaxing properties (beta-2) with little or no stimulatory effect on the cardiovascular and gastrointestinal systems (beta-1). In a dental situation in which the patient's cardiovascular status is unknown, beta-2 stimulators appear more attractive for management of the acute asthmatic episode than agents such as epinephrine and isoproterenol, which have both beta-1 and beta-2 stimulating properties. As with anginal patients, most asthmatics will carry their own medication—in their case, a bronchodilator. In most cases, it will be an inhalator that dispenses a calibrated dosage of the medication. The patient inhales as the agent is dispensed, allowing the drug to reach the bronchial mucosa, where it acts directly on bronchial smooth muscle (Fig. 3-16).

Before dental therapy is begun, the asthmatic patient should place the medication on the bracket table. Metaproterenol, epinephrine, and isoproterenol must be administered precisely as directed. One to two inhalations every hour is the maximal recommended dosage for these agents. In situations in which these nebulized agents fail to terminate the attack, epinephrine must be adminis-

tered parenterally (intramuscularly or subcutaneously).

Therapeutic indications: Respiratory distress as seen in asthma (Chapter 13); allergic reactions with primary respiratory phenomena (Chapter 24)

Side effects, contraindications, and precautions: Metaproterenol, epinephrine, and isoproterenol mistometers have potential cardiovascular side effects, producing tachycardia and ventricular arrhythmias. Their use is contraindicated in patients with preexisting tachyarrhythmias from prior use of the drug (Chapter 13).

Availability: Metaproterenol inhaler (Alupent); Epinephrine mistometer (Medihaler-epi); isoproterenol mistometer (Medihaler-iso) (Fig. 3-10)

Suggested for emergency kit: One inhaler of metaproterenol

Table 3-3 summarizes the noninjectable drugs recommended for the emergency kit.

EMERGENCY EQUIPMENT

Primary emergency equipment to be considered for the dental office includes:
1. Oxygen delivery system
2. Suction and suction tips
3. Syringes for drug administration
4. Tourniquets

Secondary equipment includes the following:
5. Scalpel or cricothyrotomy needle
6. Artificial airways
7. Airway adjuncts

Table 3-3. Noninjectable drugs for the emergency drug kit

Category	Drug of choice		Suggested for emergency kit	
	Generic	Proprietary	Quantity	Availability
Primary drugs				
Oxygen	Oxygen	—	1 (minimum E cylinder)	—
Vasodilator	Nitroglycerin	Nitrolingual spray	1 spray bottle	0.4 mg
Secondary drugs				
Respiratory stimulant	Aromatic ammonia	—	6-12 vaporoles	0.3 ml
Antihypoglycemic agent	Carbohydrate	Many available	1 dose of any form	—
Bronchodilator	Metaproterenol	Alupent	1 inhaler	1-2 inhalations/hr

Table 3-4. Emergency kit equipment

Equipment	Description	Quantity
Primary emergency equipment		
Oxygen delivery system*	Positive pressure/demand valve or self-inflating bag-valve-mask *and* clear full face masks	1 small (child) and 1 large (adult)—minimum
Suction and suction tips	Large-diameter, round-ended suction tips or tonsil suction tips (high-volume suction)	Minimum 2
Syringes for drug administration	Disposable syringes	3-4 2 ml syringes with 18- or 21-gauge needle
Tourniquets	Rubber tourniquet or latex tubing or sphygmomanometer	Minimum 1, up to 3
Secondary emergency equipment		
Scalpel or cricothyrotomy device†	Scalpel and straight blade or cricothyrotomy device	1
Artificial airways†	Oropharyngeal airways Nasopharyngeal airways	1 small (child), 1 medium (adult), and 1 large (adult)—minimum
Airway adjuncts†	Laryngoscope and endotracheal tubes	1 laryngoscope and various sizes of tubes

*Advanced training is required for safe and effective use of these devices. All dental personnel should be trained in their use.
†Advanced training is required for safe and effective use of these devices. Do not include in emergency kit if personnel are not trained to use properly.

Merely having various items of emergency equipment available does not of itself make the dental office any better equipped or the staff any more prepared to manage medical emergency situations. Personnel expected to use this equipment must be well trained in the proper selection of patients and in the proper technique of use of these items. Unfortunately, many of the emergency items commonly found in dental and medical offices can prove to be useless or—more significantly—hazardous if employed improperly or on the wrong patient. Training in the proper use of some of these items, such as the laryngoscope and the oro-

pharyngeal airway, can best be obtained only by caring for patients under general anesthesia, a situation not readily available to most dental personnel. Many of the items listed in this section are therefore recommended for use only by properly trained personnel. All of the equipment listed as secondary requires special training; unfortunately, several items listed as primary also require it (such as the oxygen delivery system). Although all dentists and physicians should be trained in the use of oxygen delivery systems, courses in which these techniques are taught are particularly difficult to locate. (Readers interested in such hands-on programs should

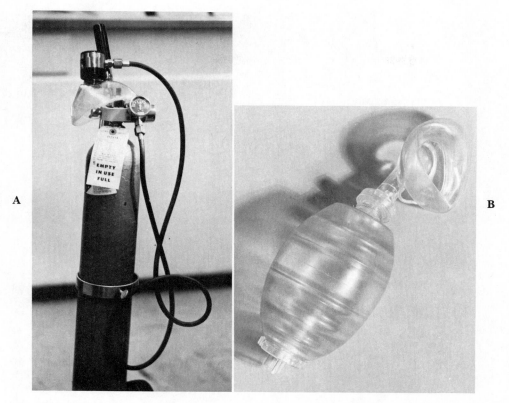

Fig. 3-17. A, Positive pressure oxygen mask (demand valve). Permits delivery of 100% oxygen. **B,** Self-inflating resuscitation bag and mask. Permits delivery of atmospheric air (20% oxygen) or oxygen-enriched air. Clear face mask is preferred to opaque.

contact their local dental society, dental school, hospital, or American Heart Association affiliate.)

It is important that dental personnel use only those pieces of emergency equipment that they are intimately familiar with and have been trained to use properly. The usefulness of the items described below will, of course, vary according to the training of the office personnel. All dental personnel should seek to become proficient in use of primary equipment. Table 3-4 summarizes the equipment recommended for the emergency kit.

Primary Emergency Equipment
Oxygen delivery system

An oxygen delivery system adaptable to the E cylinder of oxygen must allow for the delivery of positive pressure oxygen to the victim. Examples of this device include the positive pressure/demand valve (Fig. 3-17, *A*) and the reservoir bag on many inhalation units. These devices should be fitted with *clear face masks,* which allow for the efficient delivery of oxygen or air to a patient while permit-

ting the rescuer to visually inspect the mouth for the presence of foreign matter (vomitus, blood). Face masks should be available in several sizes (child, small adult, and large adult).

A portable self-inflating bag-valve-mask device (Ambu-bag; PMR), as shown in Fig. 3-17, *B* is a self-contained unit that may easily be transported to any site within the dental office. This is an important feature because not all emergencies will occur within the dental operatory, and it may become necessary to resuscitate a patient in other areas, such as the waiting room or restroom. A source of positive pressure oxygen or air must also be available in these areas. With both devices the rescuer must be able to maintain both an airtight seal and a patent airway with one hand while using the other hand to ventilate the patient (Fig. 3-18).

Suggested for emergency kit: One portable oxygen (E cylinder) with positive pressure mask and/or one portable self-inflating bag-valve-mask device

NOTE. Advanced training is required for safe and effective use of this device.

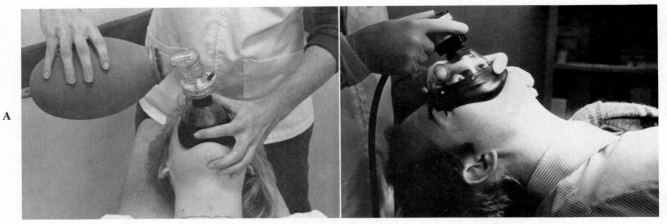

Fig. 3-18. For oxygen delivery system to be used effectively, rescuer must be capable of maintaining an airtight seal **A,** and a patent airway with one hand, **B.**

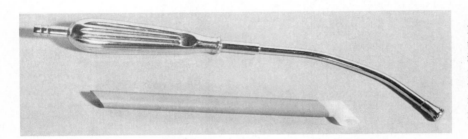

Fig. 3-19. Suction tips. Tonsil suction (*top*) has rounded ends, allowing suctioning of pharynx without producing undue bleeding. High-volume suction tip (*bottom*) is plastic; it permits removal of large material from victim's mouth.

Suction and suction tips

An essential item of emergency equipment is a strong suction system and a variety of large-diameter suction tips. The disposable saliva ejector is entirely inadequate in situations in which anything other than tiny objects must be evacuated from the mouth of a patient. Suction tips should be rounded to ensure that there is little hazard if it becomes necessary to suction the hypopharynx. Plastic evacuators and tonsil suction tips are quite adequate for this purpose (Fig. 3-19).

Suggested for emergency kit: Two plastic evacuators or tonsil suction tips

Syringes for drug administration

Plastic disposable syringes equipped with an 18- or a 21-gauge needle will be needed for drug administration. Although many sizes are available, the 2 ml syringe will be entirely adequate.

Suggested for emergency kit: Three to four 2 ml disposable syringes with an 18- or 21-gauge needle (Fig. 3-20)

Tourniquets

A tourniquet will be required if intravenous drug administration is contemplated. In addition, three tourniquets will be needed for management of the patient in acute pulmonary edema (Chapter 14). A sphygmomanometer (blood pressure cuff) may be employed as a tourniquet, as may a simple piece of latex tubing (Fig. 3-20).

Suggested for emergency kit: Three tourniquets and a sphygmomanometer

Secondary Emergency Equipment
Scalpel or cricothyrotomy device

As a final step in airway maintenance, it may become necessary to perform a cricothyrotomy. Therefore the emergency kit should contain a scalpel or a cricothyrotomy device (Fig. 3-21). The use of these items will be discussed in Chapter 11.

Suggested for emergency kit: One scalpel with disposable blade and/or one cricothyrotomy device

NOTE. Advanced training is required for safe and effective use of these devices.

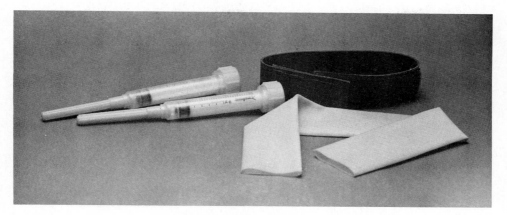

Fig. 3-20. Syringes and tourniquets.

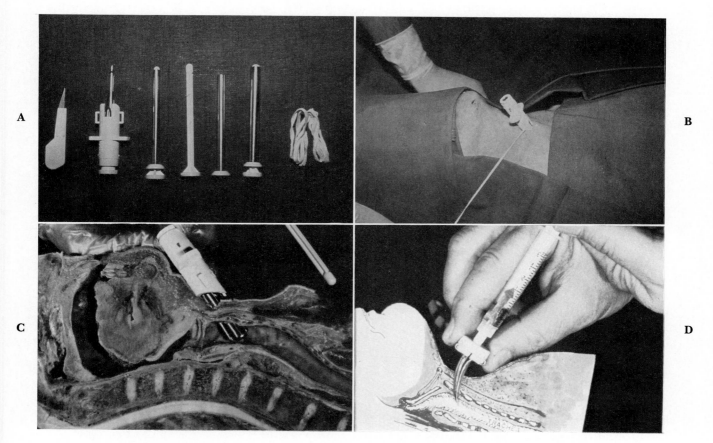

Fig. 3-21. A (Left to right), stylet; needle and housing unit; airway; coturator; airways (2); tie. **B,** Airways secured in position. **C,** Anatomical view of positioned airway. **D,** Pediatric cricothyrotomy needle.

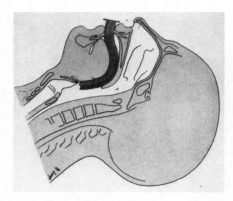

Fig. 3-22. Oral pharyngeal airway lifts base of tongue off posterior wall of pharynx.

Artificial airways

Plastic or rubber oropharyngeal or nasopharyngeal airways are used to assist in maintenance of a patent airway (Fig. 3-22). They act by lifting the base of the tongue off of the posterior pharyngeal wall. Their use is recommended by the American Heart Association (1986) only in cases where manual methods of maintaining an airway have proved ineffective. Several sizes should always be available (that is, child, small adult, normal adult) when oropharyngeal or nasopharyngeal airways are included in the emergency kit.

Suggested for emergency kit: One adult-sized and one child-sized airway (Fig. 3-23)

NOTE. Advanced training is required for safe and effective use of these devices.

Airway adjuncts

Many devices are available to aid in the management of a patent airway. These include the S tube, esophageal obturator airway, laryngoscope, and endotracheal tube. As with the other devices listed in this section, training in the use of each item is *absolutely essential.*

The S tube airway is a modification of the oropharyngeal airway that permits the rescuer to maintain a patent airway and deliver exhaled air ventilation without physically contacting the victim's mouth. Problems encountered with improper use include further obstruction of airway, vomiting, and/or laryngospasm. This device severely limits the ability of the rescuer to perform one-rescuer CPR; to ventilate the victim the rescuer must be at the head of the victim, not astride the head. Its use is not recommended.

The *esophageal obturator airway* is designed to occlude the esophagus, thus permitting air forced into the airway to enter the victim's trachea and lungs. Although it is usually easily inserted, even by untrained rescuers, problems can develop that will minimize the usefulness of this device. These include possible insertion of the tube into the trachea, thereby obstructing the airway, and the probability that the victim will vomit when the airway is removed.

Endotracheal intubation, using a *laryngoscope* (to visualize the trachea) and *endotracheal tube,* is a technique of airway maintenance that must be strictly limited to persons extremely well-trained in its use. Quite realistically, this limits its usefulness to anesthesiologists, anesthetists, trained paramedical personnel, and those few dentists and physicians who have received extensive general anesthesia training. The most common mistakes in intubation are accidental intubation of the esophagus and taking too long to intubate (it should take *no longer than 30 seconds* to intubate a patient) (Fig. 3-24).

The *McGill intubation forcep* is designed to aid in the placement of an endotracheal tube during oral or nasal intubation; this is an important reason for considering it for placement in the emergency kit. Another important use is as an aid in the removal of foreign objects (such as crowns or files) from the posterior oropharynx or hypopharynx (Fig. 3-24).

ORGANIZING THE EMERGENCY KIT

A simple means of storing emergency drugs is in a tackle box or plastic box with several compartments (Fig. 3-2, *C*). Labels should be applied to cubicles storing each drug and should give the drug's generic name (for example, epinephrine) and brand name (for example, Adrenalin) to avoid possible confusion during an emergency.

Difficulty may arise in the purchase of the small quantities of drugs required for this emergency kit. Most drug wholesalers usually sell these drugs in prepackaged boxes of 12 or 24 units, yet in most instances only two or three ampules are required for the emergency kit. This problem may be overcome by contacting a hospital pharmacy, which may dispense these drugs in smaller quantities.

Written records should be kept of the expiration date of each of the drugs in the emergency kit, and the drug should be replaced prior to its expiration

Fig. 3-23. Airway devices (top to bottom): endotracheal tube, nasopharyngeal airways (2), and oropharyngeal airway.

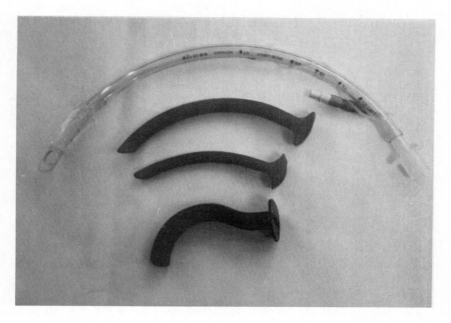

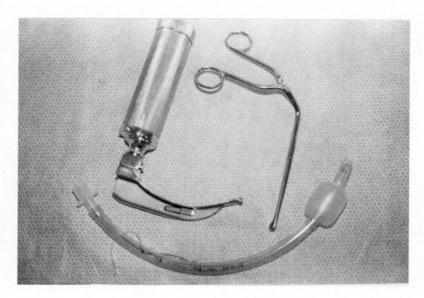

Fig. 3-24. Laryngoscope (left), Magill intubation forceps (right), and endotracheal tube (bottom).

date. Expired drugs as well as empty oxygen cylinders are ineffective in the management of any emergency situation. Office personnel should be assigned the job of regularly checking the emergency kit and all emergency equipment (especially the oxygen cylinders) at the start of every work day to ensure that all is in readiness. Records of emergency drug and equipment inspection ought to be kept in a bound, not a loose-leaf, notebook.

The emergency kit and equipment should be kept in a readily accessible area. The back of a storage closet is not the place for life-saving equipment.

Tables 3-2 through 3-4 list the components of the emergency kit. To assess whether your office is adequately prepared to manage a life-threatening situation, ask yourself the following question: If *you* were in need of emergency medical care, would you want it to be in *your* office and managed by *your* dental team?

BIBLIOGRAPHY

American Heart Association and the National Academy of Sciences, National Research Council: Standards and guidelines for cardiopulmonary resuscitation (CPR) and emergency cardiac care (ECC), JAMA **244**:453, 1980.

American Medical Association: AMA drug evaluations, ed. 5, Littleton, MA, 1985, Publishing Sciences Group, Inc.

Borth, L.L.: What you should have on hand for office emergencies, Dental Student Magazine **52**:37, 43, 61, 1974.

Burroughs Welcome Company: Methoxamine package insert, Research Triangle Park, NC, Aug., 1972.

Carden, E., and Hughes, T.: An evaluation of manually operated self-inflating resuscitation bags, Anesth. Analg. **54**:133, 1975.

Council on Dental Therapeutics: Emergency kits. J. Am. Dent. Assoc. **87**:909, 1973.

Donaldson, D., and Wood, W.W.: Recognition and control of emergencies in the dental office, J. Can. Dent. Assoc. **41**:228, 1975.

Endo Laboratories, Inc.: Naloxone package insert, Garden City, NY, 1972.

Facts and comparisons: St. Louis, 1980, Facts and Comparisons, Inc.

Freedman, S.O.: The management of acute allergic crises. Appl. Ther. **8**:126, 1966.

Goodman, L.S., and Gilman, A.: The Pharmacological Basis of Therapeutics, ed. 5, New York, 1975, Macmillan Publishing Co., Inc.

Goth, A.: Medical pharmacology, ed. 10, St. Louis, 1981, The C.V. Mosby Co.

Hendler, B.H., and Rose, L.F.: Common medical emergencies: a dilemma in dental education, J. Am. Dent. Assoc. **91**:575, 1975.

Holroyd, S.V.: Clinical pharmacology in dental practice, ed. 2, St. Louis, 1978, The C.V. Mosby Co.

Krupp, M.A., and Chatton, M.J.: Current medical diagnosis and treatment, Los Altos, Calif., 1984, Lange Medical Publications.

Levin, R.H.: The rational use of emergency medications. In Pascoe, D.J., and Grossman, M., editors: Quick reference to pediatric emergencies, ed. 3, Philadelphia, J.B. Lippincott Co., 1983.

McCarthy, F.M.: Death in the dental office: failure to administer proper aid can bring ruin to a dentist's career, Am. Dent. Assoc. News **5**:6, 1974.

McCarthy, F.M.: Emergencies in dental practice, ed. 3, Philadelphia, 1979, W.B. Saunders Co.

McCarthy, F.M.: Sudden, unexpected death in the dental office, J. Am. Dent. Assoc. **83**:109, 1971.

Malamed, S.F.: Diphenhydramine HCl: its use as a local anesthetic in dentistry, Anesth. Prog. **20**:76, 1973.

Monheim, L.M.: Emergencies in the dental office, Chicago, 1963, Year Book Medical Publishers, Inc.

Morrow, G.T.: Designing a drug kit, Dent. Clin. N. Am. **26**:21, 1982.

Nicholas, K.E.: An unnecessary hazard in dentistry, Br. Dent. J. **1**:83, 1975.

Pallasch, T.J.: Clinical drug therapy in dental practice, Philadelphia, 1973, Lea & Febiger.

Pallasch, T.J.: This emergency kit belongs in your office, Dent. Management **16**:43, 1976.

Pallasch, T.J.: Pharmacology for dental students and practitioners, Philadelphia, 1980, Lea & Febiger.

Pallasch, T.J., and Gill, C.J.: Naloxone–associated morbidity and mortality. Oral Surg. **52**:602, 1981.

Pallasch, T.J., and Oksas, F.: Synopsis of pharmacology for students in dentistry, Philadelphia, 1974, Lea & Febiger.

Parke Davis and Company: Diphenhydramine package insert, Detroit, June, 1974.

Parke Davis and Company: Epinephrine package insert, Detroit, July, 1973.

Roche Laboratories: Diazepam package insert, Nutley, NJ, April, 1974.

Sanders, K., and Dimant, J.: Barbiturates in survival kits, JAMA **234**:703, 1975.

Sudden unexpected death, editorial: JAMA **204**:1358, 1969.

United States Public Health Service, National Center for Health Statistics, Division of Vital Statistics, Washington, D.C., 1975, U.S. Government Printing Office.

Upjohn Company: Solu-Cortef package insert, Kalamazoo, MI, May, 1974.

Weiss, S.: A new emergency cricothyroidotomy instrument, J. Trauma, **23**:155, 1983.

White, R.D.: Cardiovascular pharmacology: I. In McIntyre, K.M., and Lewis, A.J., editors: Textbook of advanced cardiac life support, Dallas, 1983, American Heart Association.

White, R.D., Goldberg, A.H., and Montgomery, W.H.: Adjuncts for airway control and ventilation, In McIntyre, K.M., and Lewis, A.J., editors: Textbook of advanced cardiac life support, Dallas, 1983, American Heart Association.

Winthrop Laboratories: Pentazocine package insert, New York, May, 1974.

4 *Medical-Legal Considerations*

KENNETH S. ROBBINS

Recently, much has been written about the legal implications of practicing dentistry. There is good reason for this because each year 7% to 8% of dentists are sued. These percentages represent well over 15,000 lawsuits against dentists per year; the growing tendency of patients to sue is disquieting. The magnitude of the problem comes into sharper focus when it is discovered that these lawsuits represent only a small fraction of all claims for malpractice made against dentists; most claims are settled by insurers before they become lawsuits. As the number of dentists and attorneys continues to increase, claims and lawsuits against dentists will also continue to increase.

Most claims and lawsuits are brought against dentists because of an allegedly undesired result arising from desired treatment. Complaints of physical damage to components of the mouth are frequent, particularly nerve damage resulting in temporary or permanent loss of sensation and/or loss of control of portions of the mouth. Although malpractice complaints because of medical emergencies in dental offices constitute a minority of the total number of lawsuits against dentists, the life-and-death nature of medical emergencies makes these cases among the most serious in terms of potential injury to the patient and of the dentist's liability. As Dr. Malamed demonstrates, medical emergencies for which the dentist and dentist's staff should be prepared have substantially more serious implications to both patient and dentist than the other, less severe circumstances that (as previously mentioned) give rise to most lawsuits. Lawsuits for damages because of temporary paresthesia, a broken needle, or permanent cosmetic injuries pale in comparison to lawsuits brought because of brain damage or death from improperly administered CPR during a cardiac arrest emergency. Lawsuits resulting from medical emergencies are based on injuries and medical consequences to the patient that demand the highest jury verdicts and the highest defense costs; they are the multimillion-dollar cases. The high potential jury verdict and the high cost of defense create the maximum probability of an increase both in the individual practitioner's and the profession's dental malpractice insurance. Another potentially devastating risk to dentists in these cases is that the multimillion-dollar verdict may exceed the amount of insurance coverage available, thereby putting dentists' assets and their incomes at risk.

Therefore it is appropriate and timely to consider how dentists can avoid being sued and, if they are sued, what it will take to win.

Several forms are provided in this section; they are commonly used and have been accepted nationally. They include the ADA-recommended medical history questionnaire (Fig. 4-1), as well as the USC medical history questionnaire (p. 11). They represent forms that have been accepted throughout the profession and can be important evidence for the dentist in a lawsuit brought by a patient.

COMMONLY ASKED QUESTIONS

What is the standard of care expected when a patient or other person in the office presents the dentist with a medical emergency? Is the standard of care in a medical emergency lower than the standard of care in a nonemergency? In a genuine

**Copies of the Medical History are Available through the Order Department
of the American Dental Association**

MEDICAL HISTORY

Name .... Sex .... Date of Birth ....

Address ....

Telephone .... Height .... Weight ....

Date .... Occupation .... Marital Status ....

DIRECTIONS

If the answer is YES to the question, put a circle around "YES."
If the answer is NO to the question, put a circle around "NO."
Answer all questions by circling either YES or NO and fill in all blank spaces when indicated.

Answers to the following questions are for our records only and will be considered confidential.

1. Are you in good health	YES	NO
a. Has there been any change in your general health within the past year	YES	NO
2. My last physical examination was on		
3. Are you now under the care of a physician	YES	NO
a. If so, what is the condition being treated		
4. The name and address of my physician is		
5. Have you had any serious illness or operation	YES	NO
a. If so, what was the illness or operation		
6. Have you been hospitalized or had a serious illness within the past five (5) years	YES	NO
a. If so, what was the problem		
7. Do you have or have you had any of the following diseases or problems.		
a. Rheumatic fever or rheumatic heart disease	YES	NO
b. Congenital heart lesions	YES	NO
c. Cardiovascular disease (heart trouble, heart attack, coronary insufficiency, coronary occlusion, high blood pressure, arteriosclerosis, stroke)	YES	NO
1) Do you have pain in chest upon exertion	YES	NO
2) Are you ever short of breath after mild exercise	YES	NO
3) Do your ankles swell	YES	NO
4) Do you get short of breath when you lie down, or do you require extra pillows when you sleep	YES	NO
d. Allergy	YES	NO
e. Asthma or hay fever	YES	NO
f. Hives or a skin rash	YES	NO
g. Fainting spells or seizures	YES	NO
h. Diabetes	YES	NO
1) Do you have to urinate (pass water) more than six times a day	YES	NO
2) Are you thirsty much of the time	YES	NO
3) Does your mouth frequently become dry	YES	NO
i. Hepatitis, jaundice or liver disease	YES	NO
j. Arthritis	YES	NO
k. Inflammatory rheumatism (painful swollen joints)	YES	NO
l. Stomach ulcers	YES	NO
m. Kidney trouble	YES	NO
n. Tuberculosis	YES	NO
o. Do you have a persistent cough or cough up blood?	YES	NO
p. Low blood pressure	YES	NO
q. Venereal disease	YES	NO
r. Other		

Fig. 4-1. A.D.A. long-form medical history questionnaire. (From Emergencies, ed. 2.)

8. Have you had abnormal bleeding associated with previous extractions, surgery, or trauma . . . . YES   NO
    a. Do you bruise easily . . . . YES   NO
    b. Have you ever required a blood transfusion . . . . YES   NO

       If so, explain the circumstances _____

9. Do you have any blood disorder such as anemia . . . . YES   NO

10. Have you had surgery or x-ray treatment for a tumor, growth, or other condition of your head or neck . . . . YES   NO

11. Are you taking any drug or medicine . . . . YES   NO

     If so, what _____

12. Are you taking any of the following:
    a. Antibiotics or sulfa drugs . . . . YES   NO
    b. Anticoagulants (blood thinners) . . . . YES   NO
    c. Medicine for high blood pressure . . . . YES   NO
    d. Cortisone (steroids) . . . . YES   NO
    e. Tranquilizers . . . . YES   NO
    f. Aspirin . . . . YES   NO
    g. Insulin, tolbutamide (Orinase) or similar drug . . . . YES   NO
    h. Digitalis or drugs for heart trouble . . . . YES   NO
    i. Nitroglycerin . . . . YES   NO
    j. Antihistamine . . . . YES   NO
    k. Oral contraceptive or other hormonal therapy . . . . YES   NO
    l. Other _____
                                                   YES   NO

13. Are you allergic or have you reacted adversely to:
    a. Local anesthetics . . . . YES   NO
    b. Penicillin or other antibiotics . . . . YES   NO
    c. Sulfa drugs . . . . YES   NO
    d. Barbiturates, sedatives, or sleeping pills . . . . YES   NO
    e. Aspirin . . . . YES   NO
    f. Iodine . . . . YES   NO
    g. Codeine or other narcotics . . . . YES   NO

    h. Other_____

14. Have you had any serious trouble associated with any previous dental treatment . . . . YES   NO

    If so, explain _____

15. Do you have any disease, condition, or problem not listed above that you think I should know about? . . . . YES   NO

    If so, please explain _____

16. Are you employed in any situation which exposes you regularly to x-rays or other ionizing radiaton . . . . YES   NO

17. Are you wearing contact lenses . . . . YES   NO

WOMEN

18. Are you pregnant . . . . YES   NO

19. Do you have any problems associated with your menstrual period? . . . . YES   NO

Chief Dental Complaint:

_____

Signature of Patient

_____

Signature of Dentist

Fig. 4-1, cont'd.

medical emergency, wouldn't the Good Samaritan statute exempt the dentist from civil liability? If an emergency is truly nothing more than an unforeseen combination of circumstances, how can a dentist be held liable for it?

I am a trial-oriented defense attorney, and these are some of the questions I have been asked. Ultimately, it is a judge sitting without a jury or, more frequently, a jury that furnishes the answer to each of these questions in any given lawsuit. Therefore it is appropriate first to examine the context within which a jury answers these difficult questions.

It is hoped that a brief review of what is important at trial will provide a logical basis for understanding and applying the legal principles that pertain to medical emergencies in a dental office and legal expectations of dentists under those circumstances.

THE JURY SYSTEM—SOME IMPORTANT CONSIDERATIONS

Unless a dentist has agreed with a patient beforehand to resolve a dispute in any way other than the judicial system, such as through arbitration, the existing judicial system in each community and state is the mechanism through which a complaint of malpractice will be resolved. More particularly, if a medical emergency has arisen in a dental office and the patient claims to have been injured because of negligence during the medical emergency, and subsequently files a lawsuit, the case will be disposed of ultimately at trial by the jury.

It sometimes seems unlikely that a jury will be able to make sense of the enormous volume of evidence presented in a trial and return the proper verdict. They can, however, and they will. The result depends on the evidence, the law, and the quality of trial counsel.

Long ago, the manner in which well-heeled people resolved important disputes was by means of professionals who were adept at some form of one-on-one combat—for example, knights at a joust. Whoever hired the victorious combatant won the dispute. Those professionals of old have been replaced in the modern world by a different kind of combatant. Lawyers now oppose each other with legal, not lethal, results; the consequences, however, are just as important to those who hire them. The adversarial system between attorneys has evolved into a process that uncovers as many facts as possible to assist a nonpartisan third person (the judge) or group of third persons (the jury) in

deciding who should win and lose. Ideally, if the plaintiff's attorney and the defendant's attorney excel equally at their craft, a judge and/or jury will be provided with sufficient enlightenment to reach a just conclusion. Sadly, advocates are not equal, and frequently greater incentive to win cases is provided to patients' attorneys than to attorneys hired by insurance companies. Plaintiffs' attorneys are usually hired on a contingency fee basis; that is, they will recover a percentage of whatever they obtain for their clients (generally 25% but sometimes up to 75%). Therefore plaintiffs' attorneys have a built-in incentive to win their clients' cases. Contingency fees have not been accepted as appropriate compensation in the defense of a party to a lawsuit. Therefore virtually all dentists are defended in a lawsuit by an attorney who is paid by the hour and is generally paid the same fee, win or lose. The professionalism among defense attorneys should be sufficiently high to negate the presumption that an attorney with a vested interest in a victory will do better for his client. The primary difference between the two types of attorneys is the fact that a plaintiff-oriented attorney who chooses her cases carefully will probably generate substantially higher fee revenue than a defense attorney, who is often required to maintain highly competitive hourly rates. Thus, the insurance company, in a meritorious case, pays a fee to the plaintiff's lawyer which is usually higher than that paid to its own defense attorney. This is done to keep the carrier's expenses as low as can reasonably be expected and is particularly notable in a multimillion-dollar case, in which the patient's attorney will receive a substantial percentage of the award. Again, the professionalism and trial expertise of a community of defense attorneys should remain unaffected by the different fee arrangements, and the quality of services rendered should ideally be as high for defendants as for plaintiffs. This disparity in incentive, however, may create inequality of legal services.

A skilled attorney for the plaintiff decides to take a case based on what the attorney believes the outcome of the potential lawsuit to be. If the facts of the potential lawsuit indicate that a jury may not decide favorably for the patient, the attorney will probably not take the case at all or will accept it with the understanding that the potential lawsuit has reduced settlement value. I believe that the unhappy practice of plaintiffs' attorneys taking weak cases and settling them for reduced but substantial amounts is encouraged every time a dentist, his insurance company, and his defense attorney approve of such settlements.

An astute attorney for the plaintiff will request a copy of the patient's chart for review—by himself and probably another dentist, as well—before agreeing to accept the patient's case. A well-documented chart demonstrating satisfactory care of the patient will discourage a decision to take the case. Therefore good documentation by the dentist is not only important at trial but also extremely important in determining whether or not an attorney will represent a patient.

Once a lawsuit is filed with the court, the dentist is served by a sheriff with a complaint and a summons, either by mail or by notice in a newspaper. Within a prescribed time of service, usually 30 days or less, the dentist must file an answer or risk having a default judgment taken against him. Between the time of service and the time of answering the complaint, the dentist must secure the services of a defense attorney. Generally, the assignment of the case to a defense attorney is made by the dentist's insurance carrier. However, dentists are strongly urged to know whom they would wish to represent them before they are ever sued. Depending on the population, an insurance company usually employs one to three attorneys in any given community, to whom it gives all or most of its defense work on behalf of those insured. Sometimes the attorney selected is not the attorney whom the dentist may wish to have represent her. Therefore it is urged that a dentist familiarize herself with those attorneys in the community who excel in dental malpractice defense. The dentist should make certain when she purchases malpractice insurance that she and the insurance carrier agree on the choice of an attorney in case the dentist is sued. The worst time to make a well-reasoned decision—one that could affect the rest of the dentist's life—is when she is upset over having just been sued and has a month or less to agree on the selection of a defense attorney.

After the dentist's attorney has filed an answer to the complaint on the dentist's behalf, the process of discovery begins. There is no longer any excuse, in a case to be tried for a patient or dentist, for attorneys to be ignorant of any important facts. Liberal rules of discovery allow the use of many discovery tools. Among these are written interrogatories to be answered by each party; depositions, which are made up of testimony under oath during the discovery period; requests for production of records

by the parties; and requests to admit certain facts. The period of discovery permits both parties and their attorneys to learn as much as possible about the merits of the patient's case and the dentist's defense. The dentist should expect to be kept abreast of all important developments in the lawsuit. A feeling of teamwork should develop between dentist and attorney; each has expertise the other needs.

A clear example of good teamwork is planning for the presence of the defendant dentist during the deposition of the patient's expert witness. It is more difficult for the expert to criticize the dentist if he is sitting across the table. Often the dentist should be present during the patient's deposition, too. In addition, these depositions provide an excellent opportunity for the dentist to evaluate the quality of the attorney. Another example of teamwork is when the dentist offers assistance to his attorney on dental and medical issues. This also provides the defendant dentist with an excellent opportunity to evaluate for himself the most important evidence against him.

BURDEN OF PROOF AND *RES IPSA LOQUITUR*

With few exceptions, the plaintiff has what is called the "burden of proof" in any case, including a lawsuit against a dentist. This means that for a patient to win her case against a dentist, a jury must find that the plaintiff sustained her burden of proving the following:

1. That the dentist was at fault
2. That the dentist's fault was the cause of injuries to the patient
3. That those injuries must be compensated in dollars and cents (damages), which the dentist must pay to the patient and, in serious cases, to the patient's family

Therefore, in almost all cases in which a dentist has been sued, she may take comfort in the fact that the burden is *not* on herself to disprove any of the issues; rather, it is on the plaintiff. In practical terms, however, the best defense is often the offense for the dentist's attorney. He goes on the offense by producing evidence to disprove his client's fault, that is, he proves the dentist did not injure the patient. A good defense attorney, like a good boxer, will be prepared at trial to take the lead or to counterpunch with appropriate evidence. This decision is made as late as possible.

The reader will note some qualification when I say that the patient has the burden of proof in all instances. The law has carved out an interesting and logical exception to a plaintiff's responsibility to prove fault. That exception is known as *res ipsa loquitur,* commonly shortened to *res ipsa.* Literally translated, this phrase means "the thing speaks for itself." Expressed simply, this concept applies to lawsuits in which the result itself indicates that there must have been some wrong committed by the dentist; otherwise, the harm would not have occurred. For instance, if the dentist or oral surgeon performed a surgical procedure that required the use of small sponges and a sponge were left in the gum and discovered later, the plaintiff would not have the burden of proving that the dentist was at fault. In this case, the dentist has the burden of proving that the sponge being left in the patient's tissue was not the dentist's fault. There are relatively few areas of dentistry in which the burden of proof is shifted to the dentist because of the doctrine of *res ipsa loquitur.* Few if any lawsuits arising out of medical emergencies fall into this category.

THE EXPERT WITNESS

Part of the plaintiff's burden of proving the three indispensable elements of a case against the dentist is the procurement of expert testimony. Except in cases of *res ipsa loquitur,* the plaintiff's burden of proving a case of malpractice against a dentist is accomplished through an expert witness. The expert witness, retained by the patient's lawyer, gives testimony that includes opinions on the appropriate standard of care and whether the dentist met it in treating the patient. Cases involving medical emergencies are included in those that require an expert witness. Because a lay jury is not considered competent to reach decisions without expert testimony in cases against dentists, an indispensable part of the plaintiff's case against the dentist is having an expert witness, qualified by the court as such, who will state under oath that the dentist fell below the standard of care and that the injuries complained about resulted from the dentist's breach of this standard of care. Except in cases of *res ipsa loquitur,* most courts in most states will dismiss a lawsuit against a dentist before trial if the plaintiff has not obtained expert testimony against the defendant dentist. On the other hand, the defendant dentist and his attorney may also retain an expert witness to counter the testimony of the plaintiff's expert witness. Because the plaintiff has the burden of proof, the dentist need not obtain an expert witness to testify at trial. But if a plaintiff has an expert

witness, it is rare for an experienced defense trial attorney to fail to secure an expert witness on behalf of her own client; this witness is needed to counter the adverse testimony of the plaintiff's expert. In some cases, however, an expert need not be called on behalf of the dentist. An entire book could be written on the appropriate strategies and counterstrategies of using or not using expert witnesses at trial. I have defended cases through trial that have proved the proposition that, in rare instances, the defendant dentist may well be his own best expert witness. However, the strategy must be used carefully. Of course, selection of the expert witness is extremely important. It is a rare person who can testify equally effectively at trial in many different professional and geographic areas. Selection and use of an expert witness is an example of the great care, thought, and psychology that must be exercised in case preparation and trial.

A lawsuit tried solely on the basis of the strategy of the attorneys and the credibility of expert witnesses would be much like a football game without officials. From the beginning of the lawsuit to the conclusion of trial, a judge is always available to provide answers when the lawyers cannot agree and to interject into each case the principles of law by which all cases are governed, including those regarding standard of care, negligence, proximate cause of the injuries, and guidelines for awarding damages.

Although the precise wording of these legal concepts may vary somewhat from state to state, their interpretation is sufficiently broad to allow meaningful discussions about their application in virtually all states. Discussions of several of these important concepts provide the dentist with a better understanding of what the law expects of him in terms of anticipating, preventing, or successfully treating a medical emergency in his office. These concepts are the cornerstones of a successful defense for a lawsuit resulting from a medical emergency.

THE LAW OF EACH CASE—
THE STANDARD OF CARE

A jury must find the dentist negligent before the patient can recover damages. "Negligence" and "malpractice" are used synonymously in lawsuits against health care providers. In defining "negligence," a judge will usually tell the jury that negligence is (1) doing something that an ordinarily prudent person would not do under the same or similar circumstances or (2) not doing something that a reasonably prudent person would do under the same or similar circumstances. A judge will instruct the jury that negligence is the failure to use ordinary care. This seems easy enough to determine as it applies to an automobile driver or a shop owner who leaves a slippery substance on the floor of the shop. However, how does a jury apply the principle of negligence to a dentist?

This is where the testimony of the expert witness enters the picture. The judge's instructions will guide the jury with regard to the indispensable expert testimony in almost all cases against dentists; the judge will instruct the jury that in a case against the dentist, each side is permitted to call an expert witness to define the standard of care and testify about whether the defendant met the standard. The judge will inform the jury that people ordinarily are not permitted to come into the courtroom and offer opinions. Usually, witnesses may only testify to facts: what they saw or heard or what documents or other information they have that may assist the jury. However, the procedure differs in a lawsuit in which a jury must determine whether a dentist is at fault. In that case, expert witnesses—witnesses who have special training and experience and are acknowledged to possess the skill or education to qualify them to offer opinions to the jury—may so testify, and the jury may consider their opinions. The judge informs the jury that they need not consider any of the opinions given and may weigh the credibility of the expert witnesses by the same criteria they use for all other witnesses. The crux of the testimony of each expert witness in a dental malpractice lawsuit is whether or not the dentist was negligent. In most states, an expert witness is not permitted to testify whether she believes that the dentist was negligent or not. However, the expert witness may give opinion testimony about whether the dentist fell within or below the acceptable standard of care. In doing so, she may not use her own personal standards but must use what she believes to be the standards of the community. In recent years, the community standard has been expanded to the national community standard. Therefore, in almost all lawsuits in all courts across the country, each defendant dentist is held to a national standard of care, which the expert witnesses establish in their testimony. However, experts frequently do not agree on what the national standard is. It should now be self-evident that expert witnesses are an indispensable part of the plaintiff's case and that without them the case must be dismissed. Without expert testimony on behalf of the plaintiff who, you will recall, has the burden of proof, there can be no evidence regarding the acceptable standard of care, which the jury must use to reach a conclusion about the dentist's treatment of the patient.

A multitude of people in different professions are qualified as experts in the proper response to medical emergencies in dental offices. They include CPR instructors, paramedics, some nurses, medical doctors, and of course dentists. This creates an abundance of potential expert witnesses to testify either against the dentist or on his behalf.

Having discussed briefly the more important judicial concepts that govern the outcome of every lawsuit against a dentist, we now turn to an evaluation of the legal duty owed or not owed by dentists in anticipating and preventing or in treating medical emergencies.

FORESEEABILITY OF THE EMERGENCY

One of the underlying principles of our legal system is the concept of foreseeability. If the consequences of an act are foreseeable and result in harm, liability may be imposed. It is arguable that a cardiac arrest or an idiosyncratic reaction to medication or anesthesia in a dental office are not foreseeable events, unless the dentist has a crystal ball in her office. However, experience tells us that, although it is impossible to predict when a particular medical emergency will arise, they do occur and therefore are foreseeable. It is probably for this reason that companies with a great number of employees and large companies that have direct contact with the public, such as department stores, hotels, and restaurants, are in the process of upgrading and maintaining higher standards for responding to medical emergencies. More and more employees of such organizations are learning how to correctly administer such procedures as CPR. At the time of publication of the third edition of this book, it is questionable whether a person could bring a successful lawsuit against department store personnel for failing to respond properly to his cardiac arrest. However, as the community standard in responding to cardiac arrests is upgraded and as expectations rise as to how department store personnel or those from similar enterprises should respond to medical emergencies, it is arguable that in years to come a department store employee may be considered negligent if he does not have the wherewithal to respond to a cardiac arrest.

There is little doubt that the expectations and therefore the anticipated standards of care in responding to a medical emergency are higher in medical facilities, including dental offices. We might ask why this is so. It is common knowledge, as has been borne out in cases that I have defended, that there are circumstances and practices within a dental office that are much more likely to precipitate a medical emergency than those within, for example, a department store. This higher likelihood of emergency, then, helps to explain higher expectations of care.

What are some of the foreseeable circumstances or factors that are likely to give rise to medical emergencies in a dental office?

Many people experience fear and anxiety at the mere thought of having to see a dentist in a day or two. By the time these people find themselves in the dentist's office and are waiting for the dentist to see them, their fear and anxiety may cause measurable metabolic changes. Sometimes, anger and frustration about having to wait for a long time to see the dentist are added, and many of these patients become prone to medical emergencies precipitated by metabolic changes. However, even patients who are seen immediately will probably be substantially more stressed than they would be in most other environments.

A highly stressed patient is not the ideal patient for administration of anesthestics or medications. Furthermore, once treatment begins, the chances of a medical emergency increase for anxious and nonanxious patients alike with the administration of anesthetics and medications, virtually all of which are known to have adverse reactions, idiosyncratic reactions, and side effects. The *Physicians' Desk Reference (PDR)* or the drug package insert accompanying each anesthetic or medication lists reactions that have been reported to be associated with all anesthetics and medications used in the dental office. Virtually every anesthetic agent and medication that a dentist uses in his office can be shown to have been associated with a bizarre medical reaction. It must be kept in mind that those reactions published in the drug package insert and the *PDR,* which are generally identical, are *associated with* the use of a particular anesthetic or medication; in fact, the use of the anesthetic or medication may have absolutely nothing to do with the ensuing medical emergency, whether it be cardiac

arrest or some other life-threatening reaction that is reported and included in the *PDR*. However, there stands the description of the reaction, in print, for an expert witness to refer to at trial. The witness can say to the jury, "The adverse reaction to the anesthetic is something the dentist knew about or should have known about; it is listed as a known side effect in the pharmaceutical bible, the *PDR*, which every prescriber and administrator of medication has or should have. The same information is included with every vial and every package of medication that is opened in the dentist's office." The *PDR* excerpt for that medication will go into evidence for the jury to read during its deliberations. It can be used as *evidence of notice* to the dentist—that is, evidence that the dentist used the anesthetic or medication daily with many patients and therefore had a duty to note all of its reported side effects and adverse reactions. Consequently, the argument goes, the dentist should have anticipated and treated correctly the adverse reaction or side effect experienced by his patient. Of course, the defense attorney can counter through his own expert witnesses, through witnesses from pharmaceutical companies or the FDA, or even from the *PDR* itself that the side effects, adverse reactions, and incidents reported in association with use of the medication are based on reports made by health care providers, many of which are never investigated and verified. However, this kind of evidence can seem to the jury to be a rationalization. The dentist's attorney must anticipate this and prepare to respond successfully. However, the reader can begin to see that the *PDR*, in presenting information that offers protection to the pharmaceutical companies, also contains information that the dentist should know and use as a tool in her practice. Keeping abreast of the *PDR* avoids being painfully confronted with it in a lawsuit. Plaintiffs' attorneys experienced in dental malpractice know that there should be a *PDR* in every dental office or, failing that, that every container of anesthetic or medication in a dental office contains a drug package insert with the very same information. If the *PDR* is not used in the dental office, the plaintiff's attorney will attempt to prove that an emergency occurred because the dentist failed to keep up with medication literature.

Therefore, know the drugs you use. Stay current with them by consulting the *PDR* and its updates throughout the year. Identify patients for whom special precautions may have to be taken. Make a note in patients' charts if reevaluation of medications or further history from the patient is required. These follow-up notations reflect excellent dentistry, and just as important at trial, they are *convincing evidence* of excellent dentistry.

DEALING WITH THE MEDICAL EMERGENCY

In the preface to this book, Dr. Malamed has said that with proper patient management all medical emergency situations can be prevented. Frankly, I believe that, within a legal and perhaps medical context, this is a rather severe standard to which the dentist is expected to adhere. I would rather say that all medical emergencies are *foreseeable* and that a dentist and his staff should therefore be properly trained and equipped to confront the medical emergency as well as can be reasonably anticipated in a dental office. A dentist can probably increase the chances of a medical emergency with poor "bedside" (actually chairside) manner, including keeping a patient waiting. A dentist and his staff can increase the chances of a medical emergency by failure to identify genuine anxiety and stress, failure to allay it, or (perhaps) failure to postpone treatment until a patient's anxiety has been allayed. As far as adverse and idiosyncratic reactions to medications are concerned, there are other preventive measures that can and probably should be taken based on the current national standard of dental practice.

HISTORY TAKING

As has been discussed in Chapter 2 and stressed elsewhere in this book, it is imperative that dentists obtain a full and complete medical history from patients before treating them. Even if the patient is in severe pain and presents what can be termed a dental emergency, there are few dental emergencies that cannot wait a few additional minutes while a thorough medical history is obtained from the patient or a person familiar with the patient, such as a spouse or parent. Knowledge of such problems as liver disorders, food and drug allergies, and heart problems is indispensable in the proper care and treatment of a patient. Failure to gather such information can be the most damaging evidence of all if an anesthetic or medication, which would have been contraindicated by a satisfactory medical history, is administered and results in a serious medical emergency. Several excellent medical history questionnaires have been presented in Chapter 2.

It is urged that, to protect himself and more importantly to protect his patient, the dentist should have each patient complete such a questionnaire before initial treatment. Because the history of some categories of patients, particularly the young and the elderly, may change markedly from year to year, dentists are urged to have patients update their medical history forms annually. If a dentist has not treated a patient for several months, it's a good idea for the dentist or an office staff member to ask the patient if she has had any medical changes or has been seen by a physician for anything other than common, garden-variety illnesses; this rules out any major problems before treatment. It is particularly important these days to note on a patient's chart that she was asked about any such medical changes or treatment since the last visit. A notation of the patient's response should also be made. To demonstrate how important this is, let us say that a patient suffers a serious adverse reaction from a medication in a dentist's office during treatment, and a lawsuit is brought and subsequently is tried. There is no way in the world that a jury will believe a dentist and his staff members if they testify that they specifically recall a patient's verbal statement that nothing of any medical consequence had happened to her (the patient) since her last visit—*unless that statement was noted in writing*. To discredit a verbal statement, a skilled plaintiff's attorney simply has to establish the fact that, in the months and years that have passed since that particular visit, the dentist has had several thousand dental visits from many, many patients. Thus the jury will be asked to view the dentist's recall of the statement with great suspicion. If in fact a significant medical event *has* occurred that the patient has not related to the dentist, and if the dentist records the question and negative response in the patient's chart, this information will support the dentist years later; it will be very difficult evidence for the patient and her attorney to rebut at trial.

If a patient's medical history requires clarification, the dentist should contact the patient's primary physician, making a notation in the patient's chart about the consultation and what was discussed. Patients' charts should include the names and phone numbers of their regular physicians for this purpose. When the dentist calls, he should indicate to the physician that he is making the note and would appreciate the physician making a notation of the same discussion in his chart for the patient. These notations may prove to be extremely important at trial.

INFORMED CONSENT

In the past two decades, a national standard pertaining to informed consent has developed. The courts of each state may vary the requirements of obtaining informed consent somewhat, but in essence informed consent requires that a dentist explain the following to a patient in sufficient detail so that the patient understands:

1. Reasons for care and treatment
2. Diagnosis
3. Prognosis
4. Alternatives
5. Nature of care and treatment
6. The risks involved (inherent risks included)
7. Expectations of success
8. Possible results if care and treatment are not undertaken or if instructions are not followed

As with other topics discussed in this chapter, informed consent could be the subject of many chapters or of an entire book. However, a brief overview indicates that within the context of a discussion of medical emergencies, the concept of informed consent has an interesting twist. It is arguable that the more thorough a dentist is in explaining the risks involved and in documenting the risks discussed with the patient, the stronger the evidence may be against the dentist if a medical emergency arises out of the treatment. For instance, let us say that an oral surgeon warns a patient that cardiac arrest is a known reaction to an anesthestic and that the patient subsequently experiences cardiac arrest under that anesthetic. It will be difficult for the oral surgeon to attempt to defend himself by saying that that reaction was an unforeseeable emergency and therefore impossible to prepare for. Consequently, the more thorough a dentist is in informing the patient of risks, the more prepared he should be to prevent or treat those risks.

To the extent that it can be shown that medical emergencies will occur with higher frequency in a dentist's office than in many other places, a dentist will be expected to be that much more prepared to prevent or treat such emergencies.

Throughout this text, Dr. Malamed has discussed what kinds of emergencies dentists should anticipate and how they should be treated; therefore that discussion need not be repeated here. It should be emphasized, however, that proper response to a medical emergency often requires effective and efficient teamwork. This is particularly true in a situation in which CPR is administered, especially on the part of the team member administering CPR. Therefore each dental office should be staffed by appropriately trained personnel who know what their assigned tasks will be in case of a medical emergency. For example, who will telephone for an ambulance? Where will the emergency response equipment, including oxygen, be kept, and whose responsibility will it be to bring that equipment to the patient? In many circumstances, CPR cannot be administered effectively by only one person; therefore it may be no excuse that the dentist alone knows CPR. Because CPR is foreseeable and will probably have to be administered at some time, it may be well for all dental office employees to be familiar with and well-rehearsed in CPR technique and to have current CPR certification. In addition, dentists ought to hold occasional CPR drills in their offices and keep records of these drills, including which staff members participated. Such records will refute very effectively the contention that a patient died during cardiac arrest because of lack of CPR training of office personnel. CPR will not always save a patient, and it would be sad for a dentist to be held liable in such instances simply because she failed to document the training of her employees, as well as practice drills held in the office.

As soon as possible after an emergency, the dentist should thoroughly note what happened to the patient in the patient's chart—from the initiation of treatment to the conclusion of the emergency, or until the patient's care has been undertaken by paramedics or a physician. If the emergency was handled correctly, these notes will be invaluable in the defense at trial.

Because the dentist is responsible for job-related negligence of her associates and employees, she must be sure that her team is well trained so that an employee's act or omission will not create liability for her. Although the dentist herself may respond superbly to a medical emergency, problems will arise if her staff is untrained.

Often, paramedics may be more expert in handling medical emergencies than dentists; they may not wish to have the dentist accompany them and the patient to the hospital. A dentist should offer assistance to the paramedics before they leave for the hospital. Whatever the paramedics decide, the dentist's offer to continue assistance on the way to the hospital and the paramedics' response to that offer should be clearly documented by the dentist.

A LOWER STANDARD IN AN EMERGENCY?

The law does not require the dentist or any other health care practitioner to respond to an emergency and a nonemergency in the same manner. In other words, the standard of care expected of a dentist in an emergency is not as high as the standard of care expected in a nonemergency. However, as discussed previously, whether or not a dentist is negligent in an emergency situation will ultimately be decided by the jury on the basis of the answer to this question: Did the dentist and his staff respond as would an ordinarily prudent dentist and staff in the same or similar circumstances? The dentist and his staff will be held to the standard of the ordinarily prudent dentist and staff to the extent that the medical emergency can be shown to have been foreseeable and to the extent that evidence shows that the dentist and staff should have been prepared. Although the standard of care in emergency situations may not be as high as the nonemergency standard, there are expected standards of conduct in emergencies. If the dentist and his staff meet these standards, there will be no liability; if they fail to meet them, there will be liability.

It should be remembered that medical emergencies resulting from dental treatment may occur after the patient has left the office. If a patient begins to experience an adverse reaction to a medication at home and calls the dental office, or if a call is placed on his behalf, the dentist and his staff should be prepared to meet these emergencies also. A preplanned response to such a situation should be discussed among staff members so that the patient or his family can be given proper and immediate instructions. A dentist's failure to respond in such a circumstance may itself precipitate a lawsuit. If a patient cannot get your attention at the time of the phone call, he certainly will with a lawsuit!

GOOD SAMARITAN CONSIDERATIONS

Good Samaritan statutes differ somewhat from state to state. However, they usually say that health care providers should not be held liable for death or injury (except for gross negligence) in cases in which they render emergency life-and-death treatment, in good faith, to people who are not their patients (that is, people for whose treatment they do not expect to be compensated). The medical emergency of a patient in a dental office probably does not constitute a situation in which a Good Samaritan defense is applicable. Because the victim of the emergency is the patient of the dentist, the dentist has an obligation to treat the patient. However, if a nonpatient of the dentist, such as a family member, happens to be in the waiting room and requires an emergency response to a medical situation, a Good Samaritan defense may well apply.

•　•　•

Establish a relationship with a good, experienced malpractice defense attorney before you ever need her. Additionally, keep in touch with that attorney and seek her advice, much as you would recommend to your patients that they have periodic checkups as a preventive measure. Urge your community dental association or society to invite attorneys who specialize in dental malpractice cases to meetings; they will be able to familiarize you with informed consent requirements and other peculiarities of the law in your state. You should know of the statutes and cases that affect your practice so that you can tailor your practice to meet the requirements of the law. Learn how other dentists are equipping and preparing their offices and staffs for medical emergencies. Make certain that your preparedness is comparable to what appears to be the standard. Remember that the standard of care is not perfection, particularly when the caregiver is responding to a medical emergency.

Although today health care professionals are defending themselves against more lawsuits than ever, lawsuits can be prevented; what's more, if they do occur, they can be defended successfully. The prevention or successful defense of lawsuits depends on how you and your staff meet the challenges of increased litigation. Don't let yourself, your staff, or your colleagues down. By preventing lawsuits or providing information leading to a successful defense, you not only protect yourself but also maintain the presumption that dentists care about their patients and take prudent precautions to protect them. If you follow the suggestions in this chapter, practice within the standard of reasonableness, maintain your continuing dental education, and document office procedures and your patients' charts, the law will support you.

One last word: courage. If you have competent, experienced counsel and a strong defense, have the courage to go through with a trial, if necessary. Settling claims or lawsuits out of court, if you should and can win in court, will only encourage additional lawsuits. By going through with a trial and winning the suit, you will not only vindicate yourself and staff and discourage similar lawsuits—you will also become a better dentist.

3/17/93

5 *Unconsciousness: General Considerations*

Loss of consciousness is not an uncommon occurrence in the dental office. Although various factors may be responsible for this, the management of all cases of unconsciousness will be essentially the same and will be directed primarily toward certain basic, life-sustaining procedures. In most instances the loss of consciousness will be transient, and carrying out these basic maneuvers will be all that is required for proper patient management. However, there are still other causes of unconsciousness that will require additional attention after these steps have been taken. This section is concerned with a number of syndromes, all of which may result in the loss of consciousness. Definitions of relevant terms follow:

anoxia Absence or lack of oxygen
coma From the Greek *koma,* meaning deep sleep; designates a state of unconsciousness from which the patient cannot be aroused, even by powerful stimulation
consciousness From the Latin *conscius,* meaning aware; implies the capability of an appropriate response to question or command and the presence of intact protective reflexes, including the ability to independently maintain an airway
faint Sudden, transient loss of consciousness
hypoxia Low oxygen content
syncope From the Greek *synkope;* a sudden, transient loss of consciousness

SYNCOPE

The terms *syncope* and *fainting* are commonly used interchangeably to describe a transient loss of consciousness caused by reversible disturbances in cerebral function. Throughout this text the term *syncope* will be employed to describe this occurrence. It must be remembered that syncope is only a symptom and that although syncopal episodes may occur in healthy persons, they may also be indicative of serious medical disorders. It must also be remembered that any loss of consciousness represents a life-threatening situation. Prompt recognition and effective management will be required whenever it occurs.

PREDISPOSING FACTORS

Table 5-1 lists many of the possible causes of unconsciousness in the dental office setting and indicates the relative frequency of their occurrence. A review of these will give the reader the impression that there are many possible causes of unconsciousness. Although this is relatively accurate, a closer examination will reveal three factors that, when present, increase the chances that loss of consciousness will occur. These factors are (1) stress, (2) impaired physical status, and (3) the administration or ingestion of drugs.

In the dental office, stress is the primary etiologic agent in most cases of unconsciousness. Vasodepressor syncope, the most common cause of unconsciousness, may be considered to be a manifestation of undue stress.

Impaired physical status (ASA III or IV) is a second factor that will make the patient more susceptible to the loss of consciousness. Many of the causes listed in Table 5-1 are not initially accompanied by a loss of consciousness but may rapidly progress to this state if not promptly recognized or if the patient is debilitated. If a patient with impaired physical status must undergo undue stress, the chances are even greater that this patient will react adversely to the situation (with possible loss of consciousness).

Table 5-1. Possible causes of unconsciousness in the dental office

Cause	Frequency	Where covered in text
Vasodepressor syncope	Most common	Unconsciousness (Section II)
Drug administration/ingestion	Common	Drug-related emergencies (Section VI)
Orthostatic hypotension	Less common	Unconsciousness (Section II)
Epilepsy	Less common	Convulsions (Section V)
Hypoglycemic reaction	Less common	Altered consciousness (Section IV)
Acute adrenal insufficiency	Rare	Unconsciousness (Section II)
Acute allergic reaction	Rare	Drug-related emergencies (Section VI)
Acute myocardial infarction	Rare	Chest pain (Section VII)
Cerebrovascular accident	Rare	Altered consciousness (Section IV)
Hyperglycemic reaction	Rare	Altered consciousness (Section IV)
Hyperventilation syndrome	Rare	Altered consciousness (Section IV)

The third factor is the administration or ingestion of drugs. Certain categories of drugs are commonly used in dentistry. The three major categories are analgesics (nonnarcotics, narcotics, and local anesthetics), antianxiety agents (sedative-hypnotics and tranquilizers), and antibiotics. The first two categories may readily cause loss of consciousness in the dental patient. Various agents, primarily the narcotic analgesics, will predispose the dental patient to orthostatic hypotension (Chapter 7), whereas narcotics and other agents (such as barbiturates and other sedative-hypnotics), if administered in adequate dosages, may lead to loss of consciousness through entry into the second or third stages of general anesthesia (Guedel's classification).*

---

*The stages of anesthesia may best be understood by explaining the basic pattern of action of general anesthetic agents (and all other CNS depressant drugs). This pattern consists of a progressive depression of the central nervous system. Central nervous system depressants (general anesthetics, tranquilizers, sedative-hypnotics, and alcohol) first depress the cerebral cortex, producing a loss of sensory function, followed by loss of motor function. Then the basal ganglia and cerebellum are depressed, followed by the spinal cord and, lastly, the medulla. Medullary depression leads to depression of the respiratory and cardiovascular systems and is the usual cause of death from drug overdose. Guedel (1951) described four stages of general anesthesia based on this information. Stage 1, analgesia or altered consciousness, corresponds to the action of the drugs on the higher cortical centers (sensory). The various techniques of psychosedation are in this stage. Stage 2, delirium or excitement, corresponds to the depressant action of drugs on higher motor centers. The patient is unconscious at this stage. Stages 1 and 2 comprise the induction phase of anesthesia. In stage 3, surgical anesthesia, spinal reflexes are depressed, producing skeletal muscle relaxation. Stage 4, medullary paralysis, corresponds to the depression of the respiratory and cardiovascular centers of the medulla, first producing respiratory arrest and then cardiovascular collapse.

Local anesthetics are the most commonly employed drugs in dentistry and are a major predisposing factor for syncope. It is estimated that in excess of 6,000,000 cartridges of local anesthetic solution are injected each week by dentists in the United States, yet the morbidity and mortality rates from these agents are incredibly low. However, life-threatening situations can develop in conjunction with the use of these agents. The majority of local anesthetic reactions will be precipitated by stress (fear and anxiety); however, various reactions can develop that are related directly to the agents themselves. These include the overdose reaction and the acute allergic reaction (anaphylactic reaction). Local anesthetic reactions will be discussed more fully in Section VII of this text.

PREVENTION

Loss of consciousness can be prevented in many instances by a thorough preliminary medical and dental evaluation of the prospective patient. Important elements in the preliminary evaluation of the patient include determination of the patient's ability to tolerate, both physically and psychologically, the stresses of dental therapy. An adequate medical history questionnaire and physical examination of the patient followed by the dialogue history will usually uncover medical and/or psychologic disability, allowing the doctor to modify the treatment plan to accommodate the impaired physical or psychologic status of the patient. Determination of fear and anxiety related to dentistry is a more difficult task. A method of determining this has been successfully employed at the School of Dentistry of the University of Southern California since 1973. It consists of a short anxiety questionnaire (see p. 35), which is included in the medical history that each patient is required to complete before dental therapy. This has been patterned after the questionnaire devised by Corah (1969), which presents the patient with a series of questions related to attitudes toward various aspects of dental therapy.

Once a fear of dentistry has been determined, the dental practitioner can use any of the psychosedative techniques to reduce stress. These include nondrug techniques such as iatrosedation and hypnosis; pharmacosedative procedures including oral, rectal, and intramuscular sedation; inhalation sedation with nitrous oxide and oxygen; and intravenous sedation. When properly used, these procedures can greatly reduce the medical and psychologic risks of dental procedures. However, as mentioned earlier, the use of drugs has associated risk factors that the doctor employing the agents must be aware of and capable of managing.

According to McCarthy (1972), 90% of potential emergency situations can be prevented through proper use of preliminary patient evaluation and appropriate use of conscious sedation and pain control.

Another major factor in preventing loss of consciousness is the introduction of sit-down dentistry with treatment of patients when they are in the supine (horizontal) position. The supine position prevents the development of cerebral anoxia, the most common mechanism of unconsciousness, and has been responsible for a great decrease in the number of episodes of unconsciousness occurring in dental offices.

CLINICAL MANIFESTATIONS

A definition of unconsciousness will be taken from our earlier definition of consciousness: an unconscious patient is incapable of responding to sensory stimulation and has lost the protective reflexes (swallowing, coughing) with an attendant lack of ability to maintain a patent airway. Basic management of unconsciousness is directed at reversing these clinical manifestations. Clinical signs and symptoms of impending unconsciousness (presyncope) and the actual state of unconsciousness (syncope) will vary slightly according to the primary cause. For this reason, the precise clinical manifestations of unconsciousness will be discussed in detail under specific situations (in Chapters 6 through 9).

PATHOPHYSIOLOGY
Mechanisms of Unconsciousness

Engel (1962), in his classic text on fainting, classified the mechanisms that produce unconsciousness in four categories: (1) reduced cerebral metabolism resulting from inadequate delivery of blood or oxygen to the brain, (2) reduced cerebral metabolism resulting from general or local metabolic deficiencies, (3) direct or reflex effects on systems of the central nervous system concerned with regulation of consciousness and equilibrium, and (4) psychic mechanisms affecting levels of consciousness with their respective mechanism or mechanisms (1 to 3, above) of action (Table 5-2). Lack of oxygen (hypoxia/anoxia) and lack of adequate blood sugar (hypoglycemia) are the two most often noted causes of unconsciousness in both adult and pediatric patients.

1. Inadequate cerebral circulation

The most common mechanism of unconsciousness is a sudden decrease in the supply of blood to the brain. Vasodepressor syncope (common faint) and orthostatic hypotension will be the most commonly encountered clinical examples of this. Physiologic disturbances that result in a decrease in blood supply to the brain include (1) dilation of the peripheral arterioles, (2) failure of normal peripheral vasoconstrictor activity (orthostatic hypotension), (3) a sharp fall in cardiac output (from heart disease or decreased blood volume), (4) constriction of cerebral vessels as CO_2 is lost through hyperventilation, (5) occlusion or narrowing of the internal carotid or other arteries to the brain, and (6) ventricular asystole. The first four factors rarely produce unconsciousness when the patient is in the supine position. Management of these factors will be directed at increasing the supply of oxygenated blood to the brain.

2. General or local metabolic change

Changes in the quality of blood perfusing the brain that are caused by chemical or metabolic derangements may also be associated with unconsciousness or may predispose an individual to its occurrence. Clinical situations most frequently encountered that may lead to unconsciousness through this mechanism include hyperventilation, hyperglycemia, hypoglycemia, the administration or ingestion of drugs, and acute allergic reaction. In these cases, consciousness will not be regained until the chemical or metabolic cause is corrected.

3. Actions on the central nervous system

Loss of consciousness associated with alterations within the brain itself or through reflex effects on the central nervous system are manifested clinically as convulsive episodes and cerebrovascular accident.

4. Psychic mechanisms

Psychic mechanisms such as emotional disturbances are the most common causes of unconsciousness in the dental environment and include several clinical situations discussed previously. Vasodepressor syncope and the hyperventilation syndrome are in this category.

Oxygen Deprivation

With loss of consciousness there is a generalized decrease in muscle tone in the body equivalent to that occurring in Guedel's stage 3 of anesthesia. The tongue, being a muscle, loses tone and, because of the effect of gravity, falls back into the hypopharynx, producing either a complete or a partial airway obstruction (Fig. 5-1). In the unconscious patient hypopharyngeal obstruction by the base of the relaxed tongue always occurs when the head is flexed and almost always when the head is in the mid-position. Relief of this obstruction will thus become the primary objective in management of the unconscious patient. Until the obstruction is removed, the patient will receive hypoxic levels of oxygen (partial obstruction) or will be anoxic (total obstruction) and thus will remain unconscious. The vital importance of oxygen in the maintenance of consciousness may be seen from the following: Under normal conditions the brain derives most of its energy from the oxidation of glucose. To maintain this energy source, a continuous supply of glucose and oxygen must be delivered to the brain. Without oxygen some glucose can still be metabolized to lactic acid with some energy being provided, but this source will not fulfill the brain's requirements for more than a few seconds, rapidly leading to the loss of consciousness.

The human brain, which accounts for only 2% of the total body mass, uses approximately 20% of the total oxygen and 65% of the total glucose consumed by the body. To do this, approximately 20% of the total blood circulation per minute must reach the brain. When the supply of either of these fuels is cut off, brain functioning is rapidly affected. It is estimated that the cerebral blood flow of a normal human in the supine position is 750 ml per min-

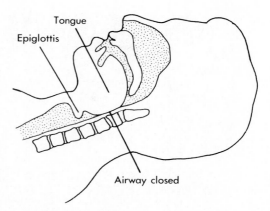

Fig. 5-1. Unconscious victim. Tongue falls backward against posterior wall of pharynx, producing airway obstruction.

Table 5-2. Classification of causes of unconsciousness by mechanism

Mechanism	Clinical example
Inadequate delivery of blood or oxygen to the brain	Acute adrenal insufficiency Orthostatic hypotension Vasodepressor syncope

Systemic or local metabolic deficiencies	Acute allergic reaction
	Drug ingestion and administration
	   Nitrites and nitrates
	   Diuretics
	   Sedatives-narcotics
	   Local anesthetics
	Hyperglycemia
	Hyperventilation
	Hypoglycemia

Direct or reflex effects on nervous system	Cerebrovascular accident Convulsive episodes
Psychic mechanisms	Emotional disturbances Hyperventilation Vasodepressor syncope

ute. At any moment, then, the blood circulating through the brain contains 7 ml of oxygen, an amount sufficient to supply the brain's requirements for less than 10 seconds. Rossen and coworkers (1943) carried out experiments in which the human brain was deprived of oxygen by sudden and complete arrest of cerebral circulation. Consciousness was lost in 6 seconds.

Complete airway obstruction, with the victim anoxic, will lead to permanent brain damage within

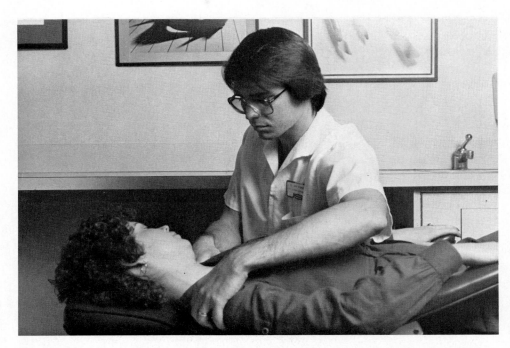

Fig. 5-2. Unconsciousness is determined by gently shaking shoulders and calling victim's name: the "shake and shout" technique.

4 to 6 minutes and to cardiac arrest within 5 to 10 minutes. Some authorities contend that anoxic periods of as little as 3 minutes' duration will cause permanent brain damage (Goldberg, 1974). Partial airway obstruction in which the victim receives hypoxic levels of oxygen may lead to the same result, although more slowly and through other, more complex pathways. In either case it is quite evident that the doctor and staff must be able to rapidly and effectively institute the steps of basic life support. Once a patent airway has been secured, and only then, can the doctor proceed to more definitive life support measures (chest compression or drug administration).

MANAGEMENT—BASIC LIFE SUPPORT

Immediate management of the unconscious victim will be predicated on two objectives:
1. Recognition of unconsciousness
2. Management of unconsciousness
   a. Recognition of airway obstruction
   b. Management of airway obstruction

Recognition of Unconsciousness

Step 1. Assessment: Identify that patient is unconscious. It is important to be able to recognize unconsciousness because many of the steps of basic

life support that follow should not be carried out on a conscious person. For this reason, we set certain criteria for unconsciousness based on the previously presented definition of unconsciousness as the state of being incapable of responding to sensory stimulation, with the loss of protective reflexes, and an attendant lack of ability to maintain a patent airway. Thus we have three criteria to aid us in the recognition of unconsciousness: (1) lack of response to sensory stimulation, (2) loss of protective reflexes, and (3) inability to maintain a patent airway.

The first of these criteria is the most useful to the rescuer seeking to rapidly assess the victim's state of consciousness. Criteria 2 and 3 are also clinical manifestations of unconsciousness but are less frequently employed than the lack of response to sensory stimulation.

To determine a lack of response to sensory stimulation, the American Heart Association (1986) recommends that the rescuer gently shake the patient's shoulder and shout loudly, "Are you all right?" to arouse him. If the patient does not respond to this "shake and shout" maneuver, the rescuer should immediately proceed to the steps of basic life support (Fig. 5-2).

Pain is another stimulus to determine the level of

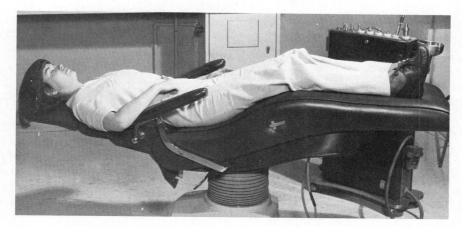

Fig. 5-3. Positioning of unconscious victim. Thorax and brain are at same level with feet elevated slightly (by 10 degrees), aiding return of venous blood to heart.

consciousness. Peripheral pain (such as pinching the suprascapular region) will usually evoke a motor response from the patient such as movement of a limb, furrowing of the forehead, or auditory responses. Lack of response to this stimulus is another indicator of unconsciousness. If the patient does not respond, the doctor should begin basic life support procedures.

Step 2. Call for help. If the victim does not respond to the "shake and shout," immediately call for assistance by activating the dental office emergency system.

Management of Unconsciousness

Loss of consciousness depresses many of the vital functions of the body, including the protective reflexes—choking, coughing, sneezing, and swallowing—and the ability of the patient to maintain a patent airway. The steps to be presented will permit the rescuer to maintain these vital functions until the victim recovers spontaneously or is transported to a hospital where definitive therapy is available.

Step 3. Position patient. As soon as unconsciousness is recognized the patient should be placed in the supine (horizontal) position with the brain at the same level as the heart and the feet elevated slightly (at a 10- to 15-degree angle). The head-down (Trendelenburg) position should be avoided because gravity will act to force the abdominal viscera superiorly into the diaphragm, thus restricting respiratory movements. The primary objective in managing unconsciousness includes the delivery of oxygen to the brain, and the supine position enables the heart to accomplish this. A slight elevation

of the feet to approximately 10 degrees will further augment the return of blood to the heart. With a contoured dental chair the patient easily may be placed in this position (Fig. 5-3).

One situation requiring modification of this basic positioning is loss of consciousness in a pregnant woman near term. Positioning a woman who is in the later stages of pregnancy in the supine position may actually produce a decrease in the return of venous blood to the heart, thereby decreasing the supply of blood available to be pumped to the brain. The gravid uterus may actually obstruct blood flow through the inferior vena cava on the right side of the abdomen, thereby trapping large volumes of blood in the legs. Normal, healthy pregnant women have actually lost consciousness by simply lying on their back on a hard surface. Should a pregnant woman (third trimester) lose consciousness in the dental office, the back of the dental chair should be quickly lowered to the supine position and the patient turned toward her right side, with a blanket or pillow under her back on her left to maintain that position. The uterus will no longer lie directly on the vena cava, and the return of blood from the legs will be unimpeded.

Step 4. Open airway. In all instances of loss of consciousness, some degree of airway obstruction will be present. For this reason, the first maneuver to be used after positioning of the patient will be the establishment of a patent airway. Opening the airway and the restoration of breathing constitute the basic steps of life support. They may be performed quickly under most circumstances and without adjunctive equipment or assistance from other persons. *Any type of head support on the dental chair should be removed* because such supports flex the neck, thus making airway maintenance more difficult to perform.

Head tilt. The initial and most important step in providing a patent airway is the head tilt procedure. This technique is usually augmented with either the chin lift or neck lift technique.

The head tilt procedure is accomplished by placing the (rescuer's) hand on the victim's forehead and applying a firm, backward pressure with the palm. In situations in which some degree of muscle tonus remains, head tilt by itself may adequately provide a patent airway. When a lesser degree of muscle tonus is present, the use of chin lift, neck lift, or jaw thrust techniques in conjunction with the head tilt technique will be necessary.

When there is any suspicion of possible neck injury (although this is unlikely to occur in the dental office), the chin lift or jaw thrust technique WITHOUT head tilt is the recommended procedure. Either of these techniques may provide a patent airway without extending the neck.

Head tilt–chin lift. To maintain an airway using the head tilt–chin lift technique (Fig. 5-4), the fingers of one hand are placed under the bony symphysis region of the mandible to lift the tip of the mandible up, bringing the chin forward. Because the tongue is attached to the mandible, it (the tongue) is thereby pulled forward and off of the posterior pharyngeal wall. Lifting the mandible forward also tilts the head backwards, aiding in head tilt.

It is vitally important to remember that the tips of the rescuer's fingers should be placed ON BONE, not on the soft tissues of the chin. Compressing these tissues will further obstruct the airway by pushing the tongue upward into the oral cavity.

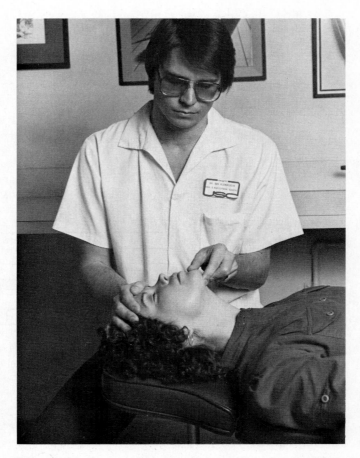

Fig. 5-4. Head tilt, chin lift. Rescuer places fingers of one hand on bony anterior portion of victim's mandible; other hand is placed on victim's forehead and rotates the head back. This is the preferred airway maintenance technique.

The chin should be lifted so that the teeth are almost brought into contact with each other. Try to avoid completely closing the mouth.

Research conducted during the past 10 years has provided significant evidence that the head tilt–chin lift technique of airway maintenance provides the most consistently reliable airway. The head tilt–neck lift technique (see below) offers no advantage over this technique. For this reason, in 1986 the American Heart Association (AHA) changed its guidelines for teaching airway management to state that the head tilt–chin lift technique was preferred.

Head tilt–neck lift. Until 1980 the head tilt–neck lift technique of airway maintenance was the technique recommended by the AHA. In 1980, after evidence surfaced that the head tilt–chin lift technique was at least equally effective, the AHA suggested that these two procedures could be used interchangeably. As mentioned above, in 1986 the recommendation was again changed to read that the head tilt–chin lift was to be the preferred method.

In the head tilt–neck lift procedure, one hand of the rescuer is placed on the forehead of the victim, and the other hand is placed beneath the victim's neck to lift and support it (Fig. 5-5). When excessive force is applied to the neck in this technique, injury to the cervical spine can occur. Because the desired movement in this technique is a rotation of the victim's head backward rather than the neck being lifted, the rescuer's hand supporting the neck should be placed as close to the base of the skull as possible to minimize the risk of hyperextension. Gentleness is very important when performing the head tilt–neck lift procedure.

Another maneuver for maintaining patency of the airway, the jaw thrust, is described on p. 96.

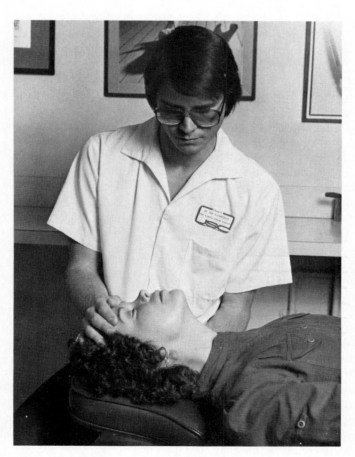

Fig. 5-5. Head tilt, neck lift. Rescuer places one hand beneath victim's neck; other hand is placed on forehead and rotates the head back.

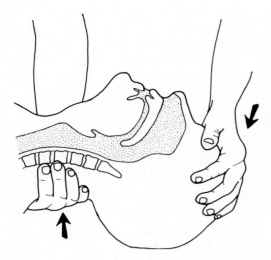

Fig. 5-6. Head tilt. Head tilt stretches soft tissues of the neck, lifting the victim's tongue off the pharynx and opening the airway.

In summary, at the present time recommendations for airway management techniques overwhelmingly favor the head tilt–chin lift procedure.

All of these maneuvers stretch the tissues between the larynx and mandible, lifting the base of the tongue from the posterior pharyngeal wall (Fig. 5-6). Anatomic obstruction of the airway caused by the tongue is relieved by these maneuvers in approximately 80% of unconscious patients. The head of the patient must be maintained in this position at all times until consciousness returns.

To what degree should the head of the victim be extended? It is important to extend the head sufficiently to elevate the tongue, thus establishing a patent airway, but it is equally important that the head not be extended too far (possibly producing damage to the vertebrae and spinal cord). One method of gauging this in the adult is the relationship of the tip of the chin to the earlobes of the victim. When the head is not extended, the unconscious victim's airway is obstructed and the tip of the chin will be well below the earlobes (Fig. 5-7). When the head is properly extended in either head tilt method, this relationship is altered so that the tip of the chin is pointing up in the air and is on line with the earlobes. This line should be perpendicular to the surface on which the victim is lying (Fig. 5-8). In an adult it is unlikely that the head will be overextended; the problem is usually the opposite—failure to extend the head far enough.

In the infant or child, however, overextension of the head may produce airway obstruction. Because of anatomic differences in the size of the trachea in children and adults,* extension of a child's head in head tilt need not be quite as great as in an adult. Extension of the child's head to the same degree as that of an adult may lead to airway obstruction as the narrow portion of the trachea is compressed even further. Although the degree of extension mentioned above will usually produce a patent airway, it is not an absolute guideline and must be altered as the need arises.

Step 5. Assess airway patency and breathing. Following performance of head tilt, the rescuer must assess the patency of the airway (Table 5-3). The victim may begin to breathe spontaneously, may be breathing but not adequately, or may not be breathing at all. During this assessment the victim's head must be maintained in the extended position previously established. To properly carry out this step, the rescuer must lean over the victim and put an ear about 1 inch from the victim's nose and mouth, at the same time looking toward the victim's chest (Fig. 5-9). Whether or not the victim is breathing is determined by *feeling, listening, and seeing.* Seeing the chest and/or abdomen move is an indication that the victim is attempting to breathe but not necessarily an indication that she is exchanging air; feeling and hearing air at the nose and mouth are also necessary to confirm airway patency. In addition, it is possible that chest and abdominal movement will not be noticed if the victim is fully clothed. However, if the victim's breath can be felt and heard, visual signs of chest movement are not necessary.

If the victim is effectively exchanging air, the airway must be maintained, and the dental team should proceed with additional therapy, including the administration of oxygen and the monitoring of vital signs (blood pressure, heart rate, and respiratory rate). If no air can be felt or heard at the mouth and nose and there is no evidence of chest or abdominal movement, a tentative diagnosis of respiratory arrest is made and artificial ventilation must be started immediately (step 8).

If no air can be felt or heard at the mouth and nose or if minimal air flow is detected along with noisy air flow in conjunction with erratic labored chest or abdominal movements, airway obstruction,

---

*At 1 year of age, the tracheal diameter is less than the width of a pencil; at 2 years of age, the glottic opening is only 6.5 mm.

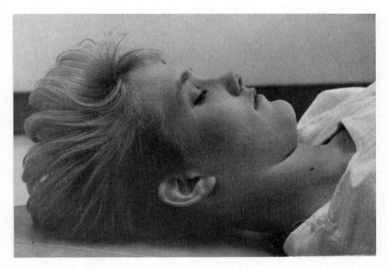

Fig. 5-7. Obstructed airway. Chin, mandible, and tongue are forced into airway, producing obstruction.

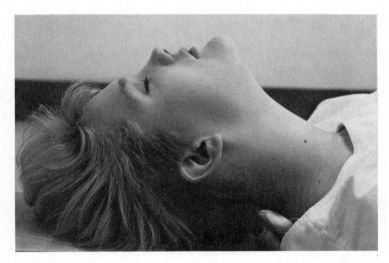

Fig. 5-8. Adequate extension of adult airway. Tip of chin extended, lifting mandible and tongue off wall of pharynx.

Table 5-3. Determination of airway patency and breathing

Clinical signs	Diagnosis	Management
Feel and hear air at nose and mouth *and* see chest and abdominal movement	Airway patent; patient is breathing	Maintain airway
Feel and hear air at nose and mouth *but see no* chest and abdominal movement	Airway patent; patient is breathing	Maintain airway
Cannot feel or hear air at mouth and nose *and* chest and abdominal movements are heaving and erratic	Patient is attempting to breathe, but airway obstruction is still present	Repeat head tilt, then if necessary proceed to step 6 of airway maintenance
Cannot feel or hear air at mouth and nose *and* no chest and abdominal movements are evident	Respiratory arrest has occurred	Proceed to step 8, begin artificial ventilation

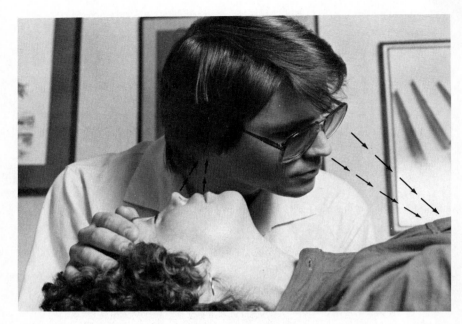

Fig. 5-9. Hear, feel, and see. Maintaining head tilt, rescuer assesses airway patency by placing ear approximately 1 inch from victim's mouth and nose, *hearing* and *feeling* any exhaled air while observing the victim's chest for spontaneous respiratory movements.

Table 5-4. Causes of partial airway obstruction

Sound heard	Probable cause	Management
Snoring	Hypopharyngeal obstruction by the tongue	Repeat head tilt; then proceed to triple airway maneuver, if necessary
Gurgling	Foreign matter (blood, water, vomitus) in airway	Suction airway
Wheezing	Bronchial obstruction (asthma)	Administer bronchodilator (via inhalation, only if conscious; IM or IV, if unconscious)
Crowing	Laryngospasm (partial)	Suction airway; positive pressure O_2

either complete or partial, is still present. Repeat head tilt (see step 4) and recheck for effectiveness (see step 5). If airway obstruction is still present, the rescuer must proceed to the next step of airway maintenance with utmost speed. The various causes of partial airway obstruction will produce sounds that may prove to be diagnostic (Table 5-4).

Foreign material in airway. If there is evidence of foreign matter in the airway following a check for airway patency, the rescuer should immediately take steps to remove the material before attempting to perform artificial ventilation (if necessary). Partial airway obstruction produces noise; complete airway obstruction produces silence, an ominous "sound."

The presence of foreign matter, primarily liquid, in the hypopharynx produces a gurgling sound similar to that produced when air bubbles through water. Most commonly the materials present are blood, water, or vomitus. Regardless of the nature of this material, it must be removed from the airway as quickly as possible. If present in large volume, it may lead to complete airway obstruction. In addition, if particulate material is present (vomitus), it may enter the trachea, creating complete obstruction of the respiratory tract, which can lead to asphyxiation and death of the patient unless corrected (Chapter 10).

The unconscious patient should have previously been placed in the supine position. As soon as for-

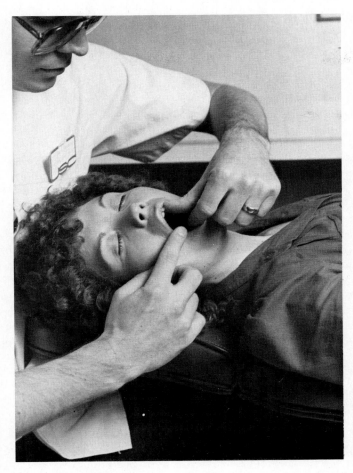

Fig. 5-10. Removal of foreign material from mouth. Fingers of rescuer's hand maintain open mouth while fingers of other hand sweep through oral cavity, removing any foreign material; suction may also be used.

eign material is thought to be present in the airway, the dental chair should be tilted back even further so that the patient's head is below the level of the heart (the Trendelenburg position), and the patient's head should be turned to one side.

Lowering the patient's head will allow the foreign material to pool in the upper segments of the airway, which are more readily accessible to the rescuer. Turning the patient's head to the side will place the material in the most dependent side of the mouth, facilitating its removal and leaving the upper side free of material, thus creating a patent airway.

Immediately after carrying out these two steps the rescuer should place two fingers in the patient's mouth and remove anything in the entire oral cavity that can be removed. The sweeping motion of the fingers should begin in the upper portion of the mouth, moving posteriorly and finally downward and anteriorly (Fig. 5-10). A high-volume suction may be used instead of fingers. The suction tips should be rounded so that they may be placed blindly, if necessary, into the posterior parts of the mouth or hypopharynx without fear of causing bleeding (from the delicate pharyngeal mucosa), which might compound the problem of airway obstruction. Suctioning should continue until all foreign material has been removed from the patient's airway, and the basic steps of airway maintenance should follow.

Step 6. Jaw thrust maneuver (if needed). Although head tilt will be effective in reestablishing airway patency in most cases, on occasion an airway will remain obstructed and additional procedures will be required. In most instances additional displacement of the mandible will be adequate to remove the obstruction. This may be accomplished by the jaw thrust maneuver (Fig. 5-11), in which the rescuer places the fingers behind the posterior border of the ramus of the mandible and (1) displaces the mandible forward, dislocating it while (2) tilting the head backward and (3) using the thumbs to retract the lower lip to allow breathing through the mouth, as well as the nose. To properly carry out the jaw thrust maneuver, it will be necessary for the rescuer to stand behind the top of the victim's (supine) head. The rescuer's elbows should rest on the surface on which the victim is lying.

Carrying out the jaw thrust maneuver will also provide the rescuer with a gauge of the depth of unconsciousness. As previously mentioned, pain is a potent sensory stimulus, and dislocation of the mandible is a painful procedure. Thus the response of the victim to this procedure will aid the rescuer in determining the level of unconsciousness. A victim's movement and audible response must be considered as positive signs, whereas lack of such response is an indication of a deeper level of unconsciousness. In addition, it has been my experience that the ease with which the mandible is dislocated is another gauge of depth of unconsciousness. With profound unconsciousness there is a marked loss of muscle tone throughout the body, and dislocation of the mandible may be easily carried out. This is in sharp contrast to attempts at dislocation of the mandible in a conscious patient or in one with a lesser degree of unconsciousness. In these instances, some degree of muscle tone remains, making it difficult to carry out this procedure.

The modified jaw thrust technique (without head tilt) is the safest initial approach to opening the airway of a victim with a suspected neck injury because it can be accomplished without extending the neck. The neck must be carefully supported without tilting it backward or turning it from side to side.

Step 7. Assess airway patency and breathing. After carrying out the jaw thrust maneuver, the rescuer must again assess the adequacy of breathing (see step 5). Once airway patency has been ensured, the rescuer or a member of the team should loosen any constricting clothing, such as belts, ties, and collars, that might interfere with breathing and blood circulation. Vital signs must be monitored and, if necessary, oxygen administered.

Step 8. Artificial ventilation (if needed). If respiratory arrest occurs, the dental team must be able to ventilate the victim so that adequate oxygen is supplied to the brain. (Refer to Table 5-3 for the criteria for initiating artificial ventilation.) Artificial ventilation may be provided in one of three ways: (1) exhaled air ventilation, (2) atmospheric air ventilation, and (3) oxygen-enriched ventilation.

Exhaled air ventilation. Exhaled air from the rescuer may be delivered to the lungs of the victim as one source of oxygen. Exhaled air is approximately 16% oxygen, which is quite adequate to maintain life. The two basic types of exhaled air ventilation are mouth-to-mouth breathing and mouth-to-nose breathing. Because no adjunctive equipment is required for these techniques, they may be carried out in any situation. For this reason they still remain the basic techniques of artificial ventilation.

To perform *mouth-to-mouth ventilation,* the rescuer uses the head tilt position (step 4) to maintain the victim's head in an optimal backward tilt. The hand that is on the forehead continues to provide a backward tilt at the same time the thumb and index fingers pinch the victim's nostrils closed (Fig. 5-12). With mouth opened widely, the rescuer takes a deep breath, makes a tight seal around the victim's mouth, and blows into the victim's mouth. The first ventilatory cycle should consist of two full breaths allowing 1 to 1.5 seconds per inspiration. Exhalation occurs passively when the rescuer's mouth is removed from the victim's, allowing gravity to deflate the lungs. Artificial ventilation in the adult must be repeated *once every 5 seconds (12 times per minute) for as long as is necessary.* In the child the ventilatory rate is once every 4 seconds (15 times per minute), whereas the infant is ventilated at a rate of once every 3 seconds (20 times per minute).

Adequacy of ventilatory efforts for patients of any size or age may be gauged by the following: feeling air going into the patient as the rescuer exhales and seeing the rise and fall of the chest of the patient. The latter is the more important factor.

Gastric distention may occur during artificial ventilation. Much more common in children than in adults, the major cause of gastric distention is overinflation during ventilation. Other causes are ventilating against a partially or totally obstructed

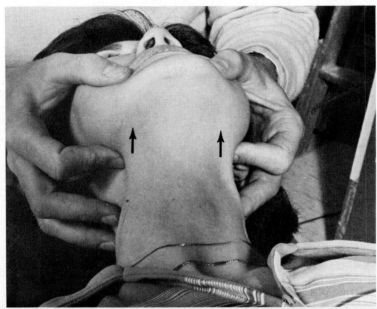

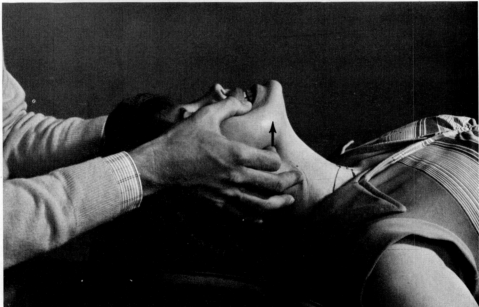

Fig. 5-11. Jaw thrust maneuver. Fingers placed behind ramus of mandible force mandible forward (top) while thumbs are placed in corners of mouth, opening it (bottom). Head is also extended at this time.

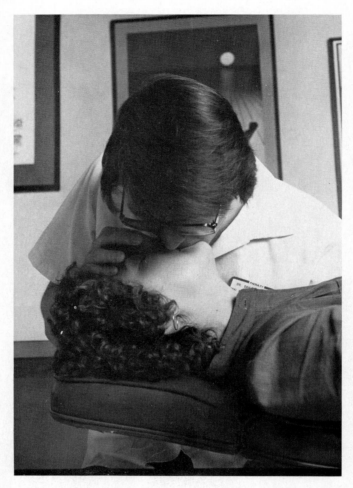

Fig. 5-12. Mouth-to-mouth ventilation. Rescuer maintains head tilt, pinches victim's nostrils closed, and blows into victim's mouth. Adequate ventilation is assessed by watching victim's chest rise with each ventilatory effort.

airway, thereby forcing air into the esophagus and GI tract. Gastric distention is dangerous for two reasons: (1) it increases the incidence of regurgitation during resuscitation, and (2) by increasing intra-abdominal pressure, it limits movement of the diaphragm, thereby reducing lung volume. Gastric distention can be minimized by limiting ventilatory efforts to the point at which the chest rises.

In some instances, *mouth-to-nose ventilation* is more effective. This is especially true when it is impossible to open a victim's mouth, when it is impossible to ventilate through the victim's mouth, or if the rescuer is unable to adequately seal the mouth of the victim. In the mouth-to-nose technique (Fig. 5-13) the rescuer keeps the head tilted backward, with one hand on the forehead; the other hand lifts the victim's mandible, sealing the lips. Taking a deep breath, the rescuer seals his lips around the victim's nose and blows in until he feels and sees the victim's lungs expand. Exhalation, as in the mouth-to-mouth technique, is passive. The same rates—12, 15, and 20 breaths per minute—are employed in this method for the adult, child, and infant, respectively, as are employed in mouth-to-mouth ventilation.

Modifications must be made if the victim is an infant or a young child. (See discussion of the head tilt procedure.) Opening of the airway and the method of artificial ventilation are essentially the same. However, when the victim is small, the

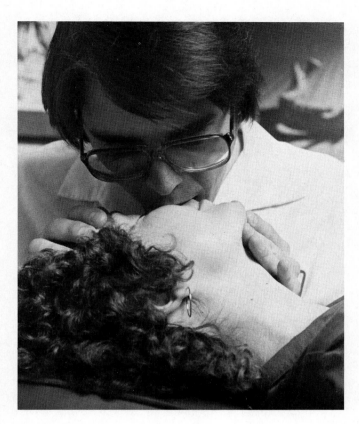

Fig. 5-13. Mouth-to-nose ventilation. Maintaining head tilt, chin lift, rescuer closes victim's mouth, sealing his lips around victim's nose.

Fig. 5-14. Atmospheric air ventilation. Head tilt is maintained, and face mask is held securely in place. Chest of victim must rise with each compression of self-inflating bag-valve-mask device.

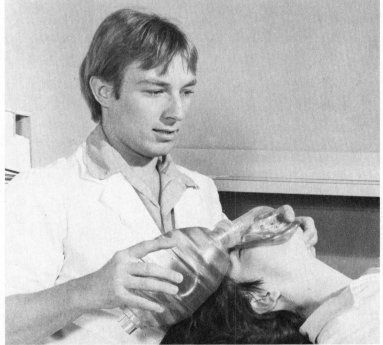
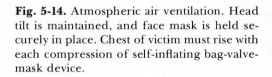

mouth *and* nose of the victim may be covered with the rescuer's mouth. The respiratory rate is increased to once every 3 seconds (infant), using smaller breaths with less volume. In addition, the neck of the child is more flexible than that of the adult; therefore care should be taken not to overextend the neck, thus further increasing airway obstruction.

When properly performed, artificial ventilation using either method may be continued for long periods without the rescuer becoming fatigued.

Atmospheric air ventilation. The air we breathe is approximately 21% oxygen. Devices are available that allow the rescuer to deliver atmospheric air to the lungs of the victim; however, *all such devices will work only if basic airway maneuvers are continually carried out.*

Self-inflating bag-valve-mask devices (Fig. 5-14). Self-filling devices such as the Ambu-Bag and Pulmonary Manual Resuscitator (PMR) usually provide less ventilatory volume than mouth-to-mouth or mouth-to-nose ventilation because of the difficulty in maintaining an airtight seal. For this reason, the American Heart Association recommends that manually operated, self-inflating bag-valve-mask units be used only by well-trained and experienced personnel such as anesthesiologists and paramedics. To use these units properly, the rescuer must be positioned near the top of the victim's head, making it virtually impossible to perform single-rescuer CPR (see Section VII).

An adequate bag-valve-mask unit must fulfill certain criteria:

1. Self-refilling but without sponge rubber inside
2. Transparent, plastic face mask with an air-filled or contoured resilient cuff
3. System for delivery of high concentrations of oxygen through ancillary oxygen inlet at the back of the bag or by means of an oxygen reservoir
4. Nonrebreathing valve
5. Available in adult and pediatric sizes
6. Standard $^{15\,mm}/_{22\,mm}$ fittings (for endotracheal tubes)
7. Easy to clean
8. Minimal dead space

Before considering the purchase of this device, the doctor should enroll in a program of advanced airway maintenance and should become thoroughly trained in the proper use of this and other adjunctive equipment.

Artificial airways. Artificial airways (Fig. 5-15) may be used whenever a bag-valve-mask device is employed but only by an individual properly trained in their use. Artificial airways should be used only on deeply unconscious persons when it is difficult to maintain an adequate airway with conventional (manual) techniques. If used on a conscious or stuporous patient, artificial airways may provoke vomiting or laryngospasm, causing a delay in obtaining adequate ventilation. An *oropharyngeal airway* must be carefully placed because, if it is improperly positioned, it may displace the tongue further back into the pharynx and add to the airway obstruction. The *nasopharyngeal airway* is of use when it is difficult to enter the patient's mouth. In addition, the nasopharyngeal airway is less likely to stimulate vomiting in the unconscious patient than is the oropharyngeal airway. However, insertion of the nasopharyngeal airway is more likely to produce significant bleeding as the delicate and highly vascular nasal mucosa is traumatized.

A variation of the oropharyngeal airway is the S *tube.* Advantages of the S tube are that it overcomes certain aesthetic considerations of direct mouth-to-mouth contact, assists in maintaining a patent airway, and helps to maintain the mouth in an open position. Disadvantages include the fact that it does not provide as effective a seal as does direct mouth-to-mouth ventilation, it may induce vomiting if used improperly, it prevents effective single-rescuer CPR, and it requires training for safe and effective use.

Many studies have demonstrated that direct mouth-to-mouth ventilation provides more effective artificial ventilation than that obtained through the use of adjunctive devices such as those mentioned here. Other devices and techniques of airway maintenance, including the esophageal obturator airway and tracheal intubation, are recommended for use only by well-trained personnel. Dentists who are properly trained through advanced cardiac life support courses or training in anesthesiology are capable of using such devices safely and effectively.

Enriched-oxygen ventilation. Wherever possible, artificial ventilation with supplemental oxygen should be employed. Exhaled air ventilation delivers 16% oxygen, whereas atmospheric air provides 21% oxygen. Because the object of basic life support is to provide the brain with oxygen, the use of supplemental oxygen must be considered as soon as it becomes available. However, *artificial ventilation*

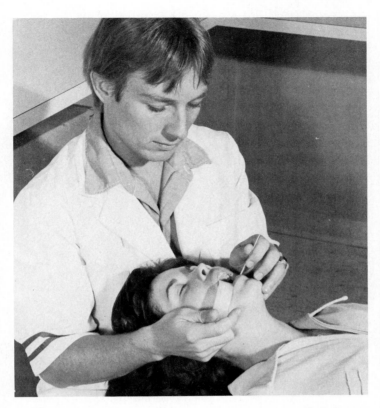

Fig. 5-15. Insertion of oropharyngeal airway. It is recommended that oropharyngeal airways not be employed without advanced training.

must never be delayed until oxygen becomes available. As recommended in Chapter 3, on the emergency kit, every doctor's office should have available a compressed oxygen cylinder no smaller than an E size. In situations in which artificial ventilation is required, an E cylinder will provide approximately 30 minutes of oxygen; smaller cylinders will provide lesser amounts and are entirely inadequate. Sources of oxygen in the dental office may include the portable E cylinder with adjustable oxygen flow (10 to 15 liters per minute) and face mask, an E cylinder with demand valve-mask unit (Fig. 5-16), or the inhalation sedation unit. If the inhalation sedation unit is to be used for artificial ventilation, the nasal hood must be discarded and replaced by a full face mask. The reservoir bag will be compressed to provide oxygen to the victim's lungs. Sources of oxygen from other than compressed gas cylinders (such as from canisters which produce oxygen via chemical reaction) will not be considered, for they are entirely inadequate for artificial ventilation.

Although oxygen benefits the unconscious patient, it behooves the doctor to receive adequate training in airway maintenance through mouth-to-mouth ventilation, because administration of enriched oxygen will be effective only as long as the oxygen cylinder remains filled. When the cylinder is empty or if one is not initially available, the rescuer must revert to the basic technique of artificial respiration.

Step 9. Assess circulation. After establishing a patent airway, the rescuer must determine the adequacy of the patient's circulation. This will include monitoring the patient's pulse rate and blood pressure. Several sites are available for recording pulse rate, including the brachial and radial arteries in the arm and the carotid artery in the neck. In nonemergency situations, either artery in the arm is an adequate indication of the heart rate; however, when a patient is unconscious, and particularly if respiratory movements have ceased, the carotid artery in the adult is a very reliable indicator of cardiovascular activity. Proper location of the ca-

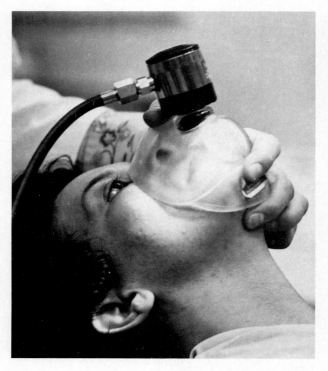

Fig. 5-16. Enriched oxygen ventilation. Demand-valve mask unit can provide up to 100% oxygen to the conscious or unconscious patient.

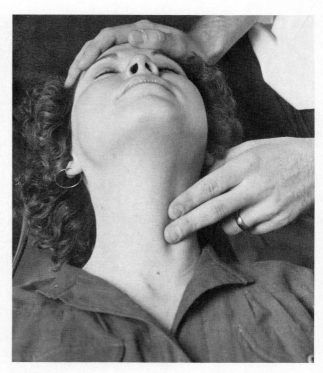

Fig. 5-17. Location of carotid pulse. Rescuer's fingers (not thumb) are placed on thyroid cartilage (Adam's apple), then moved laterally into groove formed by sternocleidomastoid muscle.

MANAGEMENT OF THE UNCONSCIOUS PATIENT

Step 1 Recognition of unconsciousness
"Shake and shout"
Painful stimuli
2 Call for help
3 Position patient
Supine position
4 Open airway
Head tilt–chin lift
5 Assess airway patency and breathing
Place ear 1 inch from patient's nose/
mouth
Hear and feel air from lungs
Look at patient's chest/abdomen
See movement of chest/abdomen
6 Jaw thrust maneuver (if needed)
Dislocation of mandible
Tilting head backward
Opening mouth with fingers
7 Assess airway patency and breathing
Place ear 1 inch from patient's mouth/
nose
Hear and feel air from lungs

Look at patient's chest/abdomen
See movement of chest/abdomen
8 Artificial ventilation
Exhaled air ventilation (16%)
Mouth-to-mouth ventilation
Mouth-to-nose ventilation
Atmospheric air (21%)
Bag-valve-mask units
Artificial airways
Oropharyngeal
Nasopharyngeal
S tubes
Enriched oxygen (up to 100%)
E cylinder with face mask
Demand/positive pressure valve
Inhalation sedation unit
9 Assess circulation
Carotid artery (adult/child)
Brachial artery (infant)
10 Definitive management of unconsciousness

rotid artery is important (Fig. 5-17). It may be found in the following manner: Place the hand supporting the patient's chin or neck on the thyroid cartilage (Adam's apple). On the side on which the rescuer is positioned, allow the fingers to slide into the groove between the thyroid cartilage and the sternocleidomastoid muscle band in the neck. The carotid artery will be located in this groove. Allow 5 to 10 seconds to feel a pulse before commencing with external chest compression if the pulse is absent. If a pulse is evident, however weak, the victim should continue to be maintained (steps 1 to 8) until recovery occurs or further medical assistance is available. In the child victim (aged 1-8 years) the carotid artery is also employed, whereas in the infant of less than a year old the brachial artery in the upper arm is recommended.

Step 10. Definitive management of unconsciousness. Once a patent airway has been provided and adequacy of circulation is ensured, the dental team may proceed to the definitive management of the unconscious patient. These procedures will be discussed in each of the three chapters to follow. The steps described in this chapter comprise the A and B segments of the ABCs of basic life support. A stands for airway, B for breathing, and C for circulation. In every instance in which a patient loses consciousness these steps must be carried out in precisely the order in which they were described. In most instances of unconsciousness, fulfillment of the A and B of basic life support will suffice. However, circulatory adequacy, or C, must be determined; if it is not present, external chest compression must begin immediately. This important aspect of basic life support will be discussed in Chapter 30.

The boxed material at left summarizes the management of the unconscious patient.

Further airway management procedures will be discussed in the section on respiratory difficulty. The preceding discussion was based on the fact that hypopharyngeal obstruction by the tongue is the most common cause of airway obstruction in the unconscious patient. The problem of lower airway (tracheal and bronchial) obstruction will be considered later in the text (Chapter 10).

BIBLIOGRAPHY

American Heart Association and National Academy of Sciences, National Research Council: Standards and guidelines for cardiopulmonary resuscitation (CPR) and emergency cardiac care (ECC), JAMA **244:**453, 1980.

American Heart Association and National Academy of Sciences, National Research Council: Standards and guidelines for cardiopulmonary resuscitation (CPR) and emergency cardiac care (ECC), JAMA **255:**2905, 1986.

American Heart Association: Instructor's manual for basic life support, Dallas, 1985, The Association.

Bercaw, B.L.: When loss of consciousness is not caused by epilepsy, Geriatrics **31:**95, 1976.

Brown, H.G.: The applied anatomy of vomiting, Brit. J. Anaesth. **35:**136, 1963.

Chue, P.W.Y.: Transient loss of consciousness: common faint or serious symptom? Dental Survey **51:**40, 1975.

Corah, N.: Development of a dental anxiety scale, J. Dent. Res. **48:**596, 1969.

Engel, L.L.: Fainting, ed. 2, Springfield, IL, 1962, Charles C Thomas, Publisher.

Goldberg, A.H.: Cardiopulmonary arrest, N. Engl. J. Med. **290:**381, 1974.

Greene, D.G., Elam, J.O., and Dobkin, A.B.: Cinefluorographic study of hyperextension of the neck and upper airway patency, JAMA **176:**570, 1961.

Gregory, G.A.: Assisted and controlled ventilation. In Pascoe, D.J., and Grossman, M., editors: Quick reference to pediatric emergencies, ed. 3, Philadelphia, 1984, J.B. Lippincott Co.

Guedel, A.E.: Inhalation anesthesia: a fundamental guide, ed. 2, New York, 1952, Macmillan Publishing Co., Inc.

Guildner, C.W.: Resuscitation—opening the airway: a comparative study of techniques for opening an airway obstructed by the tongue, JACEP **5:**588, 1976.

Harrison, J.B.: Faints and spells, Dent. Clin. North Am. **17:**461, 1973.

MacBryde, C.M., and Blacklow, R.S., editors: Signs and symptoms, ed. 5, Philadelphia, 1970, J.B. Lippincott Co.

McCarthy, F.M.: Emergencies in dental practice, ed. 3, Philadelphia, 1979, W.B. Saunders Company.

Pascoe, D.J.: Upper airway obstruction. In Pascoe, D.J., and Grossman, M., editors: Quick reference to pediatric emergencies, ed. 3, Philadelphia, 1984, J.B. Lippincott Co.

Pascoe, D.J.: Foreign bodies. In Pascoe, D.J., and Grossman, M., editors: Quick reference to pediatric emergencies, ed. 3, Philadelphia, 1984, J.B. Lippincott Co.

Ruben, H., Knudsen, E.J., and Carugati, G.: Gastric inflation in relation to airway pressure, Acta Anaesthesiol. Scand. **5:**107, 1961.

Ruben, H.M., and others: Investigation of upper airway problems in resuscitation. I. Studies of pharyngeal x-rays and performance by laymen. Anesthesiology **22:**271, 1961.

Safar, P.: Recognition and management of airway obstruction, JAMA **208:**1008, 1969.

Safar, P.: Cardiopulmonary-cerebral resuscitation including emergency airway control. In Swartz, G.R., editor: Principles and practice of emergency medicine, Philadelphia, 1980, W.B. Saunders Co.

Safar, P., and Elam, J.O.: Advances in cardiopulmonary resuscitation, New York, 1977, Springer-Verlag.

Sharpe, J.C., and Marx, F.W., Jr., editors: Management of medical emergencies, ed. 2, New York, 1969, McGraw-Hill Book Co.

Taylor, R.B.: A primer of clinical symptoms, Hagerstown, MD, 1973, Harper & Row, Publishers.

3/17/93

6 *Vasodepressor Syncope*

Vasodepressor syncope, more commonly referred to as *simple faint,* is a frequently observed, potentially life-threatening situation. Dental patients have fainted during all phases of dental therapy: during tooth extraction, other surgery, and local anesthetic injections, on first sitting in the dental chair, and even on first entering the dental office. As described in the preceding chapter, syncope is a general term referring to a sudden, transient loss of consciousness, usually secondary to cerebral ischemia. Synonyms for this clinical entity include simple faint, benign faint, swoon, atrial bradycardia, vasovagal syncope, psychogenic syncope, neurogenic syncope, and vasodepressor syncope. The last term, vasodepressor syncope, is the most descriptive and accurate and will be the term employed throughout this chapter.

Vasodepressor syncope is ordinarily a relatively harmless situation: the victim either falls gently to the floor or is laid down by a second party, regains consciousness almost immediately, and within a short period of time appears to be completely recovered. The relative benignity of this situation is borne out by statistics from Great Britain. During World War II, over 25,000 blood donors fainted, and all recovered. Yet despite its seemingly innocuous nature, vasodepressor syncope does lead to the loss of consciousness, and any loss of consciousness, however brief, produces physiologic alterations in the victim's body that are deleterious to the normal continuation of life. Examples of these are the cardiopulmonary changes, occurring secondary to hypoxia or anoxia, that are produced by airway obstruction in the unconscious patient. Although vasodepressor syncope is a fairly common emergency situation, it is one that usually can be prevented. It is also one that, when promptly

recognized and properly managed, is associated with low morbidity and mortality rates.

PREDISPOSING FACTORS

Factors that can precipitate vasodepressor syncope may be divided into two groups. The first group consists of *psychogenic* factors such as fright, anxiety, emotional stress, and receiving unwelcome news. Two other factors that may be included in this group are pain, especially of a sudden and unexpected nature, and the sight of blood or of surgical or other dental instruments (such as a local anesthetic syringe). As will be seen, these situations lead to the development of the "fight-or-flight" response and in the absence of muscular activity are manifest clinically as a transient loss of consciousness (vasodepressor syncope).

The second group consists of *nonpsychogenic* factors. These include sitting in an upright position or standing, which permits blood to pool in the periphery, thereby decreasing blood flow to the brain; hunger from dieting or a missed meal, which decreases the glucose supply to the brain below minimal levels; exhaustion; poor physical condition; and a hot, humid, crowded environment.

Vasodepressor syncope will occur more commonly in young adults, but by no means exclusively in this group. In addition, men have a higher incidence of vasodepressor syncope than do women. Indeed, men between the ages of 16 and 35 may be the most likely candidates for vasodepressor syncope, probably because of the image of the male as someone who can "take it," that is, tolerate pain or anxiety without showing any emotion. Our society does not permit men to readily express fear, and fear that is thus repressed manifests itself in a higher incidence of vasodepressor syncope. It is for

104

precisely this reason that vasodepressor syncope is such a rare occurrence in pediatric patients. Children do not hide their fears—they yell, cry, and move about, unlike the more mature and usually more inhibited typical adult male.

Within the dental office setting, the most commonly encountered precipitating factors will be those of a psychogenic nature. If one commonly encountered dental situation had to be selected as the most likely cause of vasodepressor syncope, it would be the administration of a local anesthetic agent to an anxious male patient under the age of 35, seated upright in the dental chair. Table 6-1 summarizes predisposing factors to vasodepressor syncope.

PREVENTION

Prevention of vasodepressor syncope is directed at elimination of the predisposing factors. Most dental offices are not hot, humid, crowded rooms and are commonly air conditioned, so that factor is eliminated. Hunger resulting from dieting or a missed meal before the dental appointment must be considered. Especially with an anxious patient, the dentist should request that the patient eat a light snack or meal before a dental appointment. (Hypoglycemia will be discussed further in Chapter 17.) Impaired physical status will increase the possibility of life-threatening situations developing; dental management of physically impaired individuals must therefore be modified to accommodate for their impairments.

Proper Positioning of Patient

An important contributing factor in the precipitation of most instances of vasodepressor syncope is the position of the patient in the dental chair. If the patient is standing up or is seated upright in the dental chair, the risk of vasodepressor syncope is greatly increased. With the introduction of the contoured dental chair and the advent of sit-down dentistry, most doctors no longer treat patients in the upright position. Commonly the dental patient will be in a supine or semisupine (30 to 45 degrees) position, a practice that has greatly reduced the incidence of vasodepressor syncope.

For the dental practitioner who manages patients in the upright position and cannot make the change to sit-down dentistry for dental procedures, it might still be possible to minimize this cause of vasodepressor syncope. The injection of local anesthetics is the dental procedure that most commonly

Table 6-1. Predisposing factors to vasodepressor syncope

Psychogenic factors

Fright
Anxiety
Emotional stress
Unwelcome news
Pain (sudden, unexpected)
Sight of blood
Sight of surgical and other dental instruments

site of needle (should recline before shot)

Nonpsychogenic factors

Upright or standing position
Hunger
Exhaustion
Poor physical condition
Hot, humid, crowded environment
Being an adult male
Age between 16 and 35 (approximately)

precipitates vasodepressor syncope. If the dental practitioner administers local anesthetics to the patient while she is in the supine position, vasodepressor syncope will rarely if ever occur. Following the administration of the local anesthetic, the patient may be repositioned and treatment resumed in the usual manner.

Relief of Anxiety

The most frequently encountered factors leading to vasodepressor syncope in dentistry are psychogenic. For this reason every potential dental patient must be evaluated for anxiety concerning dentistry. If anxiety is present, dental therapy may be modified to minimize or eliminate it. The recognition of anxiety will not always be an easy task. Women as well as men do not consider admitting fear the "adult" thing to do. The anxiety questionnaire developed by Corah (1969) has proved to be a big asset in recognizing anxiety (p. 35). Although patients will not admit to being fearful in an oral interview, experience with the anxiety questionnaire shows that they will express their feelings on paper. Therefore the inclusion of this short survey in the medical history questionnaire is worthwhile. Conversely, anxiety and fear in children are usually not difficult to recognize. Children do not have the inhibitions of adults and usually make their feelings known to the doctor and all others present. For this reason, as mentioned previously, vasodepressor syncope is rarely observed in children.

Medical history questionnaire

The USC medical history questionnaire (Figs. 2-1 and 2-2) provides the doctor with some information concerning anxiety. Question 2 ("Do you feel very nervous about having dentistry treatment?") and Question 3 ("Have you ever had a bad experience in the dentistry office?") permit the patient to volunteer information concerning dental attitudes. An affirmative response to either or both questions should result in a thorough dialogue history.

Dental Therapy Considerations

After anxiety is recognized, it must be managed. Along with proper positioning of the patient in the dental chair, the increased use of various modalities of psychosedation has been responsible for greatly decreasing the incidence of vasodepressor syncope. Techniques of administration include oral, rectal, and intramuscular sedation; inhalation sedation with nitrous oxide and oxygen; and intravenous sedation. Intraoperative use of psychosedation is only one of a number of stress-reducing factors discussed in Chapter 2. The concept of total patient care has led to the development of these stress-reducing protocols and has been responsible for the decreasing number of stress-related, life-threatening situations arising in dental practices. Use of these protocols will virtually eliminate the occurrence of vasodepressor syncope.

CLINICAL MANIFESTATIONS

Clinical signs and symptoms of vasodepressor syncope usually arise rapidly in the presence of an appropriate stimulus; however, the actual loss of consciousness does not usually occur for a period of time. It is for this reason that persons who experience vasodepressor syncope while alone are rarely seriously injured, since there is usually adequate time for them to sit or lie down before losing consciousness. The clinical manifestations of vasodepressor syncope may be grouped into three definite phases: presyncope, syncope, and the recovery period.

Presyncope

The clinical manifestations of vasodepressor syncope are well known. The patient in the erect or sitting position complains of a feeling of warmth in the neck and face, loses color (becomes pale or ashen-gray), and is bathed in beads of cold sweat (noted primarily on the forehead). During this time the patient will usually complain of "feeling bad" or "feeling faint." Nausea may also be present. Blood pressure monitored at this time is at baseline or slightly lower than baseline level, while the heart rate increases significantly (for example, to 120 beats per minute).

As the process continues, pupillary dilation, yawning, hyperpnea (increased depth of respiration), and a coldness in the hands and feet are noted. The blood pressure and the heart rate become acutely depressed (hypotension, bradycardia) just before loss of consciousness. At this time vision will become disturbed, the patient will feel dizzy, and unconsciousness will occur. If the patient is erect, presyncope may lead to syncope in a relatively short time (approximately 30 seconds); if the patient is supine, the presyncopal phase may not pass into the syncopal phase at all. Table 6-2 summarizes presyncopal signs and symptoms.

Syncope

With loss of consciousness, breathing may become irregular, jerky, and gasping; it may be quiet, shallow, and scarcely perceptible; or it may cease entirely (respiratory arrest, apnea). The pupils of the eyes dilate, and the patient has a deathlike appearance. Convulsive movements or muscular twitchings of the hands, legs, or facial muscles are common when consciousness is lost and the brain is hypoxic, even for as short a period as 10 seconds.

Bradycardia, which developed during the late presyncopal phase, continues. A heart rate of less than 50 beats per minute is not uncommon during the syncopal phase. In a severe episode, periods of complete ventricular asystole have been recorded even in normal healthy persons. The blood pressure, which falls precipitously to an extremely low level (30/15 torr is not uncommon), also remains low during this phase and is often difficult to measure. The pulse becomes weak and thready. With loss of consciousness there is a generalized muscular relaxation that quite commonly produces partial or complete airway obstruction.

The duration of unconsciousness will be extremely brief once the patient is positioned in the supine position, ranging from seconds to several minutes. If unconsciousness persists for more than 5 minutes after positioning and management, or if complete clinical recovery is not evident in 15 to 20 minutes, other causes for the unconsciousness must be considered.

Postsyncope (Recovery)

With proper positioning of the patient, recovery (return of consciousness) usually occurs rapidly. In the postsyncopal phase the patient may exhibit pallor, nausea, weakness, and sweating, which may persist for a few minutes to several hours. Occasionally symptoms persist for 24 hours. During the immediate postsyncopal period there may be a short period of mental confusion or disorientation. The arterial blood pressure begins to rise during this time; however, its return to baseline levels may not occur for several hours following the episode. The heart rate, which is depressed, also returns slowly towards baseline, and the quality of the pulse becomes stronger. It is important to bear in mind that once vasodepressor syncope has occurred, the tendency for the patient to faint again if raised into the sitting position or if allowed to stand too soon may persist for several hours.

PATHOPHYSIOLOGY

Vasodepressor syncope is most commonly caused by a decrease in cerebral blood flow below a critical level and is usually characterized by a sudden fall in blood pressure and a slowing of the heart rate. In the presence of predisposing factors, the following pattern of events usually develops.

Presyncope   *fight or flight syndrome*

Stress, whether emotionally triggered (fear) or sensorially triggered (unexpected pain), causes the body to release increased amounts of the catecholamines epinephrine and norepinephrine into the circulatory system. This is a part of the body's adaptation to stress, commonly called the "fight or flight" response. Changes in tissue blood perfusion occur that prepare the individual for muscular activity. Among the many responses to this catecholamine release are a decrease in peripheral vascular resistance and an increase in the blood flow to many tissues, particularly in the peripheral skeletal muscles. In situations in which muscular activity occurs, the blood volume that has been diverted to the muscles in anticipation of this movement is pumped by the muscles back to the heart. Therefore no pooling of blood occurs in the periphery in these cases. The blood pressure remains at or above baseline level, and no signs and symptoms of vasodepressor syncope develop.

By contrast, in situations in which this anticipated muscular activity does not take place (such as sitting

Table 6-2. Clinical manifestations of vasodepressor syncope: presyncopal signs and symptoms

---

Early

Feeling of warmth
Loss of color: pale or ashen-gray skin tone
Heavy perspiration
Complaints of feeling "bad" or "faint"
Nausea
Blood pressure approximately baseline
Rapid heart rate

Late

Pupillary dilation
Yawning
Hyperpnea *Labored deep breaths*
Coldness in hands and feet
Hypotension *LBP*
Bradycardia
Visual disturbances
Dizziness
Loss of consciousness

---

still in the dental chair), the diversion of large volumes of blood into the muscles causes a significant pooling of blood in the muscles, which is not returned to the heart. This leads to a relative decrease in circulating blood volume, a drop in the arterial blood pressure, and a decrease in cerebral blood flow. Signs and symptoms of the presyncopal period are produced by this decreased cerebral blood flow and other physiologic alterations that are taking place.

As blood begins to pool in peripheral vessels and the arterial blood pressure begins to fall, compensatory mechanisms are activated, which attempt to maintain cerebral blood flow. These mechanisms include the baroreceptors, which reflexly constrict the peripheral blood vessels, and the carotid and aortic arch reflexes, which increase the heart rate. These mechanisms increase venous return to the heart, increase cardiac output, and are responsible for the increase in the heart rate and the maintenance of blood pressure that occur during the early presyncopal period. However, they soon fatigue (decompensate), at which time a reflex bradycardia occurs, with the heart rate not uncommonly slowing to less than 50 beats per minute. Slowing of the heart rate leads to a significant drop in the cardiac output, which is associated with a precipitous fall in blood pressure to levels below the critical level for

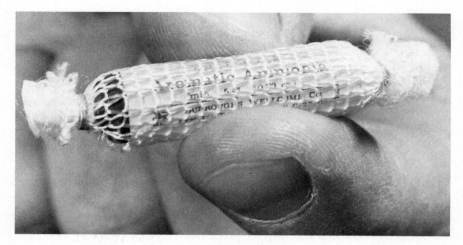

Fig. 6-1. Respiratory stimulant. Aromatic ammonia vaporole is crushed between fingers and held near victim's nose.

consciousness (see below). Cerebral ischemia results, and consciousness is lost.

Syncope

It has been estimated that the critical level of cerebral blood flow required to maintain consciousness is about 30 ml of blood per 100 g of brain tissue per minute. The human adult brain weighs approximately 1360 g (for a young adult male of medium stature). The normal value of cerebral blood flow is 50 to 55 ml per 100 g per minute. In a "fight-or-flight" situation in which muscular movement is not possible and the patient is maintained in the upright position, the ability of the heart to pump this critical supply of blood to the brain is impaired and this minimal blood flow is not reached, leading to the loss of consciousness. In a normotensive individual (systolic blood pressure below 140 torr) this minimal blood flow would be approximately equivalent to a systolic blood pressure of 70 torr. In patients with atherosclerosis and/or high blood pressure, this critical level may be reached with a systolic blood pressure considerably above 70 torr. Clinically, blood pressure recordings may be as low as 20 to 30 torr systolic during the syncopal episode, and periods of asystole may occur.

Convulsive movements, such as tonic or clonic contractions of the arms and legs or turning of the head, can occur. The degree of movement will usually depend on the degree and the duration of cerebral ischemia. When present, these movements are usually of brief duration and are rather mild.

However, cerebral ischemia for as little as 10 seconds may produce seizure activity in patients with no prior history of seizure disorders.

Recovery

Recovery is usually hastened by placing the patient in the supine position with the feet slightly elevated, thus aiding venous return to the heart and increased blood flow to the brain so that cerebral blood flow again exceeds the critical level necessary for consciousness. Signs and symptoms such as weakness, sweating, and pallor may persist for hours. The body is fatigued and will require as long as 24 hours to return to its normal functioning after the episode. An additional factor that speeds recovery is the removal of the precipitating factor (for example, a syringe or blood gauze).

MANAGEMENT
Presyncope

As soon as presyncopal signs and symptoms are noted, the dental procedure should be terminated and the patient placed in the supine position with legs elevated slightly. This will usually stop the progression of the episode. Muscular movement can also aid the return of blood from the periphery. If the patient can move his legs vigorously, pooling of blood will be less likely to occur, minimizing the severity of the reaction. The fairly common practice of placing the patient's head between his or her legs when signs and symptoms of presyncope develop should be discontinued. Bending over to

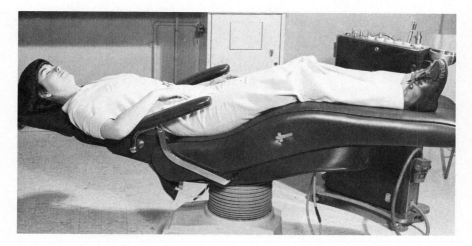

Fig. 6-2. Position of unconscious victim. Patient is placed in supine position with feet elevated slightly.

such an extreme degree may actually further impede the return of blood from the legs, by partially obstructing the inferior vena cava, causing more of a decrease of blood flow to the brain. In addition, should consciousness be lost, this patient will be in a rather awkward position for proper airway management. If considered necessary, oxygen may be administered to the patient using a full-face mask or nasal hood. An ammonia ampule may be crushed and held under the patient's nose to speed recovery (Fig. 6-1).

Syncope

Proper management of vasodepressor syncope will follow the basic management for all unconscious patients (Chapter 5). A summary is presented here.

Step 1. Position. Positioning the patient in the supine position is the first and most important step in the management of vasodepressor syncope. In addition, a slight elevation of the legs will increase the return of blood from the periphery. This step is of the utmost importance because the majority of the clinical manifestations in this situation are produced by inadequate cerebral blood flow. Failure to lower the patient into this position may lead to death or to permanent neurologic damage caused by cerebral ischemia and may occur in as little as 2 to 3 minutes if the patient is seated upright. The ancient Roman practice of crucifixion is an example of death from vasodepressor syncope when the upright position is forcibly maintained.

The supine position is therefore the preferred position for management of the unconscious patient (Fig. 6-2). An important exception to this position would be the unconscious female patient who is in the later stages of pregnancy (Chapter 5). Other alterations from this positioning will be discussed in later sections of this textbook.

Step 2. Patent airway. Establishment of a patent airway should immediately be carried out. In most instances of vasodepressor syncope, head tilt–chin lift will be the only maneuver necessary to establish a patent airway (Fig. 6-3). Adequacy of the airway should then be confirmed by looking at the chest and hearing and feeling exhaled air (Fig. 6-4). Spontaneous respiration will be evident in most of these patients; however, artificial ventilation will be necessary on those few occasions when spontaneous respiration has ceased. Positioning of the patient and establishment of a patent airway will commonly lead to the rapid recovery of consciousness.

Step 3. Additional procedures. After carrying out the preceding steps, members of the emergency team may assist the doctor with several additional procedures that can aid in recovery. These procedures include the loosening of binding clothes such as ties and collars (which if tight may decrease blood flow to the brain) and belts (which might decrease blood flow from the legs). In addition, vital signs, including blood pressure, heart rate, and respiratory rate, should be monitored and evaluated in relation to the preoperative baseline

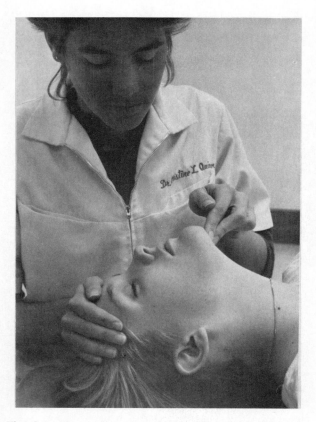

Fig. 6-3. Airway patency using head tilt–chin lift technique.

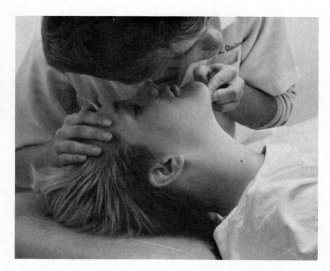

Fig. 6-4. Adequacy of airway is determined by look, listen, and feel technique.

MANAGEMENT OF VASODEPRESSOR SYNCOPE

Step 1 Place patient in supine position with feet slightly elevated

    2 Establish patent airway
        Head tilt–chin lift method
    Check breathing
    Jaw thrust maneuver if necessary
        Recheck breathing if necessary
    Artificial ventilation if necessary
    Check circulation

    3 Monitor vital signs
        Blood pressure
        Heart rate
        Respiratory rate
    Support patient
        Ammonia vaporole crushed under nose of patient
        Cold towel to forehead
        Blankets if cold or shivering
        Reassure patient

    4 Maintain *your* composure

    5 Follow-up treatment
    Determine factors causing unconsciousness
    Prevent recurrence of vasodepressor syncope
    Arrange for patient to be taken home by friend or relative
    No further dental treatment for 24 hours

---

values for the patient to determine the severity of the reaction. Oxygen can be administered to the patient at any time during the episode. A respiratory stimulant such as aromatic spirits of ammonia may be crushed between the fingers and the patient allowed to inhale it; this acts as a chemical stimulus to breathing. If the vaporole has been taped to the back of the dental unit, where the doctor may readily reach it without having to wait for the emergency kit, syncope may be terminated before assistance even arrives. A cold towel can be placed on the patient's forehead, and if the patient complains of feeling cold or is shivering, blankets can be placed over him. In lieu of blankets, a plastic patient drape of the type commonly found in dental offices may be used.

Step 4. Maintenance of composure. As the patient regains consciousness, it is important for the doctor and the entire emergency team to maintain their composure. In addition, the stimulus that precipitated the episode (syringe, instrument, bloody gauze) must be removed. The presence of a terrified dental staff or of the precipitating agent may very well cause a second episode of vasodepressor syncope.

Step 5. Delayed recovery. In the event that recovery of consciousness takes more than 5 minutes after positioning or if complete recovery has not occurred in 15 to 20 minutes, another cause for the episode should be considered. The steps of basic life support must be continually applied while the emergency team summons and waits for medical assistance. If another cause of unconsciousness is obvious (such as hypoglycemia or acute adrenal insufficiency), definitive management may be instituted. In the absence of an obvious cause, however, continued application of basic life support is indicated. When possible, the doctor should start an intravenous infusion.

Postsyncope

Following recovery from vasodepressor syncope, the patient should not be subjected to additional dental therapy for the remainder of that day. The possibility of a second episode of syncope occurring is greater during this period of time, and it has been demonstrated that the human body requires up to 24 hours to fully regain its presyncopal state. The doctor should determine from the patient what the precipitating event was and what other factors may have been present (such as hunger or fear). With this information the doctor can formulate a treatment plan to prevent this event from occurring a second time. Arrangements should then be made for the patient to be taken home by a friend or family member. It may not be prudent to allow the patient to leave the office unescorted to drive a car because of the possibility of recurrent syncopal episodes.

The boxed material on opposite page summarizes the management of vasodepressor syncope.

BIBLIOGRAPHY

Bourne, J.G.: Studies in anesthetics, London, 1974, Lloyd-Luke Ltd.

Campbell, R.L., and others: Vasovagal response during oral surgery, J. Oral Surg. **34:**698, 1976.

Conn, H.F., and Conn, R.B., editors: Current diagnosis—6, Philadelphia, 1980, W.B. Saunders Company.

Corah, N.: Development of dental anxiety scale, J. Dent. Res. **48:**596, 1969.

Ebert, E.V.: Syncope, Circulation **27:**1148, 1963.

Friedberg, C.K.: Syncope: pathological physiology, differential diagnosis and treatment, Mod. Concepts Cardiovasc. Dis. **40:**55, 1971.

Goldberger, E.: Syncope. In Treatment of cardiac emergencies, ed. 3, St. Louis, 1977, The C.V. Mosby Co.

Krupp, M.A., and Chatton, M.J.: Current medical diagnosis and treatment, Los Altos, CA, 1985, Lange Medical Publications.

Luria, M.N.: Syncope. In Schuertz, G.R., and others, editors: Principles and practice of emergency medicine, Philadelphia, 1978, W.B. Saunders Co.

Reutz, P.P., Johnson, S.A., and Callahan, R.: Fainting: a review of its mechanism and a study in blood donors, Medicine **46:**363, 1967.

Thomas, J.E., and Rooke, E.D.: Fainting, Mayo Clin. Proc. **38:**397, 1963.

Wayne, H.H.: Syncope: physiologic considerations and an analysis of the clinical characteristics in 570 patients, Am. J. Med. **30:**418, 1961.

7 *Orthostatic Hypotension*

Following vasodepressor syncope, orthostatic hypotension—also known as postural hypotension—is the most likely cause of transient unconsciousness in the dental office. Orthostatic hypotension may be defined as a disorder of the autonomic nervous system in which syncope occurs when the patient assumes the upright position. It differs in several important respects from vasodepressor syncope and is not often associated with fear and anxiety. Awareness of predisposing factors will allow the dental practitioner to prevent this situation. A typical example of this condition is syncope that develops in a 76-year-old woman whose recumbent blood pressure is 180/100, which drops to 100/50 torr immediately upon her rising.

PREDISPOSING FACTORS

Many factors have been identified that may be responsible for the development of orthostatic hypotension, including several of importance to the practice of dentistry. They include the administration and ingestion of drugs, prolonged recumbency and convalescence, an inadequate postural reflex, pregnancy, venous defects in the legs (varicose veins), postsympathectomy for "essential" hypertension, Addison's disease, physical exhaustion and starvation, and chronic orthostatic hypotension (Shy-Drager syndrome).

In addition, the incidence of orthostatic hypotension increases with age. Over the age of 65 years, about 20% of people examined will demonstrate a postural decrease in blood pressure of 20 torr or more (systolic), whereas over the age of 75 years 30% demonstrate the 20 torr fall, and 10% demonstrate a decrease in excess of 40 torr.

Orthostatic hypotension is an uncommon finding in the infant and child.

Drug administration and ingestion

Probably the most frequently encountered cause of orthostatic hypotension in the dental office will be the use of various drugs that can produce this situation. These drugs may have been given to the patient by the doctor before, during, or after dental therapy or they may have been prescribed by the patient's physician for the management of specific physical or psychologic disorders. Table 7-1 summarizes the more commonly encountered drugs that may produce orthostatic hypotension. These agents fall into the general categories of antihypertensives, especially the sodium-depleting diuretics and the ganglionic blocking agents; sedatives and tranquilizers; narcotics; antihistaminics; and L-dopa for Parkinson's disease. In general, these agents act to produce orthostatic hypotension by diminishing the body's ability to regulate blood pressure in response to the increased force of gravity that results when the patient rises. A greatly exaggerated response is thus seen.

Medications employed in dental practice for the management of fear and anxiety are capable of producing orthostatic hypotension—especially with parenteral administration (intramuscular, submucosal, intravenous, or by inhalation). Those most often used in dentistry include nitrous oxide and oxygen (by inhalation), diazepam and pentobarbital (intravenous), and meperidine (intravenous, intramuscular, or submucosal). Positional changes of patients receiving these agents should be accomplished with care.

Prolonged Recumbency and Convalescence

Confinement to bed for as little as 1 week in a normal subject has been shown to predispose to orthostatic hypotension. This is one of the reasons hospitalized patients are encouraged to ambulate as soon as possible after surgical procedures. Although dental patients are not usually confined for periods up to a week, a recent trend in dental practice has been toward an increase in the length of appointments. It is no longer uncommon for a dental patient to be seated in a dental chair for up to 2 or 3 hours, usually in a reclining position. In these circumstances orthostatic hypotension may develop at the end of the appointment. The concomitant use of psychosedative agents during the dental appointment will further increase the incidence of orthostatic hypotension.

Inadequate Postural Reflex

Healthy young people may faint when forced to stand motionless for prolonged periods of time, such as during school assemblies, religious services, or parades. Syncope might also develop if a patient is seated upright in the dental chair for prolonged periods of time. This is more likely to occur in a hot environment, which produces concomitant peripheral vasodilation. The following, excerpted from the *Los Angeles Times,* illustrates one agency's response to this physiologic occurrence:

How to faint by the numbers

VANCOUVER (UPI)—The order has gone out: Canadian troops may no longer faint in a slovenly or unseemly way while on parade. Soldiers disobeying the order will be put on report.

. . . The memo said: "To avoid the possibility of fainting, a soldier should make sure he has had breakfast on the morning of parade day.

If worse comes to worst and he must faint, a soldier should fall to the ground under control. To do so, he must turn his body approximately 45 degrees, squat down, roll to the left, and retain control of his weapon to prevent personal injury and minimize damage to the weapon.

We must ensure that soldiers who have not complied with the above instructions be charged."

Pregnancy

The pregnant female may demonstrate two forms of hypotension. In the first, orthostatic hypotension will usually be encountered during the first trimester of pregnancy, occurring on arising from bed in the morning but not recurring again during the day. The precise cause of this phenomenon is not known. The second, known as the *supine hypotensive syndrome of pregnancy,* occurs late in the third trimester if the patient is allowed to lie in the

Table 7-1. Drugs producing orthostatic hypotension

Category	Generic name	Proprietary name
Antihypertensives	Guanethidine	Ismelin
Phenothiazines	Chlorpromazine	Thorazine
	Thioridazine	Mellaril
Tricyclic antidepressants	Doxepin	Sinequan
	Amitriptyline	Elavil
	Imipramine	Tofranil
		Presamine
Narcotics	Meperidine	Demerol
	Morphine	Morphine
Antiparkinson drugs	Levodopa (L-dopa)	Dopar
		Larodopa

supine position for more than 3 to 7 minutes. Signs and symptoms of syncope become evident in this period, with consciousness being lost shortly thereafter. It has been demonstrated that the flaccid, gravid uterus compresses the inferior vena cava, decreasing venous return from the legs. If the patient is allowed to alter her position to the lateral seated or standing position, the weight of the uterus is taken off the vena cava and the clinical symptoms are rapidly reversed.

Venous Defects in the Legs

Orthostatic hypotension has been noted in patients with varicose veins and other disorders of the vascular system of the legs. Excessive pooling of blood in the legs occurs in these patients.

Postsympathectomy for High Blood Pressure

Surgical procedures to lower blood pressure and to improve circulation to the legs may produce a greater incidence of orthostatic hypotension. This is seen usually in the immediate postsurgical period, and the symptoms usually decline spontaneously with the passage of time.

Addison's Disease

Orthostatic hypotension may be seen in patients with chronic adrenocortical insufficiency. It may be managed through the administration of corticosteroids (see Chapter 8).

Physical Exhaustion, Fatigue, and Starvation

Syncope observed during physical exhaustion, fatigue, and starvation is caused by orthostatic hypotension. This factor is not usually of importance in the dental office.

Chronic Orthostatic Hypotension (Shy-Drager Syndrome)

The Shy-Drager syndrome is also known as idiopathic orthostatic hypotension; it is an uncommon disorder, the cause of which is unknown. Its course is progressive. Severe disability or death usually occurs within 5 to 10 years of onset. Patients are usually in their fifties and are initially seen with orthostatic hypotension, urinary and fecal incontinence, sexual impotence (males), and anhidrosis (lack of sweating) in the lower trunk.

PREVENTION

The clinical manifestations of orthostatic hypotension may be prevented if the clinician is aware of the causative factors. Three preventative factors will be discussed: the medical history, a physical examination to determine whether the potential problem exists, and if it does, certain dental therapy considerations to prevent unconsciousness.

Medical History Questionnaire

The medical history questionnaire (see Fig. 2-2) is a valuable source of information. Relevant questions include the following:

QUESTION 6. Have you taken any medicine or drugs during the past 2 years?

COMMENT. Medications being taken by a patient may produce the side affect of postural hypotension. The drug package insert or an appropriate textbook should be consulted.

QUESTION 9. Do you have fainting spells or seizures?

COMMENT. A history of frequent fainting spells may indicate the presence of orthostatic hypotension. The ensuing dialogue history should seek to determine the factors involved in these episodes, the presence or absence of prodromal signs and symptoms, and any medications the patient may be taking to assist in maintaining an adequate blood pressure. Ephedrine, up to 75 mg orally per day, is commonly prescribed. Fludrocortisone acetate in doses of 0.1 mg or more daily is also effective.

In the likely event that the patient does not know the name of a drug being taken, the doctor should have available a text, such as the *Physicians' Desk Reference,* in which illustrations of many medications are shown.

Physical Examination

As a routine part of the medical evaluation of all potential dental patients, vital signs should be recorded. The vital signs include blood pressure, heart rate (pulse), respiratory rate, temperature, height, and weight.

Orthostatic hypotension may be detected if the blood pressure of the patient is recorded in the sitting and standing positions. The *normal* response of blood pressure when recorded in the sitting and then the standing position (30 seconds later) is a standing systolic blood pressure within 10 torr (higher or lower, usually higher) of the sitting blood pressure level. Decreases of systolic blood pressure in excess of 20 torr on rising that are not corrected within 30 seconds should be evaluated further. The doctor should recheck the blood pressure in each position, and if this differential is still evident, medical consultation should be considered before dental therapy.

The heart rate normally accelerates on standing and generally remains about 5 to 20 beats per minute faster than in the sitting position.

Dental Therapy Considerations

In the dental patient with a previous history of orthostatic hypotension or in a patient on psychosedative therapy (inhalation, intravenous, intramuscular, or submucosal sedation) or when terminating prolonged appointments, certain precautions should be taken to prevent hypotensive episodes from developing when positional changes are made. The patient should be cautioned against rising too rapidly from the sitting or lying position. When in the dental chair, the patient should be returned to the sitting (upright) position slowly at the conclusion of therapy. This might be accomplished by two or three positional changes over a period of a minute or two to reach the upright position. Allow the patient to remain at each level until any dizziness that might be present has passed. As the patient stands it may be prudent for the doctor or an assistant to stand in front of the patient until the patient is standing. Should the patient become faint or weak on rising, dental personnel may support and assist the patient back into the dental chair, thereby preventing possible injury.

CLINICAL MANIFESTATIONS

In patients with chronic orthostatic hypotension, positioning into a standing or sitting upright stance leads to a precipitous drop in blood pressure and to loss of consciousness, usually without any of the prodromal signs and symptoms of vasodepressor syncope such as lightheadedness, pallor, dizziness, nausea, and sweating. The patient may rapidly lose consciousness or may merely develop blurred vision or become lightheaded but not actually lose consciousness. Clinical manifestations of orthostatic hypotension seen in patients with other predisposing factors, such as administration of drugs, may include some or all of the usual prodromal signs and symptoms of vasodepressor syncope before losing consciousness.

The blood pressure of the patient during the syncopal period is quite low, as in vasodepressor syncope. Unlike vasodepressor syncope, however, the heart rate remains at the baseline level or slightly higher. The patient exhibits all of the clinical manifestations of the "typical" unconscious patient described in Chapters 5 and 6. Minor convulsive movements may be noted if unconsciousness persists for ten or more seconds. When the patient is returned to the supine position, consciousness is rapidly regained. Table 7-2 summarizes signs and symptoms associated with orthostatic hypotension.

PATHOPHYSIOLOGY
Normal Regulatory Mechanisms

When a patient's position is changed from the supine to the erect position, the effect of gravity upon the cardiovascular system is intensified. Blood being pumped from the patient's heart must now be moved against the force of gravity (upward) to reach the brain and supply it with the oxygen and glucose needed for the maintenance of consciousness. When the patient is supine, the force of gravity is equally distributed over the entire body, and blood flows more readily from the heart to the brain. In other positions (semisupine, and so on), the force of gravity is such that the systolic blood pressure is decreased by 2 torr for every inch above heart level; for every inch below the level of the heart, the blood pressure is increased by 2 torr (Fig. 7-1).

To protect the brain and to ensure an adequate and continuous supply of oxygen and glucose, several intricate mechanisms have evolved that aid in the maintenance of normal blood pressure when postural changes occur. These include (1) a reflex arteriolar constriction that is mediated through baroreceptors (pressure receptors) located in the carotid sinus and the aortic arch, (2) a reflex increase in the heart rate, which occurs simultaneously with the increase in arteriolar tone and is mediated through the same mechanisms, (3) reflex

Table 7-2. Clinical manifestations of orthostatic hypotension

Type of hypotension	Manifestations
Orthostatic	Mild to no signs and symptoms of vasodepressor syncope Low blood pressure Baseline or slightly higher heart rate
Chronic orthostatic	Loss of consciousness without signs and symptoms

venous constriction, increasing the return of venous blood to the heart, both intrinsic and sympathetically mediated, (4) an increase in muscle tonus and contraction in the legs and abdomen—the so-called venous pump—which facilitates the venous return of blood (of vital importance because at least 60% of circulating blood volume at any one moment is found in the venous circulation), (5) a reflex increase in respiration, which also aids in the return of blood to the right side of the heart via changes in intraabdominal and intrathoracic pressures, and (6) the release of various neurohumoral substances, such as norepinephrine, antidiuretic hormone, renin, and angiotensin.

The usual ("normal") reaction of the cardiovascular system when a person is tilted from the supine to the erect position is an immediate drop in the systolic blood pressure of from 5 to 40 torr, but an equally rapid rise occurs so that within 30 seconds the systolic blood pressure is equal to or slightly higher than that seen in the supine position. Thereafter the systolic blood pressure tends to remain within 10 torr higher or lower (usually higher) of the supine recording. The diastolic blood pressure is seen to rise approximately 10 to 20 torr. Heart rate (pulse) increases approximately 5 to 20 beats per minute when the patient is standing.

Orthostatic Hypotension

In patients with orthostatic hypotension, one or more of these adaptive mechanisms fails to function properly, so the body is not able to adequately adapt to the effects of gravity and the blood pressure changes dramatically when positional changes occur. The fall of blood pressure in the standing position is rapid, the systolic pressure sometimes approaching a level of 60 torr in less than 1 minute. The diastolic blood pressure also falls precipitously. Associated with this fall in blood pressure is little or no alteration in the heart rate; the car-

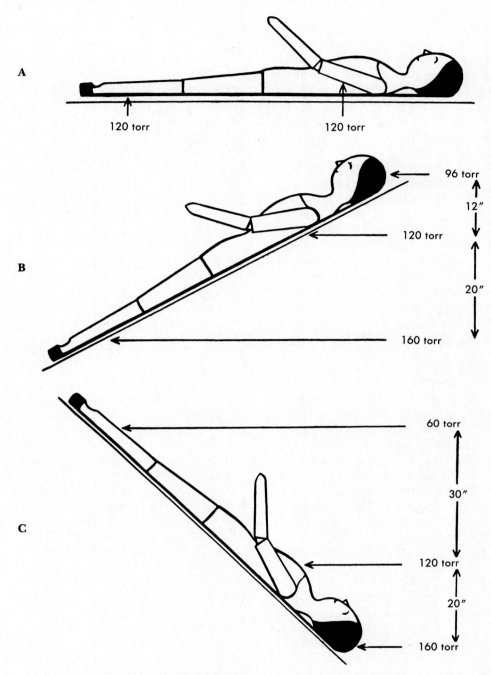

Fig. 7-1. Effect of gravity on blood pressure. **A,** Supine position. Effect of gravity is equalized over entire body. Blood pressure in legs, heart, and brain is approximately equal. **B,** Semiupright position. Blood pressure is decreased by 2 torr for every inch above level of heart. **C,** Trendelenburg (head down) position. Blood pressure increases 2 torr for every inch below level of heart. (From Enderby, G.E.H.: Lancet **1:**185, 1954.)

diovascular system is unable to react normally to the blood pressure depression. This combination of signs is pathognomonic of orthostatic hypotension. In addition, none of the usual prodromal signs of vasodepressor syncope is encountered. Consciousness will be lost when the cerebral blood flow falls below the critical level required for consciousness (approximately 30 ml per minute per 100 g of brain), equivalent to a systolic blood pressure at heart level of approximately 70 torr in a normotensive individual. Unconsciousness is short-lived once the patient is placed in the supine position because of reestablishment of adequate cerebral blood flow.

MANAGEMENT

Management of orthostatic hypotension will mimic that of vasodepressor syncope.

Step 1. Position patient. On recognition of the situation, the staff must place the unconscious patient in the proper position (supine with feet elevated) (Fig. 7-2).

Step 2. Maintain airway. After positioning the patient the steps of airway management must be followed. These include the head tilt–chin lift maneuver, checking for breathing, and possibly the jaw thrust maneuver. Oxygen may be administered to the patient, if considered necessary. Consciousness normally returns rapidly in all cases of orthostatic hypotension, but care must be taken to prevent a recurrence of the syncopal episode.

Step 3. Positional changes. Positional changes must be made carefully. It is prudent to make two or three stops over several minutes when moving the patient from the supine position to the fully erect position in the dental chair. Allow the patient's cardiovascular system to adapt to the increasing effect of gravity at each level before raising the head of the chair further. Should the patient feel dizzy or light-headed, do not raise the chair until this sensation (signs of decreased cerebral blood flow) has passed. Before allowing the patient to leave the chair, recheck the blood pressure, comparing it to the preoperative baseline levels. The doctor or an assistant should help the patient out of the chair and be available for support if necessary.

Step 4. Discharge of the patient. Patients with chronic orthostatic hypotension or orthostatic hypotension as a result of a prescribed medication (such as an antihypertensive) may be permitted to leave the dental office and drive a motor vehicle if the doctor judges that they have sufficiently recovered from the incident. This judgment of recovery might be based on a return of the vital signs to approximately the preoperative level and the ability of the patient to ambulate freely without any clinical signs and symptoms developing. When the patient's history suggests that a prescribed drug may be responsible for the episode, the doctor should consider consultation with the patient's physician if episodes recur.

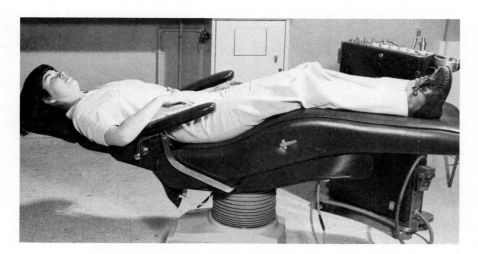

Fig. 7-2. Correct position for an unconscious patient.

MANAGEMENT OF
ORTHOSTATIC HYPOTENSION

Step 1 Place patient in supine position with feet elevated slightly (at a 10-degree angle) (NOTE: In late stages of pregnancy the lateral position is preferred)

2 Maintain airway
Head tilt–chin lift
Check breathing
Jaw thrust maneuver, if necessary
Oxygen, if necessary
Monitor vital signs

3 Make positional changes slowly

4 Discharge patient

Patients undergoing orthostatic hypotensive episodes with no prior history of such occurrences or patients who have these episodes following the administration of drugs by the doctor should be permitted to recover in the dental office while arrangements are made to have them transported home by a responsible adult. Medical consultation with the patient's physician should be considered in those cases in which there is no prior history of orthostatic hypotension.

The boxed material above summarizes the management of orthostatic hypotension.

BIBLIOGRAPHY

Barraclough, M.A., and Sharpey-Schafer, E.P.: Hypotension from absent circulatory reflexes: effects of alcohol, barbiturates, psychotherapeutic drugs, and other mechanisms, Lancet 1:1121, 1963.

Bourne, J.G.: Studies in anaesthetics, London, 1973, Lloyd-Luke Ltd.

Caird, F.I., Andrews, G.R., and Kennedy, R.D.: Effect of posture on blood pressure in the elderly, Br. Heart J. 35:527, 1973.

Chue, P.W.Y.: Transient loss of consciousness: common faint or serious symptom, Dent. Survey 51:40, 1975.

Conn, H.F., Conn, R.B., editors: Current diagnosis—6, Philadelphia, 1980, W.B. Saunders Company.

Duke, P.C., and others: The effects of age on baroreceptor reflex function in man, Can. Anaesth. Soc. J. 23:111, 1976.

Engel, G.L.: Fainting, ed. 2, Springfield, IL, 1962, Charles C. Thomas, Publisher.

Harrison, J.B.: Faints and spells, Dent. Clin. North Am. 17:461, 1973.

Heyman, A.: Syncope. In Beeson, P.B., and McDermott, W., editors: Textbook of medicine, ed. 15, Philadelphia, 1979, W.B. Saunders Co.

Hughes, R.C., Cartledge, N.E.F., and Milac, P.: Primary neurogenic orthostatic hypotension, J. Neurol. Neurosurg. Psychiatry 33:363, 1970.

Jefferson, J.W.: Hypotension from drugs, Dis. Nerv. Syst. 35:66, 1974.

Krupp, M.A., and Chatton, M.J.: Current medical diagnosis and treatment, Los Altos, CA, 1985, Lange Medical Publications.

Lorentz, I.T.: Postural hypotension, Med. J. Aust. 2:816, 1974.

Luria, M.N.: Syncope. In Schwartz, G.R., and others, editors: Principles and practice of emergency medicine, Philadelphia, 1978, W.B. Saunders Co.

Norriš, A.H., Shock, N.W., and Yiengst, M.J.: Age changes in heart rate and blood pressure responses to tilting and standardized exercise, Circulation 8:521, 1953.

O'Leary, J.L., and Landau, W.M.: Coma and convulsions. In MacBryde, C.M., and Blacklow, R.S., editors: Signs and symptoms, ed. 5, Philadelphia, 1970, J.B. Lippincott Company.

Roessman, U., van den Noort, S., and McFarland, D.E.: Idiopathic orthostatic hypotension, Arch. Neurol. 24:403, 1971.

Stead, E.A., Jr.: Fainting (syncope). In MacBryde, C.M., and Blacklow, R.S., editors: Signs and symptoms, ed. 5, Philadelphia, 1970, J.B. Lippincott Company.

Thomas, J.E., and Schirger, A.: Orthostatic hypotension: etiologic considerations, diagnosis, and treatment, Med. Clin. North Am. 52:809, 1968.

Thomas, J.E., and Schirger, A.: Idiopathic orthostatic hypotension, Arch. Neurol. 22:289, 1970.

8 *Acute Adrenal Insufficiency*

A third life-threatening situation that may result in the loss of consciousness is acute adrenal insufficiency (adrenal crisis). Of the three factors discussed in this section—vasodepressor syncope, orthostatic hypotension, and adrenal insufficiency—adrenal insufficiency is the least common. This is fortunate because adrenal insufficiency is an emergency situation with significant potential for serious morbidity and mortality.

The adrenal gland is a combination of two glands, the cortex and the medulla, which are fused together yet remain distinct and identifiable.

The adrenal cortex produces and secretes over 30 steroid hormones, most of which lack (at present) any identifiable biologic activity of importance. *Cortisol,* one of the glucocorticoids, is considered to be the most important product of the adrenal cortex. It allows the body to adapt to stress and is thereby extremely vital to survival. Hypersecretion of cortisol leads to increased fat deposition in certain areas (the face and a "buffalo hump" on the back), increases the blood pressure, and produces alterations in blood cell distribution (eosinopenia and lymphopenia). Hypersecretion of cortisol will not usually produce the acute life-threatening situation seen with cortisol deficiency. Clinically, cortisol hypersecretion is referred to as *Cushing's syndrome* and is usually readily corrected through surgical removal of a part or all of the adrenal gland. Renal and adrenal surgery today rate as important factors in the development of primary adrenal cortical insufficiency.

Cortisol deficiency, on the other hand, may lead to a relatively rapid onset of clinical symptoms including the loss of consciousness and quite possibly the patient's death. Primary adrenocortical insuffi-

ciency is termed *Addison's disease,* an insidious and usually progressive disease. The incidence of Addison's disease is estimated to be between 0.3 and 1.0 per 100,000 persons, occurring equally in both sexes and in all age groups including infants and children. Although all corticosteroids may be deficient in this disease state, it is important to note that the administration of physiologic doses of cortisol will correct most of the pathophysiologic effects.

Clinical manifestations of adrenal insufficiency usually do not develop until at least 90% of the adrenal cortex has been destroyed. Because this destruction occurs slowly, it may be several months before the diagnosis of insufficiency is made and therapy (exogenous cortisol) is instituted. During this time the patient is in constant jeopardy from acute adrenal insufficiency. The patient is able to produce endogenous cortisol levels adequate to meet the requirements of day-to-day living; however, in stressful situations (for example, a dental appointment), the adrenal cortex is unable to produce the additional cortisol required, and signs and symptoms of acute insufficiency develop.

A second form of adrenocortical hypofunction may be produced by the administration of exogenous glucocorticosteroids to a patient with normal adrenal cortices. In the development of acute adrenal crisis, secondary adrenal insufficiency is today a much greater potential threat than is Addison's disease. Glucocorticosteroid drugs are widely prescribed in pharmacologic doses for the symptomatic relief of a wide variety of disorders (Table 8-1). When used in this manner, glucocorticosteroid administration produces a disuse atrophy of the adrenal cortex, thereby deceasing the ability of the adrenal cortex to produce the levels of cortico-

Table 8-1. Clinical indications for adrenocortical steroids

Allergic disease
Angioedema
Asthma, acute and chronic
Dermatitis, contact
Dermatitis venenata
Insect bites
Pollinosis (hay fever)
Rhinitis, allergic
Serum reaction, drug and foreign, acute and delayed
Status asthmaticus
Transfusion reactions
Urticaria

Cardiovascular disease
Postpericardiotomy syndrome
Shock, toxic (septic)

Eye disease
Blepharoconjunctivitis
Burns, chemical and thermal
Conjunctivitis, allergic, catarrhal
Corneal injuries
Glaucoma, secondary
Herpes zoster
Iritis
Keratitis
Neuritis, optic, acute
Retinitis centralis
Scleritis; episcleritis

Gastrointestinal disease
Colitis, ulcerative
Enteritis, regional
Hepatitis, viral
Sprue

Genitourinary disease
Hunner's ulcer
Nephrotic syndrome

Hemopoietic disorders
Anemia, acquired hemolytic
Leukemia, acute and chronic
Lymphoma
Purpura, idiopathic thrombocytopenic

Infections and inflammation
Meningitis
Thyroiditis, acute
Typhoid fever
Waterhouse-Friderichsen syndrome

Injected locally
Arthritis, traumatic
Bursitis
Osteoarthritis
Tendinitis

Mesenchymal disease
Arthritis, rheumatoid
Dermatomyositis
Lupus erythematosus, systemic
Polyarteritis
Rheumatic fever, acute

Metabolic disease
Arthritis, gouty acute
Thyroid crisis, acute

Miscellaneous conditions
Bell's palsy
Dental surgical procedures

Pulmonary disease
Emphysema, pulmonary
Fibrosis, pulmonary
Sarcoidosis
Silicosis

Skin disease
Dermatitis
Drug eruptions
Eczema, chronic
Erythema multiforme
Herpes zoster
Lichen planus
Pemphigus vulgaris
Pityriasis rosea
Purpura, allergic
Sunburn, severe

steroid necessary to meet stressful situations, which in turn leads to the development of signs and symptoms of acute insufficiency.

Acute adrenal insufficiency is a true medical emergency in which the patient is in immediate danger of death because of glucocorticoid (cortisol) insufficiency. Death usually results from peripheral vascular collapse (shock) and ventricular asystole (cardiac arrest).

The dental practitioner is in the unenviable position of being a major stressful factor in the lives of many patients. Because of this, all dental office personnel must become capable of recognizing and managing the acute adrenal crisis; even more importantly they must be capable of preventing this situation from developing.

PREDISPOSING FACTORS

Before the availability of glucocorticosteroid therapy, acute adrenal insufficiency was the terminal stage of Addison's disease. With therapy, however, addisonian patients may lead relatively normal lives. Unusual stress requires the patient to modify steroid doses to prevent the development of acute insufficiency. The major predisposing factor in all cases of adrenal insufficiency is the lack of glucocorticosteroid hormones, which develop through several mechanisms:

1. Following *sudden* withdrawal of steroid hormones in a patient who has primary adrenal insufficiency
2. Following *sudden* withdrawal in a patient with normal adrenal cortices but with a temporary insufficiency resulting from cortical suppression by exogenous corticosteroid administration (secondary insufficiency)

COMMENT. Patients with primary and secondary adrenocortical insufficiency are dependent on exogenous steroids. Abrupt withdrawal from therapy leaves the patient with a lack of glucocorticosteroid hormones, making the patient unable to adapt normally to stress (stress-intolerant). Evidence has indicated (Graber and others, 1965) that it may take up to 9 months for full recovery of adrenal cortex function following exogenous steroid therapy in patients with normal cortices. (Others have estimated that normal function may not return for as long as 2 years.) Patients with Addison's disease will require these drugs for the rest of their lives. Withdrawal of nonaddisonian patients from exogenous corticosteroids will occur over a long period of time during which the production of endogenous gluco-

corticosteroids in the adrenal gland will increase as the level of exogenous steroids decreases. The duration of this withdrawal will vary according to several factors, including (1) dose of glucocorticosteroid administered, (2) duration of the course of therapy, (3) frequency of administration, (4) time of administration, and (5) route of administration. Protocols have been designed (Byyny, 1975) that permit withdrawal from glucocorticosteroids with minimal symptoms and relative convenience and safety for the patient.

The widespread use of glucocorticosteroids in nonaddisonian patients has become the most common cause of adrenal insufficiency. Suppression of the hypothalamic-pituitary-adrenocortical axis generally does not appear unless the glucocorticoid therapy has been of long duration or in nonphysiologic (that is, pharmacologic) doses or both. For most of the uses of glucocorticosteroids listed in Table 8-1 pharmacologic doses are required that are generally greatly in excess of physiologic doses.*

3. Following *stress* such as physiologic or psychologic stress

COMMENT. Physiologic stresses may include traumatic injuries, surgery (including oral and periodontal surgery), extensive dental procedures, infection, acute changes in environmental temperature, severe muscular exercise, and burns. Psychologic stress such as that seen in the anxious dental patient may also precipitate the adrenal crisis.

In stressful situations there is normally an increased liberation of glucocorticoids. This increase is mediated through the hypothalamic-pituitary-adrenocortical axis and normally results in rapid elevation in the blood levels of glucocorticosteroids. If the adrenal gland is unable to meet this increased demand, clinical signs and symptoms of adrenal insufficiency develop. In dental situations stress will be the most common immediate precipitating factor producing acute insufficiency.

4. Following bilateral adrenalectomy or removal of a functioning adrenal tumor that had been suppressing the other adrenal gland
5. Following sudden destruction of the pituitary gland

---

*Physiologic or replacement doses are equal to the normal daily production of a functioning adrenal cortex. This is equivalent to approximately 20 mg cortisol. Pharmacologic doses, on the other hand, are commonly four to five times (or more) the physiologic dose.

6. Following injury to both adrenal glands by trauma, hemorrhage, infection, thrombosis, or tumor

COMMENT. The last three causes of adrenal crisis will be observed most commonly in the hospitalized patient and will therefore not be of immediate concern to the dental practitioner. The first three precipitating factors will be the major causes of the development of acute adrenal insufficiency in dental situations and will therefore be discussed more fully in the sections to follow.

PREVENTION

Acute adrenal insufficiency is best managed through its prevention, which is based on the medical history questionnaire completed by the patient and the ensuing dialogue history between the doctor and patient. In many instances, specific dental therapy considerations will be necessary for the patient at risk of adrenal insufficiency.

QUESTION 6. Have you taken any medicine or drugs during the past two years?

COMMENT. "During the past two years" has been added to this question because of the probability of development of adrenocortical suppression following the long-term use of pharmacologic doses of glucocorticosteroids. Table 8-2 lists many of the generic and proprietary names of commonly prescribed corticosteroid drugs. In many instances, the patient may only know the proprietary name of the drug. Reference to this list or to the *Physicians' Desk Reference* will aid in precisely identifying the medication.

Table 8-2. Systemic corticosteroids

Generic name	Proprietary name	Generic name	Proprietary name
Hydrocortisone	A-hydroCort	Methylprednisolone	BayMep-40
	Biosone		Depoject
	Cortef		Depo-Medrol
	Fernisone		Depopred
	Hydrocortone		Duralone-80
	Lifocort		Medrol
	Solu-Cortef		Mepred-40
Cortisone	Cortone		Solu-Medrol
Prednisolone	Articulose	Triamcinolone	Aristocort, Aristospan
	Cortalone		Articulose-L.A.
	Deltasone		Cenocort
	Fernisolone-P		Kenacort, Kenalog
	Hydeltra		Tracilon
	Key-Pred-25		Trilog
	Metalone		Trilone
	Meticorten	Paramethasone	Haldrone
	Niscort	Dexamethasone	Baydex
	Predaject		Baycadron
	Predcor-25		Dalalone
	Savacort		Decadron
	Solupredalone		Dexone
Prednisone	Cortan		Dezone
	Delta-Cortef		Hexadrol
	Hydeltrasol		Savacort
	Orasone		Solurex
	Panasol	Betamethasone	Betameth
	Prednicen-M		Celestone
	Sterone		Selestoject
		Fludrocortisone	Florinef

QUESTION 9. *Circle any of the following which you have had or have at present:*
- **Rheumatic fever**
- **Asthma**
- **Hay fever**
- **Allergies or hives**
- **Arthritis**
- **Rheumatism**
- **Cortisone medicine**

COMMENT. The specific diseases or medication listed in question 9 represent only a small part of the total number of clinical uses of glucocorticosteroids (Table 8-1). In all of these situations, pharmacologic doses of the drugs are employed. If the patient has a positive history of any of these diseases, the doctor should follow with a dialogue history seeking to determine the following:

1. What drugs were used in the management of the disorder
2. Drug dose
3. Route of administration
4. Duration of time that the drug was taken
5. Length of time elapsed since drug therapy was terminated

Dialogue History

With an affirmative response to the preceding questions the doctor must vigorously pursue a dialogue history, seeking additional relevant information.

QUESTION. *What drug(s) were used in management of the disorder?*

COMMENT. As previously mentioned, the diseases indicated in question 9 are frequently managed in part through the administration of glucocorticosteroids. The doctor must determine the name of the specific agent(s) involved in this therapy. Tables 8-1 and 8-2 may help in seeking this information.

QUESTION. *What was the dose of the drug (daily)?*

COMMENT. The specific dose of glucocorticosteroid is important as one measure of the degree of cortical suppression that has occurred. The equivalent therapeutic dose of various glucocorticosteroids varies from agent to agent (Table 8-3). For example, 20 mg of hydrocortisone is equivalent to 5 mg of prednisolone, methylprednisone, and prednisone; to 4 mg of methylprednisolone and triamcinolone; and to 0.75 mg of dexamethasone.

Patients with primary adrenocortical insufficiency (Addison's disease) receive replacement (physiologic) doses of glucocorticosteroids. This usually requires the administration of approximately 10 to 20 mg of hydrocortisone (or its equivalent) on arising in the morning, 10 mg at 12 to 1 PM and 5 mg at 5 to 6 PM, in addition to 0.1 mg (approximately) of fludrocortisone each morning. These doses satisfactorily "replace" the normal output of the adrenal cortex (approximately 20 mg of cortisol daily).

Patients receiving glucocorticosteroid therapy for symptomatic treatment of their disorders (Table 8-1) commonly receive large (pharmacologic or therapeutic) doses. In the management of rheumatoid arthritis, a daily oral dose of 10 to 15 mg of prednisone is frequently administered. This is equivalent in effect to approximately 50 to 75 mg of cortisone. Prednisone is also administered orally to asthmatic patients whose acute episodes do not respond readily to bronchodilator therapy. Divided doses totaling 40 to 60 mg/day are employed. This is equivalent to 200 to 300 mg of cortisone. Doses such as these may readily cause suppression of the normal adrenal cortex if they are continued for a length of time.

The "Rule of Two's" (see box on p. 124) is extremely helpful in determining the risk factor of patients who are currently taking or previously have taken glucocorticosteroids. The first of the three factors in the Rule of Two's is the daily administration of 20 mg or more of cortisone or its equivalent.

QUESTION. *By what route was the drug administered?*

COMMENT. Glucocorticosteroids may be administered by a variety of routes. Parenteral administra-

Table 8-3. Equivalent doses of corticosteroids

Agent	Equivalent dose (mg)
Cortisone	25
Hydrocortisone	20
Prednisolone	5
Prednisone	5
Methylprednisone	5
Methylprednisolone	4
Triamcinolone	4
Dexamethasone	0.75
Betamethasone	0.6

RULE OF TWO'S

Adrenocortical suppression should be suspected if a patient has received gluco-corticosteroid therapy:
1. In a dose of 20 mg or more of cortisone or its equivalent, daily
2. Via the oral or parenteral route for a continuous period of 2 weeks or longer
3. Within 2 years of dental therapy

---

tion (intramuscular, intravenous, and subcutaneous) and enteral administration (oral) may lead to suppression of a normal adrenal cortex with decrease in production of endogenous glucocorticosteroids. Drugs administered topically (ophthalmic, dermatologic, intranasal, tracheobronchial, vaginal, or rectal) and by intra-articular application usually do not cause adrenal cortical suppression because of the relatively poor systemic absorption by these routes.

QUESTION. *How long did the glucocorticosteroid therapy last?*

COMMENT. Although the exact length of time required for the development of significant cortical suppression varies from patient to patient, it has been demonstrated that uninterrupted glucocorticosteroid therapy for as little as 2 weeks may produce this phenomenon. Any dental patient who has received glucocorticosteroid therapy for 2 weeks or longer is a potential candidate for adrenal insufficiency. This constitutes the second important factor in the Rule of Two's.

QUESTION. *How long has it been since glucocorticosteroid therapy was terminated?*

COMMENT. This question is applicable to patients who had a normal adrenal cortex at the time of the start of glucocorticosteroid therapy, underwent therapy (probably at pharmacologic dose levels) until the underlying disorder was controlled, and were then gradually withdrawn from it. The atrophic adrenal cortex does not begin to function normally for a variable period of time following termination of therapy. During this time the cortex is usually capable of producing minimal daily levels of endogenous steroids, but in stressful situations it may be unable to meet the demand, thus inducing

signs and symptoms of acute adrenal insufficiency. The length of time required for full regeneration of normal cortical function varies according to the dosage and length of therapy but is normally at least 9 to 12 months (Graber and others, 1965). Instances of acute adrenal insufficiency lasting as long as 2 years have been reported following termination of therapy. The third factor in the Rule of Two's relates to patients who have received glucocorticoid therapy within 2 years of dental therapy. The Rule of Two's allows the doctor to reliably predict which patients are at increased risk of developing acute adrenal insufficiency.

Dental Therapy Considerations

Possible modification in dental therapy is in order for patients who are currently receiving glucocorticosteroid therapy or who have received such therapy and meet the criteria of the Rule of Two's. In such circumstances the following should be considered: medical and dental evaluation should be completed, a provisional dental treatment plan drawn up, and the patient's physician consulted before any dental therapy. A patient with Addison's disease or a person on long-term pharmacologic-dose corticosteroid therapy will usually have an ASA II– or ASA III–level risk.

Glucocorticosteroid coverage

Because patients with adrenocortical insufficiency are unable to adapt to stress in a normal manner, their blood steroid levels must be increased through the administration of exogenous glucocorticosteroids before, during, and possibly after the stressful situation. The choice of a therapeutic regimen depends on the physician's evaluation of the patient's physical status and on the dentist's evaluation of the stress involved in the planned dental procedure. Many nondental practitioners (physicians) tend to underestimate the degree of stress associated with nonsurgical dental procedures. The dentist must carefully evaluate this vitally important factor. In extreme instances, such as the patient with Addison's disease who has extreme apprehension, the patient may be hospitalized and given 200 to 500 mg of cortisone per day. This is equivalent to the maximal response of the normal pituitary-adrenal system to extreme stress. In mild stress, as most dental procedures might be classified, or with moderate anxiety towards dentistry, the needed increase in glucocorticosteroid level is less. Usually a two- or fourfold increase in gluco-

---

Card for Patient on Corticosteroid Therapy

Mr.
Mrs.
Miss _ _ _ _ _ _ _ _ _ is being treated for _ _ _ (disorder) _ _

with _ (corticosteroid) _ in a dose of_ _ _ (dose) _ _ _. In the

event of "stress", the steroid dosage should be increased thus:

    1. Mild "Stress" (eg, common cold, single dental extraction,

mild trauma): use double doses daily.

    2. Moderate "Stress" (eg, flu, surgery under local anesthesia,

several dental extractions): use hydrocortisone, 100 mg, or

prednisolone, 20 mg, or dexamethasone, 4 mg daily.

    3. Severe "Stress" (eg, general surgery, pneumonia or other

systemic infections, high fever, severe trauma): use hydro-

cortisone, 200 mg, or prednisolone, 40 mg, or dexamethasone

8 mg daily.

    When vomiting or diarrhea precludes absorption of oral doses,

give dexamethasone 1 to 4 mg intramuscularly every 6 hours.

        (Signed) _____ M.D.

        (Address) _____

Fig. 8-1. Sample corticosteroid coverage protocol for patient receiving corticosteroid therapy. (From Streeten, D.H.P.: JAMA **232**:944, 1975.)

corticoid treatment on the day of the stress (the appointment day) is adequate to prepare the patient. The adrenal cortices of normal adults secrete about 20 mg of cortisol daily, which is the daily maintenance level required by most addisonian patients. Oral medications may be given. Fig. 8-1 is a sample of a corticosteroid coverage protocol.

Stress Reduction Protocol

In addition to medical consultation and the possible use of exogenous corticosteroid medications during the period of dental therapy, the Stress Reduction Protocol (p. 41) is an extremely valuable adjunct to the proper management of this patient.

Additional considerations

Many patients with Addison's disease wear an identification bracelet stating their name, the name and telephone number of a close relative, and their physician's name and telephone number. The bracelet also states, "I have adrenal insufficiency. In any emergency involving injury, vomiting, or loss of consciousness, the hydrocortisone in my possession should be injected under my skin, and my physician should be notified." Such patients carry small, clearly labeled kits containing 100 mg of hydrocortisone phosphate solution in a sterile syringe ready for use. Even if never needed, this kit is a constant reminder to the patient that survival may depend on the timely use of this medication. The kit should be taken from the high-risk patient at the time of the dental appointment and placed on the bracket table or elsewhere within ready reach of the doctor during therapy.

CLINICAL MANIFESTATIONS

In stressful situations such as might be experienced during dental therapy the patient with hypofunctioning adrenal cortices may demonstrate clinical signs and symptoms of acute insufficiency of glucocorticosteroids. The result of this acute insufficiency may be loss of consciousness and coma.

Initial signs and symptoms may include the following: mental confusion, muscle weakness, and extreme fatigue. Nausea and vomiting may develop, along with hypotension and syncopal episodes. In adrenal insufficiency of a more chronic nature, there is also hyperpigmentation, hypoglycemia, a steady loss of weight, and a craving for salt and water as dehydration and hypotension become more and more severe.

In the dental office the acute episode will be marked most notably by a progressively severe mental confusion. Intense pain develops in the abdomen, lower back, and legs, and a progressive deterioration of the cardiovascular system is noted. This latter symptom may lead to the loss of consciousness and onset of coma. Coma has been defined as a state in which a patient is totally unresponsive or is unresponsive to all except very painful stimuli and immediately returns to the state of unresponsiveness when the stimulus is terminated.

If unmanaged, acute adrenal insufficiency may lead to the death of the patient.

Loss of consciousness does not occur immediately in most instances. The progressive mental confusion and other clinical symptoms will usually permit prompt recognition of a "problem" and institution of basic steps of management. Table 8-4 summarizes signs and symptoms of acute adrenal insufficiency.

Table 8-4. Clinical manifestations of acute adrenal insufficiency

Mental confusion
Muscle weakness
Intense pain in abdomen, lower back, and legs
Hypoglycemia
Extreme fatigue
Nausea and vomiting
Hypotension
Syncopal episodes
Coma

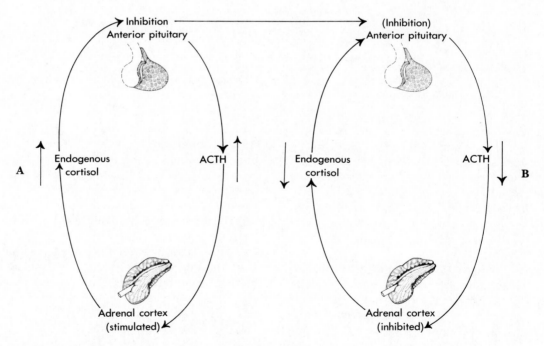

Fig. 8-2. Mechanism of glucocorticosteroid availability (normal adrenal cortex). **A,** Anterior pituitary gland increases production of ACTH, which leads to adrenocortical stimulation and increased adrenal secretion of endogenous glucocorticosteroid. This increased blood level leads to inhibition of the anterior pituitary gland. **B,** Inhibited anterior pituitary produces less ACTH. Decreased blood level of ACTH leads to inhibition of adrenal cortex and decreased production of glucocorticosteroids. Decreased blood level of glucocorticosteroids leads to stimulation of anterior pituitary (see **A**).

PATHOPHYSIOLOGY
Review of Normal Adrenal Function

The actions of adrenocortical steroid hormones affect all bodily tissues and organs and aid in keeping the internal environment of the body constant (homeostasis) through their actions on the metabolism of carbohydrates, fats, proteins, water, and electrolytes. The body provides a minimal supply of glucocorticosteroid hormones (approximately 20 mg daily in the nonstressed adult) through the actions of adrenocorticotrophic hormone (ACTH),

which is released by the anterior portion of the pituitary gland. ACTH levels in the blood plasma control the adrenal cortex and the production of all steroids except aldosterone.

In nonstress situations the rate of ACTH secretion is regulated by the level of circulating cortisol; a high level suppresses ACTH secretion, whereas a low level permits its more rapid secretion (Fig. 8-2, *A* and *B*). The mechanism is relatively slow acting and does not account for the rapid increase in blood ACTH levels observed in more stressful

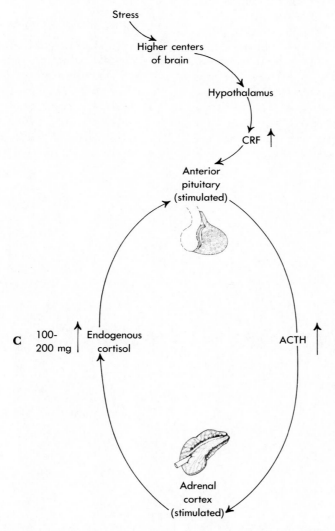

Fig. 8-2, cont'd. C, Mechanism of glucocorticosteroid availability. Normal adrenal cortex (stress situations). In stressful situations the hypothalamus receives stimuli from higher centers of the brain. Corticotrophin-releasing factor (CRF) is released, which stimulates production of ACTH by anterior pituitary. Increased blood levels of ACTH stimulate adrenal cortex to produce increased quantities of endogenous glucocorticosteroids (100 to 200 mg cortisol) required for stress adaptation.

situations. A second factor that regulates the secretion of ACTH is an individual's sleep schedule. In persons who sleep at night, plasma ACTH levels begin to rise at 2 AM, reaching their peak at the time of awakening. They fall during the day, reaching their ebb during the evening. This factor again is of primary value during nonstressful times. Cortisol blood levels mimic those of ACTH.

Under stress the pituitary gland rapidly increases the release of ACTH into the circulation, and the adrenal cortex responds within minutes by synthesizing and secreting increased amounts of various steroids. The sum total of this increased steroid production is to prepare the body to successfully manage a stressful situation by increasing the metabolic rate, increasing retention of sodium (Na+) and water, and making small blood vessels increasingly responsive to the actions of norepinephrine. A third mechanism must be activated (Fig. 8-2, *C*) to rapidly raise the levels of cortical steroids in the blood. When stressful stimuli are received by the central nervous system, they reach the level of the hypothalamus, which releases a substance known as corticotrophin-releasing factor (CRF). CRF is transported by means of the hypothalamic-hypophyseal portal venous system to the anterior lobes of the pituitary gland, where CRF stimulates the secretion of ACTH into the circulation, which then allows the adrenal cortex to increase secretion of corticosteroids. The cortisol secretion begins within minutes and continues as long as the plasma ACTH level is maintained. Once ACTH secretion ceases (with removal of stress), plasma ACTH concentration has a half-life of 10 minutes; once cortisol secretion ceases, the plasma cortisol level falls during a half-life of 1 to 2 hours.

Pathophysiology of Adrenal Insufficiency

In the patient with primary adrenocortical insufficiency (Addison's disease), the adrenal cortex is hypofunctioning and is unable to provide the necessary blood levels of corticosteroids required to maintain life even at nonstressful levels. For this reason, replacement therapy must be provided by means of oral or parenteral corticosteroids. Fig. 8-3 shows the feedback mechanisms operating in the

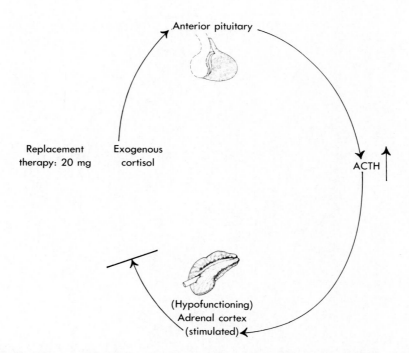

Fig. 8-3. Corticosteroid levels—primary insufficiency (Addison's disease). Anterior pituitary gland secretes ACTH, which stimulates adrenal cortex. Hypofunctioning adrenal cortex is unable to synthesize and secrete required cortisol. Blood levels of glucocorticosteroids do not fluctuate in response to ACTH levels, being fixed by exogenous doses of approximately 20 mg.

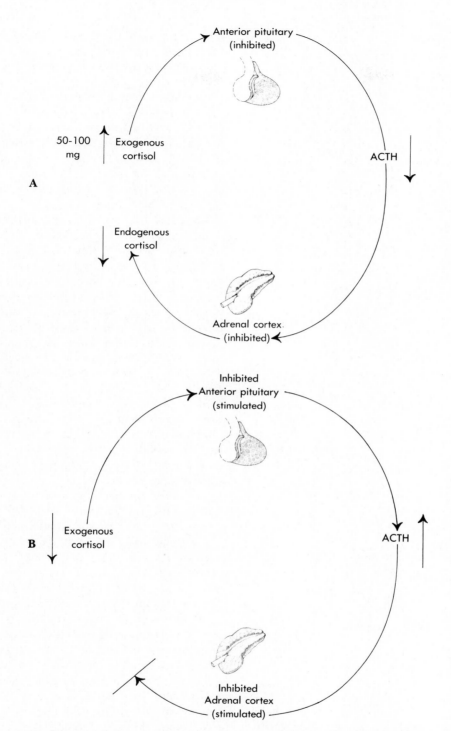

Fig. 8-4. Glucocorticosteroid levels, secondary insufficiency (exogenous therapy). **A,** In presence of normal adrenal cortex and additional exogenous glucocorticosteroid administration, blood levels are greatly increased. ACTH production by anterior pituitary is inhibited, leading to inhibition of adrenal cortical function. Inhibition of both ACTH and glucocorticosteroid production continues for duration of exogenous therapy. **B,** Exogenous therapy. Disuse atrophy of adrenal cortex and anterior pituitary develops with prolonged (2 weeks or longer) glucocorticosteroid therapy. At termination of therapy, blood levels of corticosteroids fall, stimulating anterior pituitary to produce ACTH. ACTH production may be subnormal, or even if normal, response of adrenal cortex may be inadequate. Blood cortisol levels are inadequate with patient in a stress-intolerant state.

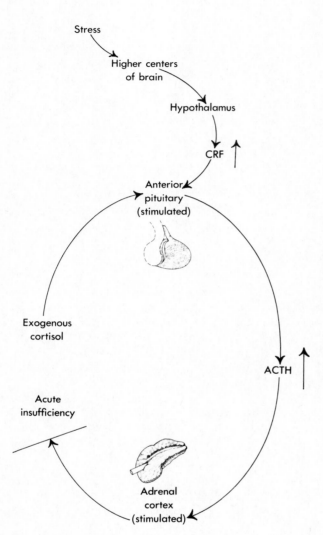

Fig. 8-5. Hypofunctioning adrenal cortex with exogenous cortisol (Addison's disease and nonendocrine cortisol). Blood level of glucocorticosteroid is fixed by exogenous doses. In stressful situation, CRF secreted by hypothalamus induces ACTH secretion by anterior pituitary, which in turn stimulates the adrenal cortex. The anterior pituitary and/or the adrenal cortex may be incapable of proper functioning, leading to cortisol blood levels inadequate to adapt the body to stress. Acute insufficiency results.

addisonian patient. Corticosteroid blood level is fixed, depending on the total milligram dosage administered during the day. As a general rule, a normal adult secretes 20 mg of cortisol per day; thus replacement therapy in Addison's disease consists of approximately 20 mg of exogenous cortisol (hydrocortisone) daily. It may be administered either orally or parenterally, in single or more usually in divided doses. The adrenal cortex is unable to respond to increases or decreases in the blood levels of ACTH, which continues to be secreted by the anterior pituitary.

In the patient with a normal adrenal cortex who is receiving glucocorticosteroid therapy for a non-endocrine disorder, the blood level of cortisol is determined by the total quantity of endogenous and exogenous glucocorticosteroid. Initially, the adrenal cortex will continue to secrete approximately 20 mg of endogenous cortisol daily, to which may be added doses in excess of 50 mg through the administration of exogenous corticosteroids. The effect of this elevated blood level of glucocorticosteroids is to inhibit the secretion of ACTH by the anterior pituitary gland. This decrease in ACTH inhibits the adrenal cortex from secreting endogenous cortisol. As exogenous therapy continues, the ability of the pituitary gland to secrete ACTH and of the adrenal cortex to produce endogenous glucocorticoids decreases, and a variable degree of disuse atrophy develops (Fig. 8-4, *A*). If exogenous steroid therapy terminates abruptly, or on rare occasions, even after the slow withdrawal of these drugs, the blood level of cortisol falls, stimulating the anterior pituitary to produce higher blood levels of ACTH, which acts to stimulate the adrenal cortex to produce endogenous cortisol. ACTH and endogenous corticosteroid levels may prove deficient at this time (Fig. 8-4, *B*). The adrenal cortex is unable to produce the required cortisol levels, and the patient is in a hypoadrenal state. Any increased requirement for cortisol, as in stressful situations, may produce an acute insufficiency. Although the adrenal cortex usually regains normal function within 2 to 4 weeks, it may require longer than a year in other instances. The longer the duration of exogenous therapy and the larger the doses received, the longer the recovery period will be.

In stressful situations the patient with adrenal hypofunction (either primary [Addison's disease] or secondary [exogenous steroids]) receives a fixed level of exogenous corticosteroid (Fig. 8-5). The patient is unable to increase this level in response to the increasing ACTH levels present in the blood (produced as a result of CRF released from the hypothalamus), and thus the clinical manifestations of acute adrenal insufficiency develop. Management of this situation requires replacement of the low blood levels of steroids.

MANAGEMENT

Acute adrenal insufficiency is a truly life-threatening situation. Effective management of this situation requires the doctor to follow the steps of basic life support and to administer glucocorticosteroids to the patient. The patient with acute adrenal insufficiency is in immediate danger because of glucocorticoid deficiency, depletion of extracellular fluid, and hyperkalemia. Treatment is based on the correction of these conditions.

Conscious Patient

Step 1. Terminate dental therapy. As soon as the doctor recognizes signs and symptoms of acute insufficiency, dental therapy must immediately be halted. Acute insufficiency should be suspected in patients who develop symptoms of mental confusion, nausea, vomiting, and abdominal pain and who are currently receiving glucocorticosteroids or have received 20 mg or more of cortisone (or its equivalent) by oral or parenteral administration for a period of 2 weeks or longer within 2 years of dental therapy (Rule of Two's).

Step 2. Monitor vital signs. Blood pressure and heart rate should be monitored. The blood pressure will be depressed and the heart rate elevated.

Step 3. Position patient. If the blood pressure is depressed, the patient should be placed in the supine position with the legs elevated slightly.

Step 4. Emergency kit (oxygen). Immediately call for the emergency kit and oxygen. Oxygen may be administered by means of a full face mask or nasal hood. A flow of approximately 5 to 10 liters per minute will be adequate.

Step 5. Administer glucocorticosteroid. Remove the glucocorticosteroid and a syringe from the emergency kit, or use the patient's medication that was previously placed on the tray. Hydrocortisone sodium succinate (Solu-Cortef) is contained as an unmixed powder and liquid in the 2 ml Mix-o-vial (Fig. 8-6). When mixed, each milliliter will contain 50 mg of hydrocortisone. To mix the solution, the plastic top cap is removed and the rubber plunger is depressed. This forces the powder and liquid to combine. Shake the vial until a clear solution has formed. Insert the syringe through the rubber stopper and withdraw the solution.

If possible, the 100 mg of hydrocortisone should be administered intravenously over 30 seconds. The intramuscular route may be employed instead of intravenous administration, 100 mg (2 ml) being injected into a suitable muscle mass.

Step 6. Summon medical assistance. Medical assistance should be summoned as early as possible. Because the victim is still conscious in this case, it may be prudent to contact the patient's physician first. In most cases the patient will be transported immediately to the physician's office or to the emergency room of a hospital, where more defini-

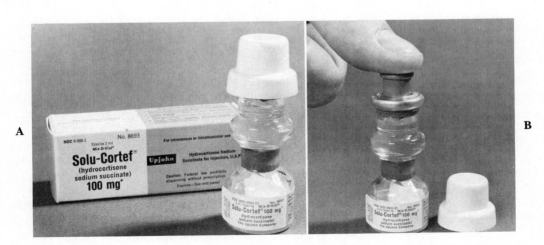

Fig. 8-6. A, Corticosteroid. **B,** Preparation of corticosteroid for use. Depressing plunger mixes powder and liquid so that fresh solution is immediately available for use.

tive management may be instituted. If this is required, the doctor should accompany the patient.

Unconscious Patient

Step 1. Recognize unconsciousness. Shake the patient and shout, "Are you all right?" Lack of response will lead to a tentative diagnosis of unconsciousness.

Step 2. Position patient. The supine position with legs elevated slightly is the preferred position for the unconscious patient.

Step 3. Basic life support. Immediate institution of the steps of basic life support (Chapter 5) is necessary. These include the use of head tilt–chin lift, assessing airway and breathing, the jaw thrust maneuver (if necessary), artificial ventilation (if necessary), and assessing circulation.

In most instances, respiration and blood pressure are depressed, and the heart rate (pulse) is rapid but weak (thready). Airway maintenance and oxygen administration are required in virtually all cases. Should the pulse be absent, external chest compression should be started immediately and continued until assistance arrives. In this case omit the following steps.

Definitive management

Step 4. Emergency kit (oxygen). Members of the emergency team bring the emergency kit and oxygen to the victim. Oxygen may be administered through a face mask or nose piece. Aromatic spirits of ammonia may be used at this time because it may be difficult to differentiate acute adrenal insufficiency from other causes of unconsciousness, including vasodepressor syncope.

Positioning the patient, adequate airway maintenance, and use of aromatic ammonia and oxygen will not lead to a noticeable improvement of the patient in acute adrenal insufficiency. If no improvement is noted, the following steps should be considered.

Step 5. Summon medical assistance. If unconsciousness continues following the preceding steps, it becomes apparent that the cause of this situation is probably not one of those more commonly encountered (vasodepressor syncope and orthostatic hypotension). Additional medical assistance should be summoned.

Step 6. Evaluate medical history. While awaiting the arrival of assistance and with the patient maintained by basic life support, a member of the emergency team should review the patient's medical

---

MANAGEMENT OF ACUTE ADRENAL INSUFFICIENCY

Conscious patient

Step 1	Terminate dental therapy
2	Monitor vital signs
3	Position patient
4	Emergency kit (oxygen)
5	Administer glucocorticosteroid
6	Summon medical assistance

Unconscious patient

Step 1	Recognize unconsciousness
2	Position patient
3	Basic life support
4	Emergency kit (oxygen)
5	Summon medical assistance
6	Evaluate medical history
7	Administer glucocorticosteroid
7a	Additional drugs (vasopressor)
8	Transfer to hospital

---

history for evidence of a possible cause of this situation. If no obvious cause is noted, the dental office team should continue to implement the steps of basic life support until assistance arrives. If evidence exists that glucocorticosteroid insufficiency is a possible or probable cause of the unconsciousness, proceed to step 7.

Step 7. Administer glucocorticosteroid. Intravenous or intramuscular administration of 100 mg of hydrocortisone is indicated in cases of suspected adrenal insufficiency. Whenever possible, 100 mg should be injected intravenously over 30 seconds. An intravenous infusion should be started, and an IV bottle to which 100 mg of hydrocortisone has been added should be administered over 2 hours. Should the intravenous route be unavailable, 100 mg of hydrocortisone may be administered intramuscularly.

Step 7a. Additional drug therapy. In the presence of a depressed blood pressure, a vasopressor may be administered (20 mg of methoxamine IM or IV) while awaiting assistance.

Step 8. Transfer to hospital. With arrival of additional medical assistance, the patient should be prepared for transfer to an emergency medical care facility. At this facility, blood samples will be taken and any existing electrolyte imbalance (such as hyperkalemia) corrected. Definitive therapy is designed to meet the needs of the individual patient but consists initially of large IV doses of glucocorticosteroids, followed by additional doses of oral or IM steroids or both.

It must again be stressed that *if there is any possibility that the loss of consciousness is in any way related to a deficiency of glucocorticosteroids, the immediate administration of 100 mg of hydrocortisone succinate may prove to be a life-saving procedure.* In the absence of such indications the doctor should continue to maintain the patient with basic life support procedures until medical assistance is available.

Management of acute adrenal insufficiency is summarized in the box at left.

BIBLIOGRAPHY

Barkin, R.M.: Endocrine disorders. In Barkin, R.M., and Rosen, P.: Emergency pediatrics, St. Louis, 1984, The C.V. Mosby Co.

Burch, P.G., and Migeon, C.J.: Systemic absorption of topical steroids, Arch. Ophthalmol. **79**:174, 1968.

Byyny, R.: Withdrawal from glucocorticoid therapy, N. Engl. J. Med. **295**:30, 1976.

Chamberlain, P., and Meyer, W.J., III: Management of pituitary-adrenal suppression secondary to corticosteroid therapy, Pediatrics **67**:245, 1981.

Conn, H.G., and Conn, R.B., editors: Current diagnosis—6, Philadelphia, 1980, W.B. Saunders Company.

Conte, F.A., and Grumbach, M.M.: Endocrine emergencies. In Pascoe, D.J., and Grossman, M., editors: Quick reference to pediatric emergencies, ed. 3, Philadelphia, 1983, J.B. Lippincott Co.

Fraser, C.G., Preuss, R.S., and Bigford, W.D.: Adrenal atrophy and irreversible shock associated with corticosteroids, JAMA **149**:1542, 1952.

Frawley, T.F.: Treatment of adrenal insufficiency states including Addison's disease, Mod. Treatm. **3**:1328, 1966.

Gonzalez, R.B.: Selected emergency endocrinologic problems. In Schwartz, G.R., and others, editors: Principles and practice of emergency medicine, Philadelphia, 1978, W.B. Saunders Co.

Graber, A.L., and others: Natural history of pituitary-adrenal recovery following long term suppression with glucocorticoids, J. Clin. Endocrinol. **25**:11, 1965.

Himathongkam, T., and others: Acute adrenal insufficiency, JAMA **230**:1317, 1974.

Krupin, T., and others: Topical corticosteroid therapy and pituitary-adrenal function, Arch. Ophthalmol. **94**:919, 1976.

Krupp, M.A., and Chatton, M.J.: Current medical diagnosis and treatment, Los Altos, CA, 1985, Lange Medical Publications.

Livanou, T., Ferriman, D., and James, V.H.T.: Recovery of hypothalamo-pituitary-adrenal function after corticosteroid therapy, Lancet **2**:856, 1967.

Plumpton, F.S., Besser, G.M., and Cole, P.V.: Corticosteroid treatment and surgery: an investigation of the indications for steroid cover, Anaesthesia **24**:3, 1969.

Plumpton, F.S., Besser, G.M., and Cole, P.V.: Corticosteroid treatment and surgery. 2. The management of steroid cover, Anaesthesia **24**:12, 1969.

Rehorst, E.D., and DeGroot, G.W.: Preoperative management of glucocorticoid dependent pedodontic patients, J. Am. Dent. Assoc. **93**:809, 1976.

Sampson, P.A., Winstone, N.E., and Brooke, B.N.: Adrenal function in surgical patients after steroid therapy, Lancet **2**:322, 1962.

Scoggins, R.B., and Kliman, B.: Percutaneous absorption of corticosteroids, J. Clin. Endocrinol. **25**:11, 1965.

Slaney, G., and Brooke, B.N.: Postoperative collapse due to adrenal insufficiency following cortisone therapy, Lancet **1**:1167, 1957.

Streeten, D.H.P.: Corticosteroid therapy. I. Pharmacological properties and principles of corticosteroid use, JAMA **232**:944, 1975.

Streeten, D.H.P.: Corticosteroid therapy. II. Complications and therapeutic indications, JAMA **232**:1046, 1975.

Treadwell, B.L.J., Savage, O., and Sever, E.D.: Pituitary adrenal function during corticosteroid therapy, Lancet **1**:355, 1963.

Trummel, C.L.: Antiinflammatory drugs. In Neidle, E.A., Kroeger, D.C., and Yagiela, J.A.: Pharmacology and therapeutics for dentistry, ed. 2, St. Louis, 1985, The C.V. Mosby Co.

Werterhof, L.: Recovery of adrenocortical function during long-term treatment with corticosteroids, Br. Med. J. **4**:534, 1970.

9 *Unconsciousness: Differential Diagnosis*

In all instances of unconsciousness the immediate response of the dental office staff to the unconscious patient should be the same: rapid initiation of the steps of basic life support. After these steps have been effectively carried out, the team should consider definitive management of the situation in accordance with the following differential diagnosis guidelines, which may assist the doctor in determining which etiologic factor(s) precipitated the loss of consciousness. Several factors are presented as aids in differential diagnosis; reference is made to Table 5-1 for the various causes of unconsciousness.

AGE OF PATIENT

The age of the unconscious patient may assist in the differential diagnosis. Unconsciousness occurring in the dental office in "normal healthy" patients *under 40 years of age* is in most instances related to psychogenic reactions such as vasodepressor syncope. Two other possible causes of unconsciousness in the under-40 age group are hypoglycemia and epilepsy. These are normally easily differentiated from the more common causes of unconsciousness and are discussed fully in other sections of the text. In patients *over the age of 40,* unconsciousness is more likely to be precipitated by cardiovascular complications (Section VII) such as acute myocardial infarction, cerebrovascular accident, valvular lesions (such as aortic stenosis) or acute cardiac arrhythmias. Psychogenic reactions are encountered much less frequently in this age group, since patients likely have "adapted" themselves to their anxieties concerning dentistry. Unconsciousness is rarely noted in young children except in the presence of specific disease states such as diabetes mellitus (hypoglycemia), epilepsy, and congenital heart lesions. Psychogenic reactions (vasodepressor syncope) are infrequent because children are vocal in expressing their feelings toward dentistry, releasing their tensions, and producing muscular movement.

CIRCUMSTANCES ASSOCIATED WITH LOSS OF CONSCIOUSNESS

Stress, whether physiologic (pain) or psychologic (anxiety), is a precipitating factor in most cases of unconsciousness that occur in dental situations. Instances in which stress may precipitate unconsciousness include vasodepressor syncope, acute adrenal insufficiency, cerebrovascular accident, hypoglycemic reaction, epilepsy, and acute myocardial infarction. Unconsciousness may also occur in the absence of obvious stress. Orthostatic hypotension will be the most common non-stress-related cause of unconsciousness. Other nonstress factors leading to the loss of consciousness include the administration or ingestion of drugs, acute allergic reactions, and the hyperglycemic reaction.

POSITION OF PATIENT

The position of the patient at the time consciousness is lost may aid in the differential diagnosis of unconsciousness. Syncope, defined as the transient loss of consciousness, rarely occurs if the patient is in the supine position. There are, however, certain instances in which consciousness may be lost when the patient is in the supine position. These include unconsciousness that develops secondary to the administration of drugs or to epileptic seizures or that develops in hypoglycemic or hyperglycemic reactions or acute adrenal insufficiency: valvular disorders, arrhythmias, acute myocardial infarction; and cerebral vascular accident. In these circumstances, positioning of the patient in the supine position does not always lead to a restoration of consciousness because the primary factor producing unconsciousness in most of these situations is not related to a simple deficiency in the cerebral blood flow. Definitive management is required in all of these cases.

Patients suffering from orthostatic hypotension do not have syncopal episodes while in the supine position; however, signs and symptoms develop rapidly when the patient is moved into a more erect position and are reversed just as rapidly when the patient is repositioned.

The hyperventilation syndrome only rarely progresses to the actual loss of consciousness and then only if the patient is permitted to remain in the upright position for long periods of time. More commonly, hyperventilation produces a state of mental confusion (light-headedness and dizziness).

PRESYNCOPAL SIGNS AND SYMPTOMS
No Clinical Symptoms

Rapid loss of consciousness without symptoms leads to a presumptive diagnosis of orthostatic hypotension if the episode occurs immediately following a change of the patient's position. It must be remembered that certain drugs used in the practice of dentistry are capable of producing orthostatic hypotension (Table 7-1). Syncope caused by cardiac arrhythmias and heart block usually is sudden in onset and may occur without warning. It may develop with the patient either sitting or standing. Cardiac arrest on rare occasion may lead to the loss of consciousness without any prodromal signs and symptoms. Diagnosis of this situation will be made during implementation of the steps of basic life support.

Pallor and Cold, "Clammy" Skin

Restlessness, pallor (loss of normal skin color), clammy (moist) skin, nausea, and vomiting are considered to be the classic signs of fainting. They are usually present in vasodepressor syncope. These signs may also be present in hypoglycemic reactions, acute adrenal insufficiency, and acute myocardial infarction.

Tingling and Numbness of Extremities

Hyperventilation, although rarely producing a loss of consciousness, may on occasion do so if the patient is allowed to remain seated upright for extended periods of time during the episode. The hyperventilation syndrome may readily be recognized by the alterations in the respiratory rate (increased) and depth of breathing (increased) that accompany it as well as by the clinical symptoms of tingling and numbness of the fingers, toes, and perioral areas.

Headache

Headache of an intense nature may be noted at the outset of a cerebrovascular accident, especially of the hemorrhagic type.

Chest Pain

Chest pain or discomfort may precede the loss of consciousness in angina pectoris (unconsciousness rarely occurring), acute myocardial infarction (loss of consciousness and cardiac arrest more likely), and on occasion in the hyperventilation syndrome.

Breath Odor

Alcohol is not uncommonly detected on the breath of dental patients and is the most frequently employed drug for anxiety reduction before dental appointments. The presence of alcohol on the breath should lead the doctor to evaluate the patient for any anxieties or fears concerning dentistry and to be extremely cautious in employing additional drugs during dental therapy that are capable of producing central nervous system depression, including local anesthetics. Unconsciousness in these situations might be produced by psychogenic factors or by profound CNS depression caused by the combination of various drugs.

The sweet, fruity odor of *acetone* is present on the breath of patients who are hyperglycemic and in ketoacidosis. In most instances, these patients are known diabetics.

Incontinence and Tonic-clonic Movements

All persons who lose consciousness may exhibit tonic and clonic movements of the upper and lower extremities. This is especially likely in patients who are not placed in the supine position but are maintained upright during the period of unconsciousness. Although tonic and clonic movements are possible during vasodepressor syncope, they are rarely observed. Seizures that arise from nonepileptic factors are usually mild and are rarely associated with sphincter muscle relaxation. However, a diagnosis of epilepsy is strongly suggested for seizure activity in which patients exhibit urinary or fecal incontinence and tongue biting.

Heart Rate and Blood Pressure

In most instances of unconsciousness the heart rate rises above the baseline level while the blood pressure decreases. For example, in a hypoglycemic or hyperglycemic reaction the blood pressure of the patient is quite low, while the heart, attempting to overcome this decrease in blood pressure, increases its rate of contraction. Exceptions do exist, including vasodepressor syncope, orthostatic hypotension, and cerebrovascular accident.

In vasodepressor syncope it is usual for blood pressure and the heart rate to decrease. A heart rate of 50 beats per minute is not uncommon during the syncopal phase of vasodepressor syncope. The heart rate during orthostatic hypotension remains at approximately the baseline level, although the blood pressure drops precipitously. The pulse, as felt in the radial, brachial, or carotid arteries, is usually described as "weak" or "thready" in persons whose blood pressure is low. In cerebrovascular accident, on the other hand, the blood pressure may be observed to be significantly elevated (systolic pressure elevated more than diastolic pressure) with the pulse quite strong, or "bounding."

Duration of Unconsciousness and Recovery

Much important diagnostic information can be obtained from the response or lack of response of the patient to the basic steps of management outlined in Chapter 5. Unconsciousness produced by vasodepressor syncope is usually reversed within a few seconds to minutes once the patient is placed in the supine position. In the recovery period the patient does not return to "normal" rapidly. More frequently, signs and symptoms such as shivering, sweating, headache, and fatigue are present. In patients with orthostatic hypotension, consciousness returns rapidly on positioning. Recovery is more complete and rapid after orthostatic hypotension than after vasodepressor syncope, residual signs and symptoms being absent or less intense. Syncope caused by cardiac arrhythmias or heart block also is quickly reversed, with the patient usually alert on recovery.

Syncope produced through mechanisms other than a lack of adequate cerebral blood flow is not readily reversed through positioning of the patient. Epileptic patients usually terminate their seizures after a few moments; however, they may remain somnolent and often develop intense headaches during recovery. Significant tonic-clonic seizure activity is not usually observed during vasodepressor syncope or orthostatic hypotension.

Unconsciousness produced through drug administration, hypoglycemia, acute adrenal insufficiency (Chapter 8), or hyperglycemia will not be reversed through basic life support. Although proper employment of these steps is absolutely vital to ensure the patient's survival, in each of these cases definitive management involving specific drug therapy is required for the patient to regain consciousness. These situations will be described in subsequent chapters.

10 *Respiratory Difficulty: General Considerations*

Difficulty in breathing can be a most disconcerting problem for a patient who is conscious yet unable to breathe normally. The most common causes of respiratory difficulty will be described in this section. Because the patient usually remains conscious throughout the episode of respiratory difficulty, the psychologic aspects of patient management are extremely important. Definitions of relevant terms follow:

anoxia No oxygen

apnea No respiratory movements

dyspnea Subjective sense of shortness of breath; "air hunger"

hyperpnea Greater than normal minute ventilation just meeting metabolic demands

hyperventilation Ventilation that exceeds metabolic demands; $Paco_2$ less than 35 torr

hypoventilation Ventilation that does not meet metabolic demands; $Paco_2$ over 45 torr

hypoxia Deficiency of oxygen in the inspired air

orthopnea Inability to breathe except in the upright position

$Paco_2$ Arterial carbon dioxide tension (normal is 35 to 45 torr)

Pao_2 Arterial oxygen tension (normal [air] is 75 to 100 torr)

respiration Process of gas exchange whereby O_2 is gained and CO_2 lost from the body

tachypnea Greater than normal respiratory rate

torr Unit of pressure equal to 1 mm Hg (named for Torricelli)

ventilation, alveolar Volume of air exchanged per minute (volume/breath − dead space × respiratory rate)

In most instances involving loss of consciousness, the primary factor producing airway obstruction is the tongue, and the steps of basic life support described in Section II are designed to eliminate this as a factor. In Section III discussion of the management of airway obstruction continues.

Respiratory difficulty will usually not present the dental office staff with an acute life-threatening situation; however, prompt recognition and management are mandatory because the patient will not be receiving a normal supply of oxygen during the episode, and it is quite possible that complications resulting from hypoxia or hypercarbia may ensue. On the other hand, lower airway obstruction is truly an acute life-threatening situation in which the patient may be receiving little or no oxygen. Recognition must be prompt and management equally prompt and effective.

PREDISPOSING FACTORS

Table 10-1 lists potential causes of respiratory difficulty. In most of these situations, however, the patient does not exhibit respiratory difficulty unless the underlying medical disorder becomes acutely exacerbated. Examples of this include acute myocardial infarction, anaphylaxis, cerebrovascular accident, hyperglycemia, and hypoglycemia. Knowledge of the primary medical disorder therefore permits the doctor to modify dental management of the patient so as to prevent the exacerbation of the underlying disorder. However, there are situations, including asthma and heart failure, in which the patient has chronic respiratory disorders. Breathing difficulty may be present at all times with these disorders, particularly heart failure, and measures must be taken by the doctor to prevent their exacerbation during dental therapy.

A major factor leading to acute exacerbation of respiratory disorders is undue stress, either physio-

137

Table 10-1. Possible causes of respiratory difficulty

Cause	Frequency	Where discussed
Hyperventilation syndrome	Most common	Respiratory difficulty (Section III)
Vasodepressor syncope	Most common	Unconsciousness (Section II)
Asthma	Common	Respiratory difficulty (Section III)
Heart failure	Common	Respiratory difficulty (Section III)
Hypoglycemia	Common	Altered consciousness (Section IV)
Overdose reaction	Less common	Drug-related emergencies (Section VI)
Acute myocardial infarction	Rare	Chest pain (Section VII)
Anaphylaxis	Rare	Allergy (Chapter 24)
Angioneurotic edema	Rare	Allergy (Chapter 24)
Cerebrovascular accident	Rare	Altered consciousness (Section IV)
Epilepsy	Rare	Seizure disorders (Chapter 21)
Hyperglycemic reaction	Rare	Altered consciousness (Section IV)

logic or psychologic. Indeed, the hyperventilation syndrome and vasodepressor syncope, which represent the most commonly encountered emergency situations in dentistry, are almost exclusively precipitated by psychologic stress. Psychologic stress in dentistry is the primary factor in the intensification of preexisting medical disorders.

Although hyperventilation and vasodepressor syncope are rarely causes of respiratory difficulty in pediatric patients, children with asthma may exhibit acute episodes of bronchospasm in stressful situations.

PREVENTION

Adequate pretreatment medical and dental evaluation of the prospective dental patient can often prevent respiratory difficulty. Once aware of medical disorders that may lead to these problems, the doctor can modify patient management to minimize the exacerbation of these conditions. When anxiety is a major factor, psychosedative procedures and stress-reduction techniques should also be employed.

CLINICAL MANIFESTATIONS

Clinical manifestations of respiratory distress vary according to the degree of breathing difficulty. In most cases the patient remains conscious throughout the episode. Although consciousness is an encouraging sign, indicating that the patient is receiving at least the minimum supply of oxygen required for consciousness, it creates an additional problem, which is the development of acute anxiety in the patient. For this reason the doctor managing the situation must at all times remain calm—or appear to be calm—and in control of the situation.

The sounds associated with distressed breathing and the clinical symptomatology vary with the cause of the problem. In asthma one can usually hear a characteristic wheezing sound produced by the turbulent flow of air through partially occluded bronchioles. In heart failure, cough may be present, as well as other sounds associated with pulmonary venous congestion. A more detailed discussion and a differential diagnosis of respiratory difficulty follows.

PATHOPHYSIOLOGY

Various parts of the respiratory system are involved in the different syndromes producing respiratory difficulty. In *asthma,* for example, the bronchioles are the primary site of the disorder. In patients with asthma the bronchi become highly reactive and demonstrate significant smooth muscle activity (bronchoconstriction) in response to various substances. The clinical signs and symptoms of asthma are therefore related in large part to the restriction of breathing produced by bronchospasm.

In *heart failure,* respiratory difficulty is usually the first sign and symptom noted. Respiratory difficulty is produced by chronic overutilization of the oxygen in the blood and an inability of the lungs to fully oxgenate venous blood. It is related to pulmonary venous engorgement with exudation of fluid into alveolar air sacs. This excess fluid prevents portions of the lung from participating in the ventilatory process, producing many of the signs and symptoms associated with heart failure.

The *hyperventilation syndrome* is a generalized problem. The primary site of the disorder is in the mind of the patient, and its clinical signs and

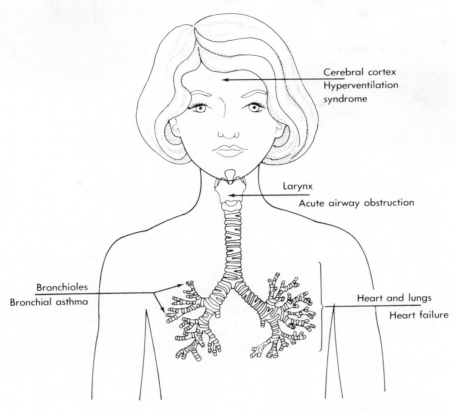

Fig. 10-1. Sites of origin of various respiratory difficulties.

symptoms are produced by an alteration in the chemical makeup of the blood. An excessive amount of carbon dioxide is eliminated through rapid breathing, which leads to a situation known as respiratory alkalosis. This in turn produces many of the clinical signs and symptoms of hyperventilation. If successfully managed, the hyperventilation syndrome produces no residual effects. However, heart failure and asthma may produce permanent changes in the respiratory system. Therefore patients subject to episodes of asthma or heart failure require special management considerations during all phases of dental therapy.

Acute lower airway obstruction is a life-threatening situation in which a foreign object becomes occluded in the respiratory tract. The level at which this object occludes the airway determines the severity of the situation and to some degree the manner in which it may be managed. If an object enters either of the mainstem bronchi, the situation is dangerous but not immediately life threatening. The chances are excellent that the foreign body will

enter the right mainstem bronchus because of the angle at which this bronchus branches off of the trachea. In this situation all or part of the right lung is cut off from ventilation, but the patient is still able to maintain adequate ventilation with the left lung. Hospitalization is required, but the patient's life is not in immediate danger. However, if the foreign object becomes impacted in the trachea, total airway obstruction ensues—an acutely life-threatening situation. Immediate recognition and management are required to prevent permanent neurologic damage and death. The management of this situation will be discussed in Chapter 11. Fig 10-1 points out the sites of various respiratory system disorders.

MANAGEMENT

Definitive management of respiratory difficulty is based on recognition of the problem and a determination of the probable cause of the situation. The following basic steps are common to the management of most cases of respiratory difficulty.

MANAGEMENT OF
RESPIRATORY DIFFICULTY

Step 1 Recognition of respiratory difficulty
Sounds (wheezing, cough)
Abnormal rate and/or depth of respiration

   2 Termination of dental procedure

   3 Position patient, implement basic life support
Unconscious—supine position
Conscious—upright position usually preferred by patient

   4 Monitor vital signs
Blood pressure, heart rate (pulse), respiratory rate

   5 Symptomatic management of patient

   6 Definitive management of respiratory difficulty

Step 1. Recognition of respiratory difficulty. Many of the disorders of respiration are associated with characteristic sounds such as the wheezing of asthma and the cough and moist respirations of heart failure. In hyperventilation there usually is no characteristic sound associated with the syndrome. However, patients appear to be and actually are acutely anxious and unable to control their breathing.

Step 2. Terminate the dental procedure. Dental therapy must be stopped as soon as the respiratory problem is recognized. Because stress is a primary precipitating factor in many of these situations, the clinical symptoms may be greatly improved merely by stopping dental treatment.

Step 3. Position patient and implement the steps of basic life support as needed. The patient presents with two major problems: the primary breathing difficulty and the superimposed problem of increased anxiety produced by the difficulty in breathing. A patient in respiratory distress who loses consciousness should immediately be placed in the supine position and managed as any other unconscious patient would be. Additional management is based on the steps of basic life support described in Chapter 5.

In most instances of acute respiratory distress, however, the flow of air into the lungs remains more than adequate to keep the victim from losing consciousness. In this situation, it is suggested that the patient assume any position that permits effective breathing. Most commonly the patient is positioned in the upright (sitting or standing) position. It is important to remember that this position can be permitted only as long as the patient remains conscious.

Step 4. Monitor vital signs. Measurement of the blood pressure, heart rate (pulse), and respiratory rate should be taken at this time and at intervals throughout the management of this situation. All measurements should be recorded for a permanent record.

Step 5. Manage signs and symptoms. The patient should be made as comfortable as possible at this time, and the doctor should begin to treat the anxiety component of this situation by speaking with the patient in a calm but firm manner. The patient's collar and other tight garments may be loosened because this enables the patient to breathe more freely.

Step 6. Definitive management of respiratory difficulty. After assessment of the cardiovascular status of the patient, the doctor may proceed to the definitive management of the situation. These procedures are described along with the major causes of respiratory difficulty in the chapters that follow. The management of respiratory difficulty is summarized in the box at left.

BIBLIOGRAPHY

Dailey, R.H., Difficulty in breathing. In Schwartz, G.R., and others, editors: Principles and practice of emergency medicine, Philadelphia, 1978, W.B. Saunders Co.

11 *Airway Obstruction*

[handwritten: asthmatic congestive heart failure]

[handwritten: primary source of hyperventilation is the mind.]

Airway obstruction must be recognized and managed as quickly as possible. For this reason, a rapid diagnosis of airway obstruction must be made and treatment initiated immediately.

In the practice of dentistry the potential is great for objects to fall into the posterior portion of the pharynx. Indeed, a great variety of devices and objects is recovered from the throats of patients every year. In my experience, items such as the head of a pedodontic handpiece, mouth mirror heads, and gold crowns have been recovered, either orally or from stool specimens, after having been swallowed accidentally. Reports in the literature have documented the retrieval of rubber dam clamps, endodontic instruments, and a post and core.

In the conscious dental patient the chances are excellent that any object "lost" in the pharynx will be swallowed by the patient and enter the esophagus or will be coughed up, so that the actual incidence of acute airway obstruction or aspiration is quite low. There is also a high probability that objects entering the trachea will be small enough to pass through the larynx without causing obstruction. In this situation the object will continue down the trachea (if gravity is assisting), coming to rest in a portion of one of the bronchi. While an acute life-threatening situation does not exist at this time, certain important steps (see below) must be carried out to ensure removal of the object and to avoid possible serious sequelae to the patient. However, the possibility that a foreign object will enter the trachea and lodge in it does exist, and for that reason the doctor must be familiar with techniques of removing such objects.

Foreign body aspiration while the patient is at home is a major cause of accidental death in chil-

dren under 6 years of age. Commonly implicated items include peanuts, uninflated balloons, and marbles. Baby aspirin, with a diameter of 7.5 mm, has caused death from an obstructed airway in several younger children. (The diameter of the glottic opening is about 6.5 mm in the 2-year-old child.)

In view of recent clinical research findings, the American Heart Association (1986) has recommended several changes in the techniques for the management of the obstructed airway in infants, children, and adults. These techniques are presented in this chapter.

In most cases the object causing the airway obstruction is firmly lodged where it cannot be seen or felt through the mouth without special equipment (laryngoscope, Magill forceps), which is not normally available. Therefore the doctor must be able to recognize the problem and act rapidly to dislodge the object from the airway.

MANAGEMENT OF "SWALLOWED" OBJECTS

In spite of our best efforts at prevention, small objects, such as inlays, alloy, burs, or pieces of debris, may fall into the oropharynx of a patient, with subsequent swallowing or aspiration. The introduction of sit-down, four-handed dentistry in which the patient is placed in a supine or semi-supine position during treatment has increased the possibility of this occurrence. Complications are associated with both swallowed and aspirated objects. Swallowed objects entering the gastrointestinal tract have produced GI blockage, abscess, perforation, and peritonitis. Objects aspirated into either the right or left bronchus can produce infection, lung abscess, pneumonia, and atelectasis.

[handwritten: Right lung has 3 lobes, left lung has 2 lobes]   *[handwritten: (wider opening)]*

141

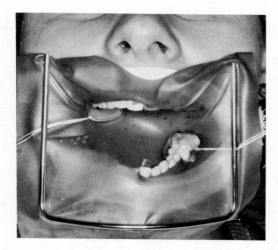

Fig. 11-1. Use of rubber dam, where possible, prevents entry of foreign objects into airway. (From Chasteen, J.: Four-handed dentistry in clinical practice, ed. 3, St. Louis, 1984, The C.V. Mosby Co.)

Barkmeier and colleagues (1978) state that two major *preventive* measures are use of a rubber dam and oral packing where applicable (Fig. 11-1). Proper use of these measures will minimize the occurrence of swallowed foreign objects.

When an object enters the oropharynx of a patient who is in a supine or semisupine position:

1. Do *not* allow the patient to sit up.
2. Position the chair into a head-down (Trendelenburg) position, permitting gravity to return the object to the oral cavity where it may be retrieved either by the patient's "coughing it up" or with an instrument such as a pick-up forceps or Magill forceps (Fig. 3-24).
3. If the object cannot be retrieved (that is, the patient "swallowed" it) radiographs are warranted to determine its location:
   a. Flat plate of abdomen, and/or
   b. Anteroposterior (AP) view of chest (Fig. 11-2), or
   c. Lateral view of chest
4. It is hoped that the object will be seen on the abdominal radiograph rather than on the chest radiograph within, for example, a bronchus.
5. If the object cannot be located or if any question exists as to its location or any potential complications, immediate consultation is recommended.

In situations in which the foreign body presumably enters the patient's trachea, the following management is recommended:

1. Do *not* allow patient to sit up.
2. Position the chair into a head-down position (Trendelenburg) with patient lying on the right side.
3. The patient may cough spontaneously; if not, encourage coughing to aid in retrieval.
4. Back blows delivered forcefully between the shoulder blades will assist in retrieval (Fig. 11-3).
5. Should the patient stop coughing and state that the object has been "swallowed," do not permit patient to leave your care until the object has been located by radiograph to ensure it is not in the trachea. *Only if the object is recovered should the patient be discharged without radiograph.*
6. If the object is not recovered, the doctor should accompany the patient to the emergency room of an acute care facility.
7. If the object is determined to be in the tracheobronchial tree, it is most often located in the right bronchus (because of the more direct path of the right bronchus compared to the left at the bifurcation of the trachea).
8. Retrieval of this object from the bronchus may involve use of the following:
   a. Fiberoptic bronchoscope to locate object
   b. Bronchoscopy to remove object
   c. Thoracotomy, if bronchoscopy is unsuccessful

In the situations just described an immediate life-threatening emergency does not exist; however, unless the object in question is retrieved, the patient must be managed carefully to prevent possibly serious sequelae.

RECOGNITION OF AIRWAY OBSTRUCTION

Total airway obstruction in the conscious patient with spontaneous respiratory movement is manifested clinically by the victim's gasping for breath with great effort, demonstrating suprasternal retraction (expansion of the thoracic cavity with the soft tissue areas—particularly the suprasternal notch and supraclavicular regions—drawn in because of the increased negative pressure in the chest). If the obstruction is total, there will be no noise associated with it. The victim usually grabs at the throat and in many instances panics and flees

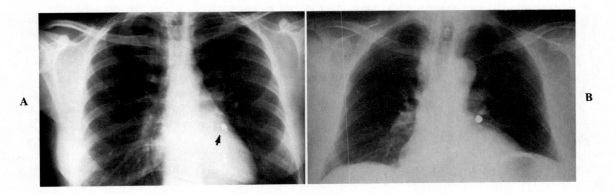

Fig. 11-2. A, Anteroposterior view of chest demonstrating rubber prophylaxis cup (arrow). **B,** Gold crown that had been aspirated into the left lung of patient.

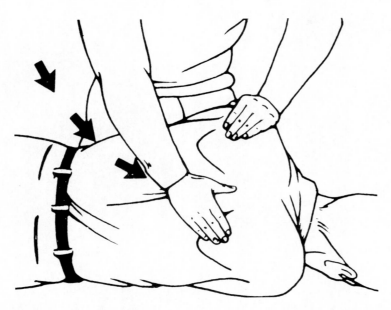

Fig. 11-3. Victim is placed on his right side, and if needed, back blows are delivered. Rescuer delivers sharp blows with open palm between shoulder blades of victim. (Reprinted from Dental Survey © 1976 by Harcourt Brace Jovanovich, Inc.)

from the scene. Because total airway obstruction usually occurs during inspiration, there is usually adequate oxygen left in the cerebral blood to permit up to 2 minutes of consciousness. If the obstruction is not recognized and managed and oxygen delivered to the victim's lungs, blood, and brain, permanent neurologic damage occurs within 3 to 5 minutes.

REVIEW OF BASIC AIRWAY MANEUVERS

Once the patient with an obstructed airway loses consciousness, the steps of basic life support, including airway maintenance (Chapter 5) must be applied. These steps are directed at the removal of the most common cause of airway obstruction—the tongue. Performance of the steps allows the rescuer to determine whether the tongue is or is not the cause of the problem and whether further steps must be taken. In those instances in which a lower airway obstruction is obvious (such as obstruction occurring immediately after a crown or a dental instrument is "swallowed"), the basic steps may be bypassed and the rescuer may proceed directly to the establishment of an emergency airway.

Step 1. Position patient. Supine position with the feet elevated slightly (Fig. 11-4).

Step 2. Head tilt. Extension of neck tissues is accomplished by head tilt–chin lift (Fig. 11-5).

Step 3. Assess airway and breathing. The rescuer's ear is placed 1 inch from the victim's mouth and nose, listening and feeling for the passage of air while looking toward the chest of the victim and watching for respiratory movement (Fig. 11-6).

Step 4. Jaw thrust maneuver (only if indicated). Rescuer places fingers behind the posterior border of the ramus of the mandible and displaces the mandible anteriorly while tilting the head back-ward and opening the mouth with other fingers (Fig. 11-7).

Step 5. Assess airway and breathing.

Step 6. Artificial ventilation (only if indicated). When the tongue is the cause of the airway obstruction, these steps usually result in a patent airway. When these steps have been carried out properly and the airway remains obstructed (diagnosed by continued lack of "hearing and seeing," aphonia, and suprasternal retraction), the rescuer should consider the possibility that the obstruction is located within the larynx or trachea and proceed to establish an emergency airway.

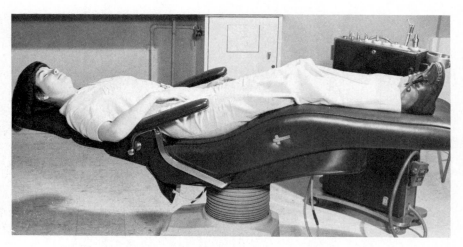

Fig. 11-4. Place patient in the supine position with feet elevated.

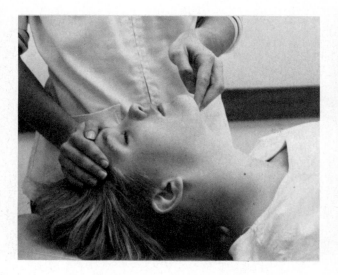

Fig. 11-5. Head tilt–chin lift.

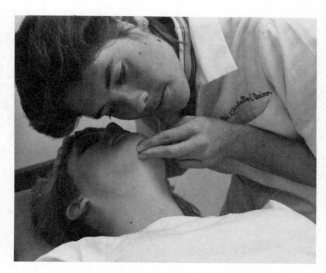

Fig. 11-6. Look, listen, and feel.

ESTABLISHMENT OF AN EMERGENCY AIRWAY

When a patient's airway is obstructed, establishment of a patent airway becomes the major goal of therapy. There are a variety of procedures available for establishing an emergency airway, and there is also a degree of controversy over some of them. Two procedures (tracheotomy and cricothyrotomy) require surgical intervention and therefore considerable knowledge and technical skill in order to be carried out effectively. A third procedure, which is nonsurgical, is the procedure of choice for the initial management of all obstructed airways when basic life support techniques for airway management prove inadequate. This is the *external subdiaphragmatic compression* technique, properly known as the abdominal thrust, or the Heimlich maneuver. Because this procedure is nonsurgical, serious complications are less likely to occur, a fact that makes it particularly useful in the dental office. The American Heart Association and the American Red Cross consider the abdominal thrust procedure to be an integral part of the emergency procedures to be followed when lower airway obstruction is a possibility, a situation responsible for 3100 deaths in 1984.

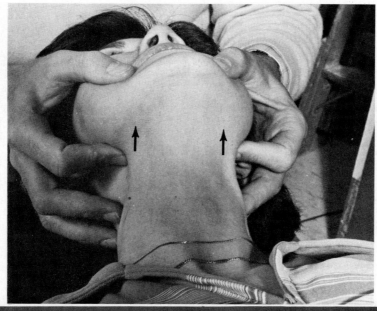

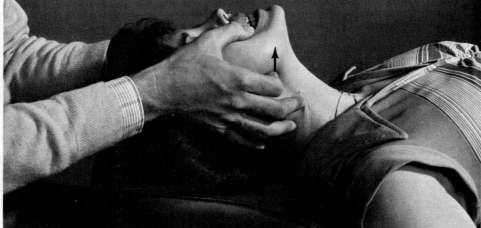

Fig. 11-7. Jaw thrust maneuver: *top,* front view; *bottom,* side view.

Table 11-1. Signs and symptoms of poor air exchange

Weak, ineffective cough
High-pitched "crowing" sound on inhalation
Increased respiratory difficulty
Ashen-gray color of skin
Possible cyanosis of nail beds and mucous membranes

Don't interrupt a coughing pt.

NONINVASIVE PROCEDURES FOR OBSTRUCTED AIRWAY

When foreign objects enter the tracheobronchial tree, a potentially life-threatening situation exists. Airway obstruction may be partial or total. Management of the situation will vary according to the degree of obstruction and the effectiveness of the patient's cough reflex. Manual, noninvasive procedures will be used wherever possible. Surgical procedures, used when all else fails, are also within the doctor's expertise and will be described.

A victim with a partial obstruction of the airway who is capable of forceful coughing and is breathing adequately (that is, no evidence of cyanosis or duskiness) should be *left alone*. Although a degree of wheezing may be evident between coughs, a forceful cough is highly effective in removing foreign objects. *Do not interfere with this victim.*

Should the victim of a partial airway obstruction demonstrate poor air exchange initially or if previously good air exchange becomes ineffective, the victim must be managed as if a complete obstruction existed. Table 11-1 lists clinical signs of poor air exchange.

In total airway obstruction the victim is unable to speak or make any sound, to breathe, or to cough. The victim will retain consciousness as long as the oxygen level of the blood is sufficiently high. This may range from 10 seconds to 2 minutes, depending on whether the obstruction occurred during inspiration (more oxygen in the blood) or expiration (less oxygen in the blood). Fortunately, most airway obstructions occur during inhalation so that the lungs are somewhat filled with oxygen and are inflated, thereby making the following procedure more effective. The victim may clutch the neck (Fig. 11-8) in the universal distress signal. Prompt management is essential, because the victim will lose consciousness and die unless a patent airway is reestablished without delay.

Several manual, noninvasive procedures are available for use in these situations. Each technique

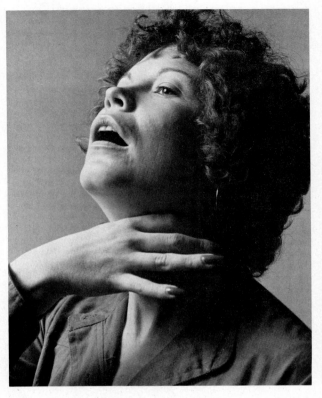

Fig. 11-8. Recommended universal distress signal for obstructed airway; victim clutches neck.

will be described, followed by the recommended sequencing of these techniques in actual situations. The manual, noninvasive techniques are as follows:
1. Back blows
2. Manual thrusts
   a. Heimlich maneuver (abdominal thrust)
   b. Chest thrust
3. Finger sweeps

Back Blows

Back blows formed an integral part of previous regimens for the removal of foreign objects from the airway. However, data presented at the 1985 National Conference on Cardiopulmonary Resuscitation and Emergency Cardiac Care suggested that, as a single method, back blows may not be as effective as the Heimlich maneuver in adults (Day et al., 1982). For this reason the Heimlich maneuver is the only method recommended at this time for the adult or child obstructed airway.

Back blows remain an integral part of the protocol for management of the obstructed airway in the infant. When back blows are performed on the infant, the patient is straddled over the rescuer's arm, with the head lower than the trunk and the head supported by firmly holding the jaw. The rescuer rests his or her hand on his or her thigh and delivers four back blows forcefully with the heel of the hand between the infant's shoulder blades (Fig. 11-9).

Manual Thrusts

Manual thrusts are a series of 6 to 10 thrusts to the upper abdomen (Heimlich maneuver or abdominal thrust) or to the lower chest (chest thrust). They function to rapidly increase intrathoracic pressure, acting as an artificial cough, which may help to dislodge a foreign body. The objective of each thrust should be to relieve the obstruction without having to complete the full series. Studies (Gordon, 1977; Guildner, 1976) have demonstrated that there are no significant differences between abdominal and chest thrusts in the amount of air flow, pressure, and volume.

There are several special situations that may indicate the use of one technique rather than the other. The *chest thrust* is indicated for use in advanced stages of pregnancy and in markedly obese individuals. The chest thrust is also less likely to cause regurgitation than the abdominal thrust. Chest thrusts are recommended in infants because of the greater possibility of organ damage (for example, the liver) with abdominal thrusts. The abdominal thrust is recommended especially in older patients, whose more brittle ribs are more likely to be fractured in chest thrust, and in children.

Internal injury is a possibility whenever the abdominal or chest thrust is employed. Injury has been reported to both thoracic and abdominal organs, including the liver, spleen, and stomach. Proper hand positioning can minimize these potential side effects. The rescuer's hands must never be located over the xiphoid process or over the lower margins of the rib cage. In the Heimlich maneuver the hands are below this area, while in chest thrust they are above it. Following successful application of a manual thrust technique, the patient should be evaluated by medical personnel for evidence of any secondary injury, such as abdominal bleeding, before the patient is discharged.

Heimlich Maneuver

The Heimlich maneuver is also known as subdiaphragmatic abdominal thrusts and the abdominal thrust. First described in 1975 by Dr. Henry J.

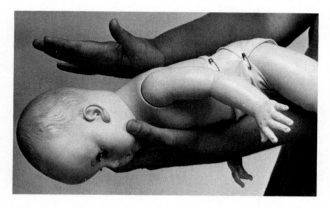

Fig. 11-9. Back blows—four back blows are delivered with heel of hand between shoulder blades of infant victim.

Heimlich, this maneuver is today recommended as the primary technique for relieving foreign-body airway obstruction in the adult and child.

TECHNIQUE. Conscious victim—standing or sitting (Figs. 11-10 and 11-11)

1. Stand behind the victim and wrap your arms around the victim's waist and under the victim's arms.
2. Grasp one fist with other hand, placing the thumb side of the fist against the victim's abdomen. The hand is held in midline slightly above the umbilicus and well below the tip of the xiphoid process (Fig. 11-10).
3. Repeat inward and upward thrusts until either the foreign body is expelled or the victim loses consciousness (Fig. 11-11).

TECHNIQUE. Unconscious victim

1. Position the victim in the supine position.
2. Open the victim's airway (head-tilt) and turn the head up. The head is turned up to (1) avoid airway obstruction by kinking the airway, (2) facilitate foreign body movement up the airway, and (3) allow the foreign body to be seen.
3. Position of rescuer:
   a. It is recommended that the rescuer straddle the victim's thighs. This position will be difficult to achieve with a victim in the dental chair.
   b. Rescuer alongside victim (Fig. 11-12). The rescuer's knees are close to the victim's hips on either the right or left side of the victim. This position, with the rescuer standing astride the victim's hips, is useful when the victim is in the dental chair (Fig. 11-13).

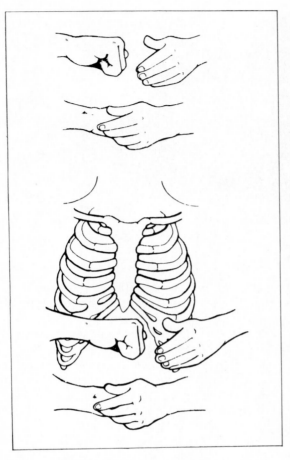

Fig. 11-10. Technique of abdominal thrust.

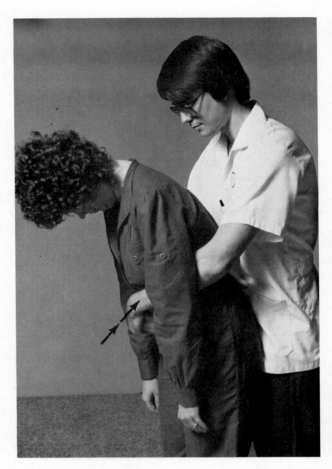

Fig. 11-11. Abdominal thrust—conscious victim.

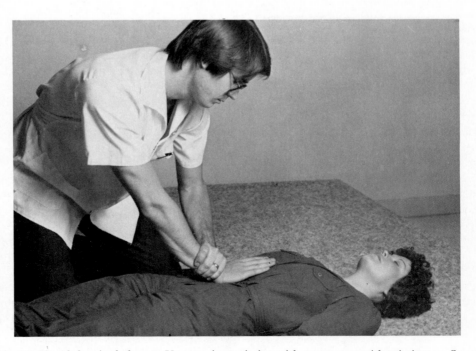

Fig. 11-12. Abdominal thrust. Unconscious victim with rescuer astride victim on floor. Victim's head is up, not turned to side.

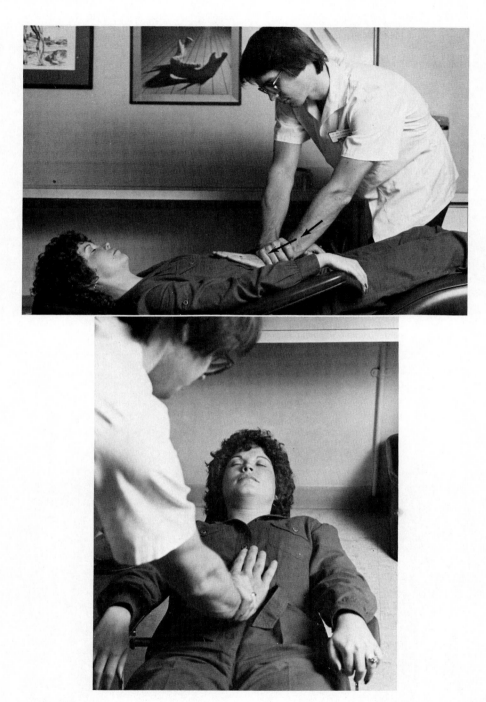

Fig. 11-13. Abdominal thrust—unconscious victim in dental chair with rescuer astride victim. Force of compression must be in upward, not lateral, direction. Victim's head is kept in "up" position.

4. Place the heel of one hand against the victim's abdomen in the midline slightly above the umbilicus and well below the tip of the xiphoid process.
5. Place the second hand directly on top of the first hand.
6. Press into the victim's abdomen with a quick inward and upward thrust. Force must *not* be directed laterally.
7. Perform 6 to 10 abdominal thrusts.

Some final points concerning the technique: this technique is exclusively a *soft tissue* procedure. No bony structures should be involved (ribs or sternum). In all cases the rescuer must apply pressure with the heel of the hand *below the rib cage*. The maneuver is not a bear hug. If carried out as one, injury to intraabdominal organs such as the liver and spleen or to the sternum and ribs could occur. After successful completion of the procedure, transport the victim to the local hospital emergency room or to his or her personal physician for evaluation.

Chest thrust

The chest thrust is an alternative to the Heimlich maneuver as a technique for opening an obstructed airway in special situations only. Studies have demonstrated that there is no substantial difference in the effectiveness of these techniques when performed properly. Table 11-2 lists the indications and contraindications for the chest thrust.

TECHNIQUE. Conscious victim—standing or sitting (Fig. 11-14)
1. Stand behind the victim; place your arms directly under the victim's armpits, encircling the victim's chest.
2. Grasp one fist with the other hand, placing the thumb side of the fist on the middle of the sternum, not on the xiphoid process or on the margins of the rib cage.
3. Perform backward thrusts until the foreign body is expelled or the victim becomes unconscious.

TECHNIQUE. Unconscious victim (Fig. 11-15)
1. Place victim in the supine position.
2. Open the victim's airway (head-tilt) and leave victim's head up.

Table 11-2. Chest thrust

Indications	Contraindications
Infant (<1 year old) and child (1 to 8 years old)	Older victim
Pregnant female	
Extreme obesity	

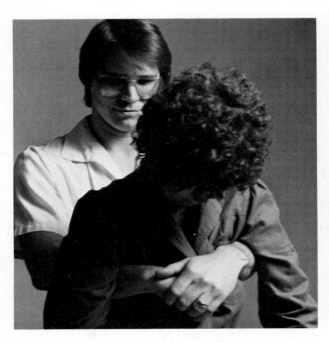

Fig. 11-14. Chest thrust—conscious victim.

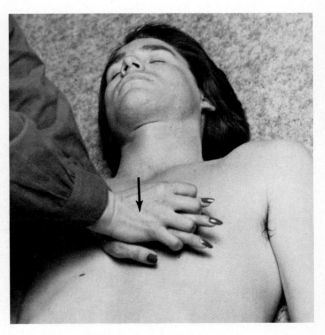

Fig. 11-15. Chest thrust—unconscious victim.

3. Either straddle or stand astride the victim, as described in abdominal thrust.
4. Hand position and technique for chest thrust are identical to those of closed chest cardiac compression (Chapter 30): Place heel of hand on lower half of sternum with second hand on top of it but not on xiphoid process.
5. Exert 6 to 10 quick, downward thrusts to compress the chest cavity.

Finger Sweep

In the conscious victim it is difficult to remove foreign bodies from the airway with fingers. When the victim loses consciousness, the muscles relax and it becomes easier for the rescuer to open the mouth and insert fingers into the oral cavity to seek and remove foreign objects. Special care must be observed when probing with a finger in an infant's or small child's airway so as not to inadvertently force the foreign body deeper into the airway. *Therefore blind finger sweeps in the infant and child are not recommended.* Foreign bodies may, however, be removed from the airway by this technique if they are located above the level of the epiglottis. Finger sweep is only performed in the unconscious person.

TECHNIQUE. Finger sweep (Fig. 11-16)
1. Place the victim in supine position with head up.
2. Grasp the victim's tongue and anterior portion of the mandible.
   a. This technique, called the *tongue-jaw lift,* pulls the tongue off the posterior wall of the pharynx, away from a foreign object that may be lodged there.
   b. If the tongue-jaw lift is ineffective, the crossed finger technique (Fig. 11-16) is used. The mouth is opened by crossing the index finger and thumb between the teeth and pushing the teeth apart.
3. Place the index finger of the other hand along the inside of the cheek, deeply into the pharynx at the base of the tongue.
4. Using a hooking movement, attempt to dislodge the foreign body and move it into the mouth where it can be removed. Care must be taken not to force the object more deeply into the airway.

Devices for removing foreign bodies, such as Kelly clamps or a Magill forceps, are recommended for use by trained rescuers only (Fig. 11-17) and only with direct visualization (for example, laryngoscope, or tongue blade and flashlight). There is no evidence, however, to support the use of devices such as the Choke Saver or Throat-E-Vac.

Recommended Sequences

The American Heart Association (1986) recommends the following sequences for removing airway obstruction.

Adult conscious victim, obstructed airway

1. Identify complete airway obstruction. Ask "Are you choking?"
2. Identify yourself as someone who will help the victim: "I can help you."
3. Apply Heimlich maneuver until either the foreign body is expelled or the victim becomes unconscious.

Adult conscious victim, known obstructed airway, who loses consciousness

1. Place victim in supine position; call for help.
2. Activate the EMS system (that is, dial the 911 number if the system is available locally), if a second person is available.
3. Open mouth using tongue-jaw lift.
4. Perform finger sweep.

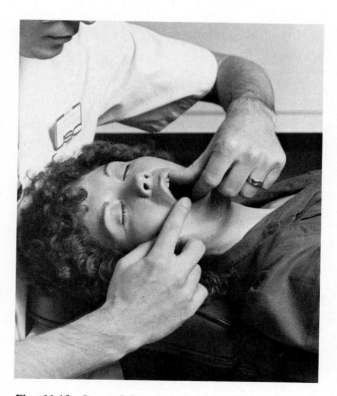

Fig. 11-16. Crossed-finger technique aids in opening mouth of unconscious victim.

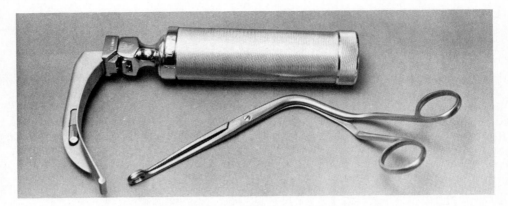

Fig. 11-17. Magill forceps and laryngoscope (*top*).

5. Attempt to ventilate. If ineffective:
6. Perform 6 to 10 abdominal thrusts.
7. Check for foreign body: finger sweep.
8. Attempt to ventilate. If ineffective:
9. Repeat steps 6 to 8 until successful.

Adult unconscious victim, cause unknown

1. Rescuer manages unconscious victim in usual manner:
   a. Assess unresponsiveness.
   b. Place victim in supine position.
   c. Call for help.
   d. Open airway.
   e. Assess breathlessness (look, listen, feel) and:
   f. Attempt to ventilate; if unsuccessful:
2. Reposition head and attempt to ventilate. If still unsuccessful, activate EMS system (call 911) and:
3. Heimlich maneuver: perform 6 to 10 abdominal thrusts.
4. Foreign body check: finger sweep.
5. Attempt to ventilate. If ineffective:
6. Repeat steps 3 to 5 until successful.

Procedures for Infants and Children

Foreign body airway obstruction in children (ages 1 to 8 years) is managed similarly to that in adults, namely with the Heimlich maneuver as a primary technique. However, in the infant victim (under the age of 1 year) the combination of back blows and chest thrusts continues to be recommended. The basic rescue procedures include the following steps:

1. Determine unresponsiveness.
2. Call for help.

3. Position the victim.
4. A (airway): Open airway (head tilt–chin lift).
5. B (breathing): Assess breathing.
6. Perform artificial ventilation. If ineffective:
7. Reattempt ventilation. If ineffective:
8. Activate EMS.
9. Manage airway obstruction (see following section).
10. C (circulation): determine presence or absence of pulse.
11. Perform external chest compression, if necessary.

Infants (Fig. 11-18)

1. Back blows:
   a. Supporting the head and neck with one hand, place the infant face down with the head lower than the trunk, straddling your forearm and supported on your thigh.
   b. Deliver four back blows forcefully between the shoulder blades with the heel of the hand.
2. Chest thrusts:
   a. While supporting the head and neck, sandwich the infant between your hands and the infant face up with the head lower than the trunk.
   b. Deliver four thrusts in the midsternal region in the same manner as external chest compressions, but at a slower rate.
3. Foreign body check:
   a. Do a tongue-jaw lift by placing a thumb in infant's mouth, over the tongue. Lift tongue and jaw with fingers wrapped over lower jaw.
   b. Remove the foreign body *if visualized*.

Don't do finger sweeps on babies + small kids.

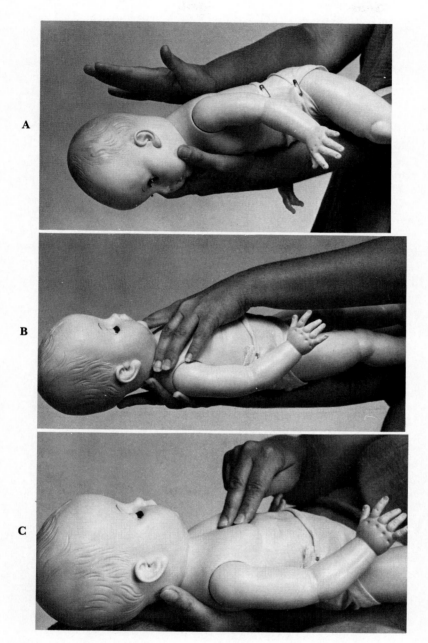

Fig. 11-18. Infant obstructed airway. **A,** Infant is supported by rescuer's forearm. Head lower than rest of body for back blows. **B,** Turning infant over, infant is supported between two arms of rescuer. **C,** Chest thrusts are applied to midsternum of victim with two fingers.

4. Attempt to ventilate:
   a. Open airway with head tilt–chin lift.
   b. Attempt to ventilate. If unsuccessful:
5. Repeat these steps until successful.

Children *(Fig. 11-19)*

The following steps are instituted when the basic procedures presented above have proved to be ineffective in reestablishing a patent airway.

1. Heimlich maneuver:
   a. Kneel at victim's feet if on floor, or stand at victim's feet if on a table.
   b. Place heel of one hand against victim's abdomen in the midline slightly above the navel and well below the tip of the xiphoid process.
   c. Place second hand directly on top of first hand.
   d. Press into abdomen with 6 to 10 abdominal thrusts.
2. Foreign body check:
   a. Keep victim's face up.
   b. Use tongue-jaw lift to open mouth.

   c. Look into mouth and remove foreign body *if visualized*.
3. Attempt to ventilate:
   a. Open airway with head tilt–chin lift.
   b. Attempt to ventilate. If unsuccessful:
4. Repeat steps 1 to 3 until successful.

The sequences presented above for the infant and child should be repeated until the foreign body has been successfully removed or until the rescuer feels that time has been exhausted. At this time a *cricothyrotomy* should be seriously considered, *if the rescuer is well trained in the procedure and has the necessary equipment available.*

INVASIVE PROCEDURES FOR OBSTRUCTED AIRWAYS
Tracheotomy versus cricothyrotomy

The techniques described previously are highly successful in removing foreign objects from the airways of most victims. However, situations have occurred in which these noninvasive techniques were ineffective in removing the object (for example, a dental cotton roll) from the victim's airway. In this situation and in others in which the airway is being obstructed by the swelling of tissues, such as

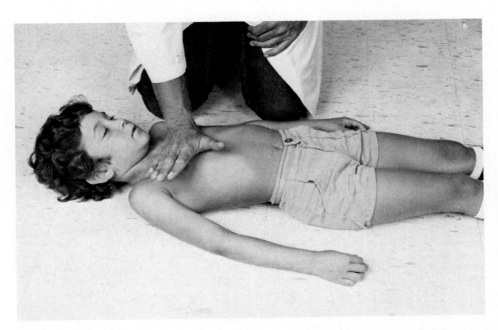

Fig. 11-19. Obstructed airway in a child. Victim placed on floor, face up. Rescuer uses heel of one hand to deliver chest thrusts on lower half of sternum.

laryngeal edema or epiglottitis caused by allergy or illness, invasive procedures may be required if a successful outcome is desired.

Surgical opening of the airway may be carried out in several ways. Two of the most commonly employed are the tracheotomy and the cricothyrotomy. Each of these techcniques has its adherents and its critics within the medical community but each is of importance, for they both permit oxygen to enter the victim's lungs. These procedures should be performed *only* by persons trained in these techniques and if *proper equipment* is available.

Tracheotomy has been used for more than 2000 years, yet its role in management of acute airway obstruction has undergone change in recent decades. It was once considered the primary technique to be employed for the relief of sudden airway embarrassment. For a variety of reasons, cricothyrotomy is now considered by many to be the surgical procedure of choice in sudden airway obstruction. In the typical dental situation there is almost no indication for tracheotomy.

Tracheotomy is a surgical procedure now usually employed for long-term airway maintenance and is not well suited for emergency airways. The tracheotomy site contains numerous anatomically important structures, such as the isthmus of the thyroid gland and several large and important blood vessels and nerves. The potential for perforating the esophagus also exists. Complications occur more commonly with tracheotomy even when it is performed slowly and meticulously under controlled conditions, such as in an oxygenated, well-ventilated patient in an operating room, than occur with cricothyrotomy. Hemorrhage and pneumothorax are major complications of tracheotomy, and there is also a risk of penetrating the isthmus of the thyroid gland. In most cases the bleeding that occurs is a major surgical complication that could not be handled satisfactorily in the dental office.

Cricothyroid membrane puncture (cricothyrotomy, cricothyroidotomy) is carried out more easily and quickly than is tracheotomy, and the incidence of complications is significantly lower. Anatomically no significant structures overlie the cricothyroid membrane. Weiss (1973) stated, "It provides the most accessible point of entry into the respiratory tree inferior to the glottis." The incision is made through skin, adipose tissue, and fascia. Bleeding is seldom encountered in cricothyrotomy (aside from minor bleeding from the skin incision). Inadvertent perforation of the posterior wall of the trachea and laceration of the underlying esophagus are prevented by the fact that the cricoid cartilage has

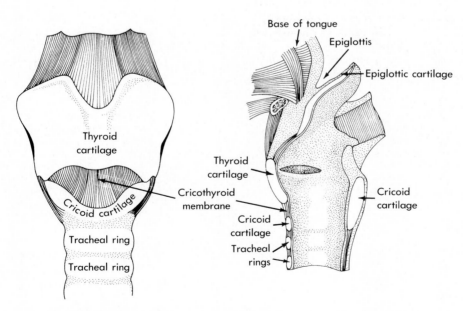

Fig. 11-20. Anatomic relationships of importance in cricothyrotomy.

an intact posterior segment (Fig. 11-20). An incision in the membrane begins to heal within a few days.

Cricothyrotomy
Anatomy

The ability to rapidly locate the proper site for the cricothyrotomy is important. The rationale behind any surgical emergency airway procedure is that the opening being made must be *below* the obstruction to be effective. Where, then, is foreign material most likely to impact in the trachea?

In the adult the narrowest portion of the trachea is located at the larynx. Most objects that produce obstruction come to rest in this area. Objects small enough to pass through the larynx and enter the trachea normally pass into one of the two mainstem bronchi, usually the right, producing an occlusion of one lung or a significant portion of it. This situation, discussed previously, is not acutely life threatening, although the victim will require hospitalization and perhaps a surgical procedure to remove the object.

In the infant the narrowest portion of the trachea occurs a short distance below the vocal cords. Obstruction is likely to occur at this site, making the cricothyrotomy ineffectual. Immediate management of this situation requires inverting the infant and applying manual thrusts and back blows.

The thyroid cartilage, largest of the tracheal cartilages, and the cricoid cartilage (the second tracheal cartilage) represent the anatomic landmarks for the cricothyrotomy (Figs. 11-20 and 11-21). The thyroid and cricoid cartilages represent the only two tracheal cartilages that are complete rings, the other tracheal rings being open on their posterior aspects. A membranous structure, the cricothyroid membrane, forms the anterior connection between these two cartilaginous rings and is the precise site for the cricothyrotomy. It may be readily located by placing a finger on the laryngeal prominence (Adam's apple) of the thyroid cartilage and moving the finger inferiorly until a slight depression is located. This is the cricothyroid membrane. Inferior to this depression is the prominence of the cricoid cartilage. The cricoid cartilage lies inferior to the incision, whereas the thyroid cartilage and vocal cords are superior to it.

Equipment

A scalpel with a straight (No. 11) blade may be employed in cricothyrotomy. Alternatively, it has been suggested that a 13-gauge, ½-inch long needle be used. Many other devices are available for use in cricothyrotomy.

One such device* that greatly facilitates the cricothyrotomy procedure is shown in Fig. 11-22. It contains the following sterile components: (a) a knife blade, (b) a puncturing mechanism, a two-part needle with a needle stylet, (c) an arcuate point

*Nu-Trake, manufactured by International Medical Devices, Inc., 19205 Parthenia, Northridge, CA 91324.

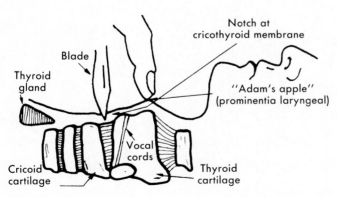

Fig. 11-21. Cricothyrotomy: incision is made inferior to the thyroid cartilage and superior to cricoid cartilage.

MANAGEMENT OF ACUTE AIRWAY OBSTRUCTION

Step 1 Recognize unconsciousness
2 Call for help
3 Position victim (supine)
4 Head tilt
5 Assess airway and breathing
6 Attempt to ventilate
7 Reposition head (head tilt) and attempt to ventilate
8 Jaw thrust maneuver
9 Attempt to ventilate
10 Activate EMS system (call 911)
11 Deliver 6 to 10 abdominal thrusts
12 Check mouth for foreign body
13 Attempt to ventilate
14 Repeat steps 11 to 13 until successful
15 Cricothyrotomy

at one end of the stylet to permit initial penetration of the cricothyroid membrane, (d) airways of 4, 6, and 8 mm diameters, and (e) obturators for the airways.

Although any of these instruments when properly used is effective in creating an emergency airway, I strongly recommend that only those devices with which the doctor is intimately familiar be considered.

Technique

The patient, unconscious yet breathing deeply, must be placed in the supine position, with a slight head-down tilt. The neck should be hyperextended (head-tilt) to permit easy identification of the thyroid and cricoid cartilages and cricothyroid membrane. A roll of material may be placed under the neck to aid hyperextension. The thyroid cartilage should be held steady between the thumb and sec-

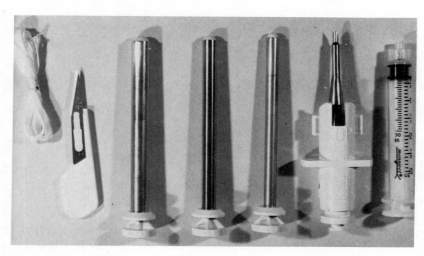

Fig. 11-22. Cricothyrotomy device (left to right): cord to secure airway; knifeblade; various size airways (3); puncturing mechanism; and syringe.

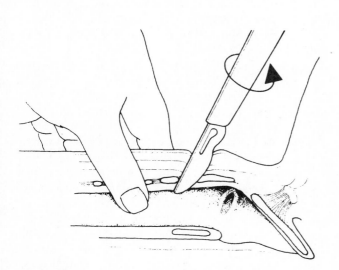

Fig. 11-23. Opening in cricothyroid space is enlarged by rotating scalpel blade 90 degrees.

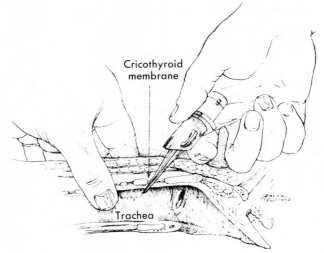

Fig. 11-24. Needle and housing unit are inserted into cricothyroid membrane with a downward thrust toward the chest.

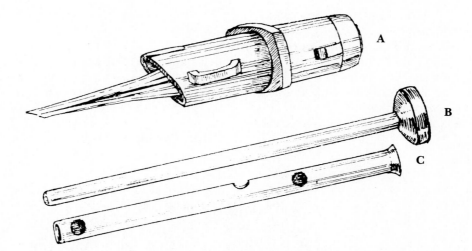

Fig. 11-25. Components of instrument for cricothyrotomy. **A,** Needle and housing unit. **B,** Obturator. **C,** Airway.

ond finger of the left hand (reverse for a left-handed operator) while the index finger identifies the cricothyroid membrane (Fig. 11-23).

A vertical skin incision is made in the midline over the thyroid and cricoid cartilages. Vessels are retracted from the midline with the thumb and index finger of the other hand. As the wound is opened by finger dissection, the cricothyroid membrane becomes readily apparent. A horizontal incision is made as close as possible to the cricoid cartilage to minimize any chance of bleeding.

Enlarge the cricothyroid space by twisting the blade of the scalpel into the horizontal incision and rotating it 90 degrees to open the airway (Fig. 11-23). If available, a cricothyroid or tracheotomy tube can be inserted temporarily. Properly performed, a cricothyrotomy can be accomplished in 15 to 30 seconds.

Anesthesia is not needed, because the patient is unconscious and unable to react to the stimulus of the scalpel incision. It is not unusual for a coughing episode to occur once the trachea is entered.

When a 13-gauge, ½-inch needle is used, the thyroid cartilage is stabilized in the same manner with the index finger identifying the cricothyroid membrane. The needle is inserted through this area until the tracheal lumen is entered. Overinsertion and perforation of the tracheoesophageal wall is prevented by the cartilagenous posterior wall of the cricoid cartilage.

When using a cricothyrotomy device the following technique is used. After the 1 to 2 cm skin incision with the scalpel (Fig. 11-21), the needle then punctures the cricothyroid membrane in the midline. This is accomplished with a downward thrust toward the chest (Fig. 11-24). A rush of air indicates successful entry into the trachea, and the obturator/airway unit is inserted (Fig. 11-25). Gently advance the blunt-edged needle farther into the trachea until its plastic hub rests on the skin. Gently rock the instrument; free movement indicates that overpenetration has not occurred (Fig. 11-26). An airway and obturators are now inserted into the distal end of the housing unit. The split end of the needle, within the trachea, is opened by the airway and obturator, after which the obturator is removed, leaving a clear passage for air to reach the lungs. This device is available in both adult and pediatric sizes. Its use, like that of all other emergency airway equipment, is recommended only for those trained in cricothyrotomy technique.

If spontaneous respiratory movements are present, the victim soon regains consciousness but is still unable to speak because of the continued presence of an obstruction at the larynx. Once this occurs it must be remembered that the opening into the trachea cannot be closed until the object producing the obstruction has been removed. In the absence of spontaneous respiratory movements artificial ventilation should be performed via the cricothy-

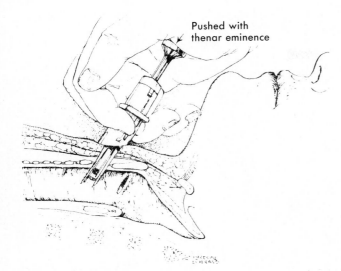

Fig. 11-26. Obturator/airway unit is inserted into needle/housing unit to open the airway. Obturator is next removed, and airway is secured.

rotomy to ensure adequate oxygenation of the blood. Adequacy of the circulation should next be determined by palpating for the carotid artery.

Additional management

Once a patent airway has been established, oxygen can be administered to the victim. A cannula or face mask can be placed over the tracheal opening. Medical assistance should also be summoned and the patient will then be transferred to an emergency medical care facility for follow-up management (removal of foreign object, closure of tracheal opening) and observation. The recommendations of the American Heart Association in management of acute airway obstruction are summarized in the box on p. 156.

BIBLIOGRAPHY

Alexander, R.E., and Delhom, J.J.: Rubber dam clamp ingestion, an operative risk, J. Am. Dent. Assoc. **82:**1387, 1971.

American Heart Association and National Academy of Sciences, National Research Council: Standards and guidelines for cardiopulmonary resuscitation (CPR) and emergency cardiac care (ECC), JAMA **244:**453, 1980.

American Heart Association and National Academy of Sciences, National Research Council: Standards and guidelines for cardiopulmonary resuscitation (CPR) and emergency cardiac care (ECC), JAMA **255:**2905, 1986.

Attia, R.R., Battit, G.E., and Murphy, J.D.: Transtracheal ventilation, JAMA **234:**1152, 1975.

Barkmeier, W.W., Cooley, R.L., and Abrams, H.: Prevention of swallowing or aspiration of foreign objects, J. Am. Dent. Assoc. **97:**473, 1978.

Brantigan, C.O., and Grow, J.B.: Cricothyroidotomy: elective use in respiratory problems requiring tracheotomy, J. Thorac. Cardiovasc. Surg. **71:**72, 1976.

Caparosa, R.J., and Zavatsky, A.R.: Practical aspects of the cricothyroid space, Laryngoscope **67:**577, 1957.

Chipps, J.E.: The dentist's role in the management of foreign bodies, Dent. Clin. North Am. **1:**393, 1957.

Committee on Emergency Medical Services, Assembly of Life Sciences, National Research Council, National Academy of Sciences: Report on emergency airway management, 1976, The Committee.

Council on Dental Therapeutics: Accepted dental therapeutics, ed. 38, Chicago, 1979, American Dental Association.

Day, R.L., Crelin, E.S., and DuBois, A.B.: Choking: the Heimlich abdominal thrust vs. back blows: an approach to the measurement of inertial and aerodynamic forces, Pediatrics **70:**113, 1982.

Gordon, A.S., Belton, M.K., and Ridolpho, R.F.: Emergency management of foreign body airway obstruction. In Safar, P., and Elam, J., editors: Advances in cardiopulmonary resuscitation, New York, 1977, Springer-Verlag, Inc.

Goultschin, J., and Heling, B.: Accidental swallowing of an endodontic instrument, Oral Surg. **32:**621, 1971.

Greene, D.A.: Tracheostomy or not? JAMA **234:**1150, 1975.

Guildner, C.W., Williams, D., and Subitch, T.: Airway obstructed by foreign material: The Heimlich maneuver, JACEP **5:**675, 1976.

Heimlich, H.J.: Pop goes the cafe coronary, Emerg. Med. **6:**154, 1974.

Heimlich, H.J.: A life-saving maneuver to prevent food-choking, JAMA **234:**398, 1975.

Henderson, J.: Emergency medical guide, ed. 3, New York, 1973, McGraw-Hill Book Co.

Korchin, L.: Establishing an emergency airway. In McCarthy, F.M.: Emergencies in dental practice, ed. 2, Philadelphia, 1972, W.B. Saunders Co.

Mitchell, S.A.: Tracheostomy: step-by-step guide, Hosp. Med. **17:**56, 1981.

Nelson, T.G., and Bowers, W.F.: Tracheotomy: indications, advantages, techniques, complications and results; analysis of 310 recent operations, JAMA **164:**1530, 1957.

Oppenheimer, R.P., and Quinn, F.B., Jr.: Quick tracheotomy, Calif. Med. **104:**51, 1966.

Oppenheimer, R.P.: Airway . . . instantly, JAMA **230:**76, 1974.

Palmer, E.: The Heimlich maneuver misused. Curr. Prescr. **5:**45, 1979.

Redding, J.S.: The choking controversy. Critique of evidence on the Heimlich maneuver, Crit. Care Med. **7:**475, 1979.

Ruben, H., and MacNaughton, F.I.: The treatment of food-choking, Practitioner **221:**725, 1978.

Safar, P.: Cardiopulmonary-cerebral resuscitation including emergency airway control. In Schwartz, G.R., editor: Principles and practice of emergency medicine, Philadelphia, 1980, W.B. Saunders Co.

Safar, P., and Penninckx, J.: Cricothyroid membrane puncture with special cannula, Anesthesiology **28:**943, 1967.

Salmon, L.F.W.: Tracheostomy, Proc. R. Soc. Med. **68:**347, 1975.

Scott, A.S., and Dooley, B.E.: Displaced post and core in epiglottic vallecula, Gen. Dent. **26:**26, 1978.

Shapiro, B.A., and Harrison, R.A.: Clinical application of respiratory care. ed. 3, Chicago, 1985, Year Book Medical Publishers.

Visintine, R.E., and Baick, C.H.: Ruptured stomach after Heimlich maneuver, JAMA **234:**415, 1975.

Watts, J.W.: Tracheostomy in modern practice, Br. J. Surg. **50:**954, 1963.

Weiss, S.: A new instrument for emergency cricothyrotomy, JACEP **23:**331, 1973.

Weiss, S.: A new emergency cricothyroidotomy instrument, J. Trauma **23:**155, 1983.

12 ★ *Hyperventilation* (excessive) *Syndrome*

Hyperventilation is defined as ventilation in excess of that required to maintain normal blood Pao_2 and $Paco_2$. It may be produced by an increase in either the frequency or depth of respiration or by a combination of the two. Although the term *hyperventilation* is of relatively recent origin, evidence of the syndrome dates back throughout history. The term *vapors* appeared in eighteenth and nineteenth century literature as a phrase for the symptomatic manifestations of anxiety. In Osler's time (the late 1800s), the terms *neurasthenia* or *psychasthenia* were in vogue. During World War I the terms *effort syndrome* and *soldier's heart* were used to describe the symptoms of anxiety encountered in the trenches of Europe.

Hyperventilation is one of the most common of the emergency situations encountered in dental practice; it is almost always a result of extreme anxiety, although organic causes for hyperventilation do exist. These include pain, metabolic acidosis, drug intoxication, hypercapnia, cirrhosis, and organic central nervous system disorders. In most instances a hyperventilating patient remains conscious throughout the episode. Indeed, unconsciousness produced by hyperventilation is an extremely rare occurrence. Hyperventilation more commonly produces impaired consciousness. The patient complains of a feeling of faintness or lightheadedness or both but does not lose consciousness.

PREDISPOSING FACTORS

The major predisposing factor in hyperventilation is the presence of acute anxiety. In the dental setting this syndrome most commonly occurs in ap-prehensive patients who attempt to hide their fear from the doctor and to "grin and bear it." Hyperventilation rarely occurs in the adult patient who admits anxiety concerning dentistry and permits the doctor to employ psychosedative techniques. Hyperventilation is rarely observed in children, primarily because children usually do not attempt to hide their anxiety. Instead, apprehensive children voice uncertainties in a manner befitting their age and the situation: crying, biting, kicking, and so on. If the anxieties of the patient are released, unpleasant situations such as hyperventilation or vasodepressor syncope rarely occur.

Hyperventilation and vasodepressor syncope seldom occur in patients over the age of 40 because these persons are usually capable of adjusting to the stresses imposed by dentistry and are more likely to admit their fears to the doctor. It has been my experience that the hyperventilation syndrome is most commonly encountered in persons from 15 years to approximately 40 years of age.

It has frequently been reported that hyperventilation occurs more commonly in women; however, recent reports (Lum, 1975) and our own experiences have demonstrated an almost equal sex incidence of this syndrome.

PREVENTION
Medical History Questionnaire

Prevention of hyperventilation is accomplished through the recognition and management of anxiety. An anxiety questionnaire (see p. 35) might be included as a part of the medical history form that the patient completes before dental therapy. With this information available the doctor can adapt the

★ common in dental office
BP will rise, rapid pulse, depths of resp. can vary

161

planned dental therapy to minimize the patient's fears. The stress reduction protocol is an invaluable asset. There are no specific questions on the long- or short-form medical histories that relate to the hyperventilation syndrome.

Physical Examination

Anxiety about dentistry can be detected through a careful examination of the patient. Shaking hands with the patient produces valuable information. Cold, wet hands usually are evidence of apprehension. In extreme instances a mild tremor of the hands may be obvious. The patient may appear quite flushed or pale. In either case the forehead is usually bathed in perspiration, and the patient may comment on the warmth of the dental office, regardless of actual temperature.

Apprehensive patients look uneasy when seated in the dental chair and will be overly concerned with everything going on around them—their eyes following every movement made by the doctor, hygienist, or assistant. Such patients appear "stiff" in the chair and, although seated, seem ready to leave quickly. The hands of the apprehensive patient may be firmly attached to the arms of the chair (the "white knuckle" syndrome), or they may be squeezing or tearing a handkerchief or tissue.

Vital signs

In the apprehensive patient the vital signs change from what is "normal" or baseline for that individual. Systolic and diastolic blood pressures will be elevated, with a greater elevation noted in the systolic. The heart rate (pulse), as recorded at the radial artery, is rapid and increases significantly above baseline for this patient. The rate of respiration in the apprehensive patient increases above the normal adult rate of 14 to 18 per minute. The depth of respiration will be either deeper or more shallow than normal.

If this apprehensive patient is being seen for the first time in the dental office, the vital signs that are recorded will be used as the baseline for all future readings. Every effort should therefore be made to minimize the anxiety of the patient at this time. (Indeed, every effort should be made to reduce the patient's anxieties at *all* times during dental therapy.) To do this the patient should be permitted to rest for a few minutes before vital signs are recorded. This is easily accomplished by starting a review of the medical history questionnaire and after a 5-minute period measuring the vital signs.

One other important factor to consider when recording baseline vital signs is that they are most likely to be "normal" for a given patient if recorded at a visit during which no dental therapy is undertaken. The patient is better able to relax, and the vital signs will be closer to "normal." At succeeding dental appointments the recording of vital signs may indeed reflect the increased apprehension of the patient.

Dental Therapy Considerations

The hyperventilation syndrome is prevented primarily through the stress reduction protocol (see p. 40). Care taken by the dental office staff to make every dental appointment a pleasant one leads to the reeducation of patients and a decrease in their anxieties. This factor is one of the most important items in proper patient management. Through the recognition and management of anxiety, the hyperventilation syndrome, vasodepressor syncope, and a host of other anxiety-related situations may be prevented.

CLINICAL MANIFESTATIONS
Signs and Symptoms

At the onset of the hyperventilation syndrome, which is quite commonly precipitated by the act of injecting a local anesthetic, the patient may complain of a feeling of tightness in the chest and of suffocation. It is not uncommon for the patient to be entirely unaware of overbreathing at this time. As hyperventilation progresses and the chemical composition of the blood continues to change, the patient becomes aware of a feeling of lightheadedness or giddiness and becomes more and more apprehensive because of it. This increased apprehension increases the severity of the situation, and a vicious cycle begins. Hyperventilation caused by anxiety of the dental situation leads to further increased anxiety when the patient becomes aware of the hyperventilation, and to a further increase in hyperventilation because of the increased anxiety. The goal of the doctor in managing this situation will be to break this cycle.

At the onset of the syndrome, symptoms related to the cardiovascular system and gastrointestinal tract often appear. These consist of palpitation (pounding of the heart), precordial discomfort, epigastric discomfort, and globus hystericus (a subjective feeling of a lump in the throat).

The syndrome may last for varying lengths of time if untreated. Patients have hyperventilated for

30 minutes or even longer and have had several recurrences a day. In instances in which hyperventilation continues for prolonged periods of time, tingling or paresthesias of the hands, feet, and perioral regions may develop. These are described by the patient as a sensation of numbness or coldness. If permitted to continue to hyperventilate, the patient may develop muscular twitching and carpopedal tetany (a syndrome manifested by flexion of the ankle joints, muscular twitchings and cramps, and convulsions). If the patient's condition is not promptly and precisely managed, the loss of consciousness may result. Table 12-1 summarizes the signs and symptoms of hyperventilation.

Vital Signs

The major clinical feature noted during the hyperventilation syndrome is the change in the rate and depth of the patient's breathing. Normal respiratory rate for an adult is from 14 to 18 breaths per minute. During hyperventilation the respiratory rate may exceed 25 to 30 breaths per minute. Along with this increased rate, an increase in the depth of breathing is usually noted. For the person who has never seen or experienced hyperventilation, the nature of the breathing is similar to that observed at the conclusion of strenuous exercise when athletes are unable to control their breathing. The rate and depth of breathing are increased as a normal physiologic adaptation to the increased metabolic rate of the body in an effort to eliminate excess carbon dioxide from the body. In the hyperventilation syndrome the nature of the breathing is similar; however, in this situation it represents an abnormal physiologic response, because there is no elevation of carbon dioxide levels in the blood.

Episodes of hyperventilation are most commonly observed in overtly apprehensive patients and are usually precipitated by obvious stress, such as many dental procedures are perceived to be by patients. However, many patients appear outwardly calm and may be totally unaware that they are hyperventilating.

Case Report

A 27-year-old female was scheduled for extraction of two third molars (nonimpacted). She appeared apprehensive when first seen and stated to the dental assistant that she was quite concerned about the procedure, particularly the local anesthetic injections. She was quite flushed and was perspiring. Blood pressure was monitored as 130/90

Table 12-1. Clinical manifestation of the hyperventilation syndrome

Body system	Manifestations
Cardiovascular	Palpitations
	Tachycardia
	Precordial discomfort
Neurologic	Dizziness
	Lightheadedness
	Disturbance of consciousness or vision
	Numbness and tingling of the extremities
	Tetany (rare)
Respiratory	Shortness of breath
	Chest pain
	Dryness of mouth
Gastrointestinal	Globus hystericus (lump in throat)
	Epigastric pain
Musculoskeletal	Muscle pains and cramps
	Tremors
	Stiffness
	Tetany
Psychologic	Tension
	Anxiety
	Nightmares

(baseline 110/70), heart rate was 110 (baseline 84), and respirations were 20 (baseline 18). No preoperative medications were prescribed. The oral surgeon elected to use nitrous oxide and oxygen inhalation sedation during the procedure. The patient was titrated to a concentration of 60% nitrous oxide and 40% oxygen, at which point the patient appeared to be adequately sedated. As the topical anesthetic was applied, the patient became visibly more tense, and her respiratory rate began to increase. During administration of the local anesthetic she began to hyperventilate (rate 28 per minute and deep), and the administration of the local anesthetic was terminated. The patient was permitted to breathe room air and was calmed by the attending oral surgeon. Slight tingling was noted in the patient's fingers, but the symptom was only of brief duration. Within 10 minutes the patient had relaxed, and her vital signs returned to approximately baseline levels. The contemplated procedure was rescheduled to be managed under intravenous sedation and local anesthetic.

The next week the patient received 30 mg flurazepam orally the evening before the dental procedure and 10 mg diazepam (Valium) orally 1 hour before the scheduled time of appointment.

loss of too much carbon-dioxide (CO_2) causes pH of blood to rise alkalinity, disrupts electrolytes,

The patient was driven to the office by a friend. An intravenous infusion was started in the right forearm with a 21-gauge scalp vein needle, and the patient was titrated to a dose of 17 mg diazepam. Local anesthesia was administered without complication or incident, and the surgical procedure was completed in 25 minutes. The patient tolerated the procedure well, commenting, "With the intravenous (drug) I didn't even need that local injection." She was discharged from the office in the company of an adult companion.

PATHOPHYSIOLOGY

The clinical signs and symptoms of hyperventilation described in the previous section are produced by several distinct causes: anxiety, respiratory alkalosis, increased blood catecholamine levels, and a decrease in the level of ionized calcium in the blood.

Anxiety is responsible for the increase in the respiratory rate and depth and also is responsible for the increase in the blood levels of circulating catecholamines (epinephrine and norepinephrine) resulting from the "fight or flight" response. The primary response to the changes in respiration is an increased exchange of oxygen and carbon dioxide in the lungs. The result is an excessive "blowing off" of carbon dioxide to a $Paco_2$ below 35 torr (hypocapnia), which results in an increase in the pH of the blood (to 7.55), a situation termed *respiratory alkalosis*. This same situation (increased ventilation) occurring at the conclusion of strenuous exercise does not produce respiratory alkalosis because the rate of metabolism of the body has increased, producing increased blood levels of carbon dioxide. Hyperventilation in this case aids in the maintenance of normal blood levels of carbon dioxide. The hyperventilating patient starting with normal levels of carbon dioxide reduces the $Paco_2$ to an abnormally low level (hypocapnia).

Hypocapnia and respiratory alkalosis are the result of hyperventilation in a nonexercising individual. Hypocapnia produces vasoconstriction in the cerebral vessels that leads to a degree of cerebral ischemia and helps to explain the symptoms of lightheadedness, dizziness, and giddiness. The degree of cerebral ischemia is usually insufficient to produce the loss of consciousness.

Hyperventilation also increases coronary artery vascular resistance. This, combined with the fact that in acute respiratory alkalosis oxygen becomes more tightly bound to hemoglobin and is less easily released to the tissues, might lead to a reduction in myocardial oxygen supply. This may prove of great clinical importance in patients with coronary disease. The chest pain commonly occurring in hyperventilating patients is usually described as shooting or stabbing in nature; however, it may also be difficult to differentiate from angina pectoris.

Anxiety is also responsible for an increase in the blood levels of catecholamines. This increase may be responsible for the symptoms of palpitations, precordial oppression, trembling, and sweating frequently observed in spontaneously hyperventilating patients. It is interesting to note that in volunteers asked to hyperventilate these symptoms, which are thought to be produced by catecholamine release, are not observed, although the symptoms relating to increased breathing rate and depth (lightheadedness, faintness) are present.

Respiratory alkalosis also has an action on the level of calcium in the blood. As the pH of the blood rises (from a normal of 7.4 to 7.55 in respiratory alkalosis) in hyperventilation, calcium metabolism is disturbed. Although the total serum level of calcium remains approximately normal, the level of ionized calcium in the blood decreases as the pH of the blood increases. Decreases in ionized calcium in the blood result in increases in neuromuscular irritability and excitability, which if permitted to progress, lead to the symptoms of tingling and paresthesia of the hands, feet, and perioral regions, carpopedal tetany, cramps, and possible convulsions.

MANAGEMENT

The management of the hyperventilation syndrome is directed at correcting the respiratory problem and in reducing the anxiety level of the patient.

Anxiety Reduction

This emergency situation has been produced by a fear of dentistry that has been kept well hidden by the patient and that is increased by the subsequent inability of the patient to regulate the breathing rate. The doctor must attempt to calm the patient, and all dental office personnel must remain calm and allow the patient to feel that the situation is well in hand.

Step 1. Terminate dental procedure. Remove the precipitating cause (syringe, handpiece, forceps, etc.) from the patient's line of vision.

Step 2. Position patient. The patient will be conscious but will demonstrate difficulty in breathing. The recommended position for this patient is sitting upright. The supine position is uncomfortable because of the diminished ventilatory volume usually observed in this position, caused by the impingement of the abdominal organs on the diaphragm. Most patients will be more comfortable if allowed to sit up.

Step 3. Remove materials from patient's mouth. Remove all foreign materials from the patient's mouth, such as the rubber dam and partial dentures; if necessary, loosen binding articles of clothing (tight collar, tight blouse, etc.), which may also impede respiration.

Step 4. Calm patient. Reassure the patient in a calm, relaxed manner that all is well. Attempt to aid the patient to regain control by breathing slowly and regularly at a rate of about 4 to 6 breaths per minute. This will permit the blood level of carbon dioxide to increase, thereby reducing the pH of the blood to normal and eliminating any symptoms produced by respiratory alkalosis. In many cases this will be all that is necessary to terminate the hyperventilation syndrome.

Step 5. Correct respiratory alkalosis. When the preceding steps do not appear to be effective, the next step is to have the patient increase the level of carbon dioxide in the blood. This may be accomplished by having the patient breathe in a gaseous mixture of 7% carbon dioxide and 93% oxygen, which is supplied in compressed gas cylinders or, more practically, by having the patient rebreathe exhaled air, which contains an increased amount of carbon dioxide. The second alternative may be ac-

complished by holding a small paper bag (Fig. 12-1) over the patient's mouth and nose and by having the patient breathe into the bag slowly (6 to 10 breaths per minute). (Note: Plastic bags should not be used, since they collapse between breaths, making breathing more difficult.) A full face mask from an oxygen delivery unit may also be used. It is important, however, that oxygen *not* be administered to the patient. The patient should breathe into the full face mask held gently but firmly over the face. If a bag or face mask is not available, the victim may cup hands together in front of the mouth and nose and breathe in and out of this reservoir of exhaled air.

Oxygen is not indicated in this emergency situation, since the symptoms of hyperventilation are produced in part by a decrease in the normal blood level of carbon dioxide and not by an increase in oxygen level. The pH of the blood rises (respiratory alkalosis), and the symptoms previously discussed are observed. For this reason a major goal of management is to produce an increase (actually a return to normal) in the blood level of carbon dioxide. The administration of 100% oxygen or any enriched oxygen mixture will further decrease the carbon dioxide level, thus delaying even longer the return to normal.

Step 6. Drug management. With a patient for whom the above steps are ineffective, it may become necessary to administer parenteral drugs to reduce anxiety. The drugs of choice are diazepam or midazolam. If possible, the agent should be ad-

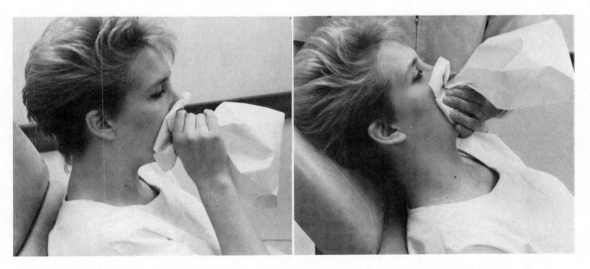

Fig. 12-1. Correction of respiratory alkalosis. Victim rebreathes exhaled air (with increased carbon dioxide content) through paper bag held gently over mouth and nose.

MANAGEMENT OF
THE HYPERVENTILATION SYNDROME

Goals: Reduce anxiety and restore chemical balance of blood

1. Anxiety reduction
   - **Step 1** Terminate dental procedure
   - **2** Position patient in any comfortable position
   - **3** Remove foreign materials from mouth
   - **4** Calm patient (iatrosedation)
2. Correct respiratory alkalosis
   - **5** Breathe CO_2-enriched air through brown paper bag, full face mask, or hands cupped over face
   - **6** Drug management
     Diazepam or midazolam
       IV (titrate)
       IM (10 mg diazepam or 5 mg midazolam deeply injected; massage)
       Oral (10 to 15 mg) diazepam
   - **7** Follow-up
     Determine cause of anxiety; treat anxiety through psychosedation

Note: Oxygen is not indicated for use in the hyperventilation syndrome.

It says "the patient is fearful of something that I am doing." It is the obligation of the doctor to then make an attempt to determine what precipitated the episode and to take measures to prevent a recurrence. Following a return of vital signs to near-baseline values, the patient may be permitted to leave the dental office. If the doctor feels that the patient should not be permitted to leave unescorted, arrangements should be made to have the patient taken home.

Hyperventilation and vasodepressor syncope ought not to occur a second time in the same patient. Proper management of the fearful patient through the use of the various techniques of psychosedation eliminates the occurrence of these two anxiety-produced, potentially life-threatening situations. Management of the hyperventilation syndrome is summarized in the box at left.

BIBLIOGRAPHY

Berger, A.J., Mitchell, R.A., and Severinghaus, J.W.: Regulation of respiration, New Engl. J. Med. **297**:92, 1977.

Brown, E.B.: Physiological effects of hyperventilation, Physiol. Rev. **33**:445, 1953.

Chue, P.W.Y.: The hyperventilation syndrome: diagnosis and management, Dent. Survey, Dec. 1975, p. 31.

Dalessio, D.J.: Hyperventilation. The vapors, effort syndrome, neurasthenia. Anxiety by any other name is just as disturbing, JAMA **239**:1401, 1978.

Heyman, A.: Hyperventilation. In Beeson, P.B., and McDermott, W., editors: Textbook of medicine, ed. 15, Philadelphia, 1979, W.B. Saunders Co.

Krupp, M.A., and Chatton, M.J.: Current medical diagnosis and treatment, Los Altos, CA, 1985, Lange Medical Publications.

Lum, L.C.: Hyperventilation: the tip and the iceberg. J. Psychosom. Res. **19**:375, 1975.

Merck manual of diagnosis and therapy, ed. 13: West Point, PA, 1980, Merck, Sharp and Dohme Research Laboratories.

Miller, F.C., and others: Hyperventilation during labor, Am. J. Obstet. Gynecol. **120**:489, 1974.

Missri, J.C., and Alexander, S.: Hyperventilation syndrome. A brief review, JAMA **240**:2093, 1978.

Neill, W.A., and Hattenhauer, M.: Impairment of myocardial oxygen supply due to hyperventilation, Circulation **52**:854, 1975.

Okel, B.B., and Hurst, J.W.: Prolonged hyperventilation in man, Arch. Intern. Med. **108**:157, 1961.

Riley, D.J.: The "oily" bag and hyperventilation, JAMA **229**:638, 1974.

Rowe, G.G., Castillo, C.A., and Crumpton, C.W.: Effects of hyperventilation on systemic and coronary hemodynamics, Am. Heart J. **63**:67, 1961.

Saltzmann, H.A., Heyman, A., and Sieker, H.O.: Correlations of clinical and physiologic manifestations of sustained hyperventilation, N. Engl. J. Med. **268**:1431, 1963.

Wheatley, C.E.: Hyperventilation syndrome: a frequent cause of chest pain, Chest **68**:195, 1975.

---

ministered intravenously, in which case the agent will be titrated until the anxiety is reduced. For an average adult this dose will approximate 10 to 15 mg of diazepam or from 5 to 7 mg of midazolam. When the intravenous route is not available, diazepam (10 mg) or midazolam (5 mg) may be administered intramuscularly, injected deeply into the muscle. The area is then massaged. When possible, the oral route should be considered for the administration of diazepam, since the latent period for this agent is actually longer following intramuscular administration than following oral administration. An oral dose of 10 to 15 mg will usually terminate the hyperventilation syndrome within 15 to 30 minutes. It must be emphasized that drug therapy to terminate hyperventilation is rarely required. Midazolam is not yet available in the United States for oral administration.

Step 7. Follow-up management. An episode of hyperventilation, like an episode of vasodepressor syncope, tells the doctor something very important.

13 *Asthma*

Asthma was defined in 1830 by Eberle, a Philadelphia physician, as a paroxysmal affection of the respiratory organs, characterized by great difficulty of breathing, tightness across the breast, and a sense of impending suffocation, without fever or local inflammation. Today asthma is defined as a clinical state of hyperreactivity of the tracheobronchial tree, characterized by recurrent paroxysms of dyspnea and wheezing, which are the result of bronchospasm, bronchial wall edema, and hypersecretion by mucous glands.

It is estimated that asthma affects 6 to 8 million Americans. A typical asthmatic patient is usually free of symptoms between acute episodes but has varying degrees of respiratory difficulty during the acute asthmatic attack. Although the degree of respiratory difficulty (dyspnea) is usually moderate, several hundred deaths each year in the United States are caused by asthma. Children with asthma represent a significant number of those making visits to emergency rooms and account for up to 8% of all admissions at one large children's hospital. Acute asthmatic episodes are usually self-limiting; however, there is a clinical entity termed *status asthmaticus,* which may be defined as a persistent exacerbation of asthma. It is potentially life threatening and initially is unresponsive to usually successful therapy, such as administration of epinephrine and theophylline.

PREDISPOSING FACTORS
Extrinsic Asthma

Asthma is usually classified according to etiologic factors into two major categories: extrinsic and intrinsic asthma. *Extrinsic asthma,* also known as allergic asthma, is more common in children and young adults. Most patients with this form of asthma demonstrate an inherited allergic predisposition. Acute asthmatic episodes may be precipitated in these individuals by the inhalation of specific allergens. These allergens may be airborne, such as house dust, feathers, animal danders, furniture stuffing, fungal spores, and a wide variety of plant pollens. Foods and drugs may also precipitate this form of asthmatic attack. Highly allergenic foods include cow's milk, eggs, fish, chocolate, shellfish, and tomatoes. Penicillin, vaccines, and aspirin are commonly implicated drugs. Bronchospasm usually develops within minutes after exposure to the allergen (antigen). This is a type I hypersensitivity reaction in which the antibodies produced in response to the allergen are of the IgE class. The allergic reaction is discussed in more detail in Chapter 24.

Extrinsic asthmatic attacks usually become less frequent and less severe during middle and late adolescence and may disappear entirely. Approximately 50% of asthmatic children become asymptomatic before adulthood. It is possible, however, for extrinsic asthma to become chronic. This apparently is much more common when the asthma originally develops in early childhood and when it is associated with eczema.

Intrinsic Asthma   *more severe*

The second major category of asthma is *intrinsic asthma,* and approximately 50% of asthmatic persons are in this category. Intrinsic asthma usually develops in adults after the age of 35. Episodes are precipitated by nonallergic factors, infection being the most common causative factor. Synonyms for this type of asthma include nonallergic asthma, idiopathic asthma, and infective asthma. There is usually a negative history to allergy, and the results of allergy testing (skin tests) are usually negative. Acute attacks may be precipitated by infection, ir-

may become chronic

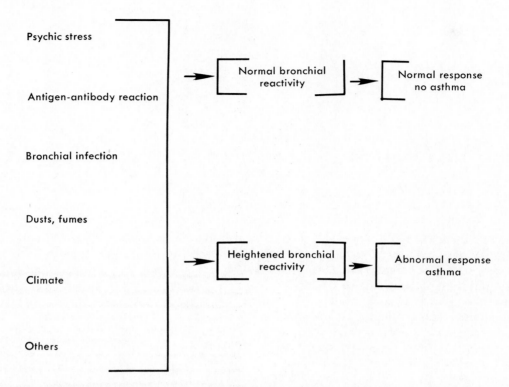

Fig. 13-1. Predisposing factors for asthma. (After Pain, M.C.F.: The treatment of asthma, Drugs **6**:118, 1973.)

ritating inhalants (air pollutants, industrial fumes, various anesthetic agents such as ether), cigarette smoke, cold air, exercise, and emotional upset.

Psychologic and physiologic stress may play important contributory roles in precipitating an asthmatic episode in susceptible individuals. In children with asthma, acute episodes are frequently seen during or after a disciplinary session with a parent. The dental office is another common site for asthmatic attacks. The asthmatic child may develop an acute episode when escorted into the treatment room. A dramatic resolution of asthmatic symptoms usually occurs if the child is simply removed from the treatment room. Psychologic factors may also be important in adult asthmatics. Stressful situations such as dental appointments produce symptoms in many adult asthmatics. Fig. 13-1 illustrates a simplified view of the mechanisms involved in asthma.

Attacks of intrinsic asthma are usually more fulminant and severe than those of allergic (extrinsic) asthma. The long-term prognosis is poorer because the disease more commonly becomes chronic and the patient eventually exhibits clinical signs and symptoms (cough and sputum production) in the intervals between acute episodes.

Mixed Asthma

Mixed asthma refers to a combination of allergic and infective asthma. In this form the major precipitating factor is the presence of infection, especially in the respiratory tract.

Status Asthmaticus

The most severe clinical form of asthma, with symptoms of wheezing, dyspnea, and others that are refractory to the usual therapy for acute asthmatic episodes, is termed *status asthmaticus.* Status asthmaticus is a true medical emergency; if not managed adequately or promptly, the patient may die from respiratory changes that develop secondary to respiratory difficulty (respiratory acidosis produced by hypoxemia and hypercapnia).

PREVENTION

The physician's goal in the long-term management of a patient with asthma is to maintain the patient with as close to normal pulmonary status as

Table 13-1. Common medications employed in long-term management of asthma

Drug group	Examples	Action
Sympathomimetic amines	Epinephrine Isoproterenol Metaproterenol Ephedrine Pseudoephedrine Terbutaline	Dilates or prevents bronchial smooth muscle constriction by stimulating conversion of adenosine triphosphate to 3'5' cyclic AMP, which in turn stabilizes cell membrane and produces muscle fiber relaxation
Xanthine derivatives	Aminophylline Theophylline Oxtriphylline Dyphylline	Inhibits the hydrolytic degradation of 3'5' cyclic AMP
Corticosteroids	Hydrocortisone Prednisone Beclometasone	Precise action unclear, but thought to lessen intensity of antigen-antibody reactions and to possess anti-inflammatory properties
Sodium cromoglycate	Cromolyn sodium	Protects against mast cell destruction and consequent release of chemical mediators of asthma due to local antigen-antibody reactions

possible, for as much of the time as possible. With the advent of long-acting medications, this goal has become more achievable. A second factor in helping to achieve this goal is the recent recognition that the pulmonary status of most asthmatic patients is far from normal in the period between acute episodes.

The goal in dental management of the patient with asthma is prevention of acute exacerbation of the disease. This is best accomplished with information taken from the patient's medical history and from the dialogue history between doctor and patient.

Medical History Questionnaire

The USC medical history questionnaire contains questions that relate to a prior history of asthma, hay fever, and allergy.

QUESTION 6. Have you taken any medicine or drugs during the past 2 years?

COMMENT. Many patients with asthma take oral drugs in the periods between acute episodes in an attempt to prevent or reduce recurrences. Some of the more commonly prescribed drugs include ephedrine HCl or sulfate, alone or in combination with phenobarbital; or combinations of ephedrine or hydroxyzine (Vistaril, Atarax), aminophylline, and a barbiturate. These agents normally have little effect on dental therapy aside from the possibility of a degree of CNS depression (sedation) caused by the barbiturate or hydroxyzine or both.

Long-term therapy with corticosteroids is employed in patients for whom acute episodes occur frequently in spite of the therapy mentioned above. These patients should be carefully evaluated for possible adrenal cortical insufficiency (see Chapter 8).

A more recent addition to the preventive management of acute asthmatic episodes is cromolyn sodium (Intal). It is used primarily in those patients with allergic asthma. It is effective only during periods of remission in preventing recurrences and decreasing the patient's requirement for corticosteroids. Cromolyn sodium is administered by inhalation as a micronized powder.

In addition, most asthmatic patients have in their possession drugs that are used to terminate an acute asthmatic episode. Most commonly, nebulized epinephrine or isoproterenol are used. These are discussed beginning on p. 175.

Table 13-1 lists medications that are commonly used by patients with asthma.

QUESTION 9. Circle any of the following which you have had or have at present:
- **Asthma**
- **Hay fever**
- **Allergy**

COMMENT. Affirmative response to any part of this question should lead to an in-depth dialogue history during which the doctor seeks more information concerning the severity of the patient's asthma.

Table 13-2. Physical status classification—asthma

Physical status	Description	Therapy modifications
II	History of asthma; acute episodes infrequent (1 per month) and readily managed by patient	Usual physical status 2 considerations
II	History of asthma; acute episodes more frequent than 1 per month but are readily managed by patient	Usual physical status 2 considerations
III	History of asthma; frequent acute episodes (1 or more per month) *or* episodes at any frequency that are difficult to manage (patient must seek medical care)	Usual physical status 3 considerations

Dialogue History

QUESTION. *Do you have asthma?*

ANSWER. *Yes.*

QUESTION. *What type of asthma do you have: allergic (extrinsic) or nonallergic (intrinsic)?*

COMMENT. Patients are usually aware of the type of asthma they have.

QUESTION. *At what age did you first develop asthma?*

COMMENT. Allergic asthma most commonly develops in children and younger adults; nonallergic asthma more commonly develops in persons over the age of 35 years.

QUESTION. *How often do you develop acute episodes?*

COMMENT. Seek to determine the frequency of acute asthmatic episodes. The more frequent the occurrence of these episodes, the greater the likelihood that such an episode will develop during dental therapy.

QUESTION. *What precipitates your acute asthmatic attacks?*

COMMENT. Knowledge of the factors involved in precipitating a patient's asthmatic attacks is valuable in preventing such episodes during dental therapy. Of particular importance is the role played by stress. If stress is indeed an important factor, the patient's attitudes regarding dentistry must be elicited and steps taken to make the dental appointments as unstressful as possible. The Stress Reduction Protocol should be used (see p. 40).

QUESTION. *How do you manage your acute asthmatic attacks?*

COMMENT. Attempt to determine what drugs or other medications the patient uses to terminate the acute episode. Most patients carry their medications with them. Have the patient show you the medications, make note of them, and direct the patient to have them available at every dental appointment. These medications, usually nebulized epinephrine or isoproterenol, should be given to the doctor before each dental appointment and kept within reach throughout the appointment.

QUESTION. *Have you ever required hospitalization for your acute asthmatic episodes?*

COMMENT. This question seeks to determine the severity of the acute episodes. Although most are readily terminated following bronchodilator administration, status asthmaticus is refractory to the usual therapy. Hospitalization of the patient is normally required in these instances.

Dental Therapy Considerations

Modifications in dental therapy depend on the severity of the asthma. Acute episodes precipitated by emotional stress in a patient with many fears of the dental situation require judicious handling by the practitioner to prevent an acute asthmatic attack. Use of the Stress Reduction Protocol minimizes the occurrence of acute episodes. There is no contraindication to the use of any conscious sedation technique in asthmatic patients except for some drug groups such as the barbiturates and narcotics (especially meperidine), which may predispose a susceptible patient toward an acute episode and are therefore relatively contraindicated.

If the dental patient has asthma of an allergic nature, care must be taken to eliminate allergens from the dental office. Any drugs that might be implicated in precipitating acute asthmatic episodes should be avoided if at all possible in these patients. Aspirin and penicillin are the most commonly prescribed drugs that can precipitate acute asthmatic episodes. Substitutes such as acetaminophen and erythromycin may be prescribed in place of these drugs.

Table 13-2 classifies asthmatic patients by ASA physical status. The typical asthmatic person carries an ASA II risk during dental treatment.

CLINICAL MANIFESTATIONS

Signs and symptoms of an asthmatic attack range in severity from acute episodes consisting of shortness of breath, wheezing, and cough, followed by complete remission, to a more chronic state in which signs and symptoms are almost continuously present and vary in intensity. An acute asthmatic attack may be an intensely terrifying experience for the patient. There is a large psychologic component in most episodes of asthma.

Usual Clinical Progression

Signs and symptoms of acute asthma may develop gradually or suddenly. In the typical episode the patient notices a sensation of thickness (congestion) in the chest. This is followed by a spell of coughing, which may or may not be associated with sputum production, and wheezing, which is audible on inspiration and expiration. These symptoms tend to increase in intensity as the episode continues. The patient experiences a variable degree of dyspnea, and it is noted that in most episodes the asthmatic patient sits up as if "fighting for air." Although the expiratory phase of the respiratory cycle is actually more difficult than the inspiratory phase for the majority of asthmatics, subjectively many asthmatics feel that inspiration is more difficult and frequently state that they do not know where their next breath is coming from.

As the degree of dyspnea increases, so do the levels of anxiety and apprehension. Breathing during an acute asthmatic attack is usually slow and labored, but the rate may increase to 25 to 30 per minute in the presence of infection or status asthmaticus. This may be the result of apprehension, airway obstruction, or a change in blood chemistry. Blood pressure may remain at approximately the baseline level, although it more commonly rises (this reflects the increased blood level of catecholamines produced by anxiety). In addition, the heart rate increases above baseline level. A rate in excess of 130 per minute may indicate severe hypoxemia.

If left untreated, the asthmatic episode just described may last for a period of minutes to several hours. Termination of the attack is usually heralded by a period of intense coughing with expectoration of a thick, tenacious mucous plug. This is followed immediately by a sensation of relief and a

Table 13-3. Clinical manifestations of asthma

Severity	Manifestations
Mild ("usual") episode	Thickness (congestion) in chest
	Spell of coughing
	Wheezing
	Dyspnea (rate normal to slow but labored)
	Increased anxiety
	Blood pressure normal to elevated
	Heart rate elevated
Severe episode	Intense dyspnea and orthopnea
	Cyanosis of mucous membranes and nailbeds
	Perspiration
	Flushing of face and torso
	Use of accessory muscles of respiration
	Soft tissue retraction
	Fatigue
	Mental confusion

"clearing" of the air passages. Prompt management with an aerosol spray usually aborts the attack within seconds.

More Severe Episodes

In the more intense asthmatic episode the patient demonstrates more pronounced dyspnea and orthopnea (difficulty in breathing except in the upright position). The patient is most comfortable if allowed to sit or stand upright with the back rounded and the chest, shoulders, and head fixed. This posture increases the effectiveness of expiratory efforts, although it reduces lung volume and vital capacity. Cyanosis of mucous membranes (lips and nailbeds) may be evident, along with perspiration and flushing of the face and upper torso. The patient uses accessory muscles of respiration (sternocleidomastoid, trapezi, and scaleni), and nasal flaring and soft tissue retraction are evident in the supraclavicular and intercostal spaces and in the epigastrium. Anxiety in this situation is usually great. If the episode continues, the patient becomes fatigued and begins to appear agitated and mentally confused; this is related to the degree of hypoxia and hypercapnia present. As previously mentioned, prompt management with medication usually terminates the episode within seconds. Table 13-3 summarizes the signs and symptoms of asthma.

Status Asthmaticus

Status asthmaticus is a state in which the acute asthmatic episode persists in spite of drug therapy. In this situation, bronchospasm may continue for hours or even days without remission. Patients with status asthmaticus most commonly exhibit signs of extreme fatigue, dehydration, severe hypoxia, cyanosis, peripheral vascular shock, and drug intoxication from intensive therapy. The patient in status asthmaticus requires hospitalization, because the condition is life threatening. Chronic partial airway obstruction may lead to death from respiratory acidosis. Status asthmaticus may occur in any asthmatic patient.

PATHOPHYSIOLOGY

In the asthmatic patient there is a continuous state of hyperreactivity of the bronchi, during which exposure to any of a wide variety of bronchial irritants may precipitate an acute episode. Numerous theories attempt to explain this state of hyperreactivity; however, none of them satisfactorily explains all types and causes of asthma. In general, the theories state that asthmatic attacks may be provoked (1) through immune (allergenic) reactions, (2) by substances directly toxic or irritating to the bronchial mucosa, or (3) through a combination of these mechanisms. In addition, contributory factors such as psychologic stress, changes in environmental temperature, or infection may be involved. Of these factors, it is felt that the immune reaction is the most significant.

Indeed, it is thought that allergic or presumed allergic factors are involved in most cases of asthma. These factors may induce bronchial hyperreactivity or trigger acute episodes or both. Extrinsic asthma is classified as a type I immune reaction, which is an immediate allergic reaction in which an antigen combines with an antibody present on the surface of bronchial mast cells, causing their degranulation and release or formation of a number of chemical mediators. These mediators include histamine, slow-reacting substance of anaphylaxis (SRS-A), bradykinin, 5-hydroxytryptamine, and others. The physiologic actions of these mediators are presented in Chapter 24. At this point it is important to note that, once released by the mast cells, the pharmacologic activity of these mediators develops rapidly so that clinical symptoms and signs of the acute asthmatic reaction are readily evident. Type I allergic reactions are characterized by rapidity of reaction time (within 15 to 30 minutes) and are associated with immunoglobulin (IgE). Clinical examples of the type I immune response include asthma, anaphylaxis, and hay fever.

In intrinsic asthma (nonallergic), although the primary provoking factor may vary (psychologic stress, physical exertion, cold, irritating inhalants, and so on), the chemical mediators and the pathologic conditions seen during the acute episode are similar to those seen in extrinsic asthma. In general, *acute episodes of either form of asthma are virtually indistinguishable clinically.*

Bronchospasm

Smooth muscle is present throughout the tracheobronchial tree. Bronchial smooth muscle tone is regulated by the vagus nerve, which, when stimulated, causes constriction, and by the sympathetic nervous system, which produces dilation. In nonasthmatic patients bronchial smooth muscle plays a role in protecting the lungs from foreign stimuli. This role involves a degree of narrowing (bronchial smooth muscle constriction) of the airways in response to these foreign stimuli. In the asthmatic patient, however, there is an exaggerated response (more intense constriction), leading to clinical signs and symptoms of respiratory difficulty. This is most prominent in the small bronchi (0.4 to 0.1 cm in diameter) and bronchioles (0.15 to 0.1 cm in diameter); however, smooth muscle constriction may occur wherever smooth muscle is present. The site of the asthmatic reaction can therefore vary, depending on the anatomic location of the bronchial smooth muscle that is stimulated.

Stimulation of irritant receptors by foreign particles (gases, pollens, and chemical mediators) initiates an autonomic (vagal) reflex. The stimulus is carried by the afferent fibers in the vagus nerve to the central nervous system and then by the efferent fibers (again in the vagus nerve) returning to the lungs; there the efferent fibers terminate on bronchial smooth muscle, producing constriction of the muscle.

Bronchial Wall Edema and Hypersecretion of Mucous Glands

In gross and microscopic sections of lungs of patients who have died during asthmatic episodes (usually status asthmaticus), the following changes are evident: mucosal and submucosal edema and thickening of the basement membrane, infiltration by leukocytes (primarily eosinophils), intraluminal mucous plugs, and bronchospasm (Fig. 13-2). When examined in gross section, the lungs appear

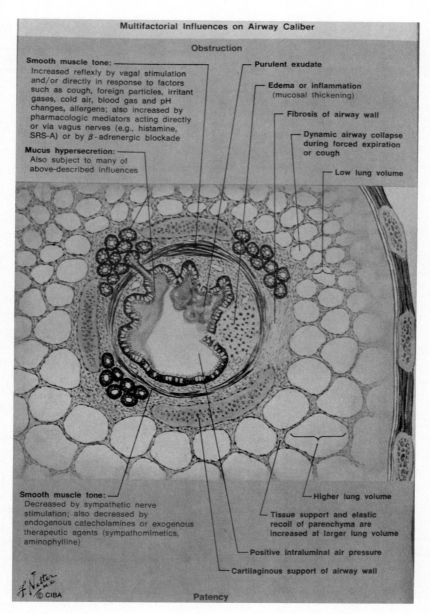

Fig. 13-2. Cross section diagram of bronchiole of patient with chronic asthmatic condition. Note mucous plugs, edema, and other changes which act to narrow lumen.

overdistended, and many of the smaller bronchi are occluded by mucous plugs. In spite of the overall appearance of overinflation, there are areas of hyperinflation alternating with areas of atelectasis produced by mucous plugs. All of these factors lead to a decrease in the size of the lumen of the airway, an increase in airway resistance, and clinical manifestations related to the degree of narrowing. Airway resistance varies inversely to the fourth power of the radius. Therefore, halving of the radius of

an airway leads to a 16-fold increase in airway resistance (according to Poiseuille's approximation). The result of this increased resistance is difficulty in breathing and, ultimately, alterations in blood chemistry and pH.

Breathing
Nonasthmatic patient

In the normal individual, breathing is composed of two phases: inspiration and expiration. The inspiratory phase is an active process. Thoracic volume increases as the diaphragm and other inspiratory muscles function. With this increase in volume the intrapleural pressure becomes more negative (going from -2 to -6 torr), and the lungs expand in an attempt to fill the increasing chest volume. Air is then drawn into the lungs until these pressures are equalized.

The expiratory phase of breathing is normally a passive process that does not require muscular energy. As the muscles of respiration relax, the elastic tissues of the lungs, which have been stretched on inspiration, are able to return to their normal unstretched state—a process termed *elastic recoil*. This shortening of fibers results in the forcing of air out of the lungs, which permits the thorax to return to its normal resting state.

Asthmatic patient

In the asthmatic patient, varying degrees of airway obstruction exist that may produce large increases in airway resistance. As airway resistance increases, air flow during inspiration and expiration is compromised. To accommodate the increased resistance during inspiration, the muscles of respiration work to produce a greater degree of chest expansion in order to allow more air to enter the lungs on inspiration.

The deleterious effects of increased airway resistance in the majority of asthmatics occur during the normally passive expiratory phase. The elastic recoil of the lungs during expiration is no longer adequate to expel air against the increased airway resistance, and air therefore is trapped in the patient's lungs (hyperinflation). To counteract this, the normally passive expiratory phase becomes an active phase with both the respiratory and accessory muscles of respiration being used to expel air from the lungs. In addition, ventilation (quantity of air exchanged per unit of time) is impaired because of increased resistance. This commonly leads to an increase in the rate of breathing (tachypnea).

As the asthmatic episode progresses and the obstruction worsens, the expiratory phase of respiration tends to become longer and air becomes increasingly trapped in the lungs. This leads to hyperinflation of alveoli, which tends to produce an increase in airway diameter (from increased tension) on the one hand and to cause increased energy utilization on the other. This increase in energy utilization is necessary during the inspiratory phase to overcome the tension of the already

Table 13-4. Clinical signs and symptoms of hypoxia and hypercarbia

Hypoxia	*Hypercarbia*
Restlessness, confusion, anxiety	Diaphoresis
Cyanosis	Hypertension (converting to hypotension if progressive)
Diaphoresis (sweating)	Hyperventilation
Tachycardia, cardiac arrhythmias	Headache
Hypertension or hypotension	Confusion, somolence
Coma	Cardiac failure
Cardiac or renal failure	

stretched elastic tissues of the lungs and to allow air to enter the lungs.

It can therefore be seen that if an asthmatic episode is permitted to continue, a great deal of energy may be expended on respiration. Fatigue occurs, further decreasing respiratory effectiveness and leading to hypoventilation of alveoli. This is seen clinically as increased dyspnea, tachypnea, and possibly cyanosis. When severe, alveolar hypoventilation produces carbon dioxide retention (hypercarbia), which is manifested by an increase in the rate and depth of respiration (hyperventilation) and a further increase in the work of breathing. Sweating (diaphoresis) is another clinical sign of hypercarbia.

This process is self-limiting. If the airway obstruction continues to worsen and the work of breathing continues to increase, increasing levels of hypercarbia and hypoxemia lead to a state of acute respiratory acidosis. Table 13-4 lists signs and symptoms associated with hypoxemia and hypercarbia. Respiratory failure may occur, and the patient will then require artificial ventilation. The mortality rate in this stage is high.

To conclude this section, let us review the pathophysiology of two degrees of asthmatic episode: mild and severe. In the milder asthmatic attack, the moderate airway obstruction present leads to a decrease in blood oxygenation. The ensuing hypoxia and increased respiratory workload lead to a heightened level of anxiety, producing hyperventilation. Hyperventilation leads to a decrease in the CO_2 level in the blood (hypocapnia) and respiratory alkalosis. (Refer to Chapter 12 for a discussion of hyperventilation.)

In the more severe asthmatic episode or in status asthmaticus, the greater degree of bronchial ob-

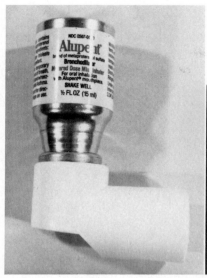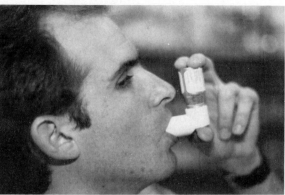

Fig. 13-3. Bronchodilator. Patient administers bronchodilator aerosol.

struction present causes a more profound decrease in blood oxgenation. The respiratory workload increases; however, these responses soon become ineffective (the asthmatic becomes fatigued) as the obstruction becomes greater, leading to inadequate ventilation and carbon dioxide retention (hypercapnia). Hypercapnia causes respiratory acidosis and may lead to respiratory failure.

MANAGEMENT
Acute Asthmatic Episode

Management of the *acute* asthmatic episode requires prompt specific drug therapy, as well as symptomatic management.

Step 1. Terminate dental therapy.

Step 2. Position patient. Upon recognition of the asthmatic episode, the patient should be positioned in any comfortable position, usually a sitting position with the arms thrown forward. Other patients may wish to stand, and still others may wish to lie down.

Step 3. Administer bronchodilator. Before the initiation of dental treatment on an asthmatic patient, the doctor should place the patient's aerosol spray of bronchodilator medication in a place within easy reach at all times during the dental appointment. When required, the patient's medication should be used in management of the acute episode.

Bronchodilators are the drugs employed to man-

age the acute asthmatic episode. The most effective bronchodilators are the adrenergic drugs such as epinephrine (Adrenalin), isoproterenol (Isuprel), and metaproterenol (Alupent), which are agonists of beta-2 receptors in the bronchial smooth muscle and act to produce dilation (muscle relaxation). These agents may be administered orally, sublingually, by aerosol inhalation, or by injection. *Rapid relief of the acute episode is most readily achieved through the oral inhalation of epinephrine, isoproterenol, or metaproterenol* (Fig. 13-3) *or the subcutaneous injection of epinephrine.* The patient should be given the inhaler of medication and be permitted to take the "usual" dose required to terminate the episode. Before administering a bronchodilator, it is important for the patient and doctor to read the package insert accompanying these medications, since there are strict limitations on the maximal quantity that may safely be administered. Untoward reactions associated with the use of these drugs relate primarily to the beta-1 and alpha receptor stimulating actions of epinephrine and isoproterenol. Metaproterenol is almost pure beta-2 with little or no beta-1 and alpha stimulating properties.* Epinephrine and isoproterenol produce

---

*Beta-1 receptors increase cardiac rate and force, relax intestinal smooth muscle, and stimulate lipolysis; *beta-2 receptors* produce relaxation of bronchial, uterine, and vascular smooth muscle and stimulation of glycogenolysis; *alpha receptors* stimulate contraction of vascular smooth muscle.

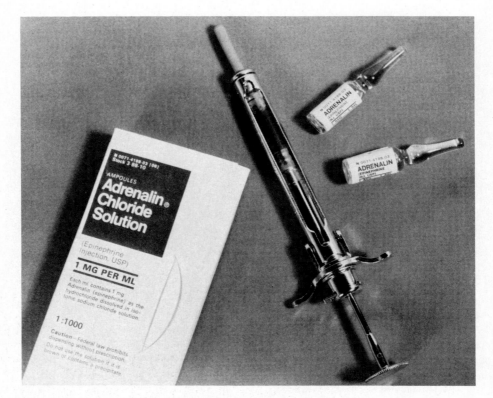

Fig. 13-4. Parenteral bronchodilator. Epinephrine (Adrenalin) is administered intramuscularly or intravenously.

palpitation, tachycardia, and disturbances of cardiac rhythm and rate. In addition, epinephrine may produce headache and increased anxiety. Epinephrine is contraindicated in asthmatic patients with concomitant high blood pressure, diabetes mellitus (since epinephrine produces hyperglycemia), hyperthyroidism, and ischemic heart disease. Metaproterenol has become much more frequently recommended for use in management of acute asthmatic attacks in patients with other medical problems. Another factor to consider when employing these medications is that their use for prolonged periods (months to years) may produce a state of refractoriness, which will lead to prolonged and not easily terminated episodes of asthma. Therefore these agents, although highly effective in managing the acute asthmatic attack, should be used judiciously.

Mild Asthmatic Episode

Management of the *mild* asthmatic attack includes the following:

Step 1. Terminate dental therpy.

Step 2. Position patient in the most comfortable position.

Step 3. Administer aerosol spray of epinephrine, isoproterenol, or metaproterenol. The onset of aerosol drug action is rapid, with relief of symptoms occurring within seconds of its administration. Epinephrine and isoproterenol are short acting (30 to 60 minutes); bronchospasm may recur as the agents are inactivated. Metaproterenol, on the other hand, has a clinical duration of effectiveness of from 2 to 6 hours. Repeated doses of the aerosol drugs should be administered cautiously (to prevent overdose reaction) and in strict adherence to the instructions on the label.

Step 4. Administer oxygen. The administration of oxygen should be considered during any acute asthmatic episode. It may be administered by means of a full face mask, nasal hood, or nasal cannula. Any clinical signs and symptoms of hypoxia and hypercarbia (Table 13-4) are indications for oxygen administration.

Step 5. Parenteral medication. For management of the more severe asthmatic episode or in those milder episodes that prove refractory to aerosol medications, the injection of aqueous epinephrine is indicated. Epinephrine in the emergency kit is available in a preloaded syringe containing 1 ml of a 1:1000 dilution. This is equivalent to 1 mg of epinephrine (Fig. 13-4).

For the adult patient, the usual SC or IM dose of epinephrine (1:1000 dilution) is 0.3 ml, which may be repeated as necessary every 30 to 60 minutes. Asthmatic children often cease to have acute symptoms when they are removed from the dental office. Should this simple measure be ineffective, the injection of 0.125 to 0.25 ml of aqueous epinephrine is indicated. Oxygen should be available and administered if considered necessary.

Step 6. Intravenous medications (optional). Patients who prove refractory to the commonly employed bronchodilators require additional drug therapy to terminate the acute asthmatic episode. Drugs employed in these circumstances include aminophylline (250 mg administered *very slowly* intravenously) and corticosteroids (hydrocortisone sodium succinate, 100 to 200 mg intravenously). If the doctor has received advanced training in emergency medicine and is able to start an IV infusion, these agents should be considered for inclusion in the office emergency kit.

Because the asthmatic patient is usually considerably anxious during an attack, the use of sedative medications during acute episodes must be considered. The more severe the asthmatic attack, however, the more potentially dangerous sedative drugs are. These agents are *absolutely contraindicated* in status asthmaticus or in very severe asthma when there is any indication of CO_2 retention. Potential respiratory depression produced by sedative agents may be accentuated by concurrent hypoxia, and respiratory arrest may occur. In less severe episodes the judicious use of sedatives (such as diazepam, 5 mg IM or IV, titrated) may be indicated to decrease the anxiety component; however, their administration is rarely indicated. Oxygen may be administered freely at all times during the asthmatic episode.

Step 6a. Summon medical assistance. Should the steps of management just discussed (steps 1 to 5) be ineffective in terminating the acute episode or if the doctor has administered the drugs in step 6, medical assistance is recommended. In either of

---

MANAGEMENT OF ASTHMA

Step 1 Terminate dental therapy
   2 Position patient
     Comfortable position
     Usually sitting with arms thrown forward
   3 Administer bronchodilator by means of aerosol spray
     Epinephrine, isoproterenol, or metaproterenol (read instructions carefully before use)
   4 Administer oxygen
   5 Parenteral medication
     If episode continues, epinephrine 1:1000 IM 0.3 ml (adult); IM 0.125 ml (infant); IM 0.25 ml (child)
   6 Intravenous medications (optional)
     If episode continues, aminophylline 250 mg by means of a very slow IV; hydrocortisone sodium succinate, 100 to 200 mg IV
  6a Summon medical assistance if step 6 is needed or if episode is refractory to management
   7 Regarding further dental therapy: terminate therapy for day
     Permit patient to recover fully before discharge

---

these situations the patient will probably require a period of hospitalization for more definitive management and observation. It should be remembered that in most acute cases of asthma the prompt administration of bronchodilating drugs terminates the response, eliminating the need for any additional assistance or hospitalization.

Step 7. Further dental therapy. Upon termination of the asthmatic episode, the patient should be reevaluated before therapy is continued. It may be prudent to forego additional therapy at that visit and reschedule the patient. Discussion of the possible psychologic component of this patient's asthmatic attack may enable the doctor to take steps (Stress Reduction Protocol) to prevent future recurrences. The patient should be permitted to rest in the dental office until all signs and symptoms have resolved before being dismissed.

The management of asthma is summarized in the box above.

BIBLIOGRAPHY

Abramowicz, M.: Drugs in asthma, Med. Lett. Drugs Ther. **24**:83, 1982.

Avner, S.E.: Beta adrenergic bronchodilators, Pediatr. Clin. North Am. **22**:129, 1975.

Bachus, B.F., and Snider, G.L.: The bronchodilator effects of aerosolized terbutaline: a controlled double-blind study, JAMA **234**:2277, 1977.

Banner, A.S., Shah, R.S., and Addington, W.W.: Rapid prediction of need for hospitalization in acute asthma, JAMA **235**:1337, 1976.

Bergner, R.K., and Bergner, A.: Rational asthma therapy for the outpatient, JAMA **235**:288, 1976.

Bierman, C.W., Pierson, W.E., and Shapiro, G.G.: Exercise induced asthma, JAMA **234**:295, 1975.

Chodosh, S.: Rational management of bronchial asthma, Arch. Intern. Med. **138**:1394, 1978.

Cotton, E.K., and Parry, W.: Treatment of status asthmaticus and respiratory failure, Pediatr. Clin. North Am. **22**:163, 1975.

Cropp, G.J.A.: Exercise induced asthma, Pediatr. Clin. North Am. **22**:63, 1975.

Dujovne, C.A., and Azarnoff, D.L.: Clinical complications of corticosteroid therapy, Med. Clin. North Am. **57**:1331, 1973.

Eberle, J.: A treatise on the practice of medicine, vol. 2, Philadelphia, 1830, John Grigg.

Flod, N.E., Franz, M.L., and Galant, S.P.: Recent advances in bronchial asthma, Am. J. Dis. Child. **130**:890, 1976.

Fraser, P.M., and others: The circumstances preceding death from asthma in young people in 1968-1969, Br. J. Dis. Chest **65**:71, 1971.

Galant, S.P.: Prognosis of asthma, Lancet **1**:437, 1972.

Hurst, A.: Metaproterenol, a potent and safe bronchodilator, Ann. Allergy **31**:460, 1973.

Imbeau, S.A., and Geller, M.: Aerosol beclomethosone treatment of chronic severe asthma: a one year experience, JAMA **240**:1260, 1978.

Leffert, F.: The management of acute severe asthma, J. Pediatr. **96**:1, 1980.

Leifer, K.N., and Wittig, H.J.: The beta-2 sympathomimetic aerosols in the treatment of asthma, Ann. Allergy **35**:69, 1975.

LeNoir, M.: Asthma and status asthmaticus. In Pascoe, D.J., and Grossman, M., editors: Quick reference to pediatric emergencies, Philadelphia, 1983, J.B. Lippincott Co.

Lulla, S., and Newcomb, R.W.: Emergency management of asthma in children, J. Pediatr. **97**:346, 1980.

Management of asthma. American Academy of Pediatrics, section on allergy and immunology, Pediatrics **68**:874, 1981.

Maselli, R., Casal, G.L., and Ellis, E.F.: Pharmacologic effects of intravenously administered aminophylline in asthmatic children, J. Pediatr. **76**:777, 1970.

McFadden, E.R., Jr.: Exertional dyspnea and cough as preludes to acute attacks of bronchial asthma, N. Engl. J. Med. **292**:555, 1973.

McFadden, E.R., Jr., Kiser, R., and DeGroot, W.J.: Acute bronchial asthma, N. Engl. J. Med. **288**:221, 1975.

Orehek, J., and others: Patient errors in use of bronchodilator metered aerosols, Br. Med. J. **1**:76, 1976.

Pain, M.C.F.: The treatment of asthma, Drugs **6**:118, 1973.

Rebuck, A.S., and Read, J.: Assessment and management of severe asthma, Am. J. Med. **51**:788, 1971.

Ryo, U.Y., Kang, B., and Townley, R.G.: Cromolyn therapy in patients with bronchial asthma, JAMA **236**:927, 1976.

Samter, M.: Intolerance to aspirin, Hosp. Pract. **8**:58, 1973.

Scheinman, H.Z., Fontana, V.J., and McKenna, P.J.: Bronchial asthma with acute respiratory failure, Mt. Sinai J. Med. **43**:268, 1976.

Segal, M.S.: Death in bronchial asthma. In Weiss, E.B., and Segal, M.S., editors: Bronchial asthma: mechanisms and therapeutics, Boston, 1976, Little, Brown & Co.

Segal, M.S., and Ishikawa, S.: Isoproterenol aerosols, Ann. Allergy **34**:205, 1975.

Sellars, W.A., and Pflanzer, J.: Cromolyn sodium in the treatment of asthma: its effectiveness and use, South. Med. J. **68**:970, 1975.

Senior, R.M., Lefrak, S.S., and Korenblat, P.E.: Status asthmaticus, JAMA **231**:1277, 1975.

Snider, G.L.: The treatment of asthma, N. Engl. J. Med. **298**:397, 1978.

Sobol, B.J., and Reed, A.: The rapidity of onset of bronchodilation: a comparison of Alupent and isoproterenol, Ann. Allergy **32**:137, 1974.

Spector, S.L., and Farr, R.S.: Bronchial inhalation procedures in asthmatics, Med. Clin. North Am. **58**:71, 1974.

Stolley, P.D.: Asthma mortality, Am. Rev. Respir. Dis. **105**:883, 1972.

Svedmyr, N., and Simonsson, B.G.: Drugs in the treatment of asthma, Pharmacol. Ther. **3**:397, 1978.

Szczeklik, A., and others: Aspirin induced asthma, J. Allergy Clin. Immunol. **58**:10, 1976.

Townley, R.G.: Progress in asthma control: pharmacological mediators in asthma, Acta Allergol. **29**(suppl. 11):15, 1974.

Weinberger, M., Hendeles, L., and Ahrens, R.: Clinical pharmacology of drugs used for asthma, Pediatr. Clin. North Amer. **28**:47, 1981.

Weisberg, S.C., and Kaiser, H.B.: New drugs in the treatment of asthma, Postgrad. Med. **60**:133, 1976.

Weiss, E.B.: Bronchial asthma, Clin. Symp. **27**:3, 1975.

Williams, M.H.: Corticosteroid aerosols for the treatment of asthma, JAMA **231**:406, 1975.

Wilson, A.F., and others: The significance of regional pulmonary function changes in bronchial asthma, Am. J. Med. **48**:216, 1970.

14 *Heart Failure and Acute Pulmonary Edema*

Heart failure is the pathophysiologic state in which an abnormality of cardiac function is responsible for failure of the heart to pump a volume of blood adequate to meet the requirements of the metabolizing tissues. Congestion develops in the pulmonary or systemic circulations or in both. *Left heart failure* is associated with signs and symptoms related to pulmonary vascular congestion; *right heart failure* commonly exhibits signs and symptoms of systemic venous and capillary engorgement. Left and right heart failure may develop independently or occur simultaneously. The term "congestive heart failure" refers to a combination of left and right heart failure, in which there is evidence of both systemic *and* pulmonary congestion. *Pulmonary edema* is usually an acute condition marked by an excess of serous fluid in the alveolar spaces or interstitial tissues of the lungs and accompanied by extreme difficulty in breathing.

The human heart functions under normal conditions as a pump, supplying the tissues and organs of the body with a supply of blood (containing oxygen and nutrients) sufficient to meet their metabolic needs at rest and during activity. When viewed as a pump, the human heart is remarkable, not only for its ability to rapidly adjust to the varying metabolic requirements of the body but also because of its extreme durability. The heart does last a lifetime—literally. As durable as the heart may be, however, it is also vulnerable to a large number of disorders that may affect its ability to function adequately. These include congenital, metabolic, inflammatory, and degenerative disorders. Dysfunction of the heart usually manifests itself clinically in one of two ways. In the first, signs and symptoms of the dysfunction are located di-

rectly at the site of the heart. These include chest pain and palpitation, which clinically are represented as angina pectoris (Chapter 27), myocardial infarction (Chapter 28), and cardiac arrhythmias. The second group includes signs and symptoms that are extracardiac and originate in organs of the body that are either hyperperfused (congested) or hypoperfused (ischemic) with blood. Heart failure is a clinical expression of the former.

Under normal circumstances the right ventricle is destined to outperform and outlast the left ventricle. This clinical fact is further accentuated by the fact that the left side of the heart is also more vulnerable to heart disease and to disorders in its blood supply and is therefore where the first expression of heart failure is usually seen. Isolated right heart failure is extremely rare. The right side of the heart commonly fails soon after left ventricular failure occurs. Cardiac function, normal and pathologic, is discussed further in the pathophysiology section of this chapter.

Heart failure therefore represents the clinical diagnosis applied to a group of signs and symptoms that occur when the heart is unable to handle its load as a pump, thus depriving the various tissues and organs of the body of an adequate supply of oxygen and nutrients. The degree of heart failure varies dramatically, from patients with only mild clinical signs and symptoms that arise solely on exertion to patients with severe heart failure who demonstrate signs and symptoms in the resting state. All patients with heart failure represent an increased risk during dental therapy. Modifications may be necessary in the dental treatment plan to accommodate their state of cardiac dysfunction. In very advanced heart failure or in patients with moderate degrees of heart failure who are faced with physiologic or psychologic stress or both, heart failure may become accentuated, producing acute pulmonary edema, in which extreme degrees of respiratory difficulty are observed. This is a medical emergency that must be managed quickly and aggressively.

Heart failure is a not uncommon finding in the general population. Most persons with progressive cardiovascular disease develop some degree of heart failure at some stage of their lives. Chapter 26 includes discussion of the etiologic factors found in the majority of these cardiovascular diseases. The dental practitioner is faced with the prospect of managing the dental needs of patients with varying degrees of heart failure. It is important to be able to adequately evaluate this patient before actual dental therapy so that measures may be taken to prevent an acute episode of heart failure (acute pulmonary edema) from occurring during therapy.

PREDISPOSING FACTORS

The tendency of heart failure to begin as left ventricular failure is related to the disproportionate workload of this side of the heart and to the prevalence of cardiac diseases in the left side of the heart. Disease produces heart failure in one of two basic ways: (1) by increasing the workload of the heart (for example, high blood pressure produces an increased resistance to ejection of blood from the left ventricle) and (2) by damaging the muscular walls of the heart (through coronary artery disease or myocardial infarction). Other causes of increased cardiac workload include cardiac valvular deficiencies (stenosis or insufficiency of the aortic, mitral, tricuspid, or pulmonary valves) and increases in the body's requirement for oxygen and nutrients (pregnancy, thyrotoxicosis, anemia). *Left ventricular failure is the leading cause of right ventricular failure.* Other causes of isolated right ventricular failure include mitral stenosis, pulmonary vascular or parenchymal disease, and pulmonary valvular stenosis.

Acute worsening of preexisting heart failure and acute pulmonary edema may be precipitated by any factor that increases the workload of the heart. Acute pulmonary edema may occur at any time, but it is commonly observed at night, after the patient has been asleep for a few hours (see the pathophysiology section later in this chapter). Other factors that increase the cardiac workload include

physical, psychologic, and climatic stress. The dental setting may easily provide these factors.

In pediatric patients heart failure may also be produced by an obstruction to the outflow of blood from the heart, such as coarctation of the aorta or pulmonary stenosis. Of all children who do develop congestive heart failure (CHF), 90% do so within the first year of life because of congenital heart lesions. Older children may also develop CHF from congenital heart lesions; however, much more common causes are acquired disease from cardiomyopathy, bacterial endocarditis, or rheumatic carditis.

PREVENTION
Medical History Questionnaire

Relevant questions from the medical history questionnaire that relate to the presence of cardiovascular disease are presented, with comments added for clarification.

QUESTION 9. Circle any of the following which you have had or have at present:

- **Heart failure**
- **Heart murmur**
- **Rheumatic fever**
- **Congenital heart lesions**
- **Scarlet fever**

COMMENT. An affirmative reply to any of the above indicates the need for further questioning (dialogue history) to determine the degree of severity and other relevant factors concerning the disease. All of the above-mentioned conditions can lead to the development of varying degrees of clinical signs and symptoms of heart failure.

QUESTION 10. When you walk up stairs or take a walk, do you ever have to stop because of pain in your chest, or shortness of breath, or because you are very tired?

COMMENT. The ability to negotiate a "normal" flight of stairs or to walk two level city blocks is an excellent gauge of cardiorespiratory fitness (see dialogue history). Shortness of breath occurring after mild exercise is termed exertional dyspnea and represents an early sign of left ventricular failure.

QUESTION 11. Do your ankles swell during the day?

COMMENT. If the answer is yes, determine at what time of night or day it develops. Dependent edema is seen in right heart failure late in the day following many hours of standing. It may be seen in other states as well, such as pregnancy, varicose veins, and renal failure.

QUESTION 12. Do you use more than two pillows to sleep?

COMMENT. Orthopnea is the inability to breathe comfortably in the supine position, requiring the use of 3 or more pillows to enable comfortable breathing. Orthopnea is a sign of left heart failure. Modifications in position and possibly in the use of a rubber dam may be desirable during dental treatment.

QUESTION 13. Have you lost or gained more than 10 pounds in the past year?

COMMENT. An affirmative reply to having gained more than 10 pounds—especially if this has occurred relatively rapidly and for no apparent reason—might indicate the development of CHF. Retention of fluid is a significant factor in the development of CHF.

QUESTION 14. Do you ever awake from sleep short of breath?

COMMENT. Termed *paroxysmal nocturnal dyspnea* (*PND*), this clinical sign is usually related to a more significant degree of left heart failure.

QUESTION 6. Have you taken any medicine or drugs during the past 2 years?

COMMENT. Patients diagnosed as having heart failure will frequently take one or more of the following medications: medications for high blood pressure and/or digitalis.

COMMENT. Patients with heart failure most commonly take drugs such as digitalis and diuretics. The fundamental action of digitalis glycosides is to increase the force and velocity of cardiac contraction whether or not the heart is failing (positive inotropic action). In congestive heart failure, digitalis significantly increases cardiac output, decreases right atrial pressure, decreases the venous pressure, and increases the excretion of sodium and water, thus correcting some of the hemodynamic and metabolic alterations in heart failure.

Diuretics are used to suppress the renal tubular reabsorption of sodium. They are commonly employed in management of diseases associated with excessive sodium and fluid retention. Table 14-1 lists some commonly employed diuretics.

Table 14-1. Commonly prescribed oral diuretics

Generic	Proprietary
Bendroflumethiazide	Benuron
	Naturetin
Benzthiazide	Exna
Chlorthalidone	Hygroton
Chlorothiazide	Diuril
Cyclothiazide	Anhydron
Ethacrynic acid	Edecrin
Flumethiazide	Ademol
Furosemide	Lasix
Hydrochlorothiazide	Esidrix
	Hydrodiuril
	Oretic
Hydroflumethiazide	Di-Ademil
	Saluron
Methyclothiazide	Enduron
Polythiazide	Renese
Quinethazone	Hydromox
Spironolactone	Aldactone
Triamterene	Dyrenium
Trichlormethiazide	Metahydrin
	Naqua

High blood pressure represents one of the leading causes of left ventricular failure. Knowing which drugs are being taken by the patient may lead the doctor to a better understanding of the degree of cardiovascular dysfunction present.

Dialogue History

Following review of the medical history questionnaire, the dialogue history is used to gather additional information concerning the degree of severity of the heart failure.

QUESTION. Are you able to carry out your normal daily activities without becoming unduly fatigued?

COMMENT. This is related to question 10 in the questionnaire; however, this question considers undue fatigue at rest, not during exercise. Undue fatigue is a common presenting symptom of left or right heart failure or both. It usually represents the first clinical manifestation of heart failure.

QUESTION. Can you climb a normal flight of stairs or walk two level city blocks without stopping?

COMMENT. Related to the preceding question, inability to climb a normal flight of stairs or walk two level city blocks is an indication of an inefficient

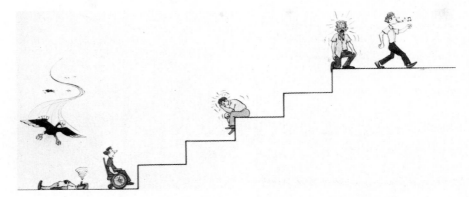

Fig. 14-1. ASA classification for CHF. (Courtesy Dr. Lawrence Day.)

cardiorespiratory system. The ASA physical status classification system (Fig. 14-1) for CHF may be linked to the patient's answers. ASA I patients will be able to climb one flight of stairs or walk two level city blocks without having to pause due to shortness of breath. ASA II patients will be able to climb one flight of stairs or walk two level city blocks but will have to stop once they are finished with either task due to shortness of breath. ASA III patients will be able to climb one flight of stairs or walk two city blocks but will have to stop before completing the task because of shortness of breath. ASA IV patients are unable to negotiate one flight of stairs or walk two level city blocks because of shortness of breath.

QUESTION. *Have you ever awakened at night short of breath?*

COMMENT. Paroxysmal nocturnal dyspnea (PND), or awakening at night short of breath, is a sign of more advanced left heart failure. If present, medical consultation should be considered before dental therapy.

• • •

Pediatric patients with CHF secondary to other etiologies will have a history of congenital or other heart problems. The parent or guardian will be able to discuss the child's status with the doctor. Consultation with the patient's primary care physician is warranted in cases of pediatric congestive heart failure.

Additionally, the doctor might encounter patients who appear to have CHF (see physical evaluation below) but who provide negative answers to the preceding questions. Please remember that people will accommodate themselves to a degree of physical disability rather well. For example, per-

sons unable to negotiate a flight of stairs or walk two level city blocks may in fact never try to do so; they may simply take an elevator or motor vehicle instead. The observant doctor will always be on the lookout for clinical clues.

Physical Evaluation

In addition to the preceding methods to aid in prevention, physical evaluation of the patient enables the doctor to determine a patient's present state of health more accurately.

Vital signs

The vital signs of the patient should be recorded. These include the blood pressure, heart rate and rhythm (pulse), respiratory rate, and weight. Patients with heart failure may demonstrate the following:

1. Blood pressure may be elevated, with the diastolic pressure elevated to a greater extent than the systolic. The pulse pressure (systolic minus diastolic) is narrowed. For example, a normal blood pressure of 130/80 yields a pulse pressure of 50; a CHF blood pressure of 130/100 yields a pulse pressure of 30.
2. Heart rate (pulse) and respiratory rate are increased.
3. Any recent, unexplained, large weight gain (more than 3 pounds in a 7-day period) may indicate the onset of acute heart failure. If noted in conjunction with clinical signs of dependent edema (such as ankle swelling), dental therapy should be withheld until medical consultation is received.

Physical examination

Physical evaluation should include a careful visual inspection of the patient by the doctor.

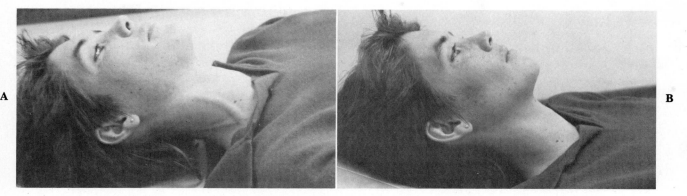

Fig. 14-2. A, Prominent jugular veins. **B,** With upright positioning, jugular vein disappears.

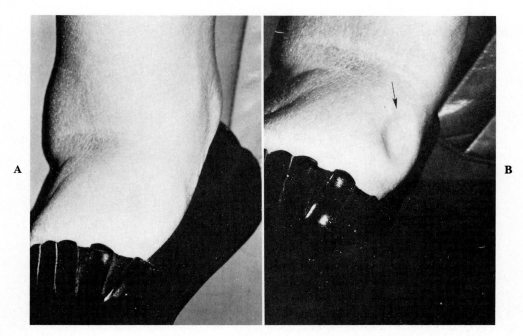

Fig. 14-3. Ankle demonstrating dependent edema. **A,** Clinical appearance of ankle before pressure application with finger. **B,** Arrows indicate "pitting" produced by pressure on right side of ankle.

Skin color. Cyanosis (a bluish tinge) is an indication of underoxygenation of the blood. Its presence should indicate the possibility of heart failure. Although skin color is important, it is perhaps more relevant to examine the patient's mucous membranes, particularly nailbeds and lips. Nail polish and lipstick may mask these areas, but the intraoral mucous membranes can always be observed.

Skin will rarely be noted to be cyanotic. More likely, the skin will appear to be ashen-gray in color. Cyanosis is much more likely to be observed in mucous membranes.

Neck. Prominent jugular veins are observable in patients with right heart failure when these patients are in the upright or semisupine position. In normal persons, jugular veins are collapsed and cannot be seen when the patient is in these positions.

Prominent jugular veins are normal when patients are placed in a supine position, but these veins will gradually "disappear" as the patient is slowly raised into a more upright position. At approximately a 30-degree angle or more, jugular veins should collapse and be undetectable (Fig. 14-2).

Ankles. Ankle swelling may be seen in patients with right heart failure (as well as in pregnant patients, those with varicose veins, and those with renal failure). If the patient follows a normal pattern of sleeping at night and being awake during the day, swelling occurs in the afternoon and disappears overnight. Edematous tissue may be differentiated from adipose tissue by a simple test. Pressure placed on edematous tissue for 30 seconds results in a "pitting" effect as the edema fluid is forced out of the area (Fig. 14-3). This pitting gradually disappears once the pressure is released. In contrast, adipose or normal tissue returns to its original dimension immediately upon release of pressure.

Dental Therapy Considerations

The information that is gathered by the methods just discussed must be formulated to enable the doctor to determine the degree of risk represented by this patient. This can be done with the following classifications:

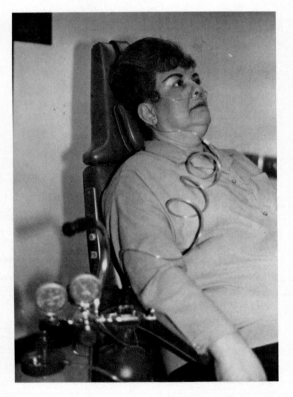

Fig. 14-4. Nasal oxygen or inhalation sedation unit used to provide supplemental oxygen to patient with CHF.

PHYSICAL STATUS ASA I. No dyspnea or undue fatigue with normal exertion

COMMENT. If all other items of the medical history are negative, this patient may be considered a normal, healthy person. No special modifications in dental therapy are indicated.

PHYSICAL STATUS ASA II. Mild dyspnea or fatigue on exertion

COMMENT. As with the class I patient, this patient may be managed in a normal manner if the rest of the medical history proves noncontributory. The Stress Reduction Protocol should be considered if any physical or psychologic stress is evident or anticipated.

PHYSICAL STATUS ASA III. Dyspnea or undue fatigue with normal activities

This patient is comfortable at rest in any position but may demonstrate a tendency toward orthopnea and have a history of paroxysmal nocturnal dyspnea.

COMMENT. The class III patient represents a greater risk during dental therapy. Before commencing dental therapy, medical consultation is recommended. The Stress Reduction Protocol and other specific modifications should be employed for this patient.

PHYSICAL STATUS ASA IV. Dyspnea, orthopnea, and undue fatigue at all times

COMMENT. The class IV patient represents a definite risk. Dental therapy should be withheld for all elective procedures until the cardiovascular disorder is corrected or controlled. Management of dental emergencies (pain and infection) should be handled with medication, and if actual physical intervention is required, the patient should be hospitalized and placed under a physician's care before, during, and immediately following the dental procedure.

With patients in any category of heart failure, and indeed with any cardiovascular disorder (angina pectoris and myocardial infarction), there is no contraindication to providing the patient with oxygen during the treatment period. A nasal cannula or nasal hood from an inhalation sedation unit may be used. A flow rate of 3 to 5 liters per minute is usually adequate (Fig. 14-4).

Positioning of the heart failure patient in the dental chair may require modification. If the patient finds it difficult to breathe in the supine position, the doctor must reposition the chair until the patient is comfortable again. As noted earlier, this is termed orthopnea and represents a class III risk, requiring medical consultation before dental therapy. The use of a rubber dam may be contraindicated in this patient, too.

CLINICAL MANIFESTATIONS

Clinical manifestations of heart failure are related to the specific portion of the heart that is failing. Varying degrees of heart failure may be present so that not all patients exhibit all of the symptoms and signs described below. In addition, most patients exhibit congestive heart failure, which is a combined failure of the left and right ventricles.

Clinical signs and symptoms are presented for each side of the heart individually and then acute pulmonary edema will be discussed. Left heart failure is clinically manifested by *symptoms* of pulmonary congestion, whereas right heart failure is dominated by *signs* of systemic venous congestion and peripheral edema. Undue fatigue and weakness are prominent symptoms in both types of heart failure.

Left Heart Failure
Symptoms

Manifestations of left heart failure are primarily associated with respiratory difficulty, with the severity of the difficulty related to the degree of heart failure. The pathophysiology of each symptom is discussed below.

Weakness and undue fatigue are usually the first symptoms of left heart failure to become evident to the patient. The patient becomes aware of them when feeling fatigued during exertion that previously caused no fatigue. As heart failure progresses, fatigue is produced with less and less exertion until it is present at rest. *Dyspnea* (difficulty in breathing) is usually evident with exertion. This is commonly associated with an increase in the rate of breathing (tachypnea). *Cough and expectoration* are present, being related to reflexes produced by the congested lungs and bronchi.

The patient with early left heart failure may report an increased frequency of urination at night (*nocturia*), a symptom produced by the mobilization of edema fluid from the extremities back into the general circulation.

Orthopnea and *paroxysmal nocturnal dyspnea* are later, more ominous signs related to left heart failure. Orthopnea is dyspnea that occurs soon after lying flat and is relieved by sitting up. The patient with orthopnea is able to alleviate this situation by supporting the head and thorax with more than 2 pillows. As heart failure progresses, this patient may be forced into the upright position (sitting in a chair) even during sleep. Positioning of this patient in the dental chair may be difficult. Orthopnea and paroxysmal nocturnal dyspnea, if present, represent a class 3 medical risk and require specific modifications in dental management of the patient. When their condition is severe, these patients may require supplemental oxygen 24 hours a day; they carry with them portable oxygen cylinders and a nasal cannula. These patients are unable to lie down when attempting to sleep, being forced to sleep in the totally erect position.

Paroxysmal nocturnal dyspnea is an exaggerated form of orthopnea. With PND, the patient is awakened from sleep, gasping for breath with a degree of respiratory difficulty verging on suffocation. The patient seeks relief desperately, usually sitting up or rushing to an open window to breathe "fresh air." For unknown reasons, these patients may exhibit inspiratory and expiratory wheezing (cardiac asthma). These episodes may pass in a few minutes or progress to become acute pulmonary edema.

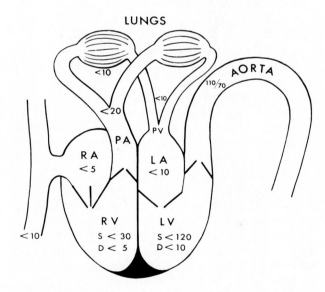

Fig. 14-5. Average blood pressures in various components of circulatory system. *LA*, left atrium; *LV*, left ventricle; *PA*, pulmonary arteries. (From Wylie, W.D., and Churchill-Davidson, H.C.: A practice of anaesthesia, ed. 3, Chicago, 1972, Year Book Medical Publishers, Inc.)

Signs

The patient with moderate-to-severe left heart failure appears pale and is usually sweating. The skin is cold to the touch, and it will be obvious to the observer that the patient is having difficulty breathing.

Monitoring of vital signs demonstrates an increase in the blood pressure, with the diastolic pressure elevated to a greater degree than the systolic. The pulse pressure (systolic pressure minus the diastolic pressure) is therefore narrowed. Heart rate is rapid. It may also be possible to detect *pulsus alternans,* which is the appearance of alternating strong and weak heart beats even though the basic rhythm of the heart remains normal; it is frequently seen in later stages of heart failure. Tachypnea (increased rate of breathing) and hyperventilation (increased depth of breathing) are commonly seen in left heart failure as a consequence of the pulmonary congestion.

Right Heart Failure
Signs

Right heart failure is characterized by signs and develops after left heart failure has been present for a short period of time. Systemic venous congestion is the chief complaint. The patient first notices signs of peripheral edema. Swelling of the feet and/or ankles develops during the day in persons with right heart failure and subsides overnight. This is referred to as dependent, or pitting, edema. If the patient is permitted to remain in the supine position for extended periods, this edema fluid will relocate in the sacral region. Dependent edema is a characteristic feature of right heart failure.

Weakness and undue fatigue are present in right heart failure as they are in left heart failure, produced by the deficient supply of oxygen and nutrients to the tissues of the body. Another result of this oxygen lack is the presence of cyanosis. Especially prominent in mucous membranes (nailbeds and lips), cyanosis is produced by the removal by the tissues of a greater than normal amount of oxygen from the arterial blood in an attempt to compensate for the decreased supply of oxygen in the blood. This decreased blood supply is also a cause of the coolness noted in the extremities.

Other signs of right heart failure include the presence of prominent jugular veins in the neck. In normal individuals the jugular veins are not evident in the erect position; with failure of the right ventricle, however, systemic blood cannot be delivered

Table 14-2. Clinical manifestations of heart failure and acute pulmonary edema

Signs	Symptoms
Heart failure	
Pallor, cool skin	Weakness and undue fatigue
Sweating	Dyspnea on exertion
Left ventricular hypertrophy	Hyperventilation
	Nocturia
Dependent edema	Orthopnea
Hepatomegaly and splenomegaly	Paroxysmal nocturnal dyspnea
Narrow pulse pressure	Wheezing (cardiac asthma)
Pulsus alternans	
Ascites	
Acute pulmonary edema	
All of the signs of heart failure	All of the symptoms of heart failure
Moist rales at base of lungs	Increased anxiety
Tachypnea	Dyspnea at rest
Dyspnea	
Cyanosis	
Frothy pink sputum	

to the heart normally, and engorgement of the jugular veins occurs.

Engorgement of the liver (hepatomegaly) and spleen (splenomegaly) also occur. On examination, the physician can palpate an enlarged liver. As right heart failure progresses, the edematous areas enlarge so that the legs, thighs, and eventually the abdomen (ascites) demonstrate clinical edema. Congestion of the gastrointestinal tract also occurs, associated with clinical signs of anorexia, nausea, and vomiting. Central nervous system signs of edema include headache, insomnia, and irritability.

In left and right heart failure there is considerable anxiety. Once difficulty in breathing manifests itself, the patient, aware of the situation, begins to hyperventilate. Indeed, patients with heart failure may hyperventilate to the point of producing respiratory alkalosis, with clinical symptoms of lightheadedness, cold hands, and tingling fingers (see Chapter 12). The workload of the heart increases even further, as does the degree of heart failure.

Acute Pulmonary Edema

Acute pulmonary edema is a disorder in which there is a sudden and rapid transudation of fluid from the pulmonary capillary bed into the alveolar spaces of the lungs. It is often precipitated by stressful situations of a physical or psychologic nature. The onset of symptoms is usually acute. A slight, dry cough is often the initial symptom; acute pulmonary edema may represent a direct extension of paroxysmal nocturnal dyspnea. Asthmatic-type wheezing may be evident at this stage (cardiac asthma). Dyspnea and orthopnea are commonly present. As the attack progresses, the patient develops a feeling of suffocation and an acute sense of anxiety that increases the rate and difficulty of breathing still further. A sense of oppression may be noted in the chest. Physical signs evident at this time include tachypnea, dyspnea, and cough. If auscultated, the lungs demonstrate moist rales at the bases, which progressively extend upward as the attack worsens.

In more severe episodes, pallor, sweating, cyanosis, and a frothy, pink (blood-tinged) sputum are present. Acute pulmonary edema is not uncommon during the period immediately following myocardial infarction if the degree of left ventricular myocardial damage has been great. Table 14-2 summarizes signs and symptoms.

PATHOPHYSIOLOGY

To view heart failure in its proper perspective, it is necessary to first review the normal function of the human heart at rest and during physical activity. The mechanisms of cardiac dysfunction then become more obvious.

The human heart is comprised of two individual pumps working together (Fig. 14-5). The right side of the heart receives venous (unoxygenated) blood from the systemic circulation and pumps this blood through the pulmonary arteries to the lungs, where it undergoes oxygenation. From the lungs, the oxygenated (arterial) blood is delivered to the left atrium and then to the left ventricle, where it is pumped to the systemic circulation. The amount of work required by each ventricle to perform its task is considerably different. The right side of the heart may be considered as the low pressure system; an average right ventricular pressure of 30 torr is required to pump blood out into the pulmonary artery. By contrast, the left side of the heart is a high pressure system; the left intraventricular pressure approximates 120/80 torr during systole (contraction). It can therefore be seen that the left ventricle performs most of the actual work of the heart. Before birth, both ventricles are taxed equally because they bear the same pressure loads. Following

Table 14-3. Minimum adult human oxygen requirements

Activity	Oxygen utilization (ml/min)
Rest	250
Standing	375
Walking	400-1000
Light work and exercise	750-1250
Intense exercise	4000 and above

birth, however, the pulmonary arterial pressure falls, the workload of the right ventricle is decreased, and its walls become thin, whereas the workload of the left ventricle increases and its walls enlarge.

The primary function of the heart is to serve as a pump, supplying blood containing oxygen and nutrients to the body. Table 14-3 lists minimal oxygen requirements per minute for the average adult performing various activities. Should the heart for whatever reason be unable to provide the body with its required oxygen supply, shortness of breath and undue fatigue result. These usually occur when oxygen transport per minute does not exceed 1000 to 1250 ml per minute. This level usually permits a person to work at a light job and enjoy light recreation and sport without discomfort but does not allow him to put forth more strenuous effort.

Normal Left Ventricular Function

The left ventricle is a thick muscular organ. At rest (diastole) the intraventricular pressure is approximately 6 to 8 torr, whereas the diastolic pressure in the aorta is approximately 80 torr. For blood to be expelled from the left ventricle into the aorta the intraventricular pressure must exceed the aortic blood pressure so that the aortic valves will open. The following is the normal sequence of left ventricular function when a person is at rest.

Maximal left ventricular filling, termed the end-diastolic volume, occurs at the instant just before the start of systole. At this moment, the muscles of the ventricle begin to contract, but no blood is being ejected from the ventricle. Instead, the size of the cavity is rapidly decreasing, producing a sharp increase in intraventricular pressure. This interval, termed the isovolemic period of systole, normally lasts 50 milliseconds (0.050 second).

In a short time the intraventricular pressure exceeds the diastolic aortic blood pressure (80 torr), the aortic valves are forced open, and the ejection of blood begins. The ventricle continues to contract for a period of time (systole), and then relaxation occurs. The blood pressure within the left ventricle falls rapidly with relaxation. Once the left-ventricular blood pressure falls below the aortic blood pressure, the aortic valve closes, signaling the end of systole and the beginning of diastole. During diastole the intra-aortic blood pressure exceeds that in the ventricle, permitting filling of the ventricle to occur.

At the time of closure of the aortic valves, the volume of blood in the left ventricle is at its lowest level. The difference in volume between end-diastolic volume (maximal volume) and end-systolic volume (minimal volume) is termed the *ejection fraction*. In a normally functioning heart at rest, this fraction is 0.56 to 0.78; in other words, from 56% to 78% of the blood present in the left ventricle at the end of diastole will be ejected into the aorta during systole. As left ventricular failure develops, the ejection fraction decreases and may be as low as 0.1 to 0.2 in severe failure.

Although this mechanism functions in normal situations, it must be remembered that the demands placed on the heart by the body change from second to second. The heart must therefore be capable of responding rapidly to these ever-changing demands by increasing or decreasing the volume of blood ejected per stroke (stroke volume). Three factors—preload, afterload, and contractility—assist in enabling the heart to meet its obligations to the tissues of the body.

Preload is the end-diastolic volume. The greater the preload, the more the myocardial muscle fibers are stretched. According to the Frank-Starling principle, the greater the myocardial muscle is stretched in diastole, the greater it will contract in systole. This may be likened to a rubber band being stretched. This principle is illustrated by the following: With a preload of 100 ml of blood and an ejection fraction of 0.6 (60%), the stroke volume will be 60 ml. Should the preload increase to 140 ml, for example, and the ejection fraction remain 0.6, the stroke volume will increase to 84 ml. In the same manner, decreased preload leads to a diminished stroke volume.

Afterload may be defined as the pressure that resists left ventricular ejection (aortic blood pressure). Increased afterload therefore makes it more difficult for the heart to eject a normal stroke volume. As an example, if the aortic blood pressure

rises rapidly (under extreme stress, for example) from 120/80 to 200/120 torr, the intraventricular pressure must rise to 120 torr (the aortic diastolic pressure) before the aortic valve will even open. This valve remains open for only a brief period before the aortic pressure once again exceeds that of the ventricle and closes the aortic valve. The ejection fraction in this instance will be very low (0.1 to 0.2). Such a stroke volume is not adequate to support the requirements of the body if permitted to continue. However, the normal heart is able to compensate for this inadequate stroke volume. The end-systolic volume is larger than normal (because of the nonejected blood). To this will be added the normal blood volume from the left atrium. This increased preload (normal volume plus large end-systolic volume) causes the myocardial fibers to stretch, thereby contracting more forcefully (Frank-Starling principle) with the next beat. Within several beats the ventricle is able to adjust the stroke volume to meet the increased blood pressure, from 120/80 to 200/120 torr. There are limits to the Frank-Starling principle in that excessive stretch or sudden increase in afterload will not be met by ever-increasing contraction of the myocardium.

If the preload and afterload of the heart are permitted to remain the same, it is still possible for the stroke volume to be increased. *Contractility* is a basic property of cardiac muscle. The sympathetic nervous system can increase the contraction of the heart through the release of epinephrine and norepinephrine. These catecholamines, which are released in increasing amounts under stress, increase the degree of myocardial fiber contraction, thus increasing the ejection fraction (from 0.6 to 0.8), and result in increased stroke volume.

Heart Failure

Heart failure may develop in any patient whose heart has been working for extended periods against an increased peripheral resistance (increased afterload), which is seen in high blood pressure, or in a patient for whom the workload of the heart has increased because of valvular defects (stenosis or insufficiency) or because of prolonged, continuous demands for increased cardiac output (as in hyperthyroidism). These states, which demand a chronic increase in cardiac workload, all lead to structural changes in the heart muscle that eventually progress to muscular weakness and the clinical symptoms and signs of heart failure.

Another major cause of myocardial weakness is the presence of disease states that directly attack the muscle, for example, coronary artery disease and myocarditis. In these conditions the myocardium is unable to respond normally to increases in afterload. The increase in fiber length that occurs will not be met with the usual increase in stroke volume, and clinical heart failure results.

The chronic progression of heart failure may best be illustrated by following the cardiac changes occurring in high blood pressure, one of the leading causes of heart failure. In response to chronic elevation of the blood pressure (afterload) the myocardium must contract more forcefully for an extended period of time to maintain an adequate stroke volume. As with other muscles doing increased work, the myocardial fibers hypertrophy (increase in diameter and length). This response is seen primarily in the left ventricle and leads to the first sign of heart failure, left ventricular hypertrophy (LVH). A normal heart weighs approximately 250 to 350 g. In mild heart failure, the heart may weigh up to 500 g; in more severe heart failure, weights of up to 1000 g have been recorded. LVH may be present for many years before being discovered, generally on a routine electrocardiogram or chest roentgenogram.

Another important feature of LVH is that, along with the increased size of muscle fibers, there is not a corresponding increase in the number of capillaries; therefore the blood supply to the myocardium becomes increasingly compromised as hypertrophy progresses. Because of the compromised blood supply seen in LVH, there comes a point at which hypertrophy alone can no longer maintain adequate stroke volume in the presence of increased blood pressure. At this point, a second mechanism aids in maintaining normal stroke volume. It is called dilation and is an increase in the capacity of the left ventricle brought about by elongation of myocardial fibers. The force of ventricular contraction of these elongated myocardial fibers increases through the Frank-Starling principle, thereby maintaining a normal stroke volume. It is evident, however, that both the end-diastolic (increased total blood volume) and the end-systolic (increased residual blood) volumes are increased. Therefore the ejection fraction is decreased (<0.56).

As the end-diastolic volume increases, the workload of the heart increases, thereby increasing the myocardial oxygen requirement. In the presence of coronary artery disease or left ventricular hypertrophy, this demand for oxygen may not be met, leading to more severe heart failure or to angina pectoris or myocardial infarction. As with left ventricular hypertrophy, dilation is evident on an ECG and chest roentgenogram.

If the blood pressure continues to rise or if the myocardium weakens, hypertrophy and dilation will be unable to maintain a stroke volume adequate to supply peripheral tissues with their required amounts of oxygen and nutrients. As this situation develops, the patient first becomes aware of the symptoms of undue fatigue and dyspnea on exertion as the left ventricle becomes unable to increase its output in response to exercise. As left heart failure progresses, dyspnea develops with less and less exertion (progressing from ASA II to III to IV risk levels). Left ventricular failure also occurs at night when the patient lies down. At this time the total blood volume is increased as venous return from the lower extremities is improved because of the decreased effects of gravity in the supine position. Patients must now elevate their head and thorax at night with pillows to breathe comfortably, because this increased fluid volume begins to produce respiratory difficulty (orthopnea).

Blood volume increases in a second and perhaps more important manner that involves the kidneys. The decrease in stroke volume leads to a decrease in renal blood flow and glomerular filtration rate (GFR), thereby decreasing the excretion of sodium. In fact, tubular reabsorption of sodium is actually stimulated through the increased secretion of renin and its attendant chemical reactions (secondary to decreased GFR). This increased sodium retention also leads to a decreased secretion of antidiuretic hormone from the pituitary, which is responsible for further water retention. These mechanisms result in an increase in total blood volume (hypervolemia).

Hypervolemia produces an increased hydrostatic pressure in the capillaries, leading at first to interstitial edema and then to an actual transudation of fluid into tissues with decreased tissue pressure. Edema of the ankles and lower extremities develops during the day when the patient is erect because of the downward force of gravity; it develops in the sacral region at night when the patient is recumbent.

Clinical signs and symptoms of left heart failure become most prominent at night when most patients assume the recumbent position. During the day when the patient is in the erect position, the force of gravity causes the excessive fluid volume to be deposited in the subcutaneous tissues of the dependent portions of the body (ankles), producing signs and symptoms of right heart failure.

With the patient in the supine position, the edematous fluid in the dependent portions of the body is mobilized, leading to a rapid increase in blood volume and venous return to the heart. This may lead to overdistention of an already weakened left ventricle, producing an acute reduction in cardiac output and a large increase in end-diastolic and end-systolic volumes. As a result, the end-diastolic pressure may also rise. A normal end-diastolic pressure of 6 to 8 torr may rise to 30 to 40 torr or greater. The increased left ventricular pressure raises the left atrial pressure. The Frank-Starling principle enables the left atrium to accommodate to this pressure, and after a few heartbeats the pressure in the left atrium increases to 30 to 40 torr or above, remaining elevated for as long as the left ventricle is in failure.

This increased left atrial pressure is next transmitted backward to the pulmonary veins and capillaries so that the pulmonary capillary pressure also increases to 30 to 40 torr. When this occurs, water and solutes diffuse out of the capillaries into the alveolar air sacs, producing paroxysmal nocturnal dyspnea or acute pulmonary edema or both. In the presence of this fluid in the alveolar air sacs, oxygen and carbon dioxide cannot be exchanged, and dyspnea is the result. Positional changes produce dramatic relief in symptoms of left heart failure by causing fluid to move from the alveolar sacs and concentrate in the lung bases.

Right ventricular and atrial failure occurs shortly after left heart failure as the increased pressures continue to back up. This results in signs and symptoms of systemic venous and capillary congestion. As this increase in pressure develops, fluid leaves the vessels in the most dependent portions of the body (ankles and feet). In addition, because of the elevated right atrial pressure, venous return from the head and upper extremities is impaired, and the jugular veins become engorged. Impaired venous return from the lower portion of the body is evident through engorgement of the liver with blood (hepatomegaly).

Nocturia, or increased frequency of urination at night, is yet another sign of heart failure. During the day with the patient awake, renal function is poor because the patient's activities increase the degree of heart failure. Therefore the patient produces less urine during the day. At night cardiac function improves, as does renal function. Increased glomerular filtration produces more urine—thus the symptom of nocturia results.

One final sign of heart failure is cyanosis. It is most evident in mucous membranes and is produced by the failure of the heart to provide an adequate stroke volume. In an effort to secure an adequate oxygen supply, the tissues of the body extract more oxygen than normal from the capillary blood. Therefore the red blood cells within the capillaries and veins are poorly oxygenated and appear a darker color, which is clinically evident as cyanosis.

MANAGEMENT

The patient with acute pulmonary edema represents a true medical emergency that must be managed quickly. In the dental office the patient who has a prior history of heart failure, be it left, right, or combined (congestive heart failure), and who is experiencing acute respiratory difficulty should be managed in the following manner.

Step 1. Position patient. As with patients with other forms of respiratory difficulty, on most occasions the patient in acute pulmonary edema remains conscious. Position the patient in the most comfortable manner, which will usually be the upright position. This position allows excess fluid within the lung tissues to concentrate at the bases of the lungs, permitting a greater exchange of oxygen to occur. Should these patients lose consciousness at any time, they must be placed in the supine position.

Step 2. Administer oxygen. Oxygen should be administered to all patients who demonstrate signs of acute pulmonary edema or congestive heart failure. High concentrations should be administered to prevent or alleviate hypoxia. Face masks and nasal hoods should be avoided if possible because they tend to exaggerate the feeling of suffocation already being experienced by the patient, thereby causing further agitation. A nasal cannula at a flow rate of 3 to 5 liters of oxygen per minute is the preferred method of administration in the dental office (Fig. 14-4). Once the patient is hospitalized, an oxygen tent can be used.

Step 3. Measure vital signs. Vital signs should be recorded. Blood pressure, heart rate, and respiratory rate will increase. Such recordings demonstrate the presence of extreme apprehension and cardiac and pulmonary congestion.

Step 4. Alleviate symptoms of respiratory distress. The immediate primary goal in the management of these patients is the alleviation of their breathing difficulty. Proper (upright) positioning of the patient is extremely important. If breathing difficulty is still evident, however, additional steps may be taken. In heart failure, the heart is unable to adequately handle the quantity of blood being delivered to it.

A procedure that may be carried out *in the hospital* is phlebotomy. Approximately 350 to 500 ml of blood is removed from the patient. Phlebotomy is sometimes rapidly effective in reducing respiratory symptoms. This effect is achieved through a reduction in the venous return to the right side of the heart while the left side is permitted to drain some of the excess fluid from the lungs.

Phlebotomy in the dental office is not often indicated. A similar effect may be achieved, however, through use of a *bloodless phlebotomy*. Tourniquets or blood pressure cuffs are applied to the extremities. (Wide, soft, rubber tubing should be used for the tourniquets.) The tourniquets are placed approximately 6 inches below the groin and approximately 4 inches below the shoulders. Tourniquets are applied to only three extremities at a time. Every 15 to 20 minutes, one of the tourniquets is released and applied to the free extremity. The tourniquets (or blood pressure cuffs) should be applied at a pressure less than the systolic blood pressure but greater than the diastolic. An arterial pulse should be palpable distal to each tourniquet or cuff. Large quantities of blood may be removed from the circulation in this manner, permitting the heart to function more effectively and dyspnea to be alleviated.

Bloodless phlebotomy actually leads to a total reduction in the circulating blood volume. While trapped in the extremities, a protein-poor filtrate is forced out of the capillaries into the tissues, where it remains for a period of time even after the tourniquet is removed.

Step 5. Alleviate apprehension. Most patients in acute pulmonary edema become acutely apprehensive. Increased apprehension leads to increases in cardiac and respiratory workload, which are absolutely contraindicated in these patients. For this reason, anxiety must be reduced.

If the preceding steps alleviated the respiratory difficulty, the patient may no longer be apprehensive. However, in the presence of continued anxiety and respiratory difficulty, drug therapy must

---

> **MANAGEMENT OF HEART FAILURE AND ACUTE PULMONARY EDEMA**
>
> *Step 1* Place patient in upright position
> *2* Administer oxygen (nasal cannula preferred)
> *3* Record vital signs
> Blood pressure
> Heart rate and rhythm
> Respiratory rate
> *4* Alleviate symptoms of respiratory difficulty
> Place patient in upright position
> Bloodless phlebotomy, rotating tourniquets
> *5* Alleviate apprehension
> Meperidine, 50 mg IM, or morphine, 10 mg IM (for adults)
> *6* Summon medical assistance

---

be considered. A narcotic agonist such as meperidine, 50 mg IM, or morphine, 10 to 15 mg IM, should be administered (adult doses). Pediatric doses of morphine in pulmonary edema are 0.1 to 0.2 mg IV per kilogram of body weight. These agents reduce anxiety and agitation and also produce vasodilation, thereby decreasing the cardiac and pulmonary workloads. An *absolute contraindication* to these agents in heart failure is the (1) clinical presence of hypoxia (Table 13-1) with cyanosis or (2) mental confusion or delirium. Narcotics further depress respiration in these individuals when they already have severely compromised respiratory function. Naloxone must be available whenever narcotic agonists are employed. Nalbuphine, a narcotic agonist-antagonist, has also been used with considerable success.

Step 6. Summon medical assistance. The patient with acute respiratory difficulty usually requires hospitalization for further medical management. At the earliest opportunity, medical assistance should be sought. When the patient is transferred to the hospital, the dentist should accompany the patient and remain until a physician takes over management of the patient. Further medical therapy in the hospital may include phlebotomy, an oxygen tent, and drugs such as digitalis and diuretics. The management of heart failure and acute pulmonary edema is summarized in the box above.

BIBLIOGRAPHY

Barkin, R.M., and Rosen, P.: Congestive heart failure. In Barkin, R.M., and Rosen, P.: Emergency pediatrics, St. Louis, 1984, The C.V. Mosby Co.

Barkin, R.M., and Rosen, P.: Pulmonary edema. In Barkin, R.M., and Rosen, P.: Emergency pediatrics, St. Louis, 1984, The C.V. Mosby Co.

Braunwald, E.: Clinical manifestations of heart failure. In Braunwald, E., editor: Heart disease, Philadelphia, 1980, W.B. Saunders Co.

Braunwald, E.: Pathophysiology of heart failure. In Braunwald, E., editor: Heart disease, Philadelphia, 1980, W.B. Saunders Co.

Burch, G.E., and DePasquale, N.P.: Congestive heart failure—acute pulmonary edema, JAMA **208:**106, 1969.

Chait, A.: Interstitial pulmonary edema, Circulation **45:**1323, 1972.

Dodge, H.T.: Hemodynamic aspects of cardiac failure, Hosp. Pract. **6:**91, 1971.

Fishman, A.P.: Pulmonary edema: The water exchanging function of the lung, Circulation **46:**390, 1972.

Goldberger, E.: Treatment of cardiac emergencies, ed. 3, St. Louis, 1982, The C.V. Mosby Co.

Hoffman, J.I.F., and Stanger, P.: Congestive heart failure. In Pascoe, D.J., and Grossman, M., editors: Quick reference to pediatric emergencies, ed. 3, Philadelphia, 1983, J.B. Lippincott Co.

Ingram, R.H., Jr., and Braunwald, E.: Pulmonary edema: cardiogenic and noncardiogenic forms. In Braunwald, E., editor: Heart disease, Philadelphia, 1980, W.B. Saunders Co.

Katz, A.M.: Congestive heart failure. N. Engl. J. Med. **293:**1184, 1975.

Laragh, J.H.: Diuretics in the management of congestive heart failure, Hosp. Pract. **5:**43, 1970.

Lassers, B.W., and others: Left ventricular failure in acute myocardial infarction, Am. J. Cardiol. **25:**511, 1970.

Levine, H.J.: Compliance of the left ventricle, Circulation **46:**423, 1972.

Mason, D.T., Zelis, R., and Wikman-Coffelt, J.: Symposium of congestive heart failure: recent advances in structure, biochemistry, physiology and pharmacology, Am. J. Cardiol. **32:**395, 1973.

McKee, P.A., and others: Natural history of congestive heart failure: the Framingham study, N. Engl. J. Med. **285:**1441, 1971.

Mescaros, W.T.: Lung changes in left heart failure, Circulation **47:**859, 1973.

Pascoe, D.J.: Pulmonary edema. In Pascoe, D.J., and Grossman, M., editors: Quick reference to pediatric emergencies, ed. 3, Philadelphia, 1983, J.B. Lippincott Co.

Ramirez, A., and Abelmann, W.H.: Cardiac decompensation, N. Engl. J. Med. **290:**499, 1974.

Robin, E.D., Cross, C.E., and Zelis, R.: Pulmonary edema, 2. N. Engl. J. Med. **288:**292, 1973.

Schlant, R.C., and Clark, D.W.: Refractory heart failure, Hosp. Med. **11:**46, 1975.

Schlant, R.C., and Hurst, J.W.: Assessment of cardiac function at the bedside, Geriatrics **30:**49, 1975.

Schreiner, B.F., Jr., Murphy, G.W., and Kramer, D.H.: The pathophysiology of pulmonary congestion, Prog. Cardiovasc. Dis. **14:**47, 1971.

Smith, T.W., and Braunwald, E.: The management of heart failure. In Braunwald, E., editor: Heart disease, Philadelphia, 1980, W.B. Saunders Co.

Smulyan, H., Gilber, R., and Eich, R.H.: Pulmonary effects of heart failure, Surg. Clin. North Am. **54:**1077, 1974.

Staub, N.C.: Pulmonary edema-hypoxia and overperfusion (editorial), N. Engl. J. Med. **302:**1085, 1980.

Talner, N.S.: Congestive heart failure in the infant: a functional approach, Pediatr. Clin. North Am. **18:**1011, 1971.

Walker, W.J.: Treatment of heart failure, JAMA **228:**1276, 1974.

15 Respiratory Difficulty: Differential Diagnosis

In most clinical situations, the etiology of respiratory difficulty is readily discernible, and definitive management of the patient is thus expedited. However, there are other situations in which the precise etiology of respiratory difficulty is less apparent. In these cases, consideration of the following factors will assist the doctor in determining the cause of the clinical problem being faced, thereby permitting definitive therapy to proceed.

Prior Medical History

The patient with respiratory difficulty almost always remains conscious during the episode. We may take advantage of this situation by asking the patient about any previous episodes of respiratory difficulty. Problems such as asthma, heart failure, or previous episodes of hyperventilation usually are noted on the medical history questionnaire, facilitating the differential diagnosis. Should this patient lose consciousness at any time, management must then proceed as with any unconscious patient (Section II).

Age of Patient

Respiratory distress in younger patients (under the age of 10) is most commonly related to asthma (usually allergic asthma); hyperventilation and heart failure are less common at this age. Between the ages of 12 and 40, the hyperventilation syndrome is the most likely cause of difficulty in breathing. Asthma may also occur in this group, but in most instances the patient will have indicated a prior awareness of its presence. Clinically significant heart failure is rarely seen before the age of 40. The peak incidence of heart failure in men is between ages 50 and 60 and in women, between ages 60 and 70.

Sex of Patient

The incidence of hyperventilation, asthma, and heart failure does not differ markedly between males and females, although the incidence of heart failure is somewhat greater in males compared to females under the age of 70.

Circumstances Associated with Respiratory Difficulty

Stress, physiologic or psychologic, is present in most instances of respiratory difficulty and in all cases increases the severity of respiratory distress. The hyperventilation syndrome is precipitated almost exclusively by extreme apprehension. Asthma, especially in children, may be acutely exacerbated in stressful situations regardless of the type of asthma (intrinsic or extrinsic). Heart failure patients undergo progressive deterioration of their physical condition when subjected to stress.

Presence of Clinical Symptoms Between Acute Episodes

The patient with heart failure may exhibit clinical signs and symptoms of the disease in periods between acute flareups. Orthopnea, dependent edema, peripheral cyanosis, dyspnea, and undue fatigue may be evident at all dental appointments, depending on the degree of pump failure present.

Adult asthmatics usually are asymptomatic in the intervals between acute episodes; however, noisy breathing and chronic cough may be present.

No clinical signs and symptoms of hyperventilation can be noted between episodes.

Position of Patient

The position of the patient at the onset of clinical symptoms of respiratory difficulty is most relevant in heart failure. Respiratory difficulty becomes progressively more severe as the dental chair approaches the supine position. Dramatic relief of symptoms can often be achieved by allowing the patient to sit upright.

Signs and symptoms of asthma and hyperventilation are not altered through positioning, although most patients experiencing respiratory difficulty are better able to breathe when sitting upright.

Sounds Associated with Respiratory Difficulty

Wheezing is usually present in patients with asthma. It may also be present in paroxysmal nocturnal dyspnea and pulmonary edema ("cardiac asthma"), although in these circumstances it is associated with other clinical symptoms of heart failure. Partial obstruction of the trachea or bronchi with a foreign object may also produce wheezing.

Moist, wet respirations may be evident in heart failure, especially acute pulmonary edema. Acute pulmonary edema is usually associated with a frothy, pink-tinged sputum and cough.

In hyperventilation, breathing is usually more rapid and deeper than normal, but no abnormal sound is associated with it.

Symptoms Associated with Respiratory Difficulty

Shortness of breath is observed in most cases of respiratory difficulty. In heart failure it becomes progressively worse on reclining (orthopnea) and increases with exertion. Shortness of breath seen in hyperventilation is related to anxiety and a feeling of suffocation and is not related to exertion. Hyperventilation is not associated with cough.

In acute asthma, shortness of breath is associated with episodic wheezing and an asymptomatic state between episodes.

Peripheral Edema and Cyanosis

Peripheral edema and cyanosis may be present in the patient with heart failure. Other possible causes of peripheral edema are renal disease, varicose veins, and pregnancy, whereas cardiorespiratory disease and polycythemia vera are causes of cyanosis. In severe asthma with hypoxia or hypercarbia, peripheral cyanosis may be present.

Paresthesia of Extremities

Tingling and numbness of the fingers, toes, and perioral region are present in the hyperventilation syndrome. In milder episodes of acute asthma and heart failure these symptoms may also be present, produced by acute anxiety.

Use of Accessory Muscles of Respiration

The patient with acute asthma demonstrates use of the accessory muscles of respiration (abdominal and neck muscles). This may also be noted in patients with acute pulmonary edema.

Chest Pain

Chest pain is commonly experienced by the hyperventilating patient. The pain is often described as a "weight" or a "pressing" sensation, or as "shooting" or "stabbing." Other clinical manifestations of cardiac disease are rarely present, however. The age of the hyperventilating patient is usually below that at which one normally expects to encounter cardiovascular disease (over 35 years).

Asthmatic and heart failure patients usually do not experience chest pain along with their other clinical symptoms.

Heart Rate and Blood Pressure

Measurement of the heart rate and blood pressure during respiratory distress usually demonstrates definite elevations of both of these vital signs. One reason for this in hyperventilation and in the acute asthmatic attack is the presence of anxiety. In these cases, blood pressure (systolic and diastolic) and heart rate are elevated.

In heart failure, although both systolic and diastolic pressures are elevated, the diastolic is usually elevated to a greater extent; therefore the pulse pressure (systolic minus diastolic) is narrowed (to less than 40). Heart rate increases in heart failure.

Duration of Respiratory Difficulty

Respiratory difficulty associated with heart failure often dramatically improves by repositioning the patient. However, if pulmonary edema is present, respiratory difficulty is not improved until definitive management is instituted (phlebotomy or anxiety control).

Most asthmatic attacks are not terminated until the patient receives proper medication (bronchodilator); status asthmaticus requires more definitive management—possibly a period of hospitalization.

The hyperventilation syndrome is usually manageable without drug intervention and rarely, if ever, necessitates the help of additional personnel or hospitalization.

The algorithm for the diagnosis and management of respiratory difficulty is found on p. 393.

16 Altered Consciousness: General Considerations

A number of systemic medical conditions may manifest themselves clinically as alterations in the victim's state of consciousness. In almost every situation listed in Table 16-1, the loss of consciousness may ultimately occur, too. However, in most cases prompt recognition of clinical signs and symptoms and the institution of corrective measures permit the victim to remain conscious until definitive management becomes available.

The following are definitions of relevant terms:

confusion A mental state marked by the mingling of ideas with consequent disturbances of comprehension and understanding, leading to bewilderment.

delirium A mental disturbance marked by illusions, delusions, cerebral excitement, physical restlessness, and incoherence.

dizziness A disturbed sense of relationship to space; a sensation of unsteadiness with a feeling of movement within the head.

Altered consciousness may be the first clinical sign of a serious medical problem that requires immediate and intensive therapy to maintain the victim's life. It is important therefore that the doctor be aware of a patient's medical background in order to recognize the developing medical problem when it arises and to manage any emergency that may develop at a later time.

PREDISPOSING FACTORS

The most common cause of altered consciousness is the ingestion or administration of drugs. With the increasing use of psychosedation in dental practice, we are likely to encounter a greater number of reports of inadvertent overadministration of these agents to patients. Proper use of these drugs will, however, minimize these incidents.

One particular psychosedative is rarely prescribed by the doctor but may well be the most commonly used drug by dental patients. The drug is alcohol, and most practicing dentists have on occasion been called on to manage the dental needs of a patient who has taken an inadvertent (or in some instances, an intentional) overdose; in other words, the patient is drunk. Proper patient management at such times is to withhold dental therapy and reschedule the patient's appointment with a strict admonition concerning the self-administration of drugs. It might be important for the doctor to seek

Table 16-1. Causes of altered consciousness

Cause	Frequency	Where discussed
Drug overdose (alcohol, barbiturates, insulin)	Most common	Drug-related emergencies (Section VI)
Hyperventilation syndrome	Common	Respiratory difficulty (Section III)
Hypoglycemia	Common	Altered consciousness (Section IV)
Hyperglycemia	Less common	Altered consciousness (Section IV)
Cerebrovascular accident, transient ischemic attack	Less common	Altered consciousness (Section IV)
Hyperthyroidism	Rare	Altered consciousness (Section IV)
Hypothyroidism	Rare	Altered consciousness (Section IV)

out the reasons behind the patient's need for alcohol before dental treatment and if necessary to take steps to alleviate the patient's dental anxiety.

The hyperventilation syndrome is the most common nondrug cause of altered consciousness. It rarely leads to loss of consciousness, but it may. Acute anxiety is the precipitating factor in almost all instances of hyperventilation. It is seen primarily in younger patients (under the age of 40 years). A full discussion of the hyperventilation syndrome is presented in Chapter 12.

Three additional systemic situations that present with clinical symptoms of altered consciousness—diabetes mellitus, cerebrovascular ischemia and infarction, and thyroid gland dysfunction—are discussed in this section. Diabetes mellitus and its associated acute clinical complications, hypoglycemia and hyperglycemia, are commonly encountered in dental patients. Inadequate medical management of the disease and the presence of stress may rapidly lead to an altered state of consciousness and possibly to the loss of consciousness. The nondiabetic patient may also be prone to episodes of hypoglycemia in certain circumstances.

Cerebrovascular ischemia and infarction (stroke) are other less common but potentially more serious causes of altered consciousness. Proper management of the post–cerebrovascular accident (CVA) patient greatly reduces the chance of a second incident precipitated by dental therapy. A prodromal form of cerebrovascular ischemia, the transient ischemic attack, is discussed along with management of this patient.

Thyroid gland dysfunction is another situation in which states of altered consciousness may develop. Although acute clinical complications from thyroid hypofunction or hyperfunction are extremely rare in dental situations, the doctor must be aware of the presence of thyroid gland dysfunction and be able to recognize signs and symptoms of thyroid complications. Of even more importance to the doctor treating a thyroid dysfunction patient is the greatly increased incidence of cardiovascular disease in these persons. In all of these situations, increased stress decreases the patient's ability to withstand dental therapy without disease-related complications.

PREVENTION

Recognition of unusually high levels of apprehension in a prospective dental patient minimizes the occurrence of vasodepressor syncope and the hyperventilation syndrome; proper use of psychosedative techniques prevents treatment-related drug overdose. In the other situations, prior awareness of a patient's medical condition allows the doctor to modify the proposed therapy to minimize the risk to the patient. The health questionnaire, physical examination, and recording of vital signs are valuable in the proper assessment of this patient. Specific questions and examinations are referred to as each potential emergency situation is discussed.

CLINICAL MANIFESTATIONS

A spectrum of signs and symptoms may be present in patients with altered consciousness: the cold, wet appearance, mental confusion, and bizarre behavior of the hypoglycemic patient contrast with the hot, dry, florid appearance of the hyperglycemic diabetic patient. The presence of "acetone breath" further aids in the clinical recognition of hyperglycemia.

Cerebrovascular accident (stroke) may occur with a sudden onset of unconsciousness (presenting an extremely poor prognosis) or a more gradual onset of symptoms related to central nervous system dysfunction. These symptoms may include variable degrees of derangement of speech, thought, motion, sensation, or vision. The state of consciousness may be unimpaired (patient alert) or the patient may demonstrate degrees of alteration of consciousness, ranging from headache, dizziness, and drowziness to mental confusion.

Hypothyroidism, if untreated, may cause symptoms of weakness, fatigue, lethargy, and slow speech, as well as many other clinical signs; untreated hyperthyroidism causes restlessness, nervousness, irritability, and degrees of motor incoordination ranging from a fine, mild tremulousness to gross tremor. A serious consequence of unmanaged hyperthyroidism is the "thyroid storm" or crisis. It may arise spontaneously but more commonly follows sudden stress in patients who are clinically hyperthyroid. The death rate associated with this complication is significant.

PATHOPHYSIOLOGY

In all three clinical situations to be discussed in this section, the clinical manifestations are evident throughout the body, even though a specific factor is responsible for the onset of symptoms and signs. Most clinical complications of diabetes mellitus are caused by a level of glucose in the blood that is too high or too low. In addition, diabetes mellitus, although usually considered a disease of impaired carbohydrate utilization, is also a disease of the blood vessels, leading to a much greater incidence of cardiovascular disease in diabetic patients than in nondiabetic patients. A change in the quality of the circulating blood is responsible for most of the acute clinical problems associated with diabetes.

Signs and symptoms of thyroid gland dysfunction are related clinically to the circulating blood level of thyroid hormone (thyroxine) and its pharmacologic actions on other parts of the body.

Inadequate blood flow to the brain also produces signs and symptoms of impaired consciousness. Temporary insufficiency leads to the clinical syndrome called transient ischemic attack; more prolonged insufficiency results in permanent neurologic changes termed cerebrovascular infarction (stroke).

MANAGEMENT

As soon as altered consciousness is recognized, several basic steps are called for in the immediate management of the patient. Definitive management of each situation is discussed in appropriate chapters.

Step 1. Recognize altered consciousness. Changes in the level of consciousness occurring during dental therapy should be a warning to the doctor to terminate the procedure. Signs and symptoms are described in the following chapters.

Step 2. Terminate dental procedure.

Step 3. Position patient. Positioning the patient with an altered state of consciousness varies according to the causative factor involved. In most instances, the patient retains consciousness; therefore the supine, semisupine, or erect position may be used. Patient comfort and vital signs (particularly blood pressure) are factors that influence what position will be used.

The conscious diabetic or thyroid patient may be most comfortable if permitted to sit up. However, should unconsciousness occur, the patient must be managed as any other unconscious patient.

Cerebrovascular accidents (CVAs) are commonly associated with extreme elevation of blood pressure. In such cases, a nonsupine position is important, because cerebral blood pressure is slightly reduced. Should the CVA lead to rapid loss of consciousness associated with a high blood pressure level, positioning of the patient is altered slightly. The supine position causes an increase in cerebral blood pressure that may not be beneficial at this time. Therefore the patient should be placed in the supine position with the head elevated slightly.

MANAGEMENT OF ALTERED CONSCIOUSNESS

Step 1 Recognition of altered consciousness
    Skin
        Cold and wet
        Hot and dry
        Hot with excessive sweating
        Cold and dry
    Breath
        "Acetone" breath
    Headache, dizziness, confusion
  2 Terminate dental procedure
  3 Position patient
    Conscious—upright position usually preferred by patient
    Unconscious—supine position
    If CVA is considered and elevated blood pressure is present, head and thorax should be elevated slightly
  4 Basic life support
  5 Monitor vital signs
    Blood pressure, heart rate (pulse), respiratory rate, and temperature
  6 Management of signs and symptoms
  7 Definitive management

Step 4. Basic life support. Institute basic life support as soon as possible: Assess airway patency and provide an airway if needed; assess spontaneous ventilation and ventilate as needed; assess circulatory adequacy and provide artificial circulation if needed.

Step 5. Monitor vital signs. Blood pressure, heart rate, respiratory rate, and temperature should be monitored throughout the crisis period, and a permanent record should be kept.

Step 6. Manage signs and symptoms. Signs and symptoms should be treated in an effort to make the patient comfortable. Blankets should be available if the patient is shivering; tight garments should be loosened to allow for ease of breathing.

Step 7. Definitive management. At this point, a decision must be made as to the definitive management of the patient. In-office management ranges from basic life support (for the cerebrovascular accident) to the administration of drugs to terminate the episode (for hypoglycemia). The following chapters detail therapy recommended for each situation.

The basic steps in management of altered consciousness are summarized in the box above.

17 Diabetes Mellitus: Hyperglycemia and Hypoglycemia

Diabetes mellitus represents a syndrome of disordered metabolism and inappropriate hyperglycemia, resulting from an absolute deficiency of insulin secretion, a reduction in its biologic effectiveness, or both. An estimated 5 million people in the United States have diabetes; about 86,000 of them are children under 15 years of age. The incidence of diabetes appears to increase with age. Table 17-1 illustrates the incidence of diabetes with age. About 80% of diabetics are over 45 years of age.

Little and Falace (1984) estimate that a dentist or dentists serving a population of 2000 people can expect to encounter 40 people with diabetes, about 20 of whom will be unaware of their condition.

ACUTE COMPLICATIONS

Hyperglycemia and its sequelae represent one of two clinical complications of importance to the doctor managing the diabetic patient. The second and normally more acutely life-threatening complication is *hypoglycemia*. Hypoglycemia may be present in diabetic and nondiabetic individuals. Blood glucose levels below 50mg/100 ml (venous blood) are usually considered to indicate hypoglycemia. Signs and symptoms of hypoglycemia may become evident within minutes and rapidly lead to the loss of consciousness. Hyperglycemia may also ultimately lead to unconsciousness (diabetic coma), but this occurrence usually represents the end of a much longer process (the amount of time from onset of symptoms to loss of consciousness is usually at least 48 hours). In either case, the doctor must be able to recognize the clinical problem and proceed to take the steps necessary to manage it properly. The differences between these two conditions are stressed in this chapter to aid in the differential diagnosis of diabetic complications.

CHRONIC COMPLICATIONS

In addition to hyperglycemia and hypoglycemia, there are other, more chronic complications to which the diabetic patient is subject. The importance of these complications is noted by the fact that most morbidity and mortality in diabetic patients occurs from them (Table 17-2).

The three major categories of complications are large blood vessel disease, small blood vessel disease (termed microangiopathy), and increased susceptibility to infection. Large blood vessel disease such as arteriosclerosis is seen frequently in the nondiabetic population; however, it is much more common in persons with diabetes and it occurs at an earlier age. The clinical manifestations observed are related to inadequate blood supply to the heart (angina pectoris, myocardial infarction, sudden death), the brain (cerebrovascular ischemia or infarction), the kidneys (glomerulosclerosis), and the lower extremities (gangrene). High blood pressure also occurs more frequently and at an earlier age in diabetic patients.

Diabetic microangiopathy (small blood vessel disease) is related to disorders affecting the arterioles, venules, and capillaries. It is thought to be specific, occurring only in diabetes mellitus, and has been

198

Table 17-1. Incidence of diabetes by age in the United States

Age group (in years)	Incidence (per 1000 people)
0-17	1.3
25-40	17.0
65 or older	79.0

Data adapted from Little, J.W., and Falace, D.A.: Dental management of the medically compromised patient, ed. 2, St. Louis, 1984, The C.V. Mosby Co.

Table 17-2. Chronic complications of diabetes mellitus

Affected part of body or condition	Complication
Vascular system	Atherosclerosis
	Large vessel disease
	Microangiopathy
Kidneys	Diabetic glomerulosclerosis
	Arteriolar nephrosclerosis
	Pyelonephritis
Nervous system	Motor, sensory, and autonomic neuropathy
Eyes	Retinopathy
	Cataract formation
	Glaucoma
	Extraocular muscle palsies
Skin	Xanthoma diabeticorum
	Necrobiosis lipoidica diabeticorum
	Pruritis
	Furunculosis
	Mycosis
Mouth	Gingivitis
	Increased incidence of dental caries and periodontal disease
	Alveolar bone loss
Pregnancy	Increased incidence of large babies, stillbirths, miscarriages, neonatal deaths, and congenital defects

the subject of much recent research. Clinical manifestations of microangiopathy are most often noted in the eye (diabetic retinopathy), kidney (arteriolar nephrosclerosis), and lower extremities (gangrene). The etiology of diabetic microangiopathy is not yet clear, but two interpretations are most often accepted. The first states that the cause is related to the carbohydrate intolerance in diabetes mellitus; however, there are instances of microangiopathy in the absence of carbohydrate intolerance. A second theory links microangiopathy to a genetic factor that also manifests diabetes.

In either case, diabetic microangiopathy may represent a more serious disease than the carbohydrate intolerance itself. Studies of the effects of blood glucose level on the progression of microangiopathy have not yet demonstrated that careful control of blood glucose levels decreases or retards small vessel disease. The extent of diabetic microangiopathy is such that diabetic retinopathy is the second leading cause of blindness in this country, and diabetic patients have 20 times the incidence of gangrene of the feet as do nondiabetics.

It is well known that diabetics are more prone to development of infection than are nondiabetics. Although the cause of this is not known, it is probably related to the combination of vascular lesions and infection. To prevent severe infection, scrupulous personal hygiene must be practiced. An increased incidence of urinary tract infections (particularly in female diabetics) may be related to the high glucose levels present in the urine, which act as excellent growth media for microorganisms.

The doctor must be aware of the acute complications of diabetes (hyperglycemia and hypoglycemia) and must take measures to avoid their occurrence. He must also look for the possible presence of chronic complications; their presence increases the medical risk to the patient during dental

therapy, which may require modification of the dental treatment plan.

PREDISPOSING FACTORS

Major factors leading to the development of diabetes mellitus are:
1. Genetic predisposition
2. Primary destruction of the islets of Langerhans in the pancreas, caused by inflammation, cancer, or surgery
3. An endocrine condition, such as hyperpituitarism or hyperthyroidism
4. Administration of steroids, resulting in iatrogenic diabetes

The most important factor in the development of diabetes mellitus is heredity. It is known that if one identical twin develops diabetes, the other twin will also become diabetic if he or she lives long enough. In addition, the offspring of two diabetic parents have almost a 100% chance of developing the disease. As illustrated in Table 17-3, it is possible to predict a risk factor for development of diabetes according to previous family history.

Table 17-3. Prediction of diabetic risk

Relative with diabetes		Diabetic relative on other side of family	Maximum risk (%)
Parent	*plus*	Grandparent and aunt or uncle	85
Parent	*plus*	Grandparent, aunt, or uncle	60
Parent	*plus*	First cousin	40
Parent			22
Grandparent			14
First cousin			9

From Steinberg, A.G.: Ann. N.Y. Acad. Sci. **82:**197, 1959.

TYPES OF DIABETES

Until recently, the classification of diabetes was based on the age of onset of the disease. In other words, the classifications were adult onset and juvenile onset diabetes (see previous editions of this book). However, the age of onset is no longer considered to be a criterion for classification of diabetic patients. Instead, the National Diabetes Data Group (1979) recommends a "therapeutic" classification, which has been endorsed by the American Diabetes Association. This classification is presented in Table 17-4.

Type I—Insulin-Dependent Diabetes Mellitus (IDDM)

Approximately 5% of diabetic patients develop insulin-dependent diabetes mellitus (IDDM). This is a more severe form of the disease characterized by ketosis in its untreated state. IDDM is seen more commonly in adolescents but may also develop in adults, usually in the nonobese and in those who are elderly when hyperglycemia first appears. In IDDM, circulating insulin is essentially absent, glucagon levels in the plasma are elevated, and pancreatic beta cells fail to respond to all insulinogenic stimuli. Exogenous insulin is required to reverse the catabolic state, prevent ketosis, reduce the hyperglucagonemia, and reduce the elevated blood glucose level.

Recent studies have demonstrated that the incidence of IDDM is linked to the presence or absence of certain genetically determined cell surface antigens found on lymphocytes. Histocompatability (HLA) antigens are strongly associated with development of type I diabetes. They are located on the sixth human chromosome, adjacent to immune response genes.

Because of the immune factors associated with development of type I IDDM, it is felt that IDDM is the result of an infectious or environmental insult to pancreatic beta cells in genetically predisposed persons. These extrinsic factors include damage produced by viruses such as mumps or coxsackie virus, B4 by toxic chemicals, or by destructive cytotoxins and antibodies released from sensitized immunocytes.

Type II—Non-Insulin-Dependent Diabetes Mellitus (NIDDM)

Type II diabetes, non-insulin-dependent diabetes mellitus (NIDDM), represents a heterogeneous group composed of milder forms of diabetes that occur most frequently in adults but are seen occasionally in children. Circulating endogenous insulin blood levels are present and adequate to prevent ketoacidosis, but insulin levels are either subnormal or relatively inadequate in the face of increased needs caused by insensitivity of the tissues.

Type II diabetes mellitus is a nonketotic form of diabetes that is not linked to HLA markers on the sixth chromosome; it has no islet cell antibodies. Those with this type of diabetes do not depend on exogenous insulin therapy to sustain life—therefore the name "non-insulin-dependent diabetes mellitus" is appropriate.

Regardless of body weight, the tissues of the NIDDM patient demonstrate a degree of insensitivity to insulin.

There are presently two subcategories of type II diabetes mellitus. These subgroups are based on the presence or absence of obesity.

Nonobese NIDDM

The person with nonobese NIDDM demonstrates either an absent or significantly blunted early phase of insulin release in response to glucose challenge. This poor insulin release may also be demonstrated in response to other insulinogenic stimuli, such as acute intravenous administration of glucagon or sulfonylureas.

Hyperglycemia noted in nonobese NIDDM often responds to oral hypoglycemic agents or, on occasion, to dietary therapy alone. On rare occasions, insulin therapy is required to achieve satisfactory control of blood sugar levels, even though it is not required to prevent ketosis.

Obese NIDDM

Obese NIDDM is secondary to extrapancreatic factors that produce insensitivity to endogenous insulin. It is characterized by nonketotic mild dia-

Table 17-4. Clinical classification of idiopathic diabetes mellitus syndromes

Type	Ketosis	Islet cell antibodies	HLA association	Treatment
Insulin-dependent (IDDM)	Present	Present at onset	Positive	Insulin (mixtures of rapid-acting and intermediate-acting insulin, at least twice daily) and diet
Non-insulin-dependent (NIDDM)				
Nonobese	Absent	Absent	Negative	1. Eucaloric diet alone 2. Diet plus insulin or sulfonylureas
Obese	Absent	Absent	Negative	1. Weight reduction 2. Hypocaloric diet plus sulfonylureas or insulin for symptomatic control only

From Karam, J.H.: Diabetes mellitus, hypoglycemia and lipoprotein disorders. In Krupp, M.A., and Chatton, M.J., editors: Current medical diagnosis and treatment, Los Altos, CA, 1984, Lange Medical Publications.

betes that occurs primarily in adults but also may be seen in children. The primary problem is a "target organ" disorder, which results in a lack of sensitivity to insulin. Hyperplasia of pancreatic B cells is often present and probably accounts for the fasting hyperinsulinism and exaggerated insulin responses to glucose and other stimuli seen in the milder forms of this disorder.

Obesity is common in this disorder because of excess caloric intake, perhaps resulting from hunger caused by mild postprandial hypoglycemia after excess insulin release. In this form of diabetes, insulin insensitivity is correlated with the presence of distended adipocytes. Liver and muscle cells also resist the deposition of additional glycogen and triglycerides in their storage depots.

Two mechanisms have been offered to explain the insensitivity of tissues to insulin in the obese form of diabetes mellitus. It is thought that chronic overfeeding may lead to either (1) sustained B cell stimulation and hyperinsulinism, which by itself may induce receptor insensitivity to insulin, or (2) a postreceptor defect associated with overdistended storage depots and a reduced ability to clear nutrients from the circulation. Consequent hyperinsulinism induces receptor insensitivity to insulin.

A reduction in overfeeding can interrupt either cycle regardless of the mechanism. In the first situation, a restricted diet would reduce islet cell stimulation of insulin release, thereby restoring insulin receptor sites and improving tissue sensitivity to insulin. In the second situation, normal tissue sensitivity would return as storage depots became less saturated.

Other possible causes of carbohydrate intolerance and hyperinsulinism in response to glucose include chronic muscle inactivity or disease and liver disease. Secondary causes of carbohydrate intolerance include endocrine disorders (for example, tumors) associated with excessive production of growth hormone, glucocorticosteroids, catecholamines, or glucagon. In these four cases, peripheral response to insulin is decreased.

The prognosis for both forms of diabetes mellitus, even in the presence of scrupulous control over blood sugar levels, is still uncertain. Recent research with pancreatic islet transplants and improved insulin delivery systems may make it possible to determine if adequate control can minimize the severity or delay the onset of complications.

In one series of 164 juvenile-onset, insulin-dependent diabetics (median age, 9 years old at onset), data were collected after 25 years. Out of every group of five from the larger group on standard dietary and insulin control, one diabetic had died and one was incapacitated with severe proliferative retinopathy and renal failure. Two others were active, contributing members of society despite mild background retinopathy, mild nephropathy, neuropathy, and some degree of ischemia of the feet. The fifth diabetic was completely free of complications (Knowles, 1971).

It appears that the period between 10 and 20 years after the onset of diabetes is a critical one. If the patient experiences no significant complications during this period, there is a strong likelihood that reasonably good health will continue. Knowledge of the type of diabetes the patient has enables the doctor to estimate the risk factor in each case. However, there are other factors, such as infection and pregnancy, that may lead to a diabetic patient's disease going "out of control."

Table 17-5 compares IDDM and NIDDM.

Table 17-5. Comparison of type I (IDDM) and type II (NIDDM) diabetes mellitus

Factors compared	Type I (IDDM)	Type II (NIDDM)
Frequency (percentage of total diabetic population)	5	85
Age at onset (years)	15	40 and over
Body build	Normal or thin	Obese
Severity	Severe	Mild
Use of insulin	Almost all	25%-30%
Oral hypoglycemic agents	Very few respond	50% respond
Ketoacidosis	Common	Uncommon
Complications	90% in 20 years	Less common than with IDDM
Rate of clinical onset	Rapid	Slow
Stability	Unstable	Stable
Family history of diabetes	Common	Less common than with IDDM
HLA antigen and abnormal autoimmune reactions	Present	Not present
Insulin receptor defects	Usually not found	—

From Little, J.W., and Falace, D.A.: Dental management of the medically compromised patient, ed. 2, St. Louis, 1984, The C.V. Mosby Co.

HYPERGLYCEMIA

Hyperglycemia may be precipitated by the following factors, all of which increase the body's requirements for insulin: weight gain, cessation of exercise, pregnancy, hyperthyroidism or thyroid medication, epinephrine therapy, corticosteroid therapy, acute infection, and fever. Although hyperglycemia itself is not usually a situation that leads to acutely life-threatening emergencies, it may, if untreated, progress to diabetic ketoacidosis and coma, which are life-threatening conditions. The most common causative factors of ketoacidosis and diabetic coma are ignorance of the disease, or neglect of therapy by the patient, or both. Infection and a secondary disease state are also common causes of hyperglycemia in diabetic patients.

HYPOGLYCEMIA

Hypoglycemia, unlike hyperglycemia, may manifest itself rapidly. This is especially true in patients receiving injectable insulin therapy, for whom loss of consciousness may occur within minutes after injection. The onset of symptoms is slower, usually over several hours, in patients on oral hypoglycemic agents. Factors that decrease a patient's insulin requirement include weight loss, increased physical exercise, termination of pregnancy, termination of other drug therapies (epinephrine, thyroid, corticosteroid), and recovery from infection and fever. Common causes of hypoglycemia are omission or delay of meals, excessive exercise before meals, and overdose of insulin. Another potential cause of hypoglycemia is accidental ingestion of the wrong medications because of the similarity of some drug names. The similarity in names of medicines has led to many instances of patients receiving the wrong medication for their medical problem. Table 17-6 lists frequently observed causes of hypoglycemia in known diabetic patients.

Dental therapy is a potential threat to the diabetic patient and to control of the disease state. First, stress—physiologic and psychologic—increases the body's requirements for insulin, so that hyperglycemia may occur in the diabetic dental patient. (Both the doctor and the patient must be aware of this so that alterations can be made in dental therapy and insulin dosage to preclude the progression of this state to diabetic coma. Second, dental therapy may require the patient to alter normal eating habits for varying periods of time. Many patients purposefully avoid eating before a dental appointment so that their teeth will be "clean." Dental patients may out of necessity be treated during a normal lunch or dinner hour, thereby delaying the meal or even causing the patient to miss the meal entirely. Third, the taking of food may be altered by the dental procedure itself. Persistent local anesthesia after therapy and extensive dental procedures (periodontal or oral surgery, or endodontics, for example) may cause the patient to avoid eating and thus precipitate hypoglycemia.

MANAGEMENT OF DIABETES

Diabetes is a fascinating disease in that it produces myriad clinical signs and symptoms. In addition, there are many factors that may affect the control of the disease on a day-to-day basis. For these reasons, diabetic patients are quite unusual in

Table 17-6. Causes of 240 consecutive cases of hypoglycemia in patients known to have diabetes mellitus*

Cause	Percent
Inadequate food (carbohydrate) intake	66
Excessive insulin dose	12
Sulfonylurea therapy	12
Strenuous exercise	4
Ethanol intake	4
Other (kidney failure, liver failure, decrease in corticosteroid dose)	2

From Davidson, J.K.: Hypoglycemia. In Schwartz, G.R., and others, editors: Principles and practice of emergency medicine, Philadelphia, 1978, W.B. Saunders Co.
*At the Grady Memorial Hospital Emergency Clinic, 1973-1975.

Table 17-7. Currently available oral hypoglycemic agents

Generic drug	Proprietary name	Equivalent doses (mg)	Doses/day
Tolbutamide	Orinase	1000	2-3
Acetohexamide	Dymelor	500	1-2
Tolazamide	Tolinase	250	1-2
Chlorpropamide	Diabinase	250	1
Glyburide	Glucotrol	5	1-2
Glipizide	DiaBeta, Mirconase	5	1-2

that they must be capable of checking the status of the disease and initiating modifications in its management as indicated.

Monitoring of blood glucose by patients has permitted a greater flexibility in management of diabetes while achieving improved glycemic control when compared to the older methods of testing urinary glucose levels. The patient must be educated to perform three essential steps. They are as follows:

1. To obtain a drop of capillary blood from a finger prick
2. To apply the blood sample to a test strip and remove the sample at the proper time
3. To accurately evaluate the color developed.

Self-monitoring of blood glucose is especially important for those with brittle diabetes (that is, those who, despite therapy, are unable to maintain a stable blood sugar level, exhibiting extremes of hyperglycemia and hypoglycemia), those attempting to maintain ideal glycemic control during pregnancy, and patients who have little or no warning of impending hypoglycemic attacks. This type of self-monitoring has proved to be a safe and reliable clinical tool in compliant patients. Diagnostic strips include Visidex and Chemstrip-bG. These permit visual estimations of glucose concentrations when compared to a series of color standards.

Capillary blood glucose levels are closer to arterial levels than are those obtained from venous blood. Normal fasting blood glucose levels for venous blood range from 60 to 100 mg/100 ml (60-100 mg%). In 1979, the National Diabetes Data Group stated that a fasting blood glucose level of 140 mg/100 ml on two or more occasions would serve as adequate criteria for the diagnosis of the presence of diabetes mellitus.

PREVENTION

The acute complications of diabetes may be averted through proper preliminary evaluation of the diabetic patient. The dental practitioner is also in a position to assist in the detection of undiagnosed diabetes. Relevant questions from the medical history questionnaire and the ensuing dialogue history follow.

Medical History Questionnaire
QUESTION 9. Circle any of the following which you have had or have at present:
• **Diabetes**
• **Cortisone medicine**

COMMENT. Knowledge of the presence of diabetes by the patient leads to a definitive dialogue history. The prolonged use of corticosteroid medications can lead to the onset of diabetes mellitus. Dialogue history must seek to determine the presence of signs and symptoms.

QUESTION 13. Have you lost or gained more than 10 pounds in the past year?

COMMENT. An affirmative response to unexplained weight loss may indicate the presence of undetected diabetes mellitus.

QUESTION 15. Are you on a special diet?

COMMENT. An affirmative response may indicate a patient with NIDDM (type II).

QUESTION 6. Have you taken any medicine or drugs during the past 2 years?

COMMENT. Table 17-7 lists many of the oral medications currently being prescribed for the management of NIDDM. It is also important for the doctor to know that other medicines being taken by a patient are capable of producing alterations in the blood sugar level. Table 17-8 lists some of these medications.

Dialogue History

In the presence of a *negative* response to diabetes mellitus (that is, when the patient indicates on the questionnaire that he or she does not have diabetes mellitus), but with affirmative responses to any or all of questions 6, 13, or 15, the following dialogue history should be considered.

QUESTIONS. Are you frequently thirsty? Are you hungry much of the time? Do you have to get up at night to void (urinate) frequently? Have you gained or lost weight recently without dieting; how many pounds?

COMMENT. These signs, although not specific for diabetes mellitus, can lead to a presumptive diagnosis of this disease. Polydipsia (increased thirst), polyphagia (increased appetite), and polyuria (increased frequency of urination), when accompanied by a loss of weight in the absence of dieting, should alert the doctor to the possible presence of

Table 17-8. Commonly used medications that lower blood glucose levels

---

Potentiate action of sulfonylureas
1. Barbiturates*
2. Bishydroxycoumarin
3. Monoamine oxidase inhibitors
4. Salicylates*
5. Thiazides

Increase insulin production
1. Alpha-adrenergic blockers
2. Beta-adrenergic stimulators
3. Monoamine oxidase inhibitors

Decrease hepatic glycogenolysis
1. Propranolol

Unknown mechanism
1. Antihistamines
   a. Tripelennamine HCl
2. Morphine*
3. Propylthiouracil
4. Tuberculostatic drugs
   a. Isoniazid
   b. Aminosalicylic acid

---

*These agents are frequently administered or prescribed in the practice of dentistry.

diabetes. If the response to the question on the history questionnaire is negative and the above questions are answered in the affirmative, the doctor should continue with the medical and dental examination and then consult with the patient's physician before dental therapy is begun.

• • •

When a *positive history* indicates the presence of diabetes mellitus, the doctor should proceed with the following dialogue history.

QUESTION. How long have you had diabetes, and what type of treatment are you taking to control it?

COMMENT. As noted earlier, the severity of the diabetes and the potential for the occurrence of acute complications are greatest in insulin-dependent and (usually) brittle non-insulin-dependent diabetics who are managed by injectable insulin plus diet control. Patients controlling their blood glucose levels through diet alone or diet plus oral hypoglycemic agents (NIDDM patients) usually have some pancreatic function remaining and are more ketosis resistant. Currently available oral hypoglycemic agents are listed in Table 17-7.

QUESTION. How often do you monitor your urine or blood glucose levels and what have been the results for the past few days?

COMMENT. For nearly four decades diabetics have tested their urine blood glucose levels. Urine tests for glucose and ketones are still an important component of many diabetics' daily routines. More recently, however, some diabetics have been measuring glucose levels in blood instead of urine, a procedure gaining increasing acceptance. Although a radical departure from accepted diabetic testing procedures in appearance, in reality blood glucose testing is a more sophisticated and logical extension of tests usually done by physicians. Many of these products are available over the counter. Proprietary names include Chemstrip bG (Bio-Dynamics), Dextrostix (Miles Labs), and Glucostix (Miles Labs). Studies have demonstrated that 8 of 10 diabetics would rather prick their finger than use a urine sample (Sonkson et al., 1980). Additionally these tests are accurate, producing results similar to those obtained by professional laboratories. Sonkson (1978) demonstrated that normal blood glucose levels can be maintained by self-assessment of blood rather than urine samples. Levels are recorded in milligrams of glucose per deciliter (100 ml) of whole blood (also read as milligrams percent). In children and adults values below 50 mg/dl indicate hypoglycemia. The upper range of values (Chemstrip bG) is 240 mg/dl for a 2-minute reading or 800 mg/dl for a 3-minute reading.

With diabetics who still monitor their urine the level of blood glucose obtained is less reliable. Readings are 0, trace, 1+, 2+, 3+, and 4+. Patients who are able to keep their glucose levels in the trace or 1+ range may be considered in good control and managed in a normal manner in the dental office. Patients with consistently negative readings are more likely to have hypoglycemic reactions.

The diabetic with 2+ readings should be carefully evaluated before dental treatment. Some physicians prefer their patients to remain in the 1+ to 2+ range where they are less likely to become hypoglycemic. If no clinical signs and symptoms of hyperglycemia or hypoglycemia are evident, dental treatment may be carried out without modification.

Readings of 3+ and 4+ indicate a lack of control of blood sugar. Stress (as in dental treatment) further elevates blood sugar and may aid in precipitating ketoacidosis and, potentially, diabetic coma. Medical consultation prior to treatment is indicated so that adjustments may be made in insulin dosages and overall diabetic management. Table 17-10 summarizes urinary glucose tests and their clinical significance.

QUESTION. How frequently (if ever) do you have hypoglycemic episodes?

COMMENT. Awareness of the problem better prepares the doctor to manage it. Patients frequently testing negative on urinary glucose or low on blood glucose are more likely to become hypoglycemic.

Physical Examination

Following the medical history questionnaire and dialogue history, the diabetic patient should be carefully evaluated for signs and symptoms of secondary disease, particularly of the cardiovascular system. Vital signs should be recorded before and after all dental procedures.

The skin of a diabetic patient may give an indication of the presence of acute complications. Hyperglycemic patients appear flushed and their skin is dry (absence of sweating); hypoglycemic patients may have a cold, moist appearance. The smell of acetone (a sweet, fruity odor) on the breath is noticeable in some hyperglycemic patients who are somewhat out of control (that is, ketoacidotic).

Dental Therapy Considerations

Following medical and dental evaluation of the diabetic patient, consideration must be given to proper patient management. If any doubt exists as to the patient's medical status, consultation with the patient's physician is indicated.

Basic procedures with the ketosis-prone diabetic patient include use of the Stress Reduction Protocol. Additional consideration should be directed toward maintenance of normal dietary habits. If the patient's eating will be restricted or impaired preoperatively or postoperatively, the insulin dosage must be adjusted accordingly. When a meal is to be missed following dental therapy, the patient should be directed to take only one half the normal insulin dose.

Diabetics are better able to withstand transient periods of hyperglycemia than they are hypoglycemia. If any doubt remains concerning adjustment of the insulin dosage, consult with the patient's physician before therapy.

After extensive dental procedures (oral or periodontal surgery), reconstruction, or endodontics, diabetic patients should be instructed to check their blood glucose levels at least four times a day for the following few days. If glucose or ketone levels are elevated, patients should initiate changes in insulin dosage or contact their physician. Tables 17-9,

Table 17-9. Status classifications of diabetic patients

Type of diabetes	Treatment	Severity	Optimal physical status
Type I—IDDM	Insulin plus diet	Severe	III
Type II—NIDDM			
1. Nonobese	Insulin plus diet	Moderate to severe	II-III
	Oral medication plus diet	Mild to moderate	II
2. Obese	Oral medication plus diet	Mild to moderate	II

Table 17-10. Physical status classification for diabetes mellitus

Glucose measurement		Change in physical status‡	Comment
Urinary*	Blood†		
0	<50 mg/dl	+1	Acceptable for treatment but more likely to be or become hypoglycemic
Trace, +, ++	80, 120, 180 mg/dl	0	Acceptable for treatment
+++	240 mg/dl	+1	Evaluate carefully prior to treatment.
++++	>400 mg/dl	+2	If consistently in this range medical consultation urged prior to treatment

*Tes-Tape.
†Chemstrip bG.
‡This table lists the change in physical status (P.S.) from the optimal presented in Table 17-9; thus if optimally a P.S. II with a 3+ urinary glucose or 240 mg/dl blood glucose, patient is treated as a P.S. III.

Table 17-11. Diabetes mellitus—dental therapy considerations*

Physical status	Consideration
II	Usual P.S. II considerations, plus: Avoid missing meals, pre- and post-operatively If omission of meal is unavoidable, preoperative insulin dose can be decreased by half
III	Usual P.S. III considerations, plus: "Brittle" diabetic—check blood or urine sugar and acetone four times daily for 4 days, and adjust insulin accordingly
IV	Usual P.S. IV considerations

*The physical status categories have been derived from Tables 17-9 and 17-10.

17-10, and 17-11 list the physical status classifications for diabetic patients.

CLINICAL MANIFESTATIONS
Hyperglycemia

Hyperglycemia may manifest itself in several different ways related to the severity of the diabetes. It may be evident in previously undiagnosed diabetic patients or in known diabetics who neglect their therapeutic regimen.

The milder form of diabetes (NIDDM) may not manifest any clinical signs or symptoms. Quite commonly, this form of diabetes is detected during a routine physical evaluation using glucose tolerance tests or urine samples tested for glycosuria. Even more frequently, diabetes mellitus is first diagnosed after a clinical episode brought about by

the advanced degree of atherosclerosis associated with the disease. Myocardial infarction in a young man or woman and/or development of peripheral vascular insufficiency at an early age may be events that eventually lead to a clinical diagnosis of diabetes mellitus.

A more severe clinical picture of hyperglycemia is seen in the insulin-dependent diabetic individual. The classic triad of "polys"—polydipsia, polyphagia, and polyuria—with a marked loss of weight is evident for *a day or more* and is associated with marked fatigue, headache, blurred vision, abdominal pain, nausea and vomiting, constipation, dyspnea, and finally mental stupor, which can progress to the state of unconsciousness known as diabetic coma.

The signs of hyperglycemia are a florid appearance of the face (bright red color) associated with hot, dry skin, both of which are indicative of dehydration. Respirations are commonly deep and rapid (signs of Kussmaul's respiration), with the fruity-sweet odor of acetone evident.

Pulse rate is rapid, and blood pressure is lower than normal. This combination of tachycardia and hypotension is yet another indication of the presence of dehydration and salt depletion (Table 17-12).

Hypoglycemia

The second of the acute complications of diabetes mellitus, hypoglycemia, may *rapidly* progress to loss of consciousness, or it may be present in a milder form, representing a less ominous clinical picture. Episodes of hypoglycemia usually occur when the patient has not eaten for several hours.

Hypoglycemia is usually evident first as a phase of

Table 17-12. Clinical manifestations of hyperglycemia

	Diabetes, type I (IDDM)	Diabetes, type II (NIDDM)
Polyuria	++	+
Polydipsia	++	+
Polyphagia with weight loss	++	−
Recurrent blurred vision	+	++
Vulvovaginitis or pruritis	+	++
Loss of strength	++	+
Nocturnal enuresis	++	−
Often asymptomatic	−	++

Other symptoms—type I
Repeated skin infections
Marked irritability
Headache
Drowsiness
Malaise
Dry mouth

Other symptoms—type II
Decreased vision
Paresthesias
Loss of sensation
Impotence
Postural hypotension

Key: −, not usually present; +, occasionally present; ++, usually present.
Derived from data in Karam, J.H.: Diabetes mellitus, hypoglycemia, and lipoprotein disorders. In Krupp, M.A., and Chatton, M.J., editors: Current medical diagnosis and treatment, Los Altos, CA, 1984, Lange Medical Publications; and Little, J.W., and Falace, D.A.: Dental management of the medically compromised patient, ed. 2, St. Louis, 1984, The C.V. Mosby Co.

Table 17-13. Clinical manifestations of hypoglycemia

Early stage—mild reaction
Diminished cerebral function
  Changes in mood
  Decreased spontaneity
Hunger
Nausea

More severe hypoglycemia
Sweating
Tachycardia
Piloerection
Increased anxiety
Bizarre behavioral patterns
  Belligerence
  Poor judgment
  Uncooperativeness

Later severe stage
Unconsciousness
Seizure activity
Hypotension
Hypothermia

diminished cerebral function, such as inability to perform simple calculations, decreased spontaneity of conversation, and changes in mood (lethargy). Signs and symptoms of central nervous system involvement follow, including hunger, nausea, and increased gastric motility.

Following this is a phase of sympathetic hyperactivity, marked clinically by signs of increased epinephrine activity that include sweating, tachycardia, piloerection, and increased anxiety. The skin is cold and wet to the touch. The patient is conscious at this time but may exhibit bizarre behavioral patterns that may lead to a suspicion of alcohol or drug intoxication. If permitted to progress, the hypoglycemic patient may lose consciousness, and seizures may occur (Table 17-13).

Because hypoglycemia is a more acute problem than hyperglycemia, diabetic patients always carry a ready source of carbohydrate, such as hard candy or a chocolate bar. In addition, diabetics will carry a card stating that they are not intoxicated but are diabetic and that, if found unconscious, a physician should be called (Fig. 17-1).

I Am a Diabetic and Take Insulin

If I am behaving peculiarly but am conscious and able to swallow, give me sugar or hard candy or orange juice slowly. If I am unconscious, call an ambulance immediately, take me to a physician or a hospital, and notify my physician. *I am not intoxicated.*

My name _____

Address _____

Telephone _____

Physician's name _____

Physician's address _____

Telephone _____

Fig. 17-1. Card carried by diabetic patients.

PATHOPHYSIOLOGY
Insulin and Blood Glucose

Glucose is a major fuel and energy source for all cells of the body. In fact, glucose is the only fuel that can be used by the brain, which requires a continuous supply of it. Too high a level of blood sugar (hyperglycemia) or too low a level (hypoglycemia) produces various degrees of central nervous system dysfunction (altered consciousness). The homeostatic mechanisms in the body are therefore aimed at maintaining the blood glucose level within the range of 50 to 150 mg/100 ml of blood (milligrams percent). The mean blood glucose level in normal persons who fast overnight is 92 mg/100 ml, with a range of from 78 to 115 mg/100 ml.

The minimal blood glucose level required by the brain for normal cerebral function is 50 mg/100 ml. When blood glucose levels exceed the saturation point of renal reabsorption (approximately 180 mg/100 ml), glucose "spills" into the urine, resulting in loss of energy and water. Insulin is the most important factor in regulation of the blood glucose level.

Insulin is synthesized in the beta cells of the pancreas and is rapidly secreted into the blood in response to elevations in blood sugar level (for example, following a meal). Insulin promotes the uptake of glucose into the cells of the body and its storage in the liver as glycogen, as well as the uptake of fatty acids and amino acids into cells and their subsequent conversion into storage forms (triglycerides and proteins). In this manner insulin produces a decrease in blood glucose levels, thereby preventing its loss through urinary excretion. In the absence of insulin, the cell membranes of many body cells are impermeable to glucose. Cells such as muscle and adipose cells are insulin dependent, requiring its presence to enable glucose to cross the cell membrane, even in hyperglycemic states. When insulin is absent, these cells break down triglycerides into fatty acids, which may be used as an alternative energy source. This gives rise to the hyperglycemic state termed ketoacidosis (diabetic acidosis). Other tissues and organs such as nerve tissue (including the brain), the kidney, and hepatic tissue are not insulin dependent, being capable of glucose transfer across cell membranes even in the absence of insulin.

In the fasting stage, decreased blood sugar levels (hypoglycemia) inhibit insulin secretion. The cells of the body continue to require glucose, however, and there are several mechanisms through which it is made available. The primary goal of these mechanisms is to provide the central nervous system with the minimal glucose level required for normal functioning.

Glycogen stored in the liver is broken down into glucose (glycogenolysis); amino acids are converted into glucose in a process termed gluconeogenesis. This newly formed glucose is available principally to the central nervous system; in fact, insulin-dependent cells actually demonstrate a decreased uptake of glucose at this time. Fuel for these cells (muscle and adipose) is provided through the breakdown of triglycerides (the storage form of fat) into free fatty acids.

In summary, insulin may be described as the body's "fed" signal. After a meal, the high blood level of insulin tells the cells of the body to take up and store any fuel that is not immediately required for metabolic needs. In the fasting state, low insulin levels tell the body that no food is entering and that storage forms of nutrients should be utilized for fuel.

Hyperglycemia, Ketosis, and Acidosis

After the diabetic patient eats a meal, hyperglycemia occurs as it does in a nondiabetic patient, but the blood glucose level remains high for a prolonged period because of a lack of insulin (type I diabetes) or a lack of response by cells to circulating insulin (type II diabetes). Other factors leading to increased blood glucose levels are an increase in the hepatic production of glucose from glycogen, as well as decreased glucose uptake by the peripheral insulin-dependent tissues (muscle and fat).

Glucose is evident in the urine when the blood glucose level exceeds the renal reabsorption threshold of approximately 180 mg/100 ml. The presence of glucose in the urine is termed glycosuria. Urinary glucose takes with it (by means of osmosis) large quantities of water and the electrolytes sodium and potassium. This, in addition to the presence of ketones, which also increase the secretion of sodium and potassium in the urine, leads to clinical symptoms of polyuria (increased frequency of urination) and polydipsia (increased thirst) and to the dehydrated state of the hyperglycemic patient, as evidenced clinically by a florid appearance and dry skin.

In the absence of insulin, the cells of the body are unable to utilize the large quantities of glucose present in the blood. Fasting state mechanisms described earlier respond to the call for required energy. Liver and muscle glycogen are converted to glucose; proteins are broken down into their component amino acids, which are then converted into glucose through the process of gluconeogenesis in the liver. Triglycerides are converted into free fatty acids in the liver. These free fatty acids, primarily acetoacetate and beta-hydroxybutyrate (ketone bodies), are used by the muscles as fuel. Acetone, evident on the breath of this patient because of its fruity, sweet odor, is a by-product of the metabolism of acetoacetate. This stage is referred to as ketosis.

If the insulin deficiency is severe, gluconeogenesis and ketogenesis continue to increase in rate, regardless of the blood glucose level. Tissue utilization of ketones, however, decreases with time so that the blood levels of acetoacetate and beta-hydroxybutyrate begin to increase markedly. This produces a decrease in the pH of the blood, a condition termed metabolic acidosis (ketoacidosis). With increased blood levels of ketones, the renal threshold is soon exceeded, and ketones too may be detected in the urine. Ketoacidosis depresses cardiac contractility and decreases the response of arterioles to the catecholamines, epinephrine and norepinephrine. More significant perhaps is the effect of metabolic acidosis on blood pH and respiration. As the blood level of the ketoacids rises, the pH of the blood falls (below 7.3). This induces hyperventilation, the body's attempt to raise the pH by means of respiratory alkalosis (see Chapter 12). When severe, this type of breathing is called Kussmaul's breathing, and may progress to the loss of consciousness (diabetic coma) if unmanaged.

Hypoglycemia

Hypoglycemia is the most commonly encountered acute complication of diabetes mellitus. It may also be seen in nondiabetic individuals. Approximately 70% of nondiabetic hypoglycemia is caused by functional hyperinsulinism. This is related to an oversecretion of insulin by beta cells of the pancreas because of an exaggerated response to glucose absorption, muscular exertion, pregnancy, or anorexia nervosa (factors that increase insulin requirements). Whatever the cause, diabetic or nondiabetic, the clinical manifestations of hypoglycemia are the same.

By arbitrary definition, hypoglycemia in adults is equated with blood glucose values below 40 mg/100 ml. It is characterized by varying degrees of neurologic dysfunction, may occur with or without signs of epinephrine overactivity, and is responsive to the administration of glucose.

Although the definition of hypoglycemia indicates a blood glucose level of less than 40 mg/100 ml, hypoglycemic reactions can occur in the presence of normal or higher than normal blood glucose levels. Indeed, reports have been published of hypoglycemia reactions in diabetic patients with blood sugars ranging from 82 to 472 mg/100 ml—the reactions occurring within 40 minutes of intravenous insulin administration. On the other hand, blood glucose levels of 25 to 30 mg/100 ml have been reported in patients without clinical evidence of hypoglycemia.

It appears that *one of the most important factors in precipitating clinical hypoglycemia is the rate of fall of the blood glucose level.* After the administration of injectable insulin, the signs and symptoms of hypoglycemia may develop within a few minutes, rapidly progressing to unconsciousness. In patients on oral hypoglycemics the onset of signs and symptoms is normally more gradual, developing over a period of hours. Clinical signs and symptoms of hypoglycemia are similar to those seen in acute anxiety states and after administration of excessive doses of epinephrine (the so-called epinephrine reactions). Lack of adequate blood glucose prevents normal functioning of the cerebral cortex, represented clinically as mental confusion and lethargy. This lack of adequate glucose further manifests itself in increased activity of the parasympathetic and sympathetic nervous systems. Part of this response is mediated by an increase in the secretion of the catecholamine epinephrine, which produces increases in the systolic and the mean blood pressures, increases sweating, and produces tachycardia.

When the blood sugar level falls still further, the patient may lose consciousness and go into a state of hypoglycemic coma (insulin shock). During this stage, tonic and clonic convulsions frequently occur, which may lead to permanent cerebral dysfunction if not treated.

MANAGEMENT

Prompt recognition of diabetes-related complications is important. Equally important is the ability to differentiate between hyperglycemia and hypoglycemia. Because of the differing rates of onset of these acute complications, it is usually stressed that diabetic patients who behave in a bizarre manner or who lose consciousness *should be managed as if they were hypoglycemic until proved otherwise.* Hyperglycemia and ketoacidosis usually develop over a period of many hours or days, and the patient will appear and behave chronically ill. Other important factors in a differential diagnosis include the hot and dry appearance of the hyperglycemic patient in contrast to the cold and wet look of the hypoglycemic patient. The presence of acetone odor on the breath further confirms a diagnosis of hyperglycemia. When doubt remains in the doctor's mind as to the cause of the clinical problem, supportive therapy is indicated until additional medical assistance becomes available.

Hyperglycemia

Overall management of hyperglycemia, ketosis, and acidosis consists of the administration of insulin to normalize body metabolism, restoration of fluid and electrolyte deficiencies, a search for the precipitating cause, and avoidance of complications. Dental office management of the hyperglycemic or ketoacidotic patient will be of a supportive nature.

Conscious patient

In the dental office, the patient with clinical signs and symptoms of hyperglycemia represents an ASA IV risk and should not receive any dental therapy until a physician has been consulted. Medical consultation in most cases leads to an immediate appointment with the physician or hospitalization if the situation appears to warrant it.

Unconscious patient

Step 1. Basic life support. If the diabetic patient loses consciousness in the dental office, the doctor should quickly implement the steps of basic life support (positioning; checking airway, breathing, and vital signs). These steps ensure an adequate cerebral blood flow. However, this patient will not regain consciousness until the underlying metabolic causes (hyperglycemia, metabolic acidosis) have been corrected. Medical assistance should be summoned if an unconscious patient demonstrates no improvement after basic life support procedures have been initiated.

Step 2. Intravenous infusion (if available). An intravenous solution of normal saline may be started, if available, before the arrival of the emergency medical team. Availability of a patent vein greatly facilitates further medical management of this patient.

Injectable insulin has no place in the emergency kit (unless the doctor or a staff member is an insulin-dependent diabetic). Insulin must be carefully administered and its effect on blood glucose monitored through blood tests. Hospitalization of the patient is required to correct the hyperglycemia and the other deficits seen in this patient.

Hypoglycemia

Management of hypoglycemia in the dental office presents more dramatic results than does management of hyperglycemia because most individuals experience a dramatic remission of symptoms in a short period of time. Choice of management is based on the patient's state of consciousness.

Conscious patient

Step 1. Recognition of hypoglycemia. Bizarre behavior (in the absence of alcohol on the patient's breath) and other clinical signs of possible glucose insufficiency should lead the doctor to suspect the presence of hypoglycemia. This may develop in both diabetic and nondiabetic individuals. Determine from the patient how long it has been since his or her last meal or insulin dose.

Step 2. Assess airway, breathing, and circulation and implement as necessary. This patient is conscious and will have adequate control over the ABCs (airway, breathing, and circulation).

Step 3. Administer oral carbohydrates. If the patient is conscious and cooperative but still demonstrating clinical symptoms of hypoglycemia, the therapy of choice is oral carbohydrate. The emergency kit contains sugar, which can be dissolved and ingested by the patient. Other available items might include orange juice, cola beverages, and candy bars. A 6 to 12 oz portion of cola soft drink contains 20 to 40 g of glucose. This should be administered in 3 or 4 oz doses every 5 to 10 minutes until symptoms are no longer present.

Step 4. Permit patient to recover. The patient should be observed for approximately 1 hour before being permitted to leave the dental office. Determine if the patient has eaten before the dental appointment, and reaffirm the importance of the patient's eating shortly before the next dental visit.

Unresponsive conscious patient

If the patient has no response to oral glucose or will not cooperate by taking oral glucose, the doctor should take the following steps.

Step 1. Recognize hypoglycemia.

Step 2. Assess ABCs.

Step 3. Administer oral carbohydrate.

Step 4. Administer parenteral carbohydrate. Should the administration of oral carbohydrate prove ineffective in reversing the signs and symptoms of hypoglycemia or should the patient become uncooperative and refuse to take oral carbohydrate, parenteral administration of drugs should be considered. Glucagon, 1 mg, may be administered intramuscularly, or if available, 50 ml of dextrose in a 50% concentration can be administered intravenously over 2 to 3 minutes (Fig. 17-2). The patient usually begins to respond within 10 to 15 minutes after IM glucagon and within 5 minutes following IV dextrose. Oral carbohydrates should be started as soon as tolerated by the patient. Small amounts of honey, syrup, or decorative icing can be placed into the buccal fold if parenteral administration is unavailable (see p. 212) and if the patient will cooperate.

Step 5. Summon medical assistance. Should parenteral medications be required, it is prudent to call for additional medical assistance. The patient should be fully evaluated before being permitted to leave the dental office. The patient may be taken to a hospital for further evaluation and management.

Unconscious patient

Step 1. Basic life support. Immediate management includes positioning (supine), airway maintenance, oxygen administration, and monitoring of vital signs. The hypoglycemic patient will not regain consciousness until the blood glucose level is elevated. The patient usually demonstrates spontaneous ventilation and circulation.

Step 2. Summon medical assistance. If the patient fails to respond following the steps of basic life support, medical assistance should be called for.

Step 3. Definitive management. An unconscious person with a prior history of diabetes mellitus is always presumed to be hypoglycemic unless other obvious causes of unconsciousness are present. Definitive management of the unconscious diabetic usually entails the administration of carbohydrate by the most effective route available. In most instances, this will be intravenously (50% dextrose solution) or intramuscularly (glucagon or epinephrine). It must be stressed that the *unconscious patient must never be given any liquid by mouth,* since this may add to the possibility of airway obstruction or pulmonary aspiration. Intravenous administration of 20 to 50 ml of a 50% glucose solution over 2 to 3 minutes restores consciousness within 5 to 10 minutes. In children, do not exceed 25 ml of 50% dextrose. The usefulness of this drug is such that it is commonly administered to unconscious persons for whom the cause of unconsciousness is unknown. It serves in these instances to rule out hypoglycemia as a possible cause of the problem, yet its administration does not increase problems if hyperglycemia is present.

Glucagon (1 mg IM) leads to an elevation of blood glucose that normally restores consciousness within 15 minutes. If glucagon and 50% dextrose are both unavailable, a 0.5 mg dose of a 1:1000 concentration

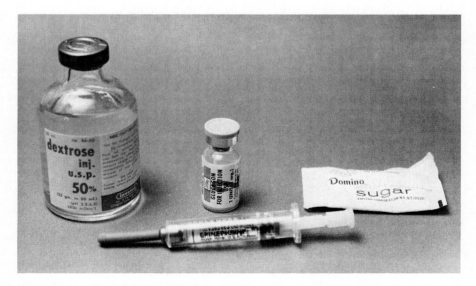

Fig. 17-2. Antihypoglycemic agents. The 50% dextrose solution must be administered IV; glucagon may be administered IM; epinephrine may be administered either IV or IM; sugar is administered orally to the conscious patient.

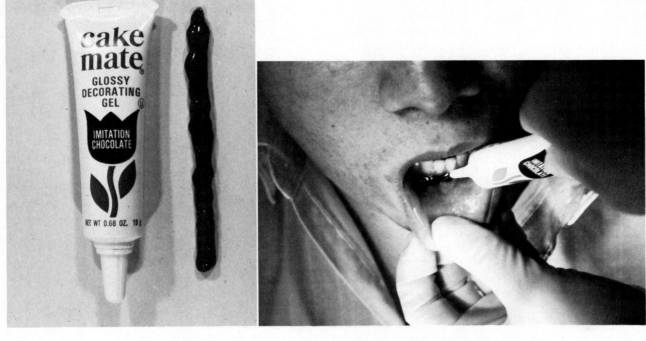

Fig. 17-3. Sugar icing placed into maxillary and mandibular folds.

Table 17-14. Management of the patient with hyperglycemia or hypoglycemia

	Hyperglycemia/diabetic acidosis	*Hypoglycemia/insulin shock*
Predisposing factors		
Onset of symptoms	Gradual (days)	Sudden (minutes to hours)
Insulin level	Insufficient	Excessive
Food intake	Normal to excessive	May be inadequate
Clinical signs and symptoms		
Skin appearance	Dry and flushed	Moist and pale
Mouth	Dry	Drooling
Thirst	Intense	Absent
Hunger	Absent	Occasional
Vomiting	Common	Rare
Abdominal pain	Frequent	Absent
Respirations	Exaggerated (Kussmaul)	Normal to shallow
Breath odor	Acetone	Normal
Blood pressure	Low	Normal
Heart rate	Weak and rapid	Full and bounding
Tremor	Absent	Frequent
Convulsions	None	In late stages
Management		
Response to treatment	Gradual	Rapid
Management	Overall—insulin	Carbohydrate: oral, IV dextrose (50%), IM
	Dental office—basic life support;	glucagon (1 mg), IM epinephrine (0.5 mg);
	medical assistance	(with unconscious patient, provide basic life
		support, medical assistance, and carbohydrate)

of epinephrine may be administered subcutaneously or intramuscularly and repeated every 15 minutes as needed. Epinephrine increases blood glucose levels. It should be used with extreme caution in patients with known cardiovascular disease. Once consciousness is restored, these patients should receive oral carbohydrates.

In the absence of the parenteral route or parenteral drugs, the doctor should maintain basic life support until medical assistance arrives. Although it is important that liquids never be placed in the mouth of an unconscious or stuporous patient—the risk of aspiration or airway obstruction is too great—a thick paste of concentrated glucose can be used with a degree of safety. Recommendations include the placement of a small amount of honey or syrup into the buccal fold. Perhaps even more effective is a small tube of decorative icing of the kind used for baked goods. Its consistency is similar to that of toothpaste. A strip of this icing can be placed in the maxillary and mandibular buccal folds (Fig. 17-3). Onset will not be rapid, but the blood sugar level will rise slowly—during which time basic life support is continued and the oral cavity is evaluated every 5 minutes and suctioned, if necessary.

Table 17-14 summarizes diagnosis and management of the patient with hyperglycemia or hypoglycemia.

BIBLIOGRAPHY

Alberti, K.G.: The management of diabetes during surgery, Br. J. Anaesth. **51:**693, 1979.

Barkin, R.M., and Rosen, P.: Endocrine disorders. In Barkin, R.M., and Rosen, P., editors: Emergency pediatrics, St. Louis, 1984, The C.V. Mosby Co.

Baruh, S., and others: Fasting hypoglycemia, Med. Clin. North Am. **57:**1441, 1973.

Beaven, D.W.: Epidemiology of diabetes mellitus, N.Z. Med. J. **8:**291, 1974.

Berger, H.: Hypoglycemia: a perspective, Postgrad. Med. **57:**81, 1975.

Bienia, R., and Ripoll, I.: Diabetic ketoacidosis, JAMA **241:**510, 1979.

Cahill, G.F., Etzwiler, D.D., and Freinkel, N.: Control and diabetes, N. Engl. J. Med. **294:**1004, 1976.

Chase, H.P.: Office management of diabetes mellitus in children, Postgrad. Med. **59:**243, 1976.

Christlieb, A.R.: Diabetes and hypertensive vascular disease: mechanisms and treatment, Am. J. Cardiol. **32:**592, 1973.

Conte, F.A., and Grumbach, M.M.: Endocrine emergencies. In Pascoe, D.J., and Grossman, M., editors: Quick reference to pediatric emergencies, ed. 2, Philadelphia, 1983, J.B. Lippincott Co.

Craighead, J.E.: Current views on the etiology of insulin-dependent diabetes, Diabetologia **22:**61, 1982.

Davidson, J.K.: Hyperglycemia. In Schwartz, G.R., and others, editors: Principles and practice of emergency medicine, Philadelphia, 1978, W.B. Saunders Co.

Davidson, J.K.: Hypoglycemia. In Schwartz, G.R., and others, editors: Principles and practice of emergency medicine, Philadelphia, 1978, W.B. Saunders Co.

Ehrlich, R.M.: Diabetes mellitus in childhood, Pediatr. Clin. North Am. **21:**871, 1974.

Extron, J.H.: Gluconeogenesis, Metabolism **21:**945, 1972.

Fajans, S.S., and Floyd, J.C., Jr.: Fasting hypoglycemia in adults, N. Engl. J. Med. **294:**766, 1976.

Felig, P.: Pathophysiology of diabetes mellitus, Med. Clin. North Am. **55:**821, 1971.

Felig, P.: Insulin: rates and routes of delivery, N. Engl. J. Med. **291:**1031, 1974.

Felig, P.: Combating diabetic ketoacidosis, Postgrad. Med. **59:**150, 1976.

Grodsky, G.M.: Insulin and the pancreas, Vitam. Horm. **28:**37, 1970.

Gross, R.C.: Emergency management of diabetes mellitus and hypoglycemia. In Warner, C.G.: Emergency care: assessment and intervention, ed. 2, St. Louis, 1978, The C.V. Mosby Co.

Hadden, D.R., and others: Maturity onset diabetes mellitus: response to intensive dietary management, Br. Med. J. **3:**276, 1975.

Hansen, B., and others: New approaches to therapy and diagnosis of diabetes, Diabetologia **22:**61, 1982.

Hockaday, T.D.R., and Alber, K.G.: Diabetic coma, Clin. Endocrinol. Metab. **1:**751, 1972.

Isaac, R.M.: Diabetic ketoacidosis. In Pascoe, D.J., and Grossman, M., editors: Quick reference to pediatric emergencies, ed. 3, Philadelphia, 1983, J.B. Lippincott Co.

Karam, J.H.: Diabetes mellitus, hypoglycemia, and lipoprotein disorders. In Krupp, M.A., and Chatton, M.J., editors: Current medical diagnosis and treatment, Los Altos, CA, 1984, Lange Medical Publications.

Kidson, W.: The emergency management of the diabetic at home, Med. J. Aust. **1:**311, 1976.

Kimble, M.A.: Diabetes, J. Am. Pharm. Assoc. **NS14:**80, 1974.

Knowles, H.C.: Diabetes mellitus in childhood and adolescence, Med. Clin. North Am. **55:**975, 1971.

Knowles, H.C., Jr.: Long-term juvenile diabetes treated with unmeasured diet, Trans. Assoc. Am. Physicians **84:**95, 1971.

Lefebvre, P.J., and Luyckx, A.S.: Glucagon and diabetes: a reappraisal, Diabetologia **16:**347, 1979.

Levine, R.: Mechanisms of insulin secretion, N. Engl. J. Med. **283:**522, 1970.

Little, J.W., and Falace, D.A.: Dental management of the medically compromised patient, ed. 2, St. Louis, 1984, The C.V. Mosby Co.

Lown, B., and others: The complications of diabetes mellitus, N. Engl. J. Med. **298:**1250, 1978.

McMillan, D.E.: Deterioration of the microcirculation in diabetes, Diabetes **24:**944, 1975.

Medalie, J.H., and others: Major factors in the development of diabetes mellitus in 10,000 men, Arch. Intern. Med. **135:**811, 1975.

National Diabetes Data Group: Classification and diagnosis of diabetes mellitus and other categories of glucose intolerance, Diabetes **28:**1039, 1979.

Oleesky, S., Shreeve, D., and Sutcliffe, C.H.: Brittle diabetes, Q. J. Med. **43:**113, 1974.

Owen, O.E., Boden, G., and Shuman, C.R.: Managing insulin-dependent diabetic patients, Postgrad. Med. **59:**127, 1976.

Owen, O.E., Trapp, V.E., and Skutches, C.L.: Acetone metabolism during diabetic ketoacidosis, Diabetes **31:**242, 1982.

Pearce, M.B., Bullock, R.T., and Kizziar, J.C.: Myocardial small vessel disease in patients with diabetes mellitus, Circulation **48:**IV-6, 1973.

Peden, N., Newton, R.W., and Feely, J.: Oral antihypoglycemic agents, Br. Med. J. **286:**1564, 1983.

Phenformin: removal from general market, FDA Drug Bull. **7:**14, 1977.

Reeves, M.L., and others: Comparison of methods for blood glucose monitoring, Diabetes Care **4:**404, 1981.

Rosenbloom, A.L., Kohrman, A., and Sperling, M.: Classification and diagnosis of diabetes mellitus in children and adolescents, J. Pediatr. **98:**320, 1981.

Rossini, A.A.: Why control blood glucose levels? Arch. Surg. **111:**229, 1976.

Saadoun, A.P.: Diabetes and periodontal disease: a review and update, Periodont. Abstr. **28:**116, 1980.

Scott, R.C.: Diabetes and the heart (editorial), Am. Heart J. **90:**283, 1975.

Scoville, A.B.: Oral therapy in diabetes mellitus—an update, South. Med. J. **69:**679, 1976.

Seltzer, H.S.: Drug induced hypoglycemia: a review based on 473 cases, Diabetes **21:**955, 1972.

Seltzer, H.S.: Efficacy and safety of oral hypoglycemic agents, Annu. Rev. Med. **31:**261, 1980.

Shen, S.W., and Bressler, R.: Clinical pharmacology of oral antidiabetic agents, N. Engl. J. Med. **296:**493, 1977.

Sonkson, P.H., Judd, S., and Lowy, C.: Home monitoring of blood glucose: new approach to management of insulin-dependent diabetic patients in Great Britain, Diabetes Care **3:**100, 1980.

Sonkson, P.H., Judd, S., and Lowy, C.: Home monitoring of blood glucose, Lancet **1:**729, 1978.

Sperling, M.A.: Diabetes mellitus, Pediatr. Clin. North Am. **26:**149, 1979.

Steinberg, A.G.: The genetics of diabetes: a review, Ann. N.Y. Acad. Sci. **82:**197, 1959.

Steinke, J.: Management of diabetes in the surgical patient, Med. Clin. North Am. **55:**939, 1971.

Timoney, F.J.: Oral hypoglycaemic drugs—our current practice, Postgrad. Med. J. **55**(suppl. 2):22, 1979.

University Group Diabetes Program: Effects of hypoglycemic agents on vascular complications in patients with adult-onset diabetes. II. Mortality results, Diabetes **19**(suppl. 2):785, 1970.

University Group Diabetes Program: Effects of hypoglycemic agents on vascular complications in patients with adult-onset diabetes. V. Evaluation of phenformin therapy, Diabetes **24**(suppl. 1):65, 1975.

University Group Diabetes Program: Effects of hypoglycemic agents on vascular complications in patients with adult-onset diabetes. VI. Supplementary report on nonfatal events in patients treated with tolbutamide, Diabetes **25:**1129, 1976.

University Group Diabetes Program: Effects of hypoglycemic agents on vascular complications in patients with adult-onset diabetes. VIII. Mortality and selected nonfatal events with insulin treatment, JAMA **240:**37, 1978.

Winegrad, A.I., and Clements, R.S., Jr.: Diabetic ketoacidosis, Med. Clin. North Am. **55:**890, 1971.

Zonana, J., and Rimoin, D.L.: Inheritance of diabetes mellitus, N. Engl. J. Med. **295:**603, 1976.

18 *Thyroid Gland Dysfunction*

The thyroid gland consists of two elongated lobes on either side of the trachea that are joined by a thin isthmus of thyroid tissue located at or below the level of the thyroid cartilage. The thyroid gland produces and secretes hormones that perform an important function in regulating the level of biochemical activity of most of the tissues of the body. Proper functioning of the thyroid gland from birth is essential for normal growth and metabolism.

Dysfunction of the thyroid gland may occur through overproduction of thyroid hormone (hyperthyroidism) or underproduction of thyroid hormone (hypothyroidism). In both instances, clinical manifestations may cover a broad spectrum, ranging from subclinical dysfunction to acute life-threatening situations. Fortunately, however, most patients with thyroid dysfunction have milder forms of the disease.

Primary emphasis in the following discussions is on the detection of clinical signs and symptoms of thyroid gland dysfunction. The life-threatening situations *myxedema coma* and *thyroid "storm" or crisis*, both of which are extremely rare, are also considered.

Hypothyroidism is a clinical state in which the tissues of the body do not receive an adequate supply of thyroid hormones. The clinical signs and symptoms of hypothyroidism are related to the age of the patient at the time of onset and to the degree and duration of hormonal deficiency. Cretinism is a clinical syndrome encountered in infants and children and results from deficiency of thyroid hormone during fetal or early life. Severe hypothyroidism developing in an adult is termed *myxedema* and refers to the appearance of mucinous infiltrates beneath the skin. Severe, unmanaged hypothyroidism may ultimately lead to the loss of consciousness that is termed myxedema coma. The mortality rate in myxedema coma is high (up to 40%) even with optimal treatment.

Hyperthyroidism is also known by several other names, including thyrotoxicosis, toxic goiter (diffuse or nodular), Basedow's disease, Graves' disease, Parry's disease, and Plummer's disease. It may be defined as a state of heightened thyroid gland activity associated with the production of excessive quantities of the thyroid hormones L-thyroxine (T_4) and L-triiodothyronine (T_3). Because the thyroid hormones affect the cellular metabolism of virtually all organ systems, the signs and symptoms of hyperthyroidism may be noted in any part of the body. Untreated hyperthyroidism may lead to the acute life-threatening situation termed thyroid storm or crisis, which manifests itself in part as severe hypermetabolism. Although uncommon today, thyroid storm still has a mortality rate of from 34% to 76% for those who experience it.

PREDISPOSING FACTORS

Dysfunction of the thyroid gland is a relatively common medical disorder. If diabetes mellitus is excluded, thyroid dysfunction accounts for 80% of all endocrine disorders.

Hypothyroidism

Hypothyroidism in the adult patient usually develops as a result of idiopathic atrophy of the thyroid gland (currently thought to occur through an autoimmune mechanism). Other causes of hypothyroidism include total thyroidectomy, ablation following radioactive iodine therapy (which are procedures frequently employed in the management of hyperfunction of the thyroid gland), and chronic thyroiditis. Thyroid hypofunction is seen more frequently in females, with its greatest incidence noted at about the time of menopause. Myxedema coma, the end stage of untreated hypothyroidism, has a mortality rate of approximately 40% but fortunately is infrequently noted clinically.

The dental practitioner should be aware of possible hypothyroid patients because, if medically untreated, they may represent an increased risk in the dental office. The hypothyroid patient is unusually sensitive to most CNS depressants including sedatives, narcotics, and antianxiety agents, which are drugs commonly employed by the dental profession. Normal therapeutic doses of these agents may result in extreme overdose reactions in clinically hypothyroid individuals.

Hyperthyroidism

Hyperthyroidism, like hypothyroidism, usually begins insidiously and if left untreated may progress to a more severe form of the disease called thyroid crisis. The incidence of thyroid gland hyperfunction is 3 out of 10,000 adults per year, and the disease is found in females in a 5:1 ratio over males. Hyperthyroidism occurs most often in patients between the ages of 20 and 40 years. Although its etiology is unknown, hyperthyroidism is more common in areas of iodine deficiency and has been shown to occur more often in people with a family history of the disease. It may manifest itself initially during periods of emotional and physical stress.

Thyroid storm or crisis, although rarely seen, occurs in patients with untreated or incompletely treated hyperfunction. On occasion, thyroid storm may occur suddenly in a patient in whom hyperthyroidism has not previously been diagnosed. Thyroid storm is a sudden, severe exacerbation of the signs and symptoms of hyperthyroidism, is usually accompanied by hyperpyrexia (elevated body temperature), and is precipitated by some intercurrent disease, infection, trauma, surgery, or physiologic stress such as pregnancy.

Thyroid gland dysfunction, whether hyperfunction or hypofunction, is associated with an increased incidence of cardiovascular disease. Milder forms of both types of dysfunction may easily pass unnoticed. Although both situations lead to an increased risk, it is the more severe, undiagnosed, or untreated individual who represents a greater potential risk during dental therapy. The doctor must be able to recognize each of these clinical entities and then take steps to decrease the potential risk.

PREVENTION

The goals in management of patients with thyroid dysfunction are (1) to prevent the occurrence of the life-threatening situations myxedema coma and thyroid storm and (2) to prevent exacerbation of the complications of thyroid dysfunction (notably cardiovascular disease).

Only one question on the USC medical history questionnaire relates to thyroid disease (Question 9). However, several other questions can provide information about potential thyroid gland dysfunction (Questions 4, 5, 6, 13, and 16). Most other medical history questionnaires have no specific mention of thyroid disease.

QUESTION 4. Have you been a patient in the hospital during the past 2 years?

QUESTION 5. Have you been under the care of a medical doctor during the past 2 years?

QUESTION 9. Circle any of the following which you have had or have at present: Thyroid disease

COMMENT. Patients with a known history of thyroid gland dysfunction will mention it in one or more of these three questions.

QUESTION 6. Have you taken any medicine or drugs during the past 2 years?

COMMENT. Patients with thyroid gland hypofunction receive thyroid extract or a synthetic preparation. The most frequently used drug and the agent considered to be the drug of choice is L-thyroxine sodium (Synthroid). Other agents used in management of hypofunction include liotrix (Euthroid, Thyrolar) and dextrothyroxine sodium (Choloxin). The goal in management of thyroid gland hypofunction or hyperfunction is to achieve a normal level of glandular functioning, termed the *euthyroid state.*

Patients with hyperfunction of the thyroid gland undergo treatment aimed at halting the excessive secretion of thyroid hormone. Management may involve surgical removal of all or part of the thyroid gland (total or subtotal thyroidectomy), long-term medical treatment with antithyroid drugs to achieve remission of the disease, or radioactive iodine therapy rather than surgical removal. Frequently prescribed antithyroid drugs include thiouracil, propylthiouracil, methimazole (Tapazole), iothiouracil (Itrumil), and iodine.

QUESTION 13. Have you lost or gained more than 10 pounds in the past year?

COMMENT. Unexplained weight loss in a patient with a ravenous appetite should alert the doctor to the possible presence of a hyperthyroid state. Conversely, an unexplained increase in weight along with other clinical signs and symptoms might indicate the possible presence of hypothyroidism.

QUESTION 16. Has your medical doctor ever said you have a cancer or a tumor?

COMMENT. Thyroid dysfunction is frequently discovered on routine examination of a patient's neck, manifesting itself as a lump or bump. This question will lead to an explanation of the type of dysfunction that was present and the mode of treatment. Total or subtotal thyroidectomy is a common mode of therapy for thyroid hyperfunction. Surgical intervention is especially common in those glands that develop benign or malignant thyroid nodules. Irradiation with radioactive iodine (^{131}I) is another commonly employed technique for destroying hyperfunctioning thyroid tissue.

QUESTION 7. Are you allergic to (i.e., itching, rash, swelling of hands, feet, or eyes) or made sick by penicillin, aspirin, codeine, or any drugs or medications?

COMMENT. Patients who are clinically hypothyroid are unusually sensitive to the pharmacologic actions of narcotics and other CNS depressants. Any adverse response to a strong analgesic (such as codeine) or CNS depressant should be carefully evaluated for precise description of the nature of the response. Overdose reactions (Chapter 23) developing after "average" doses of these agents may indicate thyroid gland hypofunction.

Dialogue History

In the presence of a positive history of thyroid disease, the following dialogue history is indicated.

QUESTION. What is (was) the nature of the thyroid dysfunction: hypofunction or hyperfunction?
QUESTION. How is it being managed?

COMMENT. These questions seek to determine general information concerning the disease state. Following dialogue history, the physical examination should seek clinical evidence of the presence of the dysfunction. In most instances, the patient is

euthyroid and will represent a normal risk during dental therapy. If there is no prior history of thyroid dysfunction but clinical evidence leads to a suspicion of its presence, the following dialogue history is recommended.

QUESTION. Have you lost or gained weight recently without dieting?

COMMENT. Recent weight gain (10 or more pounds) is commonly noted in clinical hypothyroidism, whereas weight loss in the presence of an increasing appetite is frequently noted in hyperthyroidism. Note that other medical conditions may also produce weight gain or loss (for example, congestive heart failure or malignancy).

QUESTION. Are you unusually sensitive to cold temperature or pain-relieving medications?

COMMENT. These represent commonly seen signs and symptoms of a hypofunctioning thyroid gland.

QUESTION. Are you unusually sensitive to heat?
QUESTION. Have you become increasingly irritable or tense?

COMMENT. These represent frequently seen signs and symptoms of a hyperfunctioning thyroid gland. The patient may be less aware of temperament changes; a close acquaintance is more likely to notice such changes.

Physical Examination

In most cases, the patient who has a prior history of thyroid gland dysfunction has received therapy or is currently undergoing therapy. These persons are usually in a euthyroid (normal function) state and do not represent an increased risk during dental therapy.

On the other hand, the patient with undetected thyroid gland dysfunction represents a possible significantly elevated risk during dental therapy. Clinical signs and symptoms enable the doctor to recognize these dysfunctions of the thyroid gland. The clinically *hypothyroid* patient has a large, thick tongue with atrophic papillae, and thick edematous skin with puffy hands and face. The skin is dry and sweating is usually absent. The blood pressure is approximately normal (slight elevation of diastolic), and the heart rate is slow (bradycardia). The patient appears lethargic and slow of speech.

Clinically, the *hyperthyroid* patient appears nervous, with warm sweaty hands that may exhibit a mild tremor. The blood pressure is elevated (systolic more than diastolic), and the heart rate is markedly increased (tachycardia). A very difficult differential diagnosis is between hyperthyroidism and acute anxiety. One possible clue is that the patient with hyperthyroidism has palms that are *warm* and sweaty as distinguished from the *cold* and sweaty palms of the nervous individual who is not hyperthyroid. Other signs and symptoms of thyroid dysfunction are discussed in the section on clinical manifestations.

Dental Therapy Considerations

Patients with thyroid dysfunction who are receiving or have received therapy (surgery, medications, or irradiation), who have a normal level of circulating thyroid hormone, and who are asymptomatic are considered to be euthyroid. These patients may be managed in a normal manner in the dental environment.

In the presence of mild clinical manifestations, dental therapy may also proceed in a normal manner, although certain possible modifications should be considered. If *hypothyroidism* is suspected, the following measures should be taken:

1. Medical consultation should be considered before initiating dental therapy.
2. Any CNS depressant must be used with caution. Of particular concern are the sedative-hypnotics (barbiturates), narcotic analgesics, and the antianxiety drugs. Hypothyroid patients are extremely sensitive to the depressant actions of these drugs, and administration of a "normal" dose of these agents may prove to be an overdose, leading to respiratory or cardiovascular depression or both.
3. There is an increased incidence of cardiovascular disease associated with the hypothyroid state. Barnes and Barnes (1976) have theorized that most instances of cardiovascular

disease are produced by hypofunction of the thyroid gland and that correction of the thyroid deficiency leads to elimination of the cardiovascular disease. Although controversial, this theory is intriguing.

A history of thyroid gland hypofunction should lead the doctor to seek other possible signs and symptoms of cardiovascular disease. With more intense signs and symptoms of thyroid hypofunction (mental apathy, drowsiness, or slow speech), dental therapy should be withheld until medical consultation or definitive management of the clinical disorder is accomplished.

Mild degrees of thyroid *hyperfunction* may pass for acute anxiety, with little increase in clinical risk. It must be noted that various cardiovascular disorders, primarily angina pectoris, are exaggerated in hyperthyroidism. Should these develop, management ought to proceed in the manner prescribed for such situations (Section VII). Severe hyperfunction should lead to immediate medical consultation. Dental therapy should not take place until the underlying metabolic disturbance has been corrected. It should always be remembered that thyroid crisis, although rare, may be precipitated by psychologic or physiologic stresses in untreated or incompletely treated hyperthyroid individuals.

There are additional dental therapy considerations for clinically hyperthyroid individuals. The drug atropine should not be administered. Atropine is a vagolytic agent (inhibits the vagus nerve); it increases the heart rate and may be a factor in precipitating thyroid storm. In addition, epinephrine should be used with extreme caution in these patients. Vasopressors act as cardiovascular stimulants, and when a cardiovascular system is already stimulated by the hyperthyroid state, they may precipitate cardiac arrhythmias, tachycardia, and thyroid storm. Local anesthetics may be used with vasoconstrictors if the following precautions are

Table 18-1. Physical status classifications of thyroid gland dysfunction

Degree of dysfunction	Physical status (ASA)	Considerations
Hypofunction or hyperfunction patient receiving medical therapy; no signs or symptoms of dysfunction evident	II	Usual ASA II considerations
Hypofunction or hyperfunction; signs and symptoms of dysfunction evident	III	Usual ASA III considerations: Avoidance of vasopressors (hyperfunction) or CNS depressants (hypofunction) Evaluation for cardiovascular disease

followed: the least concentrated solution that is effective should be employed, the smallest effective volume of anesthetic agent should be injected, and aspiration should be performed before every injection. (Injection technique is reviewed more thoroughly in Chapter 23.) Of greater potential risk, however, is the use of racemic epinephrine for gingival retraction. This agent is much more likely to precipitate unwanted side effects, especially in the presence of a preexisting hyperthyroid state. Its use should be avoided in these patients.

Patients who are mildly hyperthyroid might readily be mistaken for apprehensive persons. The use of conscious sedation techniques in these individuals is not contraindicated. Indeed, because the apparent nervousness is not truly dental in origin but hormonally induced, the effectiveness of sedative drugs may be less than ideal. Physical status classifications are presented in Table 18-1. Hypothyroid or hyperthyroid patients who have been treated and are presently euthyroid are ASA II risks, whereas patients with clinical manifestations of the hypothyroid or hyperthyroid state are ASA III risks.

CLINICAL MANIFESTATIONS
Hypothyroidism

Hypothyroidism may be described as a state in which all bodily functions undergo a progressive slowing caused by insufficient supply of thyroid hormones. When this deficiency occurs in childhood, alterations are noted in growth and development, and the syndrome is termed cretinism. In cretinism there has been a lack of thyroid hormone in utero or shortly after birth. The entire physical and mental development of the individual is retarded. Ossification of bone is delayed, tooth development is poor and eruption is delayed, and permanent neurologic damage is evident. Clinically, the infant is dull and apathetic, usually displaying a subnormal temperature. The tongue is enlarged, the skin and lips are thick, the face is broad and puffy, and the nose is flat (Fig. 18-1).

When hypothyroidism occurs in adults, its onset is usually insidious. The patient is often persuaded by his spouse or friends to seek medical assistance because of noticeably increased sluggishness, sudden weight gain, or an increase in sleepiness. The patient is usually unaware of these changes. Signs and symptoms that may lead to a presumptive diagnosis of hypothyroidism include abnormal weakness and fatigue, inability to tolerate cold temperatures, lethargy, and dryness of the skin. Later in the course of the disease there may be evidence of slowing of speech, hoarseness, a lack of sweating, weight gain, peripheral nonpitting edema, dyspnea, and anginal pains. Clinical signs include a puffiness of the face and eyelids, a carotenemic (orange-red) skin color with rosy cheeks, thickened tongue, and thickened edematous skin (nonpitting). Blood pressure remains approximately normal (with perhaps a slight elevation in the diastolic); however, the heart rate decreases. Congestive heart failure with pulmonary congestion may also occur in severe, untreated hypothyroidism. The most severe complication of hypothyroidism is myxedema coma. Myxedema coma has a high mortality rate and is marked by hypothermia (29.5° to 30° C), bradycardia, hypotension, and intense cerebral obtundation (loss of consciousness). Table 18-2 summarizes clinical manifestations of thyroid hypofunction.

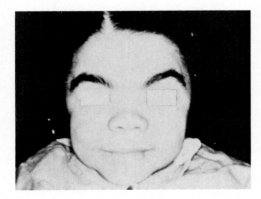

Fig. 18-1. Cretinism—clinical picture includes flat nose and broad, puffy face.

Table 18-2. Clinical manifestations of hypothyroidism (in decreasing order of occurrence)

Weakness	Thick tongue
Dry skin	Edema of face
Coarse skin	Coarseness of hair
Lethargy	Pallor of skin
Slow speech	Memory impairment
Edema of eyelids	Constipation
Sensation of cold	Gain in weight
Decreased sweating	Loss of hair
Cold skin	Pallor of lips

From Williams, R.H.: Textbook of endocrinology, ed. 5, Philadelphia, 1974, W.B. Saunders Co.

Hyperthyroidism

Hyperthyroidism, like hypothyroidism, is rarely severe at onset. In most cases, questioning of the patient reveals clinical evidence of the dysfunction over a period of months before its "discovery." As with hypofunction, the person discovering the disease frequently is not the patient but a spouse or friend who notices changes in the habits and personality of the patient. Nervousness, increasing irritability, and insomnia are usually the first clinical symptoms noted. Other clinical manifestations include an increasing intolerance to heat; hyperhidrosis (marked increase in sweating); overactivity, including quick movements with incoordination ranging from mild tremulousness to gross tremor; and rapid speech. An important sign is unexplained weight loss associated with an increased appetite. The patient fatigues easily and may be aware of heart palpitation.

Clinical signs include an increase in blood pressure (systolic pressure to a greater extent than diastolic), widening of the pulse pressure, tachycardia, and on occasion paroxysmal atrial fibrillation (or congestive heart failure). Extreme sweating is evident, and the skin appears warm and moist. The extremities, especially the hands, exhibit varying degrees of tremulousness. Exophthalmos is present in 71% of patients with hyperthyroidism and may be associated with double vision, blurred vision, burning, tearing, and diminished visual acuity (Fig. 18-2).

Untreated hyperthyroidism may progress to the life-threatening situation called thyroid storm. It is essentially an acute exacerbation of the signs and symptoms of hyperthyroidism manifested by signs of severe hypermetabolism. Clinical manifestations include hyperpyrexia (highly elevated body temperature); profuse sweating; nausea, vomiting, and abdominal pains; and cardiovascular disturbances such as tachycardia and arrhythmia, as well as congestive heart failure with possible pulmonary edema. Central nervous system manifestations usually progress from mild tremulousness to severe agitation and disorientation to frankly psychotic behavior, stupor (partial unconsciousness), and finally coma. Without management—or in many instances, even with management—thyroid storm has a high mortality rate. Fortunately, its occurrence is extremely rare. Table 18-3 summarizes signs and symptoms of thyroid hyperfunction.

PATHOPHYSIOLOGY
Hypothyroidism

The clinical signs and symptoms of hypothyroidism are produced by insufficient levels of circulating thyroid hormone. There is, in effect, a slowing down of all of the functions of the body. In addition, with chronic hypofunction there is a progressive infiltration of the skin by mucopolysaccharides and mucoproteins, giving the skin its characteristic puffy appearance. This hard (nonpitting) mucinous edema has been termed myxedema and is characteristic of hypothyroidism. This edema may also cause significant cardiac en-

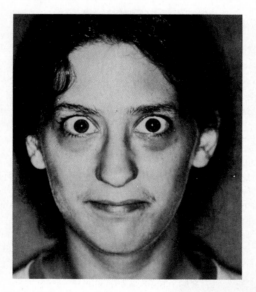

Fig. 18-2. Hyperthyroid patient exhibiting exophthalmos.

Table 18-3. Clinical manifestations of hyperthyroidism (in decreasing order of occurrence)

Symptoms	*Signs*
Nervousness	Tachycardia
Increased sweating	Goiter
Hypersensitivity to heat	Skin changes
Heart palpitation	Tremor
Fatigue	Bruit over thyroid
Weight loss	Eye signs (exophthalmos)
Tachycardia	Atrial fibrillation
Dyspnea	
Weakness	
Increased appetite	
Eye complaints	

From Williams, R.H.: Textbook of endocrinology, ed. 5, Philadelphia, 1974, W.B. Saunders Co.

largement, which leads to pericardial and pleural effusions and to the cardiovascular and respiratory difficulties associated with hypothyroidism (Barnes, 1975; Barnes and Barnes, 1976). Atherosclerosis has been demonstrated to be accelerated in clinically hypothyroid patients.

Myxedema coma is the end point in the progression of severe hypothyroidism. The actual cause of the loss of consciousness may be hypothermia, hypoglycemia, or carbon dioxide retention, all of which are present in this clinical situation.

Hyperthyroidism

Hyperthyroidism results from the excessive production of endogenous thyroid hormone by the thyroid gland or from the excessive administration of exogenous thyroid hormone (as in therapy for hypothyroid states). Clinical signs and symptoms are related to the level of these hormones in the blood.

Thyroid hormones produce an increase in energy consumption by the body and an elevation of the basal metabolic rate (BMR). Fatigue and weight loss result from this increased utilization of energy. Cardiovascular findings in hyperthyroid patients are probably related to the direct action of hormones on the myocardium. These findings include increased heart rate and increased cardiac irritability. This increased cardiac workload is probably responsible for the increased incidence of cardiac problems (angina pectoris and congestive heart failure) in hyperthyroid individuals. Subclinical cardiac disease may have been present before the onset of the hyperthyroid state or in the hypothyroid state before therapy, but with the addition of thyroid hormone, the workload and myocardial oxygen requirement of the heart are increased to the point that clinically significant cardiac disease is evident.

Liver function is diminished in hyperthyroidism; therefore all drugs and medications metabolized in the liver should be employed judiciously and in smaller than normal doses. Because of the effects of atropine and epinephrine on the heart and cardiovascular systems, these agents should not be administered to *severely* hyperthyroid individuals.

Thyroid storm or crisis is the end point of untreated hyperthyroidism. The primary differentiation of thyroid storm from severe hyperthyroidism is the presence of hyperpyrexia, which if allowed to progress may reach lethal body temperatures (105° F or higher) within 24 to 48 hours. In this state of severe hypermetabolism, the body's demand for energy overworks the cardiovascular system, leading to clinical signs and symptoms of cardiac arrhythmia, congestive heart failure, and acute pulmonary edema.

MANAGEMENT
Hypothyroidism

No special management is necessary for most patients who show clinical evidence of thyroid hypofunction. If doubt or concern is present in the doctor's mind following complete medical and dental evaluation, medical consultation before beginning dental therapy is warranted. It must always be remembered that hypothyroid patients are unusually sensitive to the following categories of drugs—sedatives (barbiturates), narcotics (meperidine, codeine), antianxiety drugs (diazepam), and most other CNS depressants (such as antihistamines). In addition, severe drug overdose may occur from "normal" doses of these agents.

Effective management of hypothyroid individuals is usually easily achieved through oral administration of desiccated thyroid hormone. In almost all cases, therapy must continue for the rest of the patient's life. Within 30 days of the start of therapy, the patient has usually returned to a normal body weight, and all clinical signs and symptoms have disappeared. Prognosis for treated hypothyroidism is a return to normal health.

Unconscious patient

Step 1. Basic life support. In the highly unlikely event that a hypothyroid individual loses consciousness, the possibility of myxedema coma must be considered. Management of this individual includes the steps of basic life support: positioning, establishing a patent airway, checking for breathing, administering oxygen, and assessing the adequacy of circulation.

Step 2. Summon medical assistance. Because the underlying cause of unconsciousness is not a lack of oxygen, this individual will not regain consciousness following these basic procedures. Therefore the doctor must summon additional medical assistance.

Step 3. Definitive management. Definitive management of this situation includes massive intravenous doses of thyroid hormones (T_3 or T_4) for several days and correction of hypothermia. Additional therapy varies according to the clinical state of the patient. The mortality rate from this illness is quite high (40%) in spite of rigorous therapy.

MANAGEMENT OF THYROID GLAND DYSFUNCTION

Hypofunction or hyperfunction under therapy (euthyroid)

Step 1 Manage normally

Clinical evidence of hypofunction or hyperfunction

Step 1 Prior medical consultation
    2 Judicious use of drugs
      CNS-depressants: sedatives, narcotics, antianxiety drugs (hypofunction)
      Atropine and epinephrine (hyperfunction)

Unconscious patient

Step 1 Basic life support
    2 Summon medical assistance if no response

Hyperthyroidism

Clinically, hyperthyroid individuals most often appear nervous and apprehensive. If clinical symptoms are intense to the point of creating doubt in the doctor's mind, medical consultation before initiating dental therapy is indicated. Although the risk of precipitating thyroid storm is low, undue stress can induce this acute life-threatening situation. The use of certain drugs, particularly atropine and epinephrine, can precipitate thyroid crisis and are therefore contraindicated for use in clinically hyperthyroid individuals.

Unconscious patient

Step 1. Basic life support.

Step 2. Summon medical assistance. A hyperthyroid individual who loses consciousness must receive prompt and efficient management. The possibility of thyroid storm occurring is not great but must always be considered, especially if the patient has an elevated temperature. Management in the dental office consists of basic life support and immediate summoning of medical assistance.

Step 3. Definitive management. Definitive therapy is usually concentrated on decreasing the body temperature and decreasing blood levels of thyroid hormones. To this end, specific therapy includes cold packs, corticosteroids, iodine and antithyroid drugs, and intravenous fluids to correct the dehy-

dration that is often present. Thyroid storm, like myxedema coma, has a poor prognosis.

Management of the patient with thyroid gland dysfunction is summarized in the box at left.

BIBLIOGRAPHY

Barkin, R.M., and Rosen, P.: Endocrine disorders. In Barkin, R.M., and Rosen, P., editors: Emergency pediatrics, St. Louis, 1984, The C.V. Mosby Co.

Barnes, B.O.: Hypertension and the thyroid gland, Clin. Exp. Pharmacol. Physiol. **2**(suppl.):167, 1975.

Barnes, B.O., and Barnes, C.W.: Solved: the riddle of heart attacks, Fort Collins, CO, 1976, Robinson Press, Inc.

Blum, M., and others: Thyroid storm after cardiac angiography with iodinated contrast medium, JAMA **235**:2324, 1976.

Bremer, W.J., and Greip, R.J.: Graves thyrotoxicosis following primary thyroid failure, JAMA **235**:1361, 1976.

Brown, J., and others: Thyroid physiology in health and disease, Ann. Intern. Med. **81**:68, 1974.

Brown, J., and others: Autoimmune thyroid diseases: Graves' and Hashimoto's, Ann. Intern. Med. **88**:379, 1978.

Camargo, C.A., and Kolb, F.O.: Endocrine disorders. In Krupp, M.A., and Chatton, M.J., editors: Current medical diagnosis and treatment, Los Altos, CA, 1984, Lange Medical Publications.

Carter, J.N., and others: Rational therapy for thyroid storm, Aust. N.Z., J. Med. **5**:458, 1975.

Dobyns, B.M.: Prevention and management of thyroid storm, World J. Surg. **2**:293, 1978.

Dorfman, S.G.: Hyperthyroidism: usual and unusual cases, Arch. Intern. Med. **137**:995, 1977.

Dorfman, S.G., Young, R.L., and Nusynowitz, M.L.: Thyroiditis and thyrotoxicosis, JAMA **240**:1520, 1978.

Eraker, S.A., Wickamasekaran, R., and Goldman, S.: Complete heart block with hyperthyroidism, JAMA **239**:1644, 1978.

Grove, A.S., Jr.: Evaluation of exophthalmos, N. Engl. J. Med. **292**:1005, 1975.

Hamburger, J.L.: The various forms of thyroiditis, N. Engl. J. Med. **294**:52, 1976.

Ingbar, S.H.: When to hospitalize the patient with thyrotoxicosis, Hosp. Pract. **45,** 1975.

Little, J.W., and Falace, D.A.: Thyroid disease. In Dental management of the medically compromised patient, ed. 2, St. Louis, 1984, The C.V. Mosby Co.

McClung, M.R., and Greer, M.A.: Treatment of hyperthyroidism, Annu. Rev. Med. **31**:385, 1980.

Menendez, C.E., and Rivlin, R.S.: Thyrotoxic crisis and myxedema coma, Med. Clin. North Am. **57**:1463, 1973.

Mitchell, M.L., and others: Screening for congenital hypothyroidism, JAMA **239**:2348, 1978.

Parker, J.Z.W., and Lawson, D.H.: Death from thyrotoxicosis, Lancet **2**:894, 1973.

Roizen, M., and Becker, C.: Thyroid storm: a review of cases at University of California, San Francisco, Calif. Med. **115**:5, 1971.

Scarpalezos, S., and others: Neural and muscular manifestations of hypothyroidism, Arch. Neurol. **29**:140, 1973.

Senior, R.M., and others: Recognition and management of myxedema coma, JAMA **217**:61, 1971.

Williams, R.H.: Textbook of endocrinology, ed. 5, Philadelphia, 1974, W.B. Saunders Co.

19 Cerebrovascular Accident

Cerebrovascular accident is a focal neurologic disorder caused by the destruction of brain substance as a result of intracerebral hemorrhage, thrombosis, embolism, or vascular insufficiency. Synonyms for cerebrovascular accident include CVA, stroke, and cerebral apoplexy. Throughout this section, the abbreviation CVA will be used to identify this disorder.

CVAs are fairly common in the adult population. In the United States, approximately 400,000 new acute CVAs are reported annually. Although mortality rates for the various forms of CVA differ considerably, the overall rate is relatively high. Approximately 200,000 deaths are reported annually from CVAs, making it the third leading cause of death in this country (heart disease and cancer are first and second). The frequency with which CVAs occur is emphasized by the fact that approximately 25% of routine autopsies (death from all causes) demonstrate evidence of CVA, even though there may have been no evidence while the patient was alive. CVAs are the most common form of brain disease. The average age of persons at the time of their first CVA is approximately 64 years. Recent evidence demonstrates that the incidence of CVA is decreasing; in the past 30 years, it has declined 25%. For every 100 first episodes of CVA that occurred in a unit of population between 1945 and 1949, only 55 first episodes of CVA occurred between 1970 and 1974. This decline is noted in both sexes and all age groups but is most noted in the elderly (Garraway. 1979; Levy, 1979; Furlan and others, 1979).

CLASSIFICATION

CVAs are usually classified by cause. Two major groups are cerebral infarction and intracranial hemorrhage. Table 19-1 presents the various forms of CVA and their relative incidence. In addition to forms of CVA listed in the table, there is a syndrome variously termed transient ischemic attack (TIA), transient cerebral ischemia (TCI), or incipient stroke. It consists of brief episodes of cerebral ischemia that result in no permanent neurologic damage, whereas a CVA results in evidence of some degree of neurologic damage.

Cerebral Ischemia and Infarction

The most prevalent form of CVA is cerebral ischemia and infarction, which accounts for over 85% of all CVAs. Atherosclerosis and thrombosis of intracranial and extracranial arteries and cerebral embolization from various origins are the primary causes of cerebral ischemia and infarction. *Cerebral infarction* may be defined as death of neural (brain) tissue from ischemia. The primary cause of ischemia is a prolonged decrease in blood flow to the brain. This form of CVA is most common between the ages of 60 and 69 years and occurs more frequently in males (2:1).

Cerebral infarction is usually accompanied by abnormalities in the arterial blood supply from the heart to the brain. In most instances, this alteration in the arterial blood supply is produced by atherosclerosis, which is commonly found in certain anatomic areas, especially at the origin of the common carotid arteries and just above the carotid bifurcation (Fig. 19-1). By the third decade of a normal adult's life, there is usually significant atherosclerotic plaque in arteries, but in most cases clinical evidence (in the form of acute myocardial infarction or cerebral infarction) is not present until the fifth and sixth decades.

Narrowing of atherosclerotic vessels must be sig-

Table 19-1. Classification of cerebrovascular disease

Etiology	Approximate percentage of all CVAs	Initial mortality rate (%)	Recurrence rate (%)
Cerebral ischemia and infarction	88	30	*
Atherosclerosis and thrombosis	81	*	20
Cerebral embolism	7	*	*
Intracranial hemorrhage	12	80	*
Arterial aneurysms	*	45	33
Hypertensive vascular disease	*	50	Rare

*Unknown.

nificant (lumenal reduction of approximately 80%) before blood flow is reduced to clinically significant levels. A second factor of importance in atherosclerotic vessels is the formation of thrombi (blood clots). Thrombus formation is much more likely to occur in atherosclerotic than in nonatherosclerotic vessels.

In either atherosclerosis or thrombosis, the blood supply to the area of brain distal to the vessel narrowing, or occlusion, is severely reduced so that a portion of brain tissue becomes ischemic and its cells become necrotic and shrunken (infarcted), producing signs and symptoms of neurologic deficit. Patients with certain diseases have been shown to be more likely to develop atherosclerosis, to develop it at an earlier age, and to have a greater degree of severity. Foremost among these diseases are high blood pressure and diabetes mellitus. Acute episodes of cerebral ischemia and infarction may develop at any time; however, approximately 20% occur during sleep.

Cerebral embolization is a causative factor in approximately 7% of CVAs. Rheumatic heart disease with mitral stenosis and atrial fibrillation is the most common cause of cerebral embolization in those under 50 years of age; other causes are acute myocardial infarction, atrial fibrillation, subacute bacterial endocarditis, and thyrotoxicosis with atrial fibrillation. Cerebral embolization occurs throughout the age spectrum of 20 to 70 years; however, it is most frequent after the age of 40 years.

The *transient ischemic attack* (TIA), also termed incipient stroke or transient cerebral ischemia, may be considered a "temporary stroke" in much the same manner that the pain of angina pectoris might be considered "temporary heart attack." TIAs are produced by periods of cerebral ischemia of varying duration. Episodes may be as short as 10 seconds or as long as 1 hour. The average episode lasts between 2 and 10 minutes. Attacks may occur many times a day or at weekly or monthly intervals. In the periods between episodes, the patient is asymptomatic. The clinical importance of TIAs is that they signal the existence of a significant degree of cerebrovascular disease and clearly demonstrate a potential danger of cerebral infarction.

The incidence of TIA in an elderly population is 1 per 1000. The risk of CVA in the elderly is four to ten times that of a control population and may reach as high as 35% incidence of CVA within a 4-year period.

Intracranial Hemorrhage

The second major category of cerebrovascular accident is intracranial hemorrhage (apoplexy). This category is responsible for approximately 10% of all acute cerebrovascular disease, and regardless of the specific cause it represents a very serious problem with a high mortality rate. It occurs most commonly in persons over the age of 50 years. Intracranial hemorrhage may develop from any blood vessel, but the usual source of bleeding is from arteries. The two major sources of intracranial hemorrhage are ruptured arterial aneurysms and hypertensive vascular disease. In both cases, the walls of the involved blood vessels are defective—with congenital defects in the former and acquired defects in the latter—producing weakened areas. The cause of the actual rupture of the vessel wall is probably an acute change (elevation) in the systolic blood pressure. Clinically, most incidents of intracranial hemorrhage occur while patients are engaged in their normal activities such as work, heavy lifting, and straining while passing stool (factors categorized as physical stress), all of which are associated with elevations in blood pressure. With this in mind, it is evident that although intracranial hemorrhage is responsible for only 10% of all CVAs, it represents more of a potential risk to the dental practitioner dealing with acutely anxious

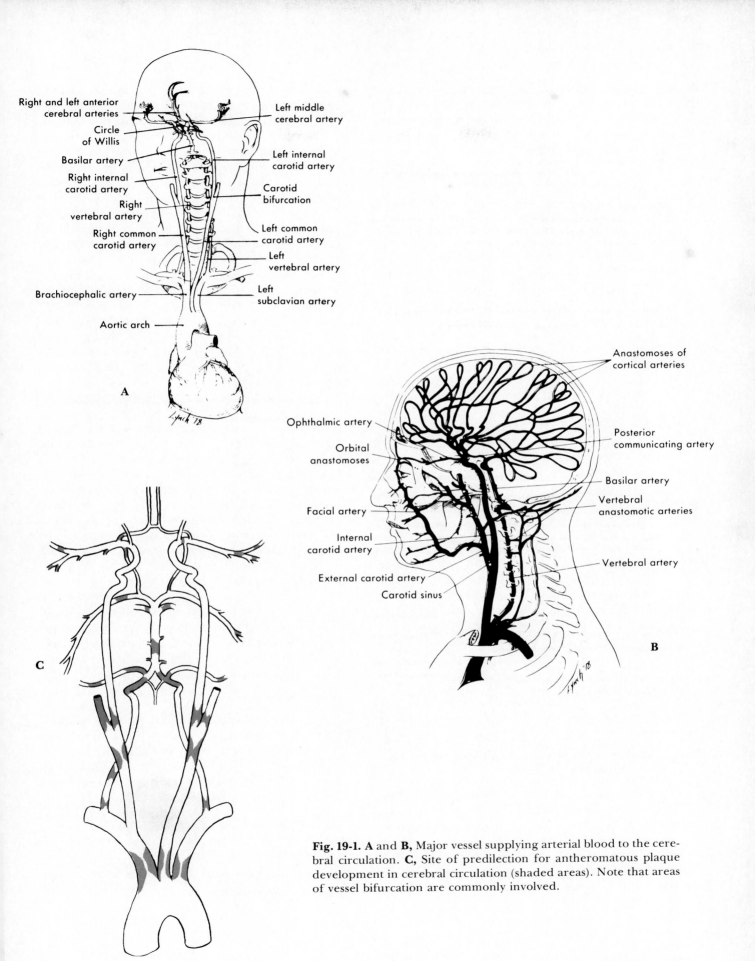

Right and left anterior
cerebral arteries

Circle
of Willis

Basilar artery

Right internal
carotid artery

Right
vertebral artery

Right common
carotid artery

Brachiocephalic artery

Aortic arch

A

Left middle
cerebral artery

Left internal
carotid artery

Carotid
bifurcation

Left common
carotid artery

Left
vertebral artery

Left
subclavian artery

Anastomoses of
cortical arteries

Ophthalmic artery

Orbital
anastomoses

Facial artery

Internal
carotid artery

External carotid artery

Carotid sinus

Posterior
communicating artery

Basilar artery

Vertebral
anastomotic arteries

Vertebral artery

B

C

Fig. 19-1. A and **B,** Major vessel supplying arterial blood to the cerebral circulation. **C,** Site of predilection for antheromatous plaque development in cerebral circulation (shaded areas). Note that areas of vessel bifurcation are commonly involved.

patients and with potentially painful procedures. Both anxiety and pain are associated with significant increases in the heart rate and blood pressure of the patient, making the development of a hemorrhagic CVA more likely.

Survivors of episodes of cerebrovascular disease have a high risk of future recurrences (Table 19-1). Within 12 to 24 months, 20% of survivors of CVAs from atherosclerotic vascular disease have a subsequent CVA; over one third of patients with ruptured aneurysms develop recurrences. However, the risk of recurrent CVA is not the major threat to survival of these patients. Cardiovascular disease is the major limiting factor for the post-CVA patient. Over 50% of these individuals die from acute myocardial infarction or heart failure. The post-CVA patient therefore represents a definite increased risk during dental therapy. Thorough evaluation of this patient before dental therapy and special considerations during therapy reduce the potential risk.

PREDISPOSING FACTORS

A number of factors have been identified that significantly increase the risk of developing a cerebrovascular accident. These factors include high blood pressure (hypertension), diabetes mellitus, cardiac enlargement (as determined with electrocardiology), hypercholesterolemia, the use of oral contraceptives, and cigarette smoking.

Consistently elevated blood pressure has been demonstrated to be a major risk factor in the development of both of the major forms of CVA. Evidence from the Framingham Study (Gresham and others, 1975) has led to the belief that high blood pressure may well be *the* major predisposing factor in the development of acute hemorrhagic CVA. It is estimated that the risk of developing an acute CVA increases by 30% for every 10 torr elevation of the systolic blood pressure above 160 torr. Prolonged periods of elevated blood pressure also produce thickening and fibrinoid degeneration of cerebral arteries. Atherosclerosis develops at an earlier age and to a more severe degree in patients with elevated blood pressure. Yet another mechanism by which high blood pressure leads to an increased incidence of CVA is through the normal response of cerebral arteries to elevations in blood pressure. Cerebral arteries, primarily the smaller cerebral arteries, constrict in response to elevations in blood pressure. This reduces the local cerebral blood flow, leading to ischemia of areas of brain tissue, which if prolonged may produce infarction.

It is worth repeating that high blood pressure represents the single greatest risk factor in the development of all forms of cerebrovascular disease. Fortunately, however, high blood pressure also represents the only major risk factor listed above that, if corrected (lowered), is *definitely* associated with a decreased incidence of CVA. This fact is of particular importance to the dental profession. So much of our dental therapy is associated with pain (either real or imagined), leading to greatly increased apprehension, that a significant percentage of dental patients exhibit signs of increased cardiovascular system activity. Clinically this is evident as elevated blood pressure recordings and an increase in heart rate. In patients with evidence of other risk factors of CVA (such as diabetes and atherosclerosis), these elevations in cardiovascular activity might well precipitate an acute cerebrovascular accident, most likely of the more ominous hemorrhagic type.

The post-CVA patient represents an even greater risk in the dental office. Survivors of CVAs have a very good chance of recovering some degree of function. In the Framingham study (Gresham and others, 1975), 84% of CVA survivors were living at home, 80% were capable of independent mobility, and 69% had total independence in the normal activities of daily living. Yet only 10% exhibited no functional deficit. These CVA survivors might correctly be termed "the walking wounded." As McCarthy (1971) has stated, they represent "accidents waiting to happen." With independent mobility, the post-CVA patient expects to receive dental care; however, it must always be remembered that the recurrence rate in CVA is high and that factors such as pain and anxiety only add to the risk presented by this patient. Proper management of pain and anxiety are therefore of the greatest importance for the post-CVA patient.

PREVENTION

Prevention of the occurrence or recurrence of CVA is based on the recognition of the risk factors discussed above and on possible alterations in dental therapy to accommodate the post-CVA patient. The medical history questionnaire and dialogue history relating to this disorder follow.

Medical History Questionnaire
QUESTION 6. Have you taken any medicine or drugs during the past 2 years?

COMMENT. In the past, all patients who survived a CVA received anticoagulant therapy. However, recent studies by several groups suggest that anticoagulant therapy helps only a few individuals in any large series of patients who have experienced a stroke. The evidence is more promising for transient ischemic attack. The risk of hemorrhage, particularly in hypertensive patients, is great.

Antiplatelet therapy, using aspirin (650 mg b.i.d.), has been shown to reduce the risk of TIA and CVA, particularly in males. The optimal aspirin dose is unknown.

Antihypertensive medications are prescribed for the 66% of post-CVA patients who have elevated blood pressure. Commonly used drugs for the management of high blood pressure include diuretics (see Table 14-1), methyldopa (Aldomet), and propranolol (Inderal). The doctor should be aware of the potential side effects of each of these agents and possible drug interactions that might be encountered with agents used in dentistry. Postural hypotension is a common side effect of many antihypertensive agents. References such as the *Physicians' Desk Reference, Facts and Comparisons, Accepted Dental Therapeutics,* and *AMA Drug Evaluations* are recommended.

QUESTION 9. Circle any of the following which you have had or have at present:
- **High blood pressure**
- **Stroke**
- **Fainting or dizzy spells**

COMMENT. High blood pressure is the single most important risk factor in causing CVAs and is the only risk factor that, if altered, results in a decreased risk of CVA. High blood pressure is present in over two thirds of the victims of CVA. Routine blood pressure screening of all potential dental patients and all medically compromised persons in particular has proved to be a significant method of minimizing the occurrence of CVA and the other major sequelae of high blood pressure (such as acute myocardial infarction and renal dysfunction).

Fainting or dizzy spells might indicate the presence of transient ischemic episodes. Further evaluation of the patient is warranted using the dialogue history.

An affirmative response regarding "stroke" requires dialogue history to determine the degree of risk.

Dialogue History

In the presence of a prior history of CVA, the following dialogue history is recommended.

QUESTION. When did you have your stroke (CVA)?

QUESTION. What type of CVA did you have?

QUESTION. Were you hospitalized? If so, for how long?

COMMENT. These questions serve to gather basic information concerning the nature and severity of the CVA. Following the CVA there is a degree of recovery of neurologic deficit. Although the length of time varies from patient to patient, maximal improvement usually occurs within 6 months. All but emergency dental therapy should be withheld during this period (physical status IV).

QUESTION. What degree of neurologic deficit (paralysis) occurred as a result of the CVA, and what degree of function has been recovered?

COMMENT. Although motor deficit (hemiplegia) may be quite obvious to the observer, minor degrees of neurologic deficit may be less obvious. The patient is normally willing to discuss these with the doctor.

QUESTION. What medication(s) are you now taking?

COMMENT. Refer to question 6 of the medical history questionnaire for discussion.

QUESTION. If high blood pressure was present at the time of CVA, what was your blood pressure when you had your CVA?

QUESTION. How often do you measure your blood pressure, and what does it normally read?

COMMENT. High blood pressure is present in most CVA victims. In many instances, it was undetected until the CVA developed. Patients who are well-motivated in management of their disease monitor their blood pressure on a regular basis. These blood pressure recordings may serve as a reference point to compare the vital signs that are recorded in the dental office. In general, the blood pressure of a post-CVA patient should not be elevated significantly. Blood pressure should be recorded routinely on post-CVA patients before every dental appointment.

In the absence of a history of prior CVA but with an affirmative response to fainting or dizzy spells, the doctor should suspect the possible presence of transient ischemic episodes. This question may also indicate the presence of anxiety toward dentistry, orthostatic hypotension, or convulsive disorders; a careful evaluation should be carried out.

QUESTION. *Have you ever experienced episodes of unexplained dizziness, numbness of the extremities, or speech defects?*

COMMENT. Transient episodes of cerebral hypoxia can produce the signs and symptoms listed in this question. These episodes may occur daily or at more infrequent intervals. In many instances, the patient is aware of the existence of TIA and is receiving drug therapy (anticoagulants, antihypertensives, aspirin) to reduce the risk of a true CVA developing. These patients should be managed in the dental office as if they have already had a CVA.

If signs and symptoms appear in a patient who has no prior knowledge of CVA occurrence, medical consultation with the patient's physician is indicated before initiation of any mode of dental therapy.

Physical Examination

Physical evaluation of the post-CVA patient should include a thorough visual examination to determine the extent of any residual neurologic deficit. The examination must include recording of the vital signs (blood pressure, pulse rate, and respiratory rate).

Vital signs

Proper technique is essential to obtain accurate blood pressure recordings (see Chapter 2). The medical risk presented by elevated blood pressure increases steadily with each elevation in blood pressure (in other words, there is no blood pressure above which an increased risk is present and below which the risk is absent). It is therefore necessary to provide guidelines for clinical use. The categorization of blood pressure used in patient screening at the University of Southern California School of Dentistry is presented on p. 16, Table 2-1. Recommended dental therapy modifications for each category are indicated.

For the doctor managing a post-CVA patient, knowledge of the patient's blood pressure before each dental treatment session is vital. Marked elevation in blood pressure is life threatening in this patient and increases the chance of a second CVA occurring. The guidelines indicate that any adult patient with a blood pressure of 200 torr systolic and/or 115 torr diastolic or above should not receive any dental therapy until the elevated blood

pressure is brought under control. This usually necessitates immediate medical consultation and a delay in dental therapy while antihypertensive therapy is started or corrected. Physical status (ASA) III blood pressure (between 160 and 200 torr systolic and/or between 95 and 115 torr diastolic) in a post-CVA patient calls for immediate medical consultation before any dental therapy is initiated.

Other factors

The presence of unusual apprehension should be determined. The physiologic response to increased anxiety includes higher circulating blood levels of the catecholamines epinephrine and norepinephrine, which increase heart rate and blood pressure.

Dental Therapy Considerations

The post-CVA patient represents a definite medical risk during dental therapy. Several basic factors are of importance in the management of this patient.

Length of time elapsed since the episode. No elective dental therapy should be considered for at least 6 months after the episode. The risk of recurrence is presumably somewhat greater during this time. Emergency therapy (for pain or infection) should be managed with medications. Actual dental therapy should be delayed if possible, or the patient should be hospitalized if dental therapy is required.

Minimizing of stress during dental treatment. The Stress Reduction Protocol should be used for the post-CVA patient. Of particular importance are short morning appointments (not to exceed the patient's tolerance), effective pain control (local anesthetics with vasoconstrictors), and the use of psychosedation during treatment.

COMMENT. All central nervous system depressants are relatively contraindicated in the post-CVA patient. Any of these agents may produce hypoxia, leading to aggravated confusion, aphasia, and other complications of CVA. In our experience, *light levels of sedation,* as produced with nitrous oxide and oxygen, have proved to be quite safe and highly effective in reducing stress in post-CVA patients. These techniques should be used only if warranted in a particular patient.

Determining when the post-CVA patient is too great a risk for dental therapy. The blood pressure and heart rate serve as indicators of cardiovascular status of the post-CVA patient at the time of dental treatment.

COMMENT. Marked elevations in blood pressure should be viewed with concern and dental therapy withheld until medical consultation or corrective therapy is accomplished. Post-CVA patients should not receive elective dental treatment for a period of 6 months after the event.

Bleeding and the post-CVA patient. Most survivors of CVAs and patients with transient ischemic attacks receive aspirin or anticoagulant therapy in an effort to reduce the morbidity and mortality associated with recurrences.

COMMENT. If a patient is receiving any of these agents and dental procedures are contemplated that may produce significant bleeding, medical consultation is indicated before the procedure. Although excessive hemorrhaging in the post-CVA patient rarely is a clinical problem in dentistry, the dentist and the physician must consider these possibilities and safeguards against it: (1) proceeding with dental therapy without altering the anticoagulant blood level, thereby possibly increasing postoperative bleeding, (2) lowering the prothrombin time (decreasing anticoagulant levels) before the procedure to decrease the risk of excessive bleeding with a possible increased risk of CVA, or (3) altering the dental treatment plan to avoid excessive bleeding in instances in which the risk of reducing the prothrombin time is too great. In most instances, dental therapy is carried out without alterations in the patient's anticoagulant drug therapy.

When dental procedures are carried out in a patient with an elevated prothrombin time, the doctor should consider precautionary steps to minimize the chance of significant postoperative hemorrhage. Among these are advising the patient and physician of the possible need for vitamin K should excessive bleeding occur; the use of hemostatic agents such as oxidized cellulose in extraction sockets; the use of multiple sutures in extraction sites and periodontal surgery; the use of pressure packs for 6 to 12 hours postoperatively (longer if necessary); and availability of the doctor by telephone for 24 hours following therapy.

In all situations, the doctor called on to manage a patient who has previously experienced a CVA should not proceed with the contemplated dental therapy until there is no doubt about the physical ability of this patient to safely tolerate the planned treatment. Whenever doubt or concern persists, discussion of the contemplated dental procedure and the physical status of the patient with a physician is indicated.

The patient with a history of transient ischemic attacks should be managed in the dental office in the same manner as the post-CVA patient. Table 19-2 presents physical status categories for CVAs and TIAs.

CLINICAL MANIFESTATIONS

Signs and symptoms of cerebrovascular disease vary depending on the area of the brain that is involved and on the type of CVA experienced. The onset may be violent; the patient may fall to the ground, unmoving, with face flushed and a bounding pulse. Respirations may be slow and one arm and leg flaccid. The onset may also be more gradual, with no alteration in consciousness and only minimal impairment of speech, thought, motor, and sensory functions.

Signs and symptoms commonly observed in CVAs include headache, dizziness and vertigo, drowsiness, sweating and chills, nausea, and vomiting. Loss of consciousness (a particularly ominous

Table 19-2. Physical status classifications of CVA and TIA

	Physical status (ASA)	Dental therapy considerations
History of one documented CVA at least 6 months before treatment; no residual neurologic deficit *or* history of TIA	II	ASA II considerations to include: Light levels of sedation only Routine postoperative follow-up by telephone
History of one or more documented CVA at least 6 months before treatment; some degree of neurologic deficit evident	III	ASA III considerations to include: Light levels of sedation only Routine follow-up by telephone
History of documented CVA within 6 months of treatment with or without residual neurologic deficit	IV	ASA IV considerations

sign) and convulsive movements are much less common. Weakness or paralysis occurs in the extremities contralateral to the CVA. Defects in speech may also be noted.

Transient Ischemic Attack

Clinical manifestations of transient ischemic attacks, as with all CVAs, vary according to the area of the brain affected. Most TIAs cause transient numbness or weakness of the contralateral extremities (legs, arms, hand, fingers), which may be described by the patient as "pins and needles." During the TIA, the level of consciousness is usually unimpaired, although the thought process may be dulled.

Transient ischemic episodes normally have a duration of 2 to 10 minutes, although they have been recorded for as long as 1 hour and as briefly as 10 seconds. Their rate of frequency varies from patient to patient.

Cerebral Infarction

In patients whose cerebral infarction is produced by atherosclerotic changes in cerebral blood vessels or thrombosis, the onset of clinical signs and symptoms is normally more gradual (neurologic signs and symptoms appearing over a period of time) and is usually preceded by episodes of TIA. Headache, if present, is usually mild and is generally limited to the side of the infarction.

Cerebral Embolism

CVAs occurring as a result of embolism differ clinically from other CVAs in that the onset of symptoms is usually abrupt. Mild headache is the first symptom, and it normally precedes the onset of neurologic symptoms by several hours. Neurologic symptoms are confined to the contralateral side of the body.

Cerebral Hemorrhage

Because of the stressful nature of dental treatment and its effects on cardiovascular function, intracerebral hemorrhage is the most likely form of CVA to develop in the dental office. Onset of clinical signs and symptoms is usually abrupt, the first manifestation being a sudden, violent headache. Victims have variously described the headache as "excruciating," "intense," and as "the worst headache I have ever experienced." The headache is at first localized but gradually becomes generalized. Other clinical signs and symptoms include nausea and vomiting, chills and sweating, dizziness, and vertigo. Signs of neurologic deficit may occur at any time but usually follow in several hours.

Hemorrhagic CVAs most commonly occur during periods of activity such as work, lifting objects, or physical and psychologic stress (as in the dental office). Over one third of patients with intracerebral hemorrhage lose consciousness within minutes of the onset. This is an ominous sign, usually indicating a large hemorrhage has occurred. Of conscious patients, 50% demonstrate a marked deterioration in consciousness and lose consciousness at a later time. The initial mortality rate from all hemorrhagic CVAs is approximately 50%, but comatose patients have a mortality rate of between 70% and 100%. Table 19-3 summarizes the signs and symptoms of CVA.

PATHOPHYSIOLOGY

Two important factors work together to produce CVA: the brain's continual requirement for oxygen and the inability of the brain to expand within its confining space, the cranium. The brain is unable to store oxygen in reserve for use in times of oxygen deprivation. Acute disruption of the oxygen supply to the brain (embolism, hemorrhage) produces alterations in brain activity (detectable by electro-

Table 19-3. Clinical manifestations of CVA

Infarction

Gradual onset of signs and symptoms
TIA frequently precedes CVA
Headache—usually mild
Neurologic signs and symptoms*

Embolism

Abrupt onset of signs and symptoms
Mild headache—precedes neurologic signs and symptoms* by several hours

Hemorrhage

Abrupt onset of signs and symptoms
Sudden, violent headache
Nausea and vomiting
Chills and sweating
Dizziness and vertigo
Neurologic signs and symptoms*
Loss of consciousness

*Neurologic signs and symptoms include paralysis on one side of the body, difficulty in breathing and swallowing, inability to speak or slurring of speech, loss of bladder and bowel control, and pupils that are unequal in size.

encephalogram) within 10 to 20 seconds and irreversible neurologic death within 3 to 10 minutes. Gradual deprivation (atherosclerotic changes) leads to the same result over a longer period of time.

Cerebrovascular Ischemia and Infarction

With the development of ischemia, changes occur in the affected neural tissues. The ischemic tissue becomes soft, and the usually well-demarcated border between the white and gray matter becomes less distinct. Under the microscope, neurons in the ischemic area appear necrotic and shrunken (Fig. 19-2).

A second factor now emerges. Edema is a normal occurrence following cerebral infarction. The degree of edema is related to the size of the infarcted

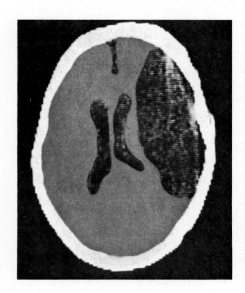

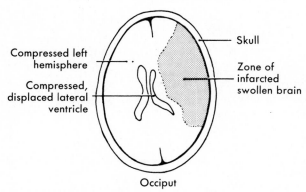

Fig. 19-2. Computerized axial tomography (CAT) scan of cranium in cerebral vascular infarction (top). Explanation of CAT scan (bottom).

area. Edema increases the mass of tissue within the confined space of the cranium and is responsible for the mild headache noted in atherosclerotic CVA. In more severe CVAs, the degree of edema may be great enough to force portions of the cerebral hemisphere down into the tentorium cerebelli, producing a further reduction in blood and cerebrospinal fluid flow to the brain. The degree of ischemia and neurologic deficit therefore increases, leading potentially to ischemia and infarction of the upper brainstem (medulla), which produces loss of consciousness and is invariably fatal.

The clinical importance of edema is noted in the fact that during the first 72 hours following a nonhemorrhagic CVA, a gradual increase in neurologic deficit and a decreasing level of consciousness are commonly observed. These changes are usually brought about by cerebral edema in and around the infarcted area. Gradual return of some neurologic function normally follows, as collateral circulation to the infarcted region improves. Maximal recovery normally occurs within 6 months.

Hemorrhagic CVA

Hemorrhagic CVAs differ clinically from non-hemorrhagic CVAs in that they have a more rapid onset and more intense symptoms and are associated with a greater risk of death. The most common source of blood in hemorrhagic CVAs is arterial. There are two primary causes of this type of CVA: ruptured aneurysms and hypertensive vascular disease. Aneurysms, which are dilations in blood vessels, have weakened muscular walls that may rupture under increased blood pressure. Hypertensive vascular disease, on the other hand, produces degenerative changes in blood vessel walls (usually smaller arteries) over a greater length of time, resulting in their weakening and possible rupture. Rupture of these vessels invariably occurs during periods of activity that result in elevations in blood pressure.

Once ruptured, the arterial blood rapidly fills the cranium, causing an increase in intracranial pressure that may produce rapid displacement of the brain into the tentorium cerebelli and ultimately death. Cerebral edema, which always develops, only serves to add to the high mortality rate of this form of CVA (Fig. 19-3).

The intense headache noted in hemorrhagic CVA is related to the irritating effects of blood and its breakdown products on the blood vessels, meninges, and neural tissues of the brain itself. The

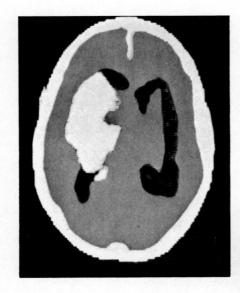

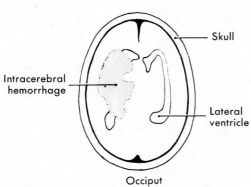

Fig. 19-3. Computerized axial tomography (CAT) scan—hemorrhagic CVA (top). Explanation of CAT scan (bottom).

headache is localized at first but becomes generalized as meningeal irritation increases because of the spread of blood. The rapid increase in intracranial pressure brought on by hemorrhage and edema is responsible for the significant clinical differences noted between hemorrhagic and nonhemorrhagic CVAs. Neurologic deficit can be determined in survivors by the area of neural tissue that has lost its blood supply and become infarcted.

MANAGEMENT

Management of the patient with an acute CVA is related to the rapidity of onset of clinical signs and to the severity of the situation. In almost all cases, supportive therapy and basic life support are indicated.

Transient Ischemic Attack

In most cases of TIA, the patient remains conscious. Indeed, it may prove to be difficult to differentiate between a TIA and a CVA. The duration of the episode is important in this regard. Most TIAs last approximately 2 to 10 minutes, whereas the signs and symptoms of a CVA do not regress. The initial management of any patient with signs and symptoms of cerebrovascular disease is of necessity identical, regardless of the ultimate cause, and includes the following:

Step 1. Terminate dental therapy.

Step 2. Initiate basic life support. Assess airway, breathing, and circulation and implement as needed.

Step 3. Manage signs and symptoms. In both TIA and CVA, most victims remain conscious. Permit the patient to remain in the upright position and attempt to comfort the patient. In the TIA, clinical signs usually disappear within 10 minutes, and there is normally no need to summon medical assistance if the patient remains conscious and symptoms disappear.

Step 4. Monitor vital signs. Blood pressure is quite elevated during the episode, and the heart rate may be normal or elevated. In most cases, either the radial or brachial arterial pulses or both are "full" or "bounding."

Step 5. Follow-up management. Following termination of the episode, the patient's physician should be contacted, and possible medical examination and alterations in future dental therapy should be discussed. The patient should not be permitted to operate a motor vehicle and should be discharged from the office in the custody of a responsible adult companion.

Cerebrovascular Accident
Conscious patient

If clinical signs and symptoms of CVA occur and do not terminate within a reasonable time (10 to 15 minutes), TIA may not be the cause, and a true CVA may be in progress. With the patient still conscious the following steps should be carried out.

Step 1. Terminate dental procedure. The patient with neurologic signs who remains conscious should be permitted to remain in the upright position.

Step 2. Initiate basic life support. Assess airway, breathing, and circulation, and implement as needed.

Step 3. Manage signs and symptoms. The patient, still conscious, should be made comfortable during the episode. Any signs or symptoms should be managed.

Step 4. Monitor vital signs. Blood pressure, heart rate, and respiratory rate should be recorded every 5 minutes during the episode.

Step 5. Summon medical assistance. Should neurologic signs and symptoms persist for 10 to 15 minutes or should clinical deterioration of the patient develop more rapidly (intense headache, progressive paralysis), medical assistance should be summoned.

Step 6. Additional measures. Oxygen need not be administered to this patient unless respiratory difficulty develops. Oxygen produces cerebral vasoconstriction, thus potentially increasing the area of ischemia and infarction. No medications should be administered to this patient. Any drugs that produce CNS depression (analgesics, antianxiety agents) may adversely affect the patient's condition.

Unconscious patient

Acute loss of consciousness has a very poor clinical prognosis (70% to 100% initial mortality rate) in CVA. The hemorrhagic type of CVA is more likely to produce unconsciousness. It is usually preceded by an intense headache, an additional indication of this problem.

Step 1. Position patient. Immediately on losing consciousness, the patient is placed in the supine position. Minor alteration in this position may be indicated later.

Step 2. Basic life support. The steps of basic life support are carried out immediately. Airway maintenance and support of respiration are critical. Oxygen should be administered if available.

Step 3. Monitor vital signs. Vital signs (blood pressure, pulse rate, and respirations) are then recorded. The heart rate in most instances is normal or slow, and the pulse may be full and bounding. Should heart rate, blood pressure, or both be absent, cardiopulmonary resuscitation is immediately initiated. The blood pressure is frequently markedly elevated (systolic in excess of 200 torr). In this instance, positioning of the unconscious CVA patient should not be in the true supine position. Because of the increase in cerebral blood flow in the supine position and the markedly elevated blood pressure observed in hemorrhagic CVA, the pa-

---

MANAGEMENT

Transient ischemic attack

Step 1 Terminate dental therapy
2 Initiate basic life support
3 Manage signs and symptoms
4 Monitor vital signs
5 Follow-up management
   Consult with physician regarding future management
   Discharge patient with adult companion

CVA in the conscious patient

Step 1 Terminate dental therapy
2 Initiate basic life support
3 Manage signs and symptoms
4 Monitor vital signs every 5 minutes
5 Summon medical assistance after 10 to 15 minutes

CVA in the unconscious patient

Step 1 Position patient (supine)
2 Basic life support
   Airway
   Breathing
3 Record vital signs
   CPR, if indicated
   Reposition patient
      Supine with head elevated slightly in presence of elevated blood pressure or signs of hemorrhagic CVA; supine if CPR is indicated
4 Summon medical assistance immediately
NOTE: 1. Any drug with potential for CNS depression should be avoided in the acute CVA patient.
   2. Oxygen should be employed in TIA and the conscious CVA patient only in the presence of respiratory difficulty. It may be freely used if unconsciousness is present.

tient may be placed in the supine position with the head elevated slightly. It *must* still be possible to maintain a patent airway and ventilate the victim adequately. If CPR is required (in the absence of pulse and blood pressure), the patient must then be repositioned (supine with feet elevated).

Step 4. Summon medical assistance. Medical assistance should be requested at the earliest possible time. Basic life support is continued during this period.

Management of CVA is summarized in the box on p. 233.

BIBLIOGRAPHY

Alter, M., and others: Cerebral infarction: clinical and angiographic correlations, Neurology **22:**590, 1972.

Bailey, W.L., and Loeser, J.D.: Intracranial aneurysms, JAMA **216:**1993, 1971.

Barrett, H.J.M.: The pathophysiology of transient cerebral ischemic attacks: therapy with platelet antiaggregants, Med. Clin. North Am. **63:**649, 1979.

Barrett, H.J.M.: Progress toward stroke prevention, Neurology **30:**1212, 1980.

Brown, M., and Glassenber, M.: Mortality factor in patients with acute stroke, JAMA **224:**1493, 1973.

Byer, J.A., and Easton, J.D.: Therapy of ischemic vascular disease, Ann. Intern. Med. **93:**742, 1980.

Canadian Cooperative Study Group: A randomized trial of aspirin and sulfinpyrazone in threatened stroke, N. Engl. J. Med. **299:**53, 1978.

Cervantes, R.D., and Schneiderman, L.J.: Anticoagulants in cerebrovascular disease, Arch. Intern. Med. **135:**875, 1975.

Chusid, J.G.: Nervous system. In Krupp, M.A., and Chatton, M.J., editors: Current medical diagnosis and treatment, Los Altos, CA, 1984, Lange Medical Publications.

Collaborative Group for the Study of Stroke in Young Women, Oral contraceptives and stroke in young women, JAMA, **231:**718, 1975.

Conneally, P.M., and others: Cooperative study of hospital frequency and character of transient ischemic attacks. VIII. Risk factors, JAMA **240:**742, 1978.

Furlan, A.J., and others: Decreasing incidence of primary intracerebral hemorrhage: a population study, Ann. Neurol. **5:**367, 1979.

Garraway, W.M., and others: The declining incidence of stroke, N. Engl. J. Med. **300:**449, 1979.

Gilroy, J.: Early manifestation and investigation of cerebral arteriosclerosis, Practitioner **217:**66, 1976.

Golden, G.S.: Strokes in children and adolescents, Curr. Concepts Cerebrovas. Dis. **12:**29, 1977.

Gresham, G.E., and others: Residual disability in survivors of stroke—the Framingham study, N. Engl. J. Med. **293:**954, 1975.

Grindal, A.G., and Toole, J.R.: Headache and transient ischemic attacks, Stroke **5:**603, 1974.

Hass, W.K.: Occlusive cerebrovascular disease, Med. Clin. North Am. **36:**1281, 1972.

Kannel, W.B., Dawber, T.R., and Cohen, M.E.: Vascular disease of the brain—epidemiologic aspects—the Framingham study, Am. J. Public Health **55:**1355, 1965.

Kannel, W.B., Wolf, P., and Dawber, T.R.: Hypertension and cardiac impairments increase stroke risk, Geriatrics **33:**71, 1978.

Kannel, W.B., and others: Systolic blood pressure, arterial rigidity and risk of stroke, JAMA **245:**1225, 1981.

Levy, R.I.: Progress in prevention of cardiovascular disease, Prev. Med. **7:**464, 1978.

Levy, R.I.: Stroke decline: implications and prospects, N. Engl. J. Med. **300:**489, 1979.

Margolis, G., and Sadowsky, C.H.: How does blood pressure cause stroke? Lancet **1:**538, 1976.

McCarthy, F.M.: Sudden, unexpected death in the dental office, J. Am. Dent. Assoc. **83:**1091, 1971.

Medina, J.L., Diamond, S., and Rubino, F.A.: Headaches in patients with transient ischemic attacks, Headache **15:**194, Oct., 1975.

Mohr, J.P.: Transient ischemic attacks and the prevention of strokes, N. Engl. J. Med. **299:**93, 1978.

Russell, R., and Green, M.: Mechanisms of transient cerebral ischemia, Br. Med. J. **1:**646, 1971.

Sedzimir, C.B., and Robinson, J.: Intracranial hemorrhage in children and adolescents, J. Neurosurg. **38:**269, 1973.

Shafer, S.Q., Bruun, B., and Richter, R.W.: The outcome of stroke at hospital discharge in New York City blacks, Stroke **4:**782, 1973.

Singer, R.A., Wasserman, R.E., and Hanna, G.R.: Associated systemic factors in cerebrovascular ischemia, South Med. J. **69:**709, 1976.

Soltero, I., Liu, K., and Cooper, R.: Trends in mortality from cerebrovascular disease in the United States, 1960-1975, Stroke **9:**549, 1978.

Tolle, J.F.: Diagnosis and management of stroke, Pub. No. 70-004B, Dallas, 1979, American Heart Association.

Torvik, A., and Skullerud, K.: How often are brain infarcts caused by hypotensive episodes?, Stroke **7:**255, 1976.

Veterans Administration Cooperative Study Group on Antihypertensive Agents: Effects of treatment on morbidity and mortality in hypertension. II. Results in patients with diastolic blood pressure averaging 90 through 114 mm Hg, JAMA **213:**1143, 1970.

Waltz, A.G.: Studies of the cerebral circulation: What have they taught us about strokes? Mayo Clin. Proc. **46:**268, 1971.

Ziegler, D.K., and Hassanein, R.S.: Prognosis in patients with transient ischemic attacks, Stroke **4:**666, 1973.

20 *Altered Consciousness: Differential Diagnosis*

A number of clinical entities are capable of producing a state of altered consciousness (see Table 16-1). In almost all of these situations, the doctor is asked to maintain the life of a patient who is still conscious yet is behaving in an unusual manner. If not recognized and managed promptly, several of these entities can progress to the loss of consciousness. Basic management of these patients is similar, yet there are several cases in which definitive management may be undertaken provided that the precise cause of the difficulty is known. The following material is provided to assist in this differential diagnosis.

PAST MEDICAL HISTORY

Several of the clinical entities discussed in this section are normally evident on review of the medical history questionnaire. The patient with diabetes mellitus or thyroid gland dysfunction or the post-CVA patient is usually aware of the presence of the disease and indicates this in the history. A thorough dialogue history should then enable the doctor to further determine the degree of risk presented by this patient. Unless it has occurred previously, the hyperventilation syndrome cannot be diagnosed from data on the medical history, nor can drug overdose.

AGE OF PATIENT

The age of a patient presenting with altered consciousness may assist in diagnosis of the cause. The hyperventilation syndrome is rarely encountered in younger or older age groups; its greatest incidence is between the ages of 15 and 40 years. Hyperthyroidism most commonly occurs between the ages of 20 and 40, while more than 80% of diabetics develop their disease after they reach the age of 35. Cerebrovascular disease is extremely rare under the age of 40 years; its incidence increases with age. Drug overdose may occur at any age.

In pediatric patients the most likely cause of altered consciousness is hypoglycemia.

SEX OF PATIENT

Hyperthyroidism (thyrotoxicosis) occurs predominantly in females, whereas the hyperventilation syndrome and the other clinical entities discussed in this section have little or no clinical differentiation between the sexes.

CIRCUMSTANCES ASSOCIATED WITH ALTERED CONSCIOUSNESS

Undue stress from anxiety and pain is an important predisposing factor in the hyperventilation syndrome. Indeed, this syndrome is primarily a clinical expression of extreme apprehension. Stress may also be related to the onset of a CVA, particularly of the hemorrhagic type. Hyperthyroid and hypoglycemic individuals may also appear to be acutely anxious; however, specific clinical signs and symptoms (see below) permit a ready differential diagnosis of these entities.

ONSET OF SYMPTOMS

Gradual onset of clinical manifestations of altered consciousness occurs in hyperglycemia (many hours to several days), in hyperthyroidism and hypothyroidism, and in CVAs produced by atherosclerotic changes in blood vessels. Patients present in the dental office with signs and symptoms of disease already evident. More rapid onset of clinical manifestations (signs and symptoms developing within the dental office) are evident in the hyperventilation syndrome, in hypoglycemia, and in CVAs produced by thrombus, embolism, and especially by intracranial hemorrhage.

PRESENCE OF SYMPTOMS BETWEEN ACUTE EPISODES

The patient with undiagnosed thyroid dysfunction or with known thyroid dysfunction that is inadequately managed has clinical evidence of the disease at all times. Post-CVA patients usually manifest a degree of residual neurologic deficit, the severity of which varies from flaccid paralysis to barely perceptible motor or sensory changes. Patients with transient ischemic attacks are clinically free of symptoms between acute episodes. Adult brittle diabetics may manifest signs and symptoms of hyperglycemia at all times.

LOSS OF CONSCIOUSNESS

Although all of the clinical entities discussed in this section manifest themselves primarily as altered states of consciousness, several of them may progress to the loss of consciousness. CVA, particularly the hemorrhagic variety, may be associated with unconsciousness, an especially ominous clinical sign. Patients with clinical evidence of thyroid dysfunction may also lose consciousness if the disease is poorly controlled. These two clinical situations, myxedema coma and thyroid crisis or storm, have significant mortality rates. Both hyperglycemic and hypoglycemic individuals may also ultimately lose consciousness; however, the hypoglycemic patient is the more likely candidate, with loss of consciousness developing much more rapidly. The hyperventilation syndrome rarely leads to unconsciousness.

SIGNS AND SYMPTOMS
Appearance of Skin (Face)

The presence or absence of sweating and the temperature of the skin may assist in the differential diagnosis. The diabetic individual who is clinically hyperglycemic appears hot and dry (dehydrated) to the touch, whereas the hypoglycemic individual appears cold and wet. The clinically hyperthyroid individual is hot and wet, and the hypothyroid individual is dry and may have a subnormal body temperature.

Appearance of Nervousness

The clinical signs of agitation, sweating, and possible fine tremor of the extremities (hands) give the appearance of nervousness and are apparent in patients with the hyperventilation syndrome, hypoglycemia, and hyperthyroidism.

Paresthesias

Paresthesias ("pins and needles") of various portions of the body are noted in several situations. Paresthesia of the perioral region, fingertips, and toes, if noted in conjunction with a rapid respiratory rate, is diagnostic of hyperventilation. Patients with transient ischemic attacks (TIA) exhibit unilateral paresthesia or muscle weakness that is unaccompanied by the respiratory change and often develop in the absence of anxiety. An acute CVA also demonstrates the above signs of TIA but continues to progress, whereas signs and symptoms of TIA normally subside within 10 minutes.

Headache

Headache may be evident in hypothyroid individuals but is much more likely to develop in the acute CVA. Severe, intense headache is an important clinical finding in intracranial hemorrhage, a form of CVA.

"Drunken" Appearance

The clinical appearance of inebriation is most commonly produced by a patient overindulging in their own premedication—alcohol. Hypoglycemia is another situation that may present this clinical picture. The patient shows signs of mental confusion and bizarre behavioral patterns that may lead to a suspicion of alcohol use. A history of diabetes or the absence of having eaten food before dental therapy will assist in this differential diagnosis.

Breath Odor

The telltale odor of alcohol on the breath aids in diagnosing "premedication," whereas patients who are severely hyperglycemic may have the characteristic fruity, sweet smell of acetone on their breath.

VITAL SIGNS
Respirations

The respiratory rate increases in hyperventilation, hyperthyroidism, and hyperglycemia. In hyperglycemia it normally is associated with acetone breath. Depressed respiration may be evident in

CVA (in the unconscious patient with slow but deep respirations), overdose of depressant drugs (alcohol, sedatives, antianxiety drugs, narcotics), and possibly in hypoglycemia.

Blood Pressure

Elevated blood pressure is found in hyperventilation, hyperthyroidism, and in many forms of CVA (intracerebral hemorrhage, subarachnoid hemorrhage, and cerebral thrombosis). The hyperglycemic individual may demonstrate a slight decrease in blood pressure, and the hypothyroid patient evidences little change in blood pressure.

Heart Rate

Rapid heart rates are noted in hyperventilation, hypoglycemia, hyperglycemia, and hyperthyroidism. A slower than normal heart rate is present in hypothyroidism.

SUMMARY

In conclusion, each of the clinical syndromes of altered consciousness is presented with relevant clinical features.

Hyperventilation. Rapid respiratory rate with deep breaths, acute anxiety, and elevated blood pressure and heart rate. Symptoms of paresthesia of extremities and mouth. Occurs primarily in patients between 15 and 40 years of age. Seldom produces unconsciousness.

Hypoglycemia. History of diabetes or lack of food ingestion. Patient appears "drunk" with "cold and wet" appearance. Rapid heart rate, possible tremor. Onset of symptoms may appear rapidly and can quickly lead to loss of consciousness.

Hyperglycemia. History of diabetes with inadequate control. Patient appears hot and dry. Probable acetone odor on breath. Rapid and deep respirations. Gradual onset of symptoms with lesser likelihood of unconsciousness.

Hypothyroidism. Patient sensitive to cold. Speech and mental capabilities appear slower than normal. No sweating, body temperature lowered. Peripheral edema (nonpitting) present, particularly noticeable around face and eyelids. Carotenemic skin color. Sensitive to CNS-depressant drugs.

Hyperthyroidism. Nervousness, hyperactivity present with elevated blood pressure, heart rate, and temperature. Patient appears "wet and warm" and is sensitive to heat. History of recent unexplained loss of weight in spite of increased appetite.

CVA. Headache, unusually intense. Onset of unilateral neurologic deficit (flaccid paralysis, speech defects). Level of consciousness normally unchanged.

21 *Seizure Disorders*

To most persons, witnessing someone having a convulsive episode is a psychologically traumatic experience. The feeling persists that a seizure constitutes a life-threatening situation, one requiring prompt intervention by a trained individual to prevent a death from occurring. Yet this is normally not the case. Most convulsive episodes, although in no sense benign, are transient alterations in brain function characterized clinically by the abrupt onset of symptoms of a motor, sensory, or psychic nature. In these instances, the prevention of injury to the victim during the actual seizure and supportive therapy during the postseizure period constitute the essentials of management. If proper management is carried out, significant morbidity and mortality related to seizures rarely occurs. A life-threatening medical emergency exists only if convulsive seizures follow one another closely or if they become continuous. In these cases, prompt action and specific therapy are required to prevent the death of the victim or significant postseizure morbidity.

The following are definitions of relevant terms:

seizure A paroxysmal disorder of cerebral function characterized by an attack involving changes in the state of consciousness, motor activity, or sensory phenomena; a seizure is sudden in onset and usually of brief duration.

epilepsy From the Greek *epilepsia,* meaning "to take hold of," a seizing; refers to any type of recurrent convulsion produced by paroxysmal excessive neuronal discharges in different parts of the brain; it is caused by a variety of cerebral and noncerebral disorders and implies chronicity of seizures.*

---

*Sutherland and Eadie (1980) have updated this definition as follows: "Epilepsy should be regarded as a symptom due to excessive temporary neuronal discharging which results from intracranial or extracranial causes; epilepsy is characterized by discrete episodes, which tend to be recurrent, in which there is a disturbance of movement, sensation, behavior, perception, and/or consciousness."

status epilepticus Rapid, repetitive recurrence of any type of seizure without recovery between attacks; a truly life-threatening situation.

tonic Describes a sustained muscular contraction; patient appears rigid ("stiff") during tonic phase of seizure.

clonic Describes intermittent muscular contraction and relaxation; the clonic phase is the actual convulsive portion of a seizure.

stertorous Characterized by snoring.

TYPES OF SEIZURE DISORDERS

The clinical manifestations of paroxysmal excessive neuronal activity in the brain span a wide range of sensory and motor activities, which may involve any or all of the following: altered visceral function; sensory, olfactory, auditory, visual, and gustatory phenomena; abnormal motor movements; changes in mental awareness and behavior; and alterations in consciousness. The box on the opposite page presents the recent classification of the epilepsies by the Commission on Classification and Terminology of the International League Against Epilepsy (1981). The incidence of epilepsy (recurrent seizures) in general populations (all age groups) is between 0.5% and 1.0%. In the United States it is estimated that more than 10 million persons have suffered at least one convulsive episode and that in excess of 2 million persons have suffered two or more episodes. In addition, it is estimated that more than 200,000 Americans have seizures more than once a month despite medical treatment. One third of epileptics are thought to have an underlying brain lesion.

The seizures that are encountered most frequently and that possess the greatest potential for morbidity and mortality are generalized seizures or seizures without local onset. Within this group are the tonic-clonic convulsive episode, which is represented clinically as grand mal epilepsy, and petit mal epilepsy, which is also termed absence attack.

CLINICAL AND ELECTROENCEPHALOGRAPHIC CLASSIFICATION OF EPILEPTIC SEIZURES*

Partial seizures (focal, local)†

Simple partial seizures
  With motor signs
  With somatosensory or special-sensory symptoms
  With autonomic symptoms or signs
  With psychic symptoms
Complex partial seizures (psychomotor, temporal lobe)
  Simple partial onset followed by impairment of consciousness‡
  With impairment of consciousness at onset
Partial seizures evolving to generalized tonic-clonic convulsions (secondarily generalized)§
  Simple partial seizures evolving to generalized tonic-clonic convulsions
  Complex partial seizures evolving to generalized tonic-clonic convulsions (including simple partial seizure to complex partial seizure to generalized tonic-clonic convulsion)

Generalized seizures (convulsive or nonconvulsive)‖

Absence seizures (true petit mal)
Atypical absence seizures
Myoclonic seizures
Clonic seizures
Tonic seizures
Tonic-clonic seizures (grand mal)
Atonic seizures
Unclassified epileptic seizures

*From Commission on Classification and Terminology of the International League Against Epilepsy.
†Partial seizures have behavioral or EEG evidence showing that the ictal discharge begins in one area of the brain. Seizures that do not alter consciousness are called simple partial; those that do are called complex partial.
‡Complex partial seizures are said to evolve from simple partial seizures when they begin without an alteration in consciousness (for example, an aura).
§Partial seizures can progress to generalized tonic-clonic convulsions and are called secondarily generalized seizures.
‖Behavioral and EEG manifestations of true generalized seizures are generalized from the start. Several types of generalized seizures are recognized; some have no known structural or chemical cause (for example, true petit mal), whereas others are associated with diffuse brain damage.

Partial or focal seizures are those that involve a specific region of the brain. Signs and symptoms of such focal seizures relate to the specific region of the brain affected. As noted in the box above, signs and symptoms may include specific motor or sensory symptoms or both or appear as "spells," with more complex symptoms involving illusions, hallucinations, or déjà vu. Focal seizures may remain localized, in which case consciousness or the awareness of the victim is normally somewhat disturbed, and variable degrees of amnesia may be evident. On the other hand, a focal seizure may spread and become a generalized seizure with loss of consciousness. Generalized seizures are of greater clinical importance to the practicing dentist than are focal seizures, because of their greater potential for injury and postseizure complications.

Generalized Seizures

The majority of patients with recurrent generalized seizures (epilepsy) develop one of three major forms: grand mal, petit mal, or psychomotor seizures. Out of all those with epilepsy, 70% have only one type of seizure disorder; the remaining 30% have two or more types.

Grand mal epilepsy is the most common form of seizure disorder (present in 90% of epileptics). Approximately 60% of epileptics have this form alone, whereas 30% have other seizure types in addition to grand mal. The tonic-clonic type of seizure disorder is what most persons characteristically think of as "epilepsy." Grand mal epilepsy may occur in any age group. The tonic-clonic type seizure may be produced by neurologic disorders or it may develop in a neurologically sound brain secondary to a systemic metabolic or toxic disturbance. Grand mal seizures (neurologically induced) usually last from 2 to 5 minutes. This type of seizure forms the basis of our discussion in this section.

Petit mal epilepsy (absence seizures) are found in 25% of epileptics. Only 4% have petit mal as the sole form of seizure disorder, the other 21% having it in combination with other forms (most commonly grand mal). Petit mal seizures almost always develop in childhood (most often in children under the age of 16 years). The incidence of petit mal seizures decreases with increasing age, and its persistence beyond the age of 30 years is rare. Clinically, the petit mal seizure consists of a brief lapse of consciousness, normally lasting from 5 to 10 seconds and only on rare occasions lasting beyond 30 seconds. The patient makes no movement during the episode (other than perhaps a cyclic blinking of the eyelids), and the termination of the episode is equally abrupt. If erect at the start of the episode the victim usually remains standing during the seizure.

A "petit mal triad" is recognized, consisting of myoclonic jerks, akinetic seizures, and brief absences (blank spells) without associated falling and body convulsion. A characteristic electroencephalographic (EEG) pattern consisting of 3 cycles per second is noted in petit mal epilepsy.

With *jacksonian epilepsy* (simple partial seizure), consciousness is often maintained. The focal convulsions of jacksonian epilepsy may be motor, sensory, or autonomic in nature. Commonly, this type of epilepsy begins in a part of a limb or the face as a localized chronic spasm and spreads in a more or less orderly manner. For example, it may start in the great toe and extend to the leg, thigh, trunk, and shoulder and may possibly involve the upper limb. If the seizure crosses to the opposite side, consciousness is likely to be lost.

Psychomotor seizures are present in approximately 18% of epileptics (6% having psychomotor seizures alone, 12% having them in combination with other forms) and are minor seizures in which the victim loses contact with the environment for approximately 1 to 2 minutes. They may develop at any age. The category of psychomotor seizures includes most seizures that do not meet the criteria described previously for grand mal, petit mal, and jacksonian seizures. Automatisms, apparently purposeful movements, incoherent speech, turning of the head, shifting of the eyes, smacking of lips, twisting and writhing movements of the extremi-

ties, clouding of consciousness, and amnesia are common.

Status epilepticus is a state in which seizures recur without recovery between episodes. Although status epilepticus may occur with any type of seizure, the term is most commonly applied to episodes of grand mal epilepsy in which the patient remains unconscious and to continuous tonic-clonic seizures for long periods (hours to days). Grand mal status is a life-threatening situation that, if not managed effectively, may progress to cerebral damage, cardiac or renal failure, and death.

CAUSES

Many factors are known to produce convulsive seizures; however, over 65% of persons with recurrent seizures (epileptics) are said to suffer from idiopathic epilepsy, in which no definite etiologic factor for the seizures can be found. Another name for idiopathic epilepsy is genetic epilepsy. Relatives of persons with idiopathic epilepsy have a 3% to 5% incidence rate, which is six to ten times the expected rate. Acquired epilepsy (symptomatic epilepsy) is present in the remaining 35% of persons with recurrent seizures. The term "symptomatic" indicates that evaluation of the patient demonstrates a probable cause or causes. Factors known to produce clinical seizure activity include congenital conditions such as maternal infection (rubella), trauma, or hypoxia-anoxia during delivery; central nervous system infection (meningitis, encephalitis); head injury (a very common cause); fever; cerebrovascular disease; and toxic and metabolic disorders. Dahlquist, Mellinger, and Klass (1983) described a phenomenon of seizures developing in children exposed to flickering lights and geometric patterns while playing video games. The introduction of new, noninvasive neurodiagnostic techniques (most significantly computerized axial tomography scans [CAT scans] and nuclear magnetic resonance [NMR]) has improved the detection of underlying lesions in persons with epileptic disorders.

Febrile convulsions are usually associated with and are precipitated by marked elevations in temperature. They occur almost exclusively in infants and young children, particularly during the first year of life. Approximately 5% of children suffer febrile convulsions. Febrile convulsions are more common in children with a family history of epilepsy. Such convulsions do not recur in more than 85% of cases; however, approximately 30% of these children may later develop psychomotor epilepsy without fever. Febrile convulsions are not a major factor in dental practice.

Cerebrovascular disease is another potential cause of seizures and is encountered most often in older age groups. Loss of consciousness progressing to convulsive seizures is produced by a decrease in cerebral blood flow (see Chapter 19).

Major factors leading to acquired epilepsy are toxic and metabolic disorders (Table 21-1). It is important to be aware of these factors, because seizures produced by them may be prevented or, should they occur, terminated through specific therapy. Management of the acute seizure is uniform regardless of the cause.

The most common of these seizure-producing factors in a dental office are overdose reactions from local anesthetics and the hypoglycemic reaction. These reactions are described elsewhere in the text.

PREDISPOSING FACTORS

Management of most patients with a history of seizure disorders is concerned with minimizing the incidence of acute seizure activity through long-term drug therapy. In spite of this therapy, acute seizure activity may still develop. In some cases, there is no apparent reason (predisposing factor) for this occurrence, the seizure episode suddenly developing without warning. There are, however, a number of factors that increase the frequency with which seizure activity develops. It is known, for instance, that the immature brain is much more susceptible to biochemical alteration in cerebral blood flow than is the adult brain. Therefore convulsions brought about by hypoxia, hypoglycemia, and hypocalcemia are more likely to occur in younger age groups. In the adult patient, a "breakthrough" of seizure activity in a well-managed patient may also occur. In these patients the onset of the acute episode has been shown in many cases to be correlated with sleep or menstrual cycles.

In a great many instances of seizure activity, there appears to be an acute triggering disturbance. These triggering factors include flickering lights (especially prominent in precipitating petit mal seizures), fatigue or decreased physical health of patient, and physical or emotional stress.

Seizures may therefore be said to be precipitated by a combination of several factors. Among these are the genetically determined predisposition to seizures (idiopathic or genetic epilepsy) and the

Table 21-1. Metabolic and toxic causes of seizure activity

Metabolic causes	Toxic causes	
	Drug overdose	Drug withdrawal
Hypoglycemia	Local anesthetics	Alcohol
Hypocalcemia	Propoxyphene	Barbiturates
Hypercapnia	Phenothiazines	Sedatives
Anoxia		Hypnotics

presence of a localized brain lesion. One or more of the following factors may also induce acute seizure activity: a generalized metabolic or toxic disturbance that produces an increase in cerebral neuronal excitation; a state of cerebrovascular insufficiency; an acute triggering disturbance such as sleep, menstrual cycle, fatigue, flickering lights, or physical or psychologic stress. Each of the factors listed above may also act individually to produce seizure activity.

PREVENTION
Nonepileptic Causes

The prevention of acute seizure activity in the dental office is indeed difficult, owing to the idiopathic nature of most seizures. However, the prevention of seizures produced by metabolic or toxic disturbances may be facilitated through adequate physical evaluation of the dental patient before therapy. The reader is referred to Chapter 17 for a discussion of the prevention of the hypoglycemic reaction.

In dental practice an overdose (toxic) reaction to local anesthetic drugs is the most likely cause of seizure activity. Adequate patient evaluation and preparation and care in selection of a local anesthetic agent go far in preventing this complication. The most important factor in preventing such a toxic reaction is the proper technique of injection of the local anesthetic agent (see Chapter 23).

Epileptic Causes

For most epileptic patients, the goal of the doctor is to determine the probability of an acute seizure developing during dental therapy and to take certain steps to minimize that possibility. In addition, the doctor and staff should prepare to manage any seizure that might arise and attempt to prevent any clinical complications (soft-tissue injury or fractures).

Medical History Questionnaire
QUESTION 9. *Circle any of the following which you have had or have at present:*
- **Epilepsy or seizures**
- **Fainting or dizzy spells**

COMMENT. Affirmative responses indicate knowledge of the disorder. Most epileptics are aware of their condition and respond accordingly on the questionnaire.

QUESTION 6. *Have you taken any medicine or drugs during the past two years?*

COMMENT. Most epileptics require long-term drug therapy to minimize recurrent seizure activity. The ideal anticonvulsant is described as long acting, nonsedating, well tolerated, useful in many types of seizures, and without substantive effect on vital organs as it restores the electroencephalogram (EEG) to normal. However, this ideal agent does not exist. A basic principle followed in use of anticonvulsants is to select a single drug first, rather than a combination, and use it either until it becomes effective or until toxic signs appear. If seizure control proves effective (no seizures occurring for a period of years), the question of terminating drug therapy is normally raised with the patient asking, "Do I still need to take those drugs every day?" Some physicians will gradually withdraw anticonvulsant medications if the patient has been free of seizures for from 2 to 4 years. However, in many cases recurrences of seizure activity do occur. Sudden withdrawal of anticonvulsant therapy is the most common cause of status epilepticus. For the average adult with grand mal epilepsy, continuous, life-long therapy is usually indicated.

Whenever possible, sedative medications that interfere with behavioral and functional aspects of a patient's life should be avoided. This is especially true with the barbiturates and the benzodiazepines. A friend recently placed on anticonvulsant medications following a first seizure complained to me that when people spoke to him, they "sounded as though they were talking under water" and that everything appeared to happen in slow motion. Because of an increased risk of learning deficit in epileptic children taking anticonvulsant drugs,

Table 21-2. Drugs used in long-term management of epilepsy

Generic name	Proprietary name	Type of seizure	Side effects
Acetazolamide	Diamox	Grand mal, petit mal	Drowsiness, paresthesia
Carbamazepine	Tegretol	Psychomotor, grand mal	Diplopia, transient blurred vision, drowsiness, ataxia, bone marrow depression
Clonazepam	Clonopin	Petit mal, atypical petit mal, myoclonic, akinetic	Drowsiness, ataxia, agitation
Ethosuximide	Zarontin	Petit mal	Drowsiness, nausea, vomiting
Methsuximide	Celontin	Petit mal, psychomotor	Ataxia, drowsiness
Mephenytoin	Mesantoin	Grand mal, some cases of psychomotor; effective when petit mal and grand mal coexist	Nervousness, ataxia, nystagmus, pancytopenia, exfoliative dermatitis
Phenacemide	Phenurone	Psychomotor	Hepatitis, benign proteinuria, dermatitis, headache, and personality changes
Phenobarbital	—	One of the safest drugs for all seizures; may aggravate psychomotor seizures	Drowsiness, dermatitis
Phenytoin sodium	Dilantin	Safest drug for grand mal and some cases of psychomotor epilepsy; may accentuate petit mal	Gingival hypertrophy, rash, nervousness, ataxia, drowsiness, nystagmus
Primidone	Mysoline	Grand mal, especially in conjunction with other drugs	Drowsiness, ataxia
Valproic acid	Depakene	Petit mal, atypical petit mal, myoclonic, akinetic	Nausea and vomiting, drowsiness; interferes with platelets (similar to aspirin) and therefore may increase bleeding

physicians usually attempt to gradually withdraw younger patients from drug therapy. When a child has been seizure free for 4 consecutive years, gradual withdrawal is usually attempted. A seizure relapse rate does occur, which varies significantly; 53% of patients with jacksonian seizure relapse, while only 8% with grand mal epilepsy and 12% with uncomplicated petit mal epilepsy relapse (Menzer and Sabin, 1978). Withdrawal is rarely attempted at puberty, especially in females; therapy is usually continued through adolescence. Drugs used in long-term management of epilepsy are listed in Table 21-2. Table 21-3 lists the drugs commonly used to manage the various types of seizures.

Dialogue History

In response to a positive history of convulsive seizures, the following information should be sought:

QUESTION. What type of seizures (epilepsy) do you have?

QUESTION. How often do you have acute seizures? When was your last seizure?

COMMENT. Grand mal epilepsy is effectively controlled in many patients. Proper treatment with drug therapy will prevent seizures in more than 70% of epileptics. These patients may have been seizure free for several years, or seizures may occur only infrequently (once or twice a year). In other patients the frequency of seizures may be greater, perhaps several times a week. Petit mal seizures may occur as frequently as every several days, or they may occur frequently in clusters of 100 or more per day. Greater frequency implies a greater likelihood of seizures developing during dental therapy.

QUESTION. What signals the onset of your seizure?

COMMENT. Patients with grand mal epilepsy have specific auras, or premonitions, that herald the onset of a seizure. The aura is commonly of brief duration and is related to the specific region of the brain in which the abnormal electrical discharge originates. The aura may be stereotyped for an individual patient. Some common auras include an "odd" sensation in the epigastric region, and unpleasant taste or smell, various visual and/or auditory hallucinations, a sense of fear, strange sensations (such as numbness) in the limbs, and motor phenomena (such as turning of the head or eyes or spasm of a limb).

QUESTION. How long do your seizures last?

COMMENT. Seizures, except for status epilepticus, are self-limiting. The tonic-clonic phase of a grand mal seizure usually lasts 2 to 5 minutes. The duration of the convulsive phase of the seizure has important implications in clinical management. Once completed, seizures do not tend to recur during the immediate postseizure period; however, relapses of seizures may occur.

QUESTION. Have you ever been hospitalized as a result of your seizures?

COMMENT. This question is asked to determine whether status epilepticus has ever occurred and whether serious injury to the patient has resulted from any previous seizures.

Physical Examination

There are no specific clinical signs or symptoms that can lead to a diagnosis of epilepsy if a patient is examined between seizures; however, over 50% of patients with recurring seizures demonstrate EEG

Table 21-3. Drug management of epilepsies by type of seizure

Type of seizure	Drugs of choice	Comments
Generalized tonic-clonic and partial seizures	Phenytoin Phenobarbital Primidone Carbamazepine Valproic acid	Phenytoin is the drug of choice in the management of grand mal. Phenobarbital is added if phenytoin alone is ineffective. Combination of two is more effective than either drug used alone.
Absence seizures	Ethosuximide Valproic acid Clonazepam	Ethosuximide is the drug of choice in the management of petit mal. Valproic acid is effective in resistant cases. Clonazepam is likely to produce drowsiness and ataxia.

abnormalities in the interictal period. No specific treatment modification is indicated aside from possible psychosedation necessitated by obvious anxiety over the dental situation. Because most anticonvulsants are CNS depressants, care must be observed whenever the use of psychosedative techniques is contemplated to avoid inadvertent oversedation.

Psychologic Implications of Epilepsy

Folklore and myths have arisen connecting epilepsy to violent behavior. Although there is very little evidence to link violence with epilepsy, many physicians and laymen retain the belief that epileptics are dangerous, potentially violent people. The incidence of epilepsy among prisoners in jails in the United States is approximately 1.8%, compared to an incidence of between 0.5% and 1% in the general population. Patients with psychomotor or grand mal seizures may exhibit signs of fright and may in fact struggle irrationally with anyone trying to help them during the seizure.

Most patients with recurrent seizures can and do adapt into the working force and social system despite occasional periods of disability caused by seizures and their immediate consequences. The most serious feature of epileptic disability is social ostracism. This ostracism is especially damaging to the school-aged child who is embarrassed by seizures and may be set apart from the other children because of fear and ignorance. Many epileptics feel rejected and withdraw. This withdrawal, combined with the prejudice that may be experienced throughout childhood and adolescence, can lead to inadequate educational, matrimonial, and employment opportunities. Because of low self-esteem, many epileptic persons may choose companions with emotional, physical, or mental handicaps of their own. Alcoholism and substance abuse may follow.

Dental Therapy Considerations

The major consideration in dental therapy for the epileptic patient is how to manage the patient if a seizure occurs. Specific modifications of therapy should be considered only if the situation warrants them.

Psychologic stress and fatigue tend to increase the probability of a seizure developing. In the presence of apprehension, psychosedation should be considered. Nitrous oxide and oxygen inhalation sedation or intravenous sedation with diazepam (Valium) or midazolam (Versed) with oxygen supplementation are commonly used. Oral premedication may be appropriate if a patient appears unduly apprehensive about an impending visit to the dental office. More profound levels of sedation should not be employed in epileptic patients because hypoxia, which may accompany such sedation, may precipitate seizure activity. Whenever possible, titration of drugs to clinical effect is preferred because of the possible interactions between anticonvulsants and those agents administered to manage anxiety and fear.

The use of alcohol is definitely contraindicated in epileptic patients because it may precipitate seizures. Therefore epileptic patients should not undergo dental therapy if it is obvious that they have recently ingested alcohol, nor should the doctor consider the use of alcohol as a sedative agent in epileptic patients. Table 21-4 lists the physical status classifications for epileptic patients. The typical well-controlled epileptic represents an ASA II risk, while less well-controlled patients may represent ASA III or ASA IV risks.

CLINICAL MANIFESTATIONS

The tonic-clonic seizure (grand mal, generalized seizure, major convulsion) will be described in depth following a brief description of other seizure types.

Partial Seizures

Partial seizures occur when an attack begins from a localized area of the brain and involves only one hemisphere. The seizure is called a simple partial when consciousness is unaltered; for example, a focal motor seizure is a simple partial in which the victim experiences jerking of a limb for several seconds while remaining fully alert and conscious. If, however, the abnormal neuronal discharge spreads to the opposite hemisphere, consciousness is altered and the ability to respond is impaired. This is called a complex partial seizure and is associated with complex behavior patterns called automatisms. An example of a typical complex partial seizure is the sudden onset of a bad taste in the mouth, which is followed by a lack of responsiveness, fumbling of hands, and smacking of lips. The patient slowly becomes reoriented in about 1 minute and is back to normal except for slight lethargy within 3 minutes. Focal status epilepticus is not common but is resistant to anticonvulsant therapy; characteristically, seizure activity lasts over a period

Table 21-4. Physical status classification of seizure disorders

	Physical status (ASA)	Considerations
History of seizure activity well controlled by medications (no seizures within past 3 months)	II	Usual ASA II considerations
History of seizure activity controlled by medications, yet seizures occurring more often than once a month	III	ASA III considerations to include preparation for management of seizure
History of status epilepticus	III-IV	Medical consultation before dental therapy
History of seizure activity poorly controlled by medication; frequency of one or more seizures per week	IV	Medical consultation and better control of seizures before routine dental therapy

of weeks despite vigorous treatment. Fortunately, this type of seizure is not life threatening.

Both simple and complex partial seizures may progress to generalized tonic-clonic seizures.

Petit Mal (Absence Attacks)

Absence attacks occur primarily in children. The victim appears confused and distracted. Intermittent blinking (at a rate of 3 cycles per second) and mouthing movements may also be observed. On occasion, the victim may speak or respond to spoken language. The absence attack may last for 5 to 30 seconds, whereas petit mal status may persist for hours or days. There is no prodromal or postictal period. The blank stare is followed by the immediate resumption of normal activity. It is not uncommon for an informal "diagnosis" of petit mal to occur when a young child first enters school. After a few weeks or months, the child's teacher may advise the parents that their child "daydreams a lot" or that he or she "goes off into their own world" for brief periods of time. Medical evaluation usually proves definitive.

Tonic-clonic Seizure

The tonic-clonic seizure may be divided into three distinct clinical phases: a prodromal phase, a convulsive or ictal phase, and a postseizure or postictal phase.

Prodromal phase

For a variable period of time (several minutes to several hours) before the occurrence of a generalized seizure, the epileptic patient exhibits subtle or obvious changes in emotional reactivity. The patient may exhibit an increase in either anxiety or depression. These changes are usually not evident to the staff of the dental office but might be detected by a close friend or relative of the patient. If such changes appear in an epileptic patient before a dental appointment, therapy might best be postponed until a later date.

The immediate onset of the seizure is marked by the appearance of an aura in most, but not all, patients. The aura is not truly a warning sign that a seizure is about to occur but is an actual part of the seizure. The same aura may recur with each seizure in an epileptic patient. Duration of the aura is quite brief, usually only a few seconds. The clinical manifestations of the aura are related to the specific area of the brain from which the seizure originates. The aura may be considered a simple partial seizure that progresses to a generalized tonic-clonic seizure. It may be olfactory, visual, gustatory, or auditory in nature.

Unfortunately, many patients are unaware of their aura because they are amnesic of this period. Most people with grand mal epilepsy remember nothing from the time immediately preceding the onset of the seizure until they fully recover, perhaps 30 or more minutes later. Patients will know their aura if a person near them when a seizure occurs tells them about it at a later time. For example, "you made certain noises or mentioned a bad taste or smell."

Convulsive (ictal) phase

Soon after the appearance of the aura, the patient loses consciousness and, if standing, falls to the floor. The so-called epileptic cry then occurs. This is a sudden vocalization produced by air expelled through a partially closed glottis as the diaphragmatic muscles go into spasm. Severe tonic contractions of skeletal muscles occur, leading to a

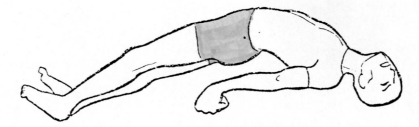

Fig. 21-1. Victim during tonic phase of generalized seizure (grand mal).

tonic extensor rigidity of the extremities and the trunk (Fig. 21-1). During this phase of the seizure the muscles of respiration are also involved, and dyspnea and cyanosis may become evident, indicating inadequate ventilation. The tonic phase usually lasts for less than 1 minute and is followed by generalized clonic movements of the body accompanied by heavy, stertorous breathing (Fig. 21-2). During the clonic phase, frothing at the mouth may be noted, because air and saliva are mixed. Blood may also appear in the mouth because the victim may bite the tongue and cheek during the clonic portion of the seizure. Clonic movements become less frequent as the seizure progresses. Usual duration of this phase of seizure activity is from 2 to 5 minutes. The convulsive phase ends as respiratory movements return to normal and the tonic-clonic movements cease. Urinary and fecal incontinence may occur at this time; these are caused by muscle (including sphincter) relaxation.

Postictal phase

With the cessation of tonic-clonic movement and the return of normal respiration, the patient is said to enter the postictal phase, during which consciousness gradually returns. The clinical manifestations of this phase largely depend on the severity of the ictal phase. Immediately following the termination of seizure activity, the patient relaxes and sleeps deeply. If the seizure was severe, the victim may be in a comatose (nonresponsive) state. As consciousness returns, patients are initially quite disoriented and confused, unaware of where they are or what day of the week it is and unable to count backward from 10 to 1 or do other simple mathematical calculations. Patients then fall into a deep sleep, and on awakening will complain of headache and muscle soreness. Following most generalized seizures there is almost total amnesia of the ictal and postictal phases. Some persons do retain memory of the prodromal phase, however.

Grand Mal Status (Status Epilepticus)

Status epilepticus is defined as the repetitive recurrence of any type of seizure without recovery between attacks. In this discussion it is considered to be a direct continuation of the tonic-clonic seizure described above. As mentioned previously, grand mal status is a life-threatening situation. Patients in status exhibit the same clinical signs and symptoms as those seen during the convulsive phase of a generalized seizure, the one major difference being their duration. Tonic-clonic seizures normally last from 2 to 5 minutes with some minor variance on either extreme of time. Grand mal status may persist for hours or days and is the major cause of mortality directly related to seizure disorders. Mortality figures range from 3% to 23%, depending on the study cited. The incidence of grand mal status has actually increased since the introduction of effective anticonvulsants. Most cases result from drug or alcohol withdrawal (barbiturate withdrawal is particularly severe), severe head injury, or metabolic derangements.

For the purposes of clinical management any continuous generalized (tonic-clonic) seizure lasting for 5 minutes or longer is classified as grand mal status. The patient is nonresponsive (unconscious), cyanotic, perspires profusely, and demonstrates generalized clonic contractions with a very brief or entirely absent tonic phase. As grand mal status progresses, the patient becomes hyperthermic (body temperature rising to 106° F or above). The cardiovascular system is greatly overworked; rapid heart rate and irregular rhythm occur, and blood pressure is quite elevated—measurements of 300/150 torr are not uncommon. Untreated grand mal status may progress to death of the victim resulting

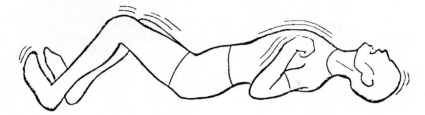

Fig. 21-2. Victim during clonic phase of generalized seizure (grand mal).

from cardiac arrest, irreversible neuronal damage from cerebral hypoxia (which occurs secondary to inadequate ventilation), the increased metabolic requirements of the entire body but the central nervous system in particular, a decrease in cerebral blood flow in response to increased intracranial pressure, and a decrease in blood glucose levels.

PATHOPHYSIOLOGY

Epilepsy is not a disease but a symptom. The symptom normally represents a primary form of brain dysfunction, although it is not possible to detect such a lesion in approximately 75% of patients with recurrent seizure disorders (idiopathic epilepsy). Adult-onset epilepsy most often indicates a structural lesion of the brain, even though the initial examination may fail to demonstrate it. Small tumors may take considerable time to enlarge to detectable size. Periodic medical examination (every 4 to 6 months) and annual EEGs are recommended. The use of the CAT scan and N.M.R. have greatly aided in detection of previously undetectable lesions. Theoretical models of epilepsy presume that there are intrinsic intracellular and extracellular metabolic disturbances in neurons of epileptics that produce excessive and prolonged membrane depolarization. These hyperexcitable neurons are located in aggregates in a seizure focus (the site or origin of the seizure) somewhere within the brain and tend toward recurrent, high frequency bursts of action potentials.

Clinical seizure activity develops if the abnormal discharge is propagated along neural pathways or if local neuron recruitment occurs (if additional neighboring neurons are stimulated to discharge). If this discharge remains localized within the focal area, a partial seizure develops with clinical signs and symptoms related to the specific focal area. If the discharge continues to spread through normal neuronal tissue and recruitment continues, generalized seizures occur. Clinical manifestations of the seizure depend on the focus of origin (partial seizures and aura of grand mal) and the region of the brain into which the discharge subsequently spreads.

That seizures can also arise in normal neurologic tissues is evidenced in clinical seizures caused by systemic metabolic and toxic disorders. Deficiencies in oxygen or glucose or decreases in calcium ions create a membrane instability that predisposes otherwise normal neurons to paroxysmal discharge. Adequate electrical stimulation may also produce clinical seizures in normal neurologic tissues.

MANAGEMENT

Management of a patient during the tonic-clonic phase of a generalized seizure is based on prevention of injury and the assurance of adequate ventilation. In most instances, the need to administer anticonvulsant medications does not arise. Should a seizure persist for an unusually long period of time, such drugs may be necessary. Following the convulsive phase of the seizure, patients exhibit variable degrees of CNS depression, which may require additional supportive management.

Petit Mal and Partial Seizures

Management of petit mal and partial seizures is of a protective nature. The rescuer merely prevents any injury to the victim. In both of these seizure types there is little or no danger to the victim, so that even without assistance from staff members, morbidity seldom occurs. However, should these seizures persist for a significant length of time (average petit mal episode is 5 to 30 seconds; partial seizure lasts from 1 to 2 minutes), medical assistance may be summoned.

MANAGEMENT OF TONIC-CLONIC SEIZURES

Convulsive (ictal) phase

Step 1 Position patient (supine)
    2 Prevent injury to patient
        Soft object under head
        Soft object between teeth, if possible
        Loosen tight clothing
    3 Initiate basic life support
    4 Monitor vital signs

Postictal phase

    5 Initiate basic life support
    6 Permit patient to recover, contact physician
    7 Discharge patient in company of responsible adult companion

Grand mal status

Step 1 Position patient (supine)
    2 Prevent injury to patient
    3 Initiate basic life support
    4 Monitor vital signs
    5 Administer anticonvulsant drug
        Diazepam, 2 mg/min slowly and intravenously (for adult)
        Pentobarbital, 25 mg/min slowly and intravenously
    6 Summon medical assistance

Generalized Tonic-clonic Seizures
Convulsive (ictal) phase

Step 1. Position patient. If a generalized tonic-clonic seizure occurs, the victim must be positioned properly. When possible, the victim should be on the floor in the supine position. Should a seizure occur in the dental chair, moving this patient may prove to be exceedingly difficult. In this situation the patient should be left in the chair, which should be placed in the supine position.

Step 2. Prevent injury. Prevention of injury to the convulsing patient is the next concern. If the victim is on a well-padded, carpeted floor in an area devoid of hard objects that may cause injury, the rescuer can permit the patient to convulse with little chance of injury occurring. *Gently* restraining the victim's arms and legs from gross movements (allowing for minor movement) prevents injury from overextension or dislocation of joints.

With the victim in the dental chair, however, there is a possibility of injury from nearby dental equipment. The headrest of most dental units is normally well padded so that no additional protection for the head is necessary. The concern therefore must be to prevent the patient from impaling the arms or legs on equipment (such as burs and hand instruments). A member of the team should move as much equipment as possible out of range of the victim while two other members stand by the patient to prevent injury from occurring. One member is positioned at the patient's head and is responsible for head and arms; the second is at the feet. The extremities should not be *forcibly* restrained, because this has led to severe injury of the victim (fractures of bones) and the rescuer.

The soft headrest on the dental chair or a pillow or folded coat (if the patient is on the floor) should be placed beneath the victim's head. *If possible,* another soft item, such as a folded handkerchief, cloth towel, or large gauze pads (4 × 4 inch or bigger) may be placed between the teeth to prevent biting of the tongue and lips. Care must be taken to be certain that objects placed in the patient's mouth do not cause airway obstruction. Under no circumstances should a rescuer's fingers be placed between the teeth of a convulsing patient. The use of hard objects such as rubber or ratchet-type mouth props and tongue depressors covered with gauze should be considered only if the other soft items are not available. Tissue injury and bleeding caused by improper placement of these devices have been reported. In most grand mal seizures only minor degrees of bleeding develop. Roberge and Maciera-Rodriguez in 1985 reporting on the incidence of seizure-related lacerations stated that 44% of seizing patients suffered intraoral lacerations, primarily of the tongue. Only two of 44 patients subsequently required surgical repair of the lacerations. In my experience, forcibly attempting to place mouth props in a victim's mouth has produced greater and potentially more dangerous degrees of hemorrhage. Placement of any object in the oral cavity is usually NOT indicated during tonic-clonic seizures.

Tight, binding clothes should be loosened to prevent possible injury caused by the straining patient and to assist in breathing. This includes opening the collar and loosening a tie or belt.

Step 3. Initiate basic life support. During seizure activity, especially the tonic phase, respirations may not be adequate. Indeed, brief periods of apnea may occur, and cyanosis may be evident. Secretions may also accumulate in the oral cavity and may, in large enough amounts, produce a degree of airway obstruction. Saliva and blood are the most common secretions.

The victim's head should be extended (head tilt) to establish airway patency, and the oral cavity should be suctioned carefully to remove secretions if they seem excessive. Suctioning is usually not required in a patient actively experiencing a seizure. Soft rubber or plastic suction catheters are preferable to metallic ones, which can produce more tissue damage (bleeding). In either case, the suction apparatus should be inserted between the buccal surface of the teeth and the cheek. It should not be inserted between the teeth of the patient. Nonpermanent dental prostheses such as removable partial dentures or full dentures should be removed from the victim's mouth as soon as possible because if they are dislodged, they may obstruct the patient's airway. Oxygen, if available and if considered necessary (as in cyanosis), may be administered to the patient having a seizure.

Step 4. Monitor vital signs. Throughout the seizure the blood pressure, pulse rate, and respiratory rate may be monitored. As mentioned previously, the blood pressure and heart rate may be markedly elevated and respiratory movements may be absent during the tonic phase. During clonic activity heavy, stertorous breathing may be present.

Postictal phase

Step 5. Basic life support. With cessation of seizure activity the patient enters the postictal phase. This is a phase of generalized depression, with the degree of depression related to the degree of stimulation experienced during the ictal phase. It is during the postictal phase that significant morbidity and even mortality may occur. The ictal phase of a seizure is a highly dramatic and emotionally charged event for the eyewitnesses, and attention is quickly focused on the patient. Once the convulsive phase ends, the patient "relaxes" and so, unfortunately, do the rescuers. This is premature because during the postictal period the patient may demonstrate significant CNS depression to such a degree that respiratory depression and/or airway obstruction may be evident. Airway maintenance and artificial ventilation may be required. Oxygen may be administered by means of a full face mask or nasal cannula, if indicated. Airway maintenance and adequacy of ventilation remain the primary consid-

erations at this time. Vital signs should be recorded at regular intervals (at least every 5 minutes). Blood pressure and respirations may be depressed in the immediate postictal period; however, they should gradually return toward the baseline level for that patient. The heart rate may be near baseline or only slightly depressed.

Step 6. Permit patient to recover. Patients should be allowed to rest until recovery is complete enough to permit them to be discharged. Recovery includes a return of the vital signs to approximately the baseline level and recovery from the confusion and disorientation present during the early postictal period. Consultation with the patient's physician is indicated while the patient is recovering. The physician may wish the patient to be examined in his office or be admitted to a hospital for further evaluation.

Step 7. Discharge from office. The patient should be discharged from the dental office in the custody of a responsible adult. A relative or close friend should be called to the office to accompany the patient. The patient must be advised against operating a motor vehicle for the remainder of that day.*

Grand Mal Status

In the event that generalized convulsive activity persists for unusually long periods (5 minutes or more), it may become necessary to terminate the seizure through the use of anticonvulsant drugs and to summon medical assistance.

Step 1. Position patient.
Step 2. Prevent injury to patient.
Step 3. Initiate basic life support.
Step 4. Monitor vital signs every 5 minutes.

In the preceding steps 1 through 4, we have been managing the patient with possible grand mal status in the same manner as a patient with generalized tonic-clonic seizure. If seizure activity continues beyond the usual duration (5 minutes), we must consider the possible presence of grand mal status and take steps to manage it.

Step 5. Administer anticonvulsant drug. Various anticonvulsant drugs may be used to terminate seizures. To be effective, these agents should be administered intravenously; the intramuscular route is highly unpredictable and the oral route is contraindicated in an unconscious, convulsing patient

---

*In most states epileptic persons are not permitted to hold valid drivers licenses.

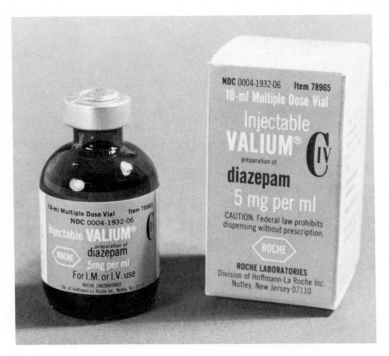

Fig. 21-3. The anticonvulsant diazepam (Valium) is the drug of choice for the management of tonic-clonic seizures. It is administered intravenously at a rate not to exceed 2 mg/minute.

in seizure. An intravenous infusion should be established, or the drugs may be injected directly into the vein of the patient. If proper equipment and adequately trained staff are not available, do not attempt intravenous injections. In these instances, it is advisable to summon assistance immediately and continue with supportive therapy until more highly trained personnel arrive (step 6).

The drug of choice for management of seizures is diazepam (Valium), pictured in Fig. 21-3. It should be administered slowly, at a rate not to exceed 2 mg per minute in the adult; 1 mg per year of age for the child patient (from the ages of 1 to 8), not to exceed 10 mg; or 0.3 mg/kg of body weight, not to exceed 5 mg, in the infant. The rate of diazepam administration in the infant and child should not exceed 1 mg per minute.

If seizures persist, the injection may be repeated every 2 minutes. Potentially serious side effects of diazepam are related to excessively rapid injection and include transient hypotension, bradycardia, respiratory depression, and cardiac arrest. These side effects are rarely observed if the agent is titrated slowly to effect.

Barbiturates may be used in place of diazepam for seizure control. Pentobarbital (Nembutal), injected intravenously at a rate of 50 mg every 2 minutes, is an effective anticonvulsant. However, barbiturates have the disturbing ability to produce significant central nervous system depression when employed in anticonvulsant doses so that the level of postictal depression may be intensified. Respiratory depression and apnea are not uncommon when barbiturates are employed as anticonvulsants. Airway maintenance and artificial ventilation *must* be provided until the patient has recovered.

Step 6. Summon medical assistance. Medical assistance should be summoned at the earliest convenient time during this episode. Most patients with grand mal status require a period of hospitalization following the episode for neurologic evaluation and initiation of a treatment protocol to minimize further episodes.

The management of tonic-clonic seizures is summarized in the box on p. 248.

DIFFERENTIAL DIAGNOSIS OF SEIZURES

The diagnosis of an epileptic seizure is not easily confused with other systemic medical conditions. There are, however, several systemic disorders that

Table 21-5. Possible causes of seizure disorders

Cause	Frequency	Where discussed in text
Epilepsy (grand mal)	Most common	Seizures (Section V)
Local anesthetic overdose reaction	Less common	Drug-related emergencies (Section VI)
Hyperventilation	Rare	Respiratory difficulty (Section III)
Cerebrovascular accident	Rare	Altered consciousness (Section IV)
Hypoglycemic reaction	Rare	Altered consciousness (Section IV)
Vasodepressor syncope	Rare	Unconsciousness (Section II)

may have seizures as a part of their clinical signs and symptoms (Table 21-5). The following discussion is presented to aid in diagnosing these possible causes of seizure activity.

Vasodepressor syncope is the most common cause of unconsciousness in the dental office. If hypoxia or anoxia persist, brief periods of seizure activity may occur. Differentiating factors indicating vasodepressor syncope include the presence of a definite precipitating factor, such as fear. Prodromal signs such as lightheadedness, nausea or vomiting, and profuse sweating are present before the loss of consciousness but are absent in epilepsy. The loss of consciousness in vasodepressor syncope is quite brief, recovery beginning once blood flow to the brain is increased. Muscles are flaccid, and there is no convulsive movement initially. The blood pressure and heart rate are depressed in vasodepressor syncope. Bladder and bowel incontinence rarely occur. On recovery of consciousness, the mental confusion and disorientation associated with epileptic convulsions are not present. The patient is alert and able to perform simple mental calculations.

CVA may lead to the loss of consciousness with possible convulsions. Aids to differential diagnosis indicating CVA include the possible presence of an intense headache before the loss of consciousness and signs of neurologic dysfunction (muscle weakness or paralysis) before unconsciousness.

Hypoglycemia may also progress to the loss of consciousness and seizures. The patient's history, in addition to prior clinical signs and symptoms (Chapter 17), will provide evidence. Additional management in this situation requires the administration of intravenous dextrose.

BIBLIOGRAPHY

Aminoff, M.J., and Simon, R.P.: Status epilepticus. Causes, clinical features, and consequences in 98 patients, Am. J. Med. **69**:657, 1980.

Atkinson, A.J.: Individualization of anticonvulsant therapy, Med. Clin. North Am. **58**:1037, 1974.

Bagley, C.: Social prejudice and the adjustment of people with epilepsy, Epilepsia **13**:33, 1972.

Barkin, R.M., and Rosen, P.: Status epilepticus. In Barkin, R.M., .nd Rosen, P., editors: Emergency pediatrics, St. Louis, 1984, The C.V. Mosby Co.

Berg, B.O.: Prognosis of childhood epilepsy: another look, N. Engl. J. Med. **386**:861, 1982.

Berg, B.O.: Convulsions. In Pascoe, D.J., and Grossman, M., editors: Quick reference to pediatric emergencies, ed. 3, Philadelphia, 1984, J.B. Lippincott Co.

Carney, L.R.: Seizures after the age of sixty, Practitioner **217**:74, 1976.

Commission on classification and terminology of the International League against Epilepsy: Proposal for revised clinical and electroencephalographic classification of epileptic seizures, Epilepsia **22**:489, 1981.

Conomy, J.P., and McNamara, J.O.: Emergency management of the patient with seizures. I. Classification and treatment system, common seizure disorders, Postgrad. Med. **55**:59, 1974.

Conomy, J.P., and McNamara, J.O.: Emergency management of the patient with seizures. II. Generalized status epilepticus, Postgrad. Med. **55**:71, 1974.

Dahlquist, N.R., Mellinger, J.F., and Klass, D.W.: Hazard of video games in patients with light-sensitive epilepsy, JAMA **249**:776, 1983.

Delgado-Escueta, A.V., and others: Current concepts in neurology: management of status epilepticus, N. Engl. J. Med. **306**:607, 1982.

Delgado-Escueta, A.V., Treiman, D.M., and Walsh, G.O.: The treatable epilepsies. (second of two parts), N. Engl. J. Med. **308**:1576, 1983.

Dreifuss, E.E.: Use of anticonvulsant drugs, JAMA **241**:607, 1979.

Engel, J., Jr., and others: Recent developments in the diagnosis and therapy of epilepsy, Ann. Intern. Med. **97**:584, 1982.

Feldman, R.G., and Paul, N.L.: Identity of emotional triggers in epilepsy, J. Nerv. Ment. Dis. **162**:345, 1976.

Ferngren, H.G.: Diazepam treatment for acute convulsions in children, Epilepsia **15**:27, 1974.

Gomez, M.R., and Klass, D.W.: Epilepsies of infancy and childhood, Ann. Neurol. **13**:113, 1983.

Grant, R.H.E.: The management of epilepsy, Scott. Med. J. **21**:11, 1976.

Gunn, J.C., and Fenton, G.: Epilepsy in prisons: a diagnostic survey, Br. Med. J. **4**:326, 1969.

Hauser, W.A., and Kurland, L.T.: The epidemiology of epilepsy in Rochester, Minnesota, 1935 through 1967, Epilepsia **16:**1, 1975.

King, L.N., and Young, Q.D.: Increased prevalence of seizure disorders among prisoners, JAMA **239:**2674, 1978.

Lemmen, L.J., Klassen, M., and Duiser, B.: Intravenous lidocaine in the treatment of convulsions, JAMA **239:**2025, 1978.

Lewis, J.A.: Violence and epilepsy, JAMA **232:**1165, 1975.

Menzer, L., and Sabin, T.D.: Convulsions. In Schwartz, G.R., and others, editors: Principles and practice of emergency medicine, Philadelphia, 1978, W.B. Saunders Co.

Nicol, C.F.: Status epilepticus, JAMA **234:**419, 1975.

Oppenheimer, E.Y., and Rosman, N.P.: Seizures in childhood: an approach to emergency management, Pediatr. Clin. North Am. **26:**837, 1979.

Parsonage, M.: Epilepsy, Practitioner **213:**552, 1974.

Penry, J.K., and Newmar, M.E.: The use of antiepileptic drugs, Ann. Intern. Med. **90:**207, 1979.

Penry, J.K., and Porter, R.J.: Epilepsy: mechanisms and therapy, Med. Clin. N. Am. **63:**801, 1979.

Plaa, G.L.: Acute toxicity of antiepileptic drugs, Epilepsia **16:**183, 1975.

Rapport, R.L., and others: Human epileptic brain, Arch. Neurol. **32:**549, 1975.

Roberge, R.J., and Maciera-Rodriguez, L.: Seizure-related oral lacerations: incidence and distribution, JADA **111:**279, 1985.

Sherwin, A.L., Eisen, A.A., and Sokolowski, C.D.: Anticonvulsant drugs in human epileptogenic brain, Arch. Neurol. **29:**73, 1974.

Smith, R.W., and Sipe, J.C.: The unconscious patient, seizures, and headache. In Warner, C.G., editor: Emergency care: assessment and intervention, ed. 2, St. Louis, 1978, The C.V. Mosby Co.

So, E.L., and Penry, J.K.: Epilepsy in adults, Ann. Neurol. **9:**3, 1981.

Sutherland, J.M., and Eadie, M.J.: The epilepsies: modern diagnosis and treatment, ed. 3, Edinburgh, 1980, Churchill Livingstone Inc.

Terrence, C.R., Wisotzkey, H.M., and Perper, J.A.: Unexpected unexplained death in epileptic patients, Neurology **25:**594, 1975.

Van Allen, M.W.: Epilepsy among persons convicted of crimes, JAMA **239:**2694, 1978.

Vinson, T.: Towards demythologizing epilepsy, Med. J. Aust. **2:**663, 1975.

Wannsamaker, B.B.: Problems in seizure management, Res. Staff Phys. **27:**43, 1981.

Woodbury, D.M., Penry, J.K., and Schmidt, R.P.: Antiepileptic drugs, New York, 1972, Raven Press.

22   *Drug-Related Emergencies: General Considerations*

The administration of drugs has become commonplace within the practice of dentistry. The administration of *local anesthetic* agents is considered an essential part of dental treatment whenever potentially painful procedures are contemplated. *Analgesic* medications are frequently prescribed for the relief of preexisting pain or for the alleviation of potential postoperative discomfort. *Antibiotics* are used whenever infection is present, and more and more commonly *antianxiety* drugs are being employed during all phases of the dental experience (preappointment, during the appointment, and postappointment). Other drugs are employed (Table 22-1), but the four categories mentioned above constitute the overwhelming majority of all drugs used in the practice of dentistry.

In all instances, it is hoped that whenever a drug is administered or prescribed to a dental patient a rational purpose exists for its administration. Indiscriminate use of drugs has become one of the major causes of the great increase in the number of serious incidents of drug-related, life-threatening emergencies that are being reported in the medical and dental literature. Most drug-related emergency situations are classified as one aspect of iatrogenic disease, a category that encompasses an entire spectrum of adverse effects produced unintentionally by physicians or dentists during the management of their patients.

The frequency of occurrence of adverse drug reactions (ADRs) has been reported in the medical literature. Such reactions have accounted for 3% to 20% of all hospital admissions in various reports.

An additional 5% to 40% of patients hospitalized for other reasons will experience an adverse drug reaction during their hospitalization. Furthermore, 10% to 18% of those patients admitted to the hospital because of an ADR have yet another drug reaction while in the hospital, which results in the length of hospitalization being doubled. In most cases, careful prescribing habits or care in administration of drugs might have prevented the adverse drug reaction from occurring.

Some general principles of toxicology must be stated at this time so that the following material may be better understood by the reader (see box on p. 254). *Toxicology* is defined as the study of the harmful effects of chemicals (drugs) on biologic systems. These harmful effects range from those that may prove inconsequential to the patient and are entirely reversible once the chemical is withdrawn, to those that prove uncomfortable but are not seriously harmful, to reactions that may seriously incapacitate the patient or cause death.

Whenever any drug is administered, two types of drug actions may be observed: desired drug actions—those that are clinically sought and are usually beneficial—and side effects, which are often undesirable drug actions. An example of a desired drug action is the relief of anxiety achieved through the administration of diazepam to a fearful dental patient. A side effect of diazepam that normally is not desired but is not usually harmful to the patient is drowsiness. This effect of diazepam can even prove beneficial in certain circumstances; for example, a degree of drowsiness in an ap-

Table 22-1. Drug-prescribing habits in a U.S. dental school from 1983 to 1985

Drug category		Number of prescriptions
Analgesics		5730
Nonnarcotic	1139	
Combined with codeine	4570	
Plain narcotic	21	
Antibiotics		3931
Penicillin	2977	
Erythromycin	637	
Tetracycline	187	
Cephalosporin	130	
Minor tranquilizers		219
Sedative-hypnotics		65
Other categories		1500
TOTAL PRESCRIPTIONS FILLED		11,445

Data from Department of Pharmacology, University of Southern California School of Dentistry, Los Angeles, CA.

GENERAL PRINCIPLES OF TOXICOLOGY

1. No drug ever exerts a single action.
2. No clinically useful drug is entirely devoid of toxicity.
3. Potential toxicity of a drug rests in the hands of the user.

---

prehensive patient can be desirable. However, that same degree of drowsiness while the patient is driving an automobile may prove hazardous. The side effect or undesired drug action may also prove to be harmful to the patient. Respiratory and cardiovascular depression, although rarely observed with proper administration, have been reported after diazepam administration both parenterally (IM or IV) and orally.

A general principle of toxicology is: *No drug ever exerts a single action.* All chemicals exert many actions, some desirable, others undesirable. Ideally, the right drug in the right dose will be administered by the right route to the right patient at the right time for the right reason, and it will not produce any unwanted effects. This clinical situation is rarely if ever attained, because no drug is so specific that it produces only the desired effects in all patients. *No clinically useful drug is entirely devoid of toxicity.* It must also be remembered that adverse drug reactions may occur when the wrong drug is administered to the wrong patient in the wrong dose by the wrong route at the wrong time and for the wrong reason.

PREVENTION

Although the preceding discussion may seem unduly pessimistic, it has not been presented with the intention of scaring dental practitioners away from the use of drugs for their patients. Indeed, it is my firm conviction that drug use within the practice of dentistry is absolutely essential for the safe

and proper management of many dental patients. For this reason, it is important for the doctor to become familiar with the pharmacologic properties of all drugs used in dental practice. Several excellent reference books are available that belong on the desk of the doctor as readily available sources of information. These include *Facts and Comparisons* (revised monthly), *Accepted Dental Therapeutics* (published biannually by the American Dental Association), and the American Medical Association's *AMA Drug Evaluations.*

As Pallasch (1980) has stated:

In most cases it is possible with sound clinical and pharmacological judgment to prevent serious toxicity from occurring. The aim of rational therapeutics is to maximize the therapeutic and minimize the toxic effects of a given drug.

No drug is "completely safe" or "completely harmful." All drugs are capable of producing harm if handled improperly, and conversely any drug may be handled safely if proper precautions are observed. *The potential toxicity of a drug rests in the hands of the user.*

A second factor in the safe use of drugs is consideration of the patient to whom the drug will be administered. Individuals may react differently to the same stimulus; patients therefore vary markedly in their reactions to drugs. Before administering any drug or prescribing any medication to a patient, the doctor must ask specific questions of the patient concerning past and present drug history.

Medical History Questionnaire
QUESTION 6. Have you taken any medicine or drugs during the past 2 years?

COMMENT. An accurate assessment of medications currently or recently taken is essential if potential drug interactions, as well as side effects, are to be prevented.

QUESTION 7. Are you allergic to (i.e., itching, rash, swelling of hands, feet, or eyes) or made sick by penicillin, aspirin, codeine, or any drugs or medications?

COMMENT. Common signs and symptoms of allergy are presented in this question along with the names of three common allergy-producing medications. An alleged history of allergy to any drug must lead the doctor to an in-depth dialogue history of the patient concerning the incident or incidents (see Chapters 23 and 24).

QUESTION 9. Circle any of the following which you have had or have at present:
Allergy or hives
Chemotherapy (cancer, leukemia)
Cortisone medicine

COMMENT. Affirmative responses should be followed by dialogue history to determine the drug(s) used, the reason for administration, and the reaction (if any) to the drug(s).

Dialogue History

Following an affirmative response to the question concerning allergy or adverse reaction, the doctor should seek to determine the following information from the patient concerning the incident:

What drug was used?

Was the patient taking any other medications at the time of the "allergy" or reaction?

Were vital signs recorded?

What was the time sequence of events?

Where was the patient when the reaction occurred?

What were the clinical manifestations of the reaction?

What therapy was given?

Has the patient received the offending agent, or any chemical related to it, since the incident?

As will become evident in the chapters to follow, most patients respond affirmatively to the question on allergy if they have experienced *any* adverse reaction to a drug in the past. In actuality, the incidence of allergic phenomena is quite low; however, the reporting of allergy on dental and medical records is significantly higher. The reason for this variance lies in the fact that to the patient any ADR is labeled an "allergy." The layperson is often not familiar with the classification of drug reactions. For this reason, "allergy to Novocain" and "allergy to codeine" are commonly found as answers on dental history questionnaires. Although allergy to these agents is not impossible, the reaction that did

occur probably was not allergic. Careful questioning by the doctor usually reveals that the "allergy to Novocain" was a psychogenic reaction such as the hyperventilation syndrome or vasodepressor syncope or an overdose (toxic) reaction to the agent; the "allergy to codeine" probably consisted of nausea or vomiting, which represents an unwanted side effect of the drug but is not an allergic reaction.

Questioning of the patient is vital to determine the precise nature of the reaction. However, there are times when the patient's responses are unable to remove doubt from the doctor's mind. In such cases, the doctor should attempt to locate and speak to the person who observed or managed the "allergic" reaction and attempt to determine the exact nature of the event.

Reactions that are often deemed to be adverse drug reactions may in fact be unrelated to the drug being administered. In a fascinating paper entitled "Adverse Nondrug Reactions," Reidenberg and Lowenthal (1968) demonstrated the occurrence of so-called drug side effects in persons who had not received any medications for a period of 2 weeks. Had they been receiving medications during this time, an ADR might have been reported.

It is important to keep in mind that whenever doubt remains concerning the safety of any drug (in other words, did an allergy occur?), it is prudent to assume the patient is *allergic* to that agent and avoid its use until the question can be definitively answered. This process may require referral of the patient to an allergist for further evaluation. In many instances, however, alternative agents are available for use that possess the same beneficial clinical effects but do not have the allergic potential of the drug in question. These agents should be employed until the question of allergy can be conclusively decided.

Even in the absence of a positive history of ADR in the medical history questionnaire, it is still recommended that the patient be questioned directly concerning any agent that is being considered for use. Therefore the doctor might ask the patient, "Have you ever taken Valium before?" and, if the answer is yes, "What effect did it have?" Common, proprietary names ought to be used because few patients are familiar with generic names of drugs.

In the absence of any prior adverse reaction to a medication, the doctor may feel more confident in administering the drug to the patient, always keeping in mind that adverse reactions can still arise despite prior administrations of the same agent without complication.

Care in Administration of Drugs

It is recognized that most instances of ADR are related to the administration of an overdose of a particular agent. Overdose of a drug may be an absolute overdose (too much of an agent), or a relative overdose (normal therapeutic dose for most patients that proves to be an overdose for an individual patient). Regardless of the type of overdose reaction encountered, most may be prevented through care in determination of dosage (oral or IM administration) or through the careful administration of the drug to the patient (titration with the IV and inhalation routes). Most responses to drugs are related to the dose administered (in other words, they are dose dependent); however, even minute quantities of a drug may precipitate a severe allergic reaction (anaphylaxis) in a previously sensitized individual.

The route of administration has an effect on the number and severity of ADRs. Two major routes of drug administration are considered: enteral and parenteral. Enteral routes of administration are those in which the drug is placed into the gastrointestinal tract, from which the drug is absorbed into the blood. Enteral administration includes the oral and rectal routes. Parenteral administration bypasses the gastrointestinal tract and includes intramuscular, submucosal, subcutaneous, intravenous, intraspinal, and intracapsular injections. Inhalation and topical application are other routes of administration that are considered by various authorities as either enteral or parenteral.

In general, serious drug reactions are observed more frequently when drugs are administered parenterally than by other routes. Intravenous administration is the most effective route because of rapid onset and high reliability, but it also has a great potential for serious drug reactions. However, when used properly, the intravenous route remains an important technique in dentistry. ADRs seen in enteral administration are fewer in number and usually of a less serious nature. However, the effectiveness of drugs administered enterally is greatly diminished compared to those administered parenterally.

When administering any drug to a patient, the choice of the proper route of administration must be carefully considered. Not all drugs can be administered by every route, and the degree of effectiveness varies considerably comparing one route to another with some agents. For example, 10 mg of diazepam administered intravenously usually pro-

vides profound sedation so that a fearful dental patient readily tolerates dental therapy; however, the level of sedation achieved when 10 mg of diazepam is administered orally is probably inadequate to permit comfortable dental therapy for the highly anxious patient. On the other hand, antibiotic prophylaxis for the patient with rheumatic heart disease may be achieved with either intramuscular injection or oral administration of penicillin 1 hour before therapy. In both instances, the blood level of antibiotic achieved is adequate to prevent transient bacteremia from producing subacute bacterial endocarditis. In this instance, however, the oral route is preferred over the parenteral route. As will be discussed later, penicillin has a high potential to cause allergy, and the route of administration may have significant bearing on the severity of any reaction that might occur.

A general rule in drug administration is: *If a drug is clinically effective by means of enteral administration, this route is preferred over parenteral administration.*

Most drug-related emergency situations can be prevented. Questioning the patient concerning prior exposure and reaction to a drug before administering it, carefully selecting the proper route of administration and applying the proper technique, and most importantly, being familiar with the pharmacology of all drugs used in the dental office greatly reduce the incidence of adverse drug reactions.

CLASSIFICATION

Classification of adverse drug reactions has become a task involving much confusion. In the past, a variety of terms such as side effects, adverse experience, drug-induced disease, diseases of medical progress, secondary effects, and intolerance were used. The approach today is more simple, and most reactions are classified as *adverse reactions*.

The classification proposed by Pallasch (1980), shown in Table 22-2, represents a simplified approach to the problem of classifying adverse drug reactions. In this classification there are three major methods by which drugs may produce adverse reactions: (1) a direct extension of a drug's pharmacologic actions, (2) a deleterious effect on a chemically, genetically, metabolically, or morphologically altered recipient (the patient), and (3) initiation of an immune (allergic) response.

Most drug reactions are not life threatening. There are, however, several potential responses that are life-threatening situations requiring immediate effective management if the patient is to fully recover. These include the overdose reaction (direct extension of the pharmacologic activity of the drug) and the allergic response. Because of the nature of these responses and their importance to the dental practitioner, they are discussed in greater detail in subsequent chapters.

In any discussion of drug-related or drug-induced emergencies there are normally three situations that are of immediate importance to the dental practitioner: overdose, allergy, and idiosyncrasy. Idiosyncrasy is discussed in this chapter; overdose and allergy are discussed more fully in later chapters but are also discussed briefly in this chapter. Approximately 85% of ADRs result from the pharmacologic effects of the drug, whereas 15% of ADRs result from immunologic reactions.

Overdose Reaction

Overdose reaction refers to symptoms resulting from an absolute or relative overadministration of a drug that produces elevated blood levels of the agent. Clinical manifestations of overdose are related to a direct extension of the normal pharmacologic actions of the agent. In therapeutic doses barbiturates, for example, produce mild depression of the central nervous system, which results in sedation or hypnosis (desired effects). Barbiturate overdose produces a more profound depression of the CNS with possible respiratory and cardiovascular depression. Local anesthetics are also CNS depressants. When administered prop-

Table 22-2. Classification of adverse drug reactions

Toxicity resulting from direct extension of pharmacologic effects

Side effects
Abnormal dosage (overdosage)
Local toxic effects

Toxicity resulting from altered recipient (patient)

Presence of pathology
Emotional disturbances
Genetic aberrations (idiosyncrasy)
Teratogenicity
Drug-drug interactions

Toxicity resulting from drug allergy

From Pallasch, T.J.: Pharmacology for dental students and practitioners, Philadelphia, 1980, Lea & Febiger.

erly and in therapeutic doses, little or no evidence of CNS depression is evident; however, with increased blood levels signs and symptoms of selective CNS depression are noted. These reactions and their management are discussed in Chapter 23.

Allergy

Allergy may be defined as a hypersensitive state acquired through exposure to a particular allergen (a substance capable of inducing allergy), reexposure to which brings about a heightened capacity to react. Clinically there are a variety of ways in which allergy expresses itself. These include drug fever, angioedema, urticaria, dermatitis, depression of the blood-forming organs, photosensitivity, and anaphylaxis (an acute systemic reaction resulting in respiratory difficulty and cardiovascular collapse). Certain drugs are more likely to cause allergic reactions than others, and allergic reaction is possible with any substance.

In contrast to the overdose reaction, in which clinical manifestations are related directly to the pharmacologic properties of the causative agent, the response observed clinically in the allergic reaction is always produced by the exaggerated response of the immune system of the body. The degree of this response determines the acuteness of the reaction. Therefore allergic responses to a barbiturate, a local anesthetic, and an antibiotic are produced by the same mechanism and may appear similar clinically. All require the same basic management, whereas overdose reactions to these three agents are quite different clinically and require entirely different modes of management.

Idiosyncratic Reaction

Idiosyncrasy, or idiosyncratic reactions, may be defined as those ADRs that cannot be explained by any known pharmacologic or biochemical mechanism. Another definition considers an idiosyncratic reaction to be any ADR that is neither an overdose nor an allergic reaction. An example of idiosyncratic reaction is CNS stimulation (excitation, agitation) produced following the administration of a known CNS-depressant agent such as a barbiturate.

Idiosyncratic reactions span an extremely wide range of clinical expression. Virtually any type of reaction may be seen; for example, reactions include depression following administration of a stimulant, stimulation following administration of a depressant, and hyperpyrexia (markedly elevated body temperature) following administration of a muscle relaxant (like succinylcholine). It is virtually impossible to predict which persons will experience such reactions or indeed the nature of the resulting idiosyncratic reactions.

Management of idiosyncracy

Because of the unpredictability of the nature and occurrence of idiosyncratic reactions, their management is, of necessity, symptomatic. Of primary importance in the management of these situations are the essentials of basic life support: maintenance of the airway, ventilation, and circulation. Should seizures occur, treatment consists of the procedures described in Chapter 21. Prevention of injury and airway management are the primary considerations. Knowledge of the basic management of the various categories of emergency situations presented in this text will enable the doctor to adequately manage the majority of idiosyncratic reactions.

It is thought today that virtually all instances of idiosyncratic reaction have an underlying genetic mechanism. These genetic aberrations remain undetected until the individual receives a specific drug, such as succinylcholine, which then produces its bizarre (nonpharmacologic) clinical expression.

DRUG-RELATED EMERGENCIES

Before discussing the drugs used in dental practice and the major adverse reactions associated with each of them, it is important to discuss a factor responsible for more drug-related emergencies than any other. In the preceding discussion of ADRs all responses were related directly to the action of a drug on a biologic system. However, many drug reactions occur *in association with* the administration of a drug but are not produced by the action of the drug on the body. Probably the major cause of drug-related emergency situations within the dental office is the administration of local anesthetics. Although it is possible for ADRs to occur from the action of local anesthetics, most reactions observed are related to the *act of administering* the local anesthetic. Psychogenic reactions, seen clinically as vasodepressor syncope and the hyperventilation syndrome, are the most common forms of drug-related emergency observed in dental practice and result from stress produced by the injection technique, not by the local anesthetic itself. Psychogenic reactions may also be observed with the parenteral administration of any drug. Whenever a needle and syringe are involved, the potential for a psy-

chogenic reaction is increased. It is rare to observe a psychogenic reaction with an enterally administered drug.

DRUG USE IN DENTISTRY

The dental profession employs four major categories of drugs to the virtual exclusion of all others in the management of patients. Table 22-1 listed the drug-prescribing habits of faculty members and students at the University of Southern California School of Dentistry over a 3-year period. The major categories of prescription drugs used in dentistry include analgesics, antibiotics, and antianxiety drugs. To these categories a fourth, local anesthetics, must be added. Local anesthetics are the most commonly employed drugs and are routinely administered whenever a dental procedure appears capable of producing an unacceptable degree of discomfort.

Examples of commonly prescribed or administered drugs and their potential adverse drug reactions are discussed in the following pages. It is recommended that the reader also consult a textbook on pharmacology when considering the use of any drug.

Local Anesthetics

Local anesthetics, the most widely used drugs in dentistry, have also proved to be among the safest agents available when properly administered. Table 22-3 lists the most commonly used local anesthetics in the United States, Canada, Europe, and Asia today. Lidocaine, mepivacaine, prilocaine, bupivacaine, etidocaine, and articaine are local anesthetics of the amide group, whereas benzocaine, propoxycaine, and procaine are agents of the ester group. Before lidocaine's introduction, the first

Table 22-3. Commonly used local anesthetics in dentistry

Generic name	Proprietary name(s)	Group
Articaine	Ultracaine	Amide
Benzocaine	—	Ester
Bupivacaine	Marcaine	Amide
Etidocaine	Duranest	Amide
Mepivacaine	Carbocaine, Isocaine, Polocaine	Amide
Prilocaine	Citanest	Amide
Procaine	Novocaine	Ester
Propoxycaine	Ravocaine	Ester

amide type of local anesthetic, in 1944, the esters were the most commonly employed agents. Although highly effective drugs, the ester type local anesthetics possess a significant allergy-producing potential. This potential was one of the reasons for the development and introduction of the amide type of local anesthetics. Allergy to these local anesthetic agents, although not impossible, is extremely rare. Reports occasionally appear in the medical and dental literature of "allergy" to an amide local anesthetic. However, with careful documentation most incidents prove to be psychogenic, overdose, or idiosyncratic reactions or are found to be the result of an allergy to some other component of the solution injected. A more detailed discussion of local anesthetic allergy is presented in Chapter 24.

The most commonly observed ADRs to local anesthetic agents of the amide type are those associated with injection of the drugs; psychogenic responses such as vasodepressor syncope and the hyperventilation syndrome comprise the greatest number of local anesthetic reactions observed today. The next most common cause of adverse response to local anesthetics is the overdose reaction, which in many instances is produced by a relative overdose (that is, caused by inadvertent intravascular injection) of the agent rather than by absolute overdose (that is, caused by injection of too great a total dose).

Topically applied local anesthetic agents are also capable of producing adverse reactions. Psychogenic responses are rare with these agents; indeed, topical anesthetics are usually employed to minimize the occurrence of psychogenic responses during the administration of local anesthetics. However, two adverse reactions to topical anesthetics are observed with a disturbing degree of frequency. The first adverse reaction results because most topical anesthetics contain local anesthetics of the ester type (for example, benzocaine) in addition to a variety of other ingredients (for example, methylparaben), which possess a relatively high allergenicity. Allergic responses, such as erythema or angioedema of mucous membranes and lips, are not uncommon when these agents are employed. The second adverse reaction from topically applied local anesthetics is the overdose reaction. This reaction is related to the extremely rapid absorption of some of these agents through the mucous membranes of the oral cavity with a consequent rapid elevation of local anesthetic blood level.

I strongly recommend the use of topical anes-

thetics before administering any local anesthetic by injection. The benefit to be gained clearly outweighs the risk. Safer use of these agents may be achieved through the use of topical anesthetics of the amide type and judicious administration of topical anesthetics to mucous membranes. A topical anesthetic can be administered by spray in a metered dose form (Fig. 22-1).

Antibiotics

Antibiotics are another frequently prescribed category of drugs in dentistry. They are properly employed in the treatment of an established active infection; they should not be prescribed prophylactically to "prevent" a possible infection from developing (except in special circumstances such as

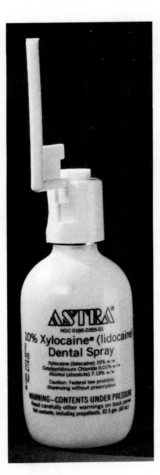

Fig. 22-1. Topical anesthetic spray, which delivers a metered dose of 10 mg with each application. High blood levels of anesthetics may be avoided through this controlled administration.

the prevention of bacterial endocarditis). Because of the potential development of resistant bacterial strains and of allergy to these agents, they should be used only when indicated. As a group, antibiotics possess the lowest incidence of adverse side effects. This fact has probably been responsible for the current overadministration of these agents with the subsequent development of resistant bacterial strains (for example, penicillin-resistant gonococcus). There is also increasing trepidation expressed by medical personnel when administering parenteral antibiotics because of their high allergic potential.

Within the practice of dentistry there is little call for the parenteral administration of antibiotics. The blood levels of drugs and therapeutic efficacy should be much the same with both parenterally and orally administered agents if proper attention is paid to dosage and sequence of administration. A major advantage of the oral form of administration is the decreased likelihood of adverse reactions. If these reactions should occur, it is probable that they will be less acute than those following parenteral

administration of the same drug, although serious reactions can develop in either case. If the parenteral administration of antibiotics (particularly penicillin) is required, I strongly recommend that the medication NOT be administered in the dental office, but rather that the patient be sent to the emergency room of a nearby hospital where the drug can be administered parenterally and the patient kept for observation for approximately 1 hour. Table 22-4 lists commonly used antibiotics and their usual oral dose. The major ADR for which the doctor must prepare when antibiotics are administered is allergy.

Analgesics

Drugs for the relief of pain comprise a significant portion of prescriptions written by dentists. Two major categories of analgesics are considered: mild analgesics (nonnarcotic) and strong analgesics (narcotics).

Aspirin and codeine are the most commonly prescribed analgesics. The major adverse effects of aspirin include a high allergic potential, with symp-

Table 22-4. Commonly used antibiotics in dentistry

Generic name	Proprietary names	Dose*
Penicillin G	Pentids Kesso-pen Pfizerpen	400,000 to 1.2 million units every 4-6 hours
Penicillin V (phenoxymethyl penicillin)	Compocillin V V-Cillin Pen·Vee K Ledercillin	250-500 mg every 4-6 hours
Ampicillin	Amcill Polycillin Principen Totacillin	250-500 mg every 4-6 hours
Erythromycin	E-Mycin Ilotycin Erythrocin Pediamycin Ilosone	250-500 mg every 6 hours
Clindamycin	Cleocin	300 mg every 6 hours
Cephalosporin	Keflex Velosef Anspor	250-500 mg every 6 hours

*The dosage forms indicated are those for a normal healthy 70 kg male. Patient response to these doses may vary; therefore the reader is advised to consult the drug insert for specific prescribing information before the administration of any drug.

toms ranging from urticaria to bronchospasm to fatal anaphylaxis (see Chapter 24) and overdose (salicylism).

Codeine is a narcotic analgesic; however, it is a mild analgesic when compared to narcotics such as morphine and meperidine. Although allergy to codeine may occur, its incidence is low. The primary ADRs to codeine are nausea, vomiting, drowsiness, and constipation. With a 60 mg oral dose, approximately 22% of patients become nauseated. Significantly lower percentages of nausea are found with decreased doses of codeine (30 mg). Codeine may produce the same clinical signs and symptoms of overdose as other, more potent narcotics (respiratory and cardiovascular depression). Thirty milligrams (orally) appears to be a highly effective analgesic dose of codeine and is associated with a minimal incidence of adverse reactions.

Propoxyphene hydrochloride, more commonly known by one of its brand names, Darvon, is useful in the management of milder forms of oral pain. Major adverse side effects of propoxyphene include nausea and vomiting, sedation, dizziness, and drowsiness. Allergy and overdose have been reported. The incidence of allergy from propoxyphene is much lower than the incidence of allergy from aspirin. Overdose of propoxyphene produces signs and symptoms similar to those seen in narcotic overdose—respiratory and cardiovascular depression.

Meperidine (Demerol) and other narcotic agonists are occasionally employed in dentistry for relief of more intense pain. As with codeine, the major ADRs observed are more annoying than life threatening. Nausea and vomiting, dizziness, ataxia, sweating, and orthostatic hypotension are the most frequently noted side effects. Overdose may occur and, as with all narcotics, results in respiratory and cardiovascular depression. Allergy, though possible, is rare. Table 22-5 lists commonly prescribed analgesic drugs.

Antianxiety Drugs

The use of drugs for the relief of anxiety during all phases of dental therapy has increased greatly in recent years. Although the enteral routes were almost the exclusive modes of administration in the past and are still commonly employed today, the current trend in management of anxiety in dentistry is toward parenteral administration of antianxiety agents. With this trend has come a greater potential for the development of ADRs because of the much greater effectiveness of parenterally administered drugs. Although a wide variety of drugs are available for use in the relief of anxiety in dental patients, the most frequently employed agents are

Table 22-5. Commonly used analgesic drugs in dentistry

Generic name	Proprietary name(s)	Dose*
Acetylsalicylic acid (aspirin)	Numerous	600 mg every 4 hours
Acetaminophen	Tylenol Datril Phenaphen	325-650 mg every 4 hours
Propoxyphene	Darvon Dolene Darvon-N Doxaphene	65 mg every 4 hours
Pentazocine	Talwin	50 mg every 3-4 hours
Meperidine	Demerol	50-100 mg every 6-8 hours
Oxycodone	Percodan Percocet	1 tablet every 6 hours (contains oxycodine and aspirin)
Ibuprofen	Motrin	400-600 mg every 4-6 hours

*The dosage forms indicated are those for a normal healthy 70 kg male. Patient response to these doses may vary; therefore the reader is advised to consult the drug insert for specific prescribing information before prescribing any drug.

barbiturates (administered orally and parenterally), nonbarbiturate antianxiety agents (administered orally and parenterally), and inhalation agents (primarily nitrous oxide and oxygen).

Barbiturates

Barbiturates are the oldest group of antianxiety drugs available (excluding alcohol). Examples of barbiturates used in the dental office are given in Table 22-6. Effective orally and parenterally, the barbiturate sedative-hypnotics were the most frequently prescribed medications in dentistry for the management of fear and anxiety until the introduction of the benzodiazepines in the 1960s. Undesirable side effects are common following barbiturate administration. One of the most annoying side effects of barbiturate administration is the "hangover" effect, consisting of lassitude, inebriation, and vertigo. Allergy to barbiturates may also occur and represents an absolute contraindication to the use of *any* barbiturate. Probably the major factor behind the growing disenchantment with barbiturates, however, is their potential for overdose, both accidental and intentional. They are the leading drug cause of suicide (carbon monoxide poisoning being the leading mode of suicide). Overdose of barbiturates causes central nervous system depression to the point that respiratory function is depressed and eventually ceases. Cardiovascular and central nervous system collapse follow, leading to death unless basic and advanced life support procedures are initiated immediately.

Nonbarbiturates

Nonbarbiturate antianxiety agents were developed in the hope of managing anxiety effectively without the unpleasant and dangerous drug reactions associated with barbiturates. The major nonbarbiturate antianxiety and sedative-hypnotic agents are listed in Table 22-6. The benzodiazepines represented a major advance in the management of anxiety; the first benzodiazepine, chlordiazepoxide (Librium), was introduced in 1960. Another benzodiazepine, diazepam (Valium), is among the most prescribed drugs in the Western world and is one of the most effective and most widely used antianxiety agents in dentistry. It is administered orally and intravenously. Benzodiazepines are a decided improvement over barbiturates because of the remarkably low incidence of side effects and overdose reactions observed with their administration. Overdose to benzodiazepines, even when administered intravenously, usually consists of oversedation, drowsiness, and ataxia. Respiratory depression, although possible, is infrequent. Flurazepam (Dalmane) and triazolam (Halcion) are benzodiazepines that are marketed as nonbarbiturate sedative-hypnotics. They are highly effective as substitutes for the barbiturates when used as "sleeping pills."

Table 22-6. Commonly used antianxiety drugs in dentistry

Drug group	Proprietary name(s)	Dose (oral)*
Barbiturates		
Hexobarbital	Presed	250-500 mg
	Sombulex	
Secobarbital	Seconal	100 mg
Pentobarbital	Nembutal	50-100 mg
Benzodiazepines		
Diazepam	Valium	5-10 mg
Flurazepam	Dalmane	15-30 mg
Oxazepam	Serax	15-30 mg
Triazolam	Halcion	0.25-0.5 mg
Others		
Chloral hydrate	Noctec	500-1000 mg
	Kessodrate	
	Felsules	
Hydroxyzine	Atarax	50-100 mg
	Vistaril	
Promethazine	Pherergan	25-50 mg

*The dosage forms indicated are those for oral administration to a normal healthy 70 kg male. Patient response to these doses may vary; therefore the reader is advised to consult the drug insert for specific prescribing information before prescribing any drug.

Inhalation sedation

Nitrous oxide and oxygen inhalation sedation is another method of anxiety control that has attracted increasing attention among those in the dental profession. Discovered in 1786 and first employed clinically in 1844, nitrous oxide is a highly effective antianxiety agent that, when employed properly, is remarkably free of unpleasant and potentially dangerous adverse reactions. Unwanted side effects from nitrous oxide and oxygen include nausea, vomiting, and oversedation. If inhalation sedation is administered with less than 20% oxygen, unconsciousness may ensue with cellular damage occurring from hypoxia but not from nitrous oxide. With the development of a new generation of inhalation sedation machines and an increasing awareness on the part of dental educators and manufacturers, safety features have been incorporated into current sedation units that make it extremely difficult to administer less than 20% oxygen to a patient receiving nitrous oxide and oxygen.

Allergy to nitrous oxide has never been reported. Overdose consists of oversedation, which may manifest itself as a loss of consciousness. Management of this situation consists of decreasing the percentage of nitrous oxide and increasing the percentage of oxygen and employing the steps of basic life support until the patient regains consciousness.

Table 22-7 summarizes the most commonly used drug categories in dentistry and lists their most likely adverse reactions. It must be remembered that all drugs are capable of producing virtually any of the three adverse reactions (allergy, overdose, and idiosyncrasy).

Table 22-7. Common drugs and most likely adverse drug reactions (ADRs)

Drug	Allergy	Overdose	Side effects
Local anesthetics			
Esters	Common, especially with topical anesthetics; manifested as localized erythema and edema	Unlikely with esters unless genetic deficiency is present (for example, atypical pseudocholinesterase)	Rare; sedation (drowsiness) most common
Amides	Rare, virtually nonexistent; most clinical reports prove alleged allergy to be overdose or allergy to other component of cartridge	Most common ADR; CNS depression; manifested as drowsiness, tremor, tonic-clonic seizures	Rare; sedation most common
Antibiotics			
	Common; high allergic potential to many antibiotics; manifested clinically over entire range of allergic phenomena	Rare; for penicillin, virtually nonexistent	Rare; gastrointestinal upset is most common
Analgesics			
Nonnarcotic	Common; high allergic potential (aspirin)	Common; salicylism	Common
Narcotic	Uncommon	Common; manifested as CNS depression (drowsiness), respiratory depression	Most common ADR; manifested clinically as nausea/vomiting, orthostatic hypotension
Antianxiety agents			
Barbiturates	Uncommon	Most common ADR; CNS depression; manifested as oversedation, loss of consciousness, respiratory and cardiovascular depression	Common; "barbiturate hangover"
Benzodiazepines	Uncommon	Uncommon; CNS depression; manifested as oversedation	Most common side effect is drowsiness
Nitrous oxide	Rare, to date never reported	Common; manifested as oversedation	Most common ADR; manifested as nausea/vomiting

BIBLIOGRAPHY

Adatia, A.K.: Intravascular injection of local anesthetics, Br. Dent. J. **138**:328, 1975.

Adriani, J.: Etiology and management of adverse reactions to local anesthetics, Int. Anesthesiol. Clin. **10**:127, 1972.

Aldrete, J.A., and Johnson, D.A.: Evaluation of intracutaneous testing for investigation of allergy to local anesthetic agents, Anesth. Analg. (Cleve) **49**:173, 1970.

Bateman, P.P.: Multiple allergies to local anesthetics including prilocaine, Med. J. Aust. **2**:449, 1974.

Caranasos, G.J., Stewart, R.B., and Cluff, L.E.: Drug-induced illness leading to hospitalization, JAMA **228**:713, 1974.

Caranasos, G.J.: Drug reactions. In Schwartz, G.R., and others, editors: Principles and practice of emergency medicine, Philadelphia, 1978, W.B. Saunders Co.

Caranasos, G.J., and others: Drug associated deaths in hospital inpatients, Arch. Intern. Med. **136**:872, 1976.

Dougherty, R.J.: Propoxyphene overdose deaths, JAMA **235**:2716, 1976.

Girwood, R.H.: Death after taking medicaments, Br. Med. J. **1**:501, 1974.

Glauda, N.M., Henefer, E.P., and Supur, S.: Nonfatal anaphylaxis caused by penicillin: report of case, J. Am. Dent. Assoc. **90**:159, 1975.

Hoddinott, B.C., and others: Drug reactions and errors in administration on a medical ward, Can. Med. Assoc. J. **97**:1001, 1967.

Hurwitz, N.: Admissions to hospitals due to drugs, Br. Med. J. **1**:539, 1969.

Hurwitz, N., and Wade, O.L.: Intensive hospital monitoring of adverse reactions to drugs, Br. Med. J. **1**:531, 1969.

Irey, N.S.: Adverse drug reactions and death, JAMA **236**:575, 1976.

Koch-Weser, J.: Fatal reactions to drug therapy, N. Engl. J. Med. **291**:302, 1974.

Kramer, H.S., and Mitton, V.A.: Complications of local anesthesia, Dent. Clin. North Am. **17**:443, 1973.

Lear, E., and others: Atypical pseudocholinesterase: a clinical report, Anesth. Analg. **55**:243, 1976.

Levy, M., and others: Adverse reactions to drugs in hospitalized patients: a comparative study, Isr. J. Med. Sci. **9**:614, 1973.

McKenney, J.M., and Harrison, W.L.: Drug-related hospital admissions, Am. J. Hosp. Pharm. **33**:792, 1976.

Michel, R.G., Hudson, W.R., and Pope, T.H.: Angioneurotic edema, Arch. Otolaryngol. **101**:544, 1975.

Miescher, P.A.: Drug induced thrombocytopenia, Semin. Hematol. **10**:311, 1973.

Miller, R.M.: Hospital admissions due to adverse drug reactions, Arch. Intern. Med. **134**:219, 1974.

Pallasch, T.J.: Pharmacology for dental students and practitioners, Philadelphia, 1980, Lea & Febiger.

Prince, L.C., Garry, P.J., and Lubin, A.H.: Silent cholinesterase gene—report of a family, Anesthesiology **37**:652, 1972.

Ravindranathan, N.: Allergic reaction to lignocaine, Br. Dent. J. **138**:101, 1975.

Reidenberg, M.M., and Lowenthal, D.T.: Adverse nondrug reactions, N. Engl. J. Med. **279**:678, 1968.

Royal, B.W.: Monitoring adverse reactions to drugs, WHO Chron. **27**:469, 1973.

Schwartz, H.C.: Allergic reaction to lignocaine, Br. Dent. J. **138**:101, 1975.

Shapiro, S., and others: Fatal drug reactions among medical in-patients, JAMA **216**:467, 1971.

Smith, J.M.: Incidence of atopic disease, Med. Clin. North Am. **58**:3, 1974.

Spark, R.P.: Fatal anaphylaxis to oral penicillin, Am. J. Clin. Pathol. **56**:406, 1971.

Spear, P.W., and Protass, L.M.: Barbiturate poisoning—an endemic disease, Med. Clin. North Am. **57**:1471, 1973.

Speer, F.: Aspirin allergy: a clinical study, South. Med. J. **68**:314, 1975.

Stetler, C.J.: Drug-induced illness, JAMA **229**:1403, 1974.

Vakil, B.J., and others: Intense surveillance of adverse drug reactions, J. Clin. Pharmacol. **15**:435, 1975.

Wells, J.H.: Understanding atopic syndromes, Postgrad. Med. **58**:67, 1975.

23 Drug Overdose Reactions

Drug overdose reaction has previously been defined as those clinical signs and symptoms resulting from overly high blood levels of a drug in various tissues and organs. Overdose reactions are the most common of all ADRs, accounting for up to 85% in some estimates. Overdose reactions represent a direct extension of the normal pharmacologic properties of the involved drug.

For an overdose to occur, the drug in question must gain access to the circulatory system in quantities sufficient to produce adverse effects on various tissues of the body. Under normal circumstances there is a constant absorption of a drug from its site of administration (digestive tract, muscles, and so on) into the circulation and a steady removal of the same agent from the blood as it undergoes redistribution (for example, to skeletal muscle) and biotransformation (metabolism, detoxification) in other parts of the body (primarily the liver). In this situation, overly high blood levels of drugs rarely occur (Fig. 23-1). However, there are a number of ways in which this "steady state" may be altered, leading to either a rapid elevation in blood level (producing a sudden onset of overdose reaction) or to a more gradual elevation of blood level (producing a slower onset of symptoms). In either case, *an overdose reaction is caused by a blood (plasma) level of a drug sufficiently high to produce adverse effects in various organs and tissues of the body.* The reaction continues only as long as the blood level of the agent remains above the threshold for overdose.

In dentistry there are four commonly employed categories of drugs with significant overdose potential: local anesthetics, vasoconstrictors (such as epinephrine), sedative-hypnotics, and narcotic analgesics. Of these, the local anesthetics are by far the most commonly used. Overdose reaction to this group may be classified as a seizure reaction; the most commonly observed overdose reaction to the sedative-hypnotics and narcotic analgesics is respiratory depression. Epinephrine, or vasoconstrictor, overdose causes an "anxiety" reaction with an increase in blood pressure and heart rate.

Because the usual route of administration, the nature of overdose reaction, and the management of the reaction differ considerably in these groups, the following discussion is divided into three sections: overdose reaction from (1) administration of local anesthetics, (2) vasoconstricting agents, and (3) sedative-hypnotic and narcotic analgesic medications.

LOCAL-ANESTHETIC OVERDOSE REACTION
General Considerations

Local anesthetics are the most commonly employed drugs in dentistry. The number of local anesthetic cartridges injected by dentists in the United States is conservatively estimated at 6 million cartridges per week, or in excess of 300 million per year. In actuality, the numbers probably greatly exceed this figure. In addition, local anesthetics are administered by many physicians and podiatrists. With the administration of this number of local anesthetics per year, it is quite remarkable that more ADRs attributed to these agents are not reported. In all probability, however, a great many reactions go unreported because they were transitory and innocuous enough to be missed by the doctor or not deemed worthy of reporting. As discussed in the preceding chapter, the most com-

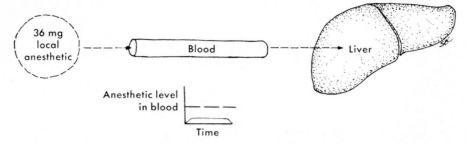

Fig. 23-1. Under normal conditions there is a constant absorption of local anesthetic from the site of deposition into the cardiovascular system and a constant removal of the agent from the blood by the liver. Local anesthetic levels in the blood remain low. (From Malamed, S.F.: Handbook of local anesthesia, ed. 2, St. Louis, 1986, The C.V. Mosby Co.)

monly observed and reported reactions to local anesthetics are normally labelled "allergic" reactions; however, after careful scrutiny most of these are determined to have been either overdose reactions or (more likely) psychogenic responses.

Predisposing Factors

Overdose reaction to a local anesthetic is related to the blood level of active local anesthetic agent occurring in certain tissues after its administration. There are many factors that can have a profound effect on the rate at which this blood level is elevated and the length of time it remains elevated. Presence of these factors predisposes the patient to the development of overdose reaction. The first group of factors is related to the patient; the second group is related to the agent and the area into which it is administered.

Patient factors

Predisposing patient factors are those factors that alter the reaction of various individuals to the same dose of drugs. This is commonly referred to as biologic or individual variation. The normal distribution curve exemplifies this variable reaction to drugs (Fig. 23-2). It explains the unpredictability observed in all drug administration and the fact that drug effects vary even in the same patient on different occasions. Predisposing patient factors that affect drug activity include age, body weight, the presence of pathology, genetics, mental attitude and environment, and sex.

Age. At either end of the age spectrum, individuals experience a higher incidence of ADRs. There are many reasons for this finding, several of which are relevant to this discussion. The functions of

absorption, metabolism, and excretion of drugs may be imperfectly developed (as in younger age groups) or may be diminished (as in older age groups). Higher blood levels may occur because of the individual's inability to transform the local anesthetic into an inactive product, this in turn resulting from undeveloped or decreased liver function. Or the individual may be unable to excrete active local anesthetic because of renal dysfunction. In geriatric patients (ages 61 to 71 years) the half-life of lidocaine was shown to be increased by approximately 70% over a control group (ages 22 to 26 years) (Nation, R.L., and others, 1977). As a general rule of thumb, doses of medications are decreased in patients under the age of 6 and over the age of 65.

Body weight. In general, the greater the body weight of the individual (within limits), the greater the dose of a drug that can be tolerated before overdose reactions occur. This is primarily related to the greater blood volume in larger (heavier, but nonobese) individuals. This relationship does not apply to obese persons compared to thin patients, since the blood supply to fat is quite sparse compared to that supplying muscle. Therefore a 200 pound obese patient cannot tolerate the same dose of local anesthetic as safely as a 200 pound muscular individual can. Since most drugs are distributed evenly throughout the entire body, the larger the individual, the lower the blood level of the agent per milliliter of blood. For example, a dose of a local anesthetic administered to a 67.5 kg (150 pound) adult produces a lower blood level than the same dose administered to a 22.5 kg (50 pound) child. Drug doses are normally calculated on the basis of milligram of drug per kilogram or pound of

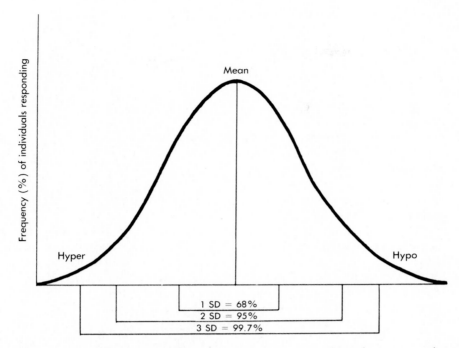

Fig. 23-2. Normal (bell-shaped) distribution curve. For any given drug, approximately 68% of patients experience desirable clinical effects with the usual adult dose; 95% exhibit desirable effects with a slightly lower or higher dose range. A small percentage of patients are hyporesponsive (right side of curve), requiring doses in excess of "normal" before clinically desirable results appear. Of more importance, however, is the small group of hyperresponsive individuals (left side of curve), who exhibit clinically desirable results at lower than "normal" dose levels. Drug overdose is more likely to develop in these patients. (From Pallasch, T.J.: Pharmacology for dental students and practitioners, Philadelphia, 1980, Lea & Febiger.)

body weight. Such considerations are especially important in pediatric patients. One of the major factors involved in local anesthetic overdose in the past was a lack of consideration of this extremely important factor.

Dosages calculated in terms of milligram per pound or per kilogram of body weight are based on the reaction of the "normal responding patient," which is calculated from the responses of thousands of patients. Individual patient responses to drug administration, however, may demonstrate significant variation. The "normal distribution curve" (Fig. 23-2) illustrates this fact. The "usual" blood level of lidocaine required to induce seizure activity is 7.5 μg of lidocaine per milliliter of blood (μg/ml) in the brain. Hyporesponding patients may not demonstrate seizures until a significantly higher brain blood level is reached, whereas others, termed hyperresponders, may exhibit seizures at a brain blood level of lidocaine considerably below 7.5 μg/ml.

Presence of pathology. The presence of preexisting disease may affect the ability of the body to biotransform a drug into an inactive product. As is explained in a later section, most local anesthetics are biotransformed in the liver into breakdown products, with a small percentage of the drug excreted unchanged through the kidneys. It is evident that liver dysfunction impairs the ability of the individual to break down and excrete the local anesthetic agent, leading to an increase in the blood level of the drug with greater likelihood of overdose reaction occurring. However, renal dysfunction appears to have little effect on local anesthetic toxicity.

Patients with cardiovascular disease, especially congestive heart failure, demonstrate blood levels of local anesthetics approximately twice those found in healthy patients receiving the same dose. This is a result of several factors, including a reduced blood volume for drug distribution and a diminished hepatic blood flow secondary to low cardiac output.

Pulmonary disease states, especially those associated with CO_2 retention, lead to an increased risk of local anesthetic overdose. Carbon dioxide retention ($>Paco_2$) leads to respiratory acidosis, which is accompanied by a decrease in local anesthetic seizure threshold.

Genetics. It has been reported with increasing frequency that certain individuals possess genetic deficiencies that alter their responses to certain drugs. A genetic deficiency in the enzyme serum cholinesterase is an important example. This enzyme, produced in the liver, circulates in the blood and is responsible for the biotransformation of two important drugs: succinylcholine and the ester type of local anesthetics.

Succinylcholine is a short-acting neuromuscular blocking agent frequently used during the induction of general anesthesia for production of skeletal muscle relaxation and respiratory arrest during intubation. In normal individuals the action of succinylcholine lasts approximately 3 minutes, the drug being metabolized by serum cholinesterase. In persons with deficient (or atypical) serum cholinesterase, however, succinylcholine is biotransformed at an extremely slow rate, with the ensuing period of apnea persisting for unacceptably long periods of time (several hours). This same enzyme is responsible for the biotransformation of the ester type of local anesthetics (Table 22-3). In the presence of atypical or deficient serum cholinesterase, the blood level of the ester type local anesthetic continues to increase along with a greatly increased likelihood of an overdose reaction.

Mental attitude and environment. The psychologic attitude of a patient greatly influences the ultimate effect of a drug. This factor is of greater importance in the use of sedative-hypnotic and narcotic analgesic drugs; what a patient expects a drug to do greatly affects the clinical efficacy of that agent. This expectation of a drug's action is termed the placebo response, and its proper use is of great benefit to the doctor.

In regard to local anesthetics, it has been shown that the local-anesthetic seizure threshold is decreased in patients who are overly stressed (for example, frightened). In addition, a patient's psychologic attitude affects the response to various stimuli. All dental personnel have encountered the apprehensive individual who overreacts to a stimulus, experiencing "pain" when gentle pressure is applied to tissues.

Table 23-1. Comparison of physicochemical properties of local anesthetics

	Lipid/ buffer partition coefficient	Protein binding (%)	Relative vasodilating values (lidocaine = 1.0)
Procaine	0.6	5.8	>2.5
Prilocaine	0.8	55	0.5
Mepivacaine	1.0	77	0.8
Lidocaine	2.9	64	1.0
Bupivacaine	28	95	2.5
Etidocaine	141	94	2.5

Sex. Differences between men and women regarding drug distribution, response, and metabolism have been described in animals but are not of major importance in humans. The only instance of sexual difference in the human species occurs in the pregnant woman. During pregnancy, renal function may be disturbed, and this may lead to impaired excretion of certain drugs and their accumulation in the blood, resulting in possible overdose. Although highly unlikely, this disturbance of renal function is a potential cause of local-anesthetic overdose.

Clinical reports have demonstrated that the incidence of ADRs is higher in women than in men. This sexual difference has not yet been explained.

Drug factors

The second group of predisposing factors in the development of overdose reactions relates to the drugs themselves and to their site of administration. Included are the vasoactivity of the drug, dose, route of administration, speed of administration, vascularity of site of administration, and the presence of vasoconstrictors.

Vasoactivity of drug. Several factors relating to the physicochemical properties of local anesthetics are important in determining whether the blood level of an agent following injection will be high or low. These include lipid solubility, protein binding, and vascular activity.

Agents that are more lipid soluble and more highly protein bound, such as etidocaine and bupivacaine, are retained by the fat and tissues at the injection site and therefore exhibit a slower net systemic absorption rate compared to agents such as lidocaine and mepivacaine. This slower systemic absorption rate is associated with increased margins of safety for these agents. The rate of absorption of local anesthetics also depends on their direct actions on blood vessels at the site of injection. All local anesthetics, with the notable exception of cocaine, have vasodilating properties. Bupivacaine and etidocaine produce more vasodilation than do prilocaine, lidocaine, and mepivacaine. Vascular regulation of absorption appears to be a more important factor for the shorter-acting agents such as lidocaine, mepivacaine, and prilocaine, whereas tissue binding is of greater significance for the longer-acting agents, bupivacaine and etidocaine. Table 23-1 compares the lipid solubility, protein binding, and vasodilating properties of commonly used local anesthetics.

Dose of drug. For many years it was thought that the concentration of an injected solution was of major importance in determining overdose potential, even though the total milligram dosage remained the same. This has been shown to be incorrect. Braid and Scott (1965) demonstrated that 3% and 2% solutions of prilocaine yield the same blood level as an equivalent dose of a 1% solution, if the same number of milligrams are administered. Jebson (1971) proved the same thing using 10% and 2% lidocaine.

Dosage, on the other hand, is a highly significant factor. Within the clinical dosage range for most local anesthetics, there is a linear relationship between dose and maximal blood concentration. Table 23-2 lists the concentrations of currently available local anesthetics.

Route of administration. Local anesthetic agents, when used for the control of pain, produce their clinical actions at the site of injection. Unlike most other drugs, it is not necessary for local anesthetics to enter into the circulation and reach a certain minimal therapeutic blood level. The greater the length of time a local anesthetic agent remains in the area where pain control is required and the greater its concentration at that site, the longer the agent's duration of action. As the drug is absorbed into the circulation, it becomes less and less effective as a pain-controlling agent. When sufficient volume has been removed from the area, painful stimuli may again be felt. At the same time, the more rapidly the agent is removed from the site of injection, the more rapidly the blood level of the drug increases toward overdose levels.

A frequent factor in overdose reaction to local anesthetics is the inadvertent intravascular injection of these drugs. In this instance, extremely high blood levels are produced in a brief period of time, producing acute overdose reactions. Absorption of topical anesthetics through the oral mucous mem-

Table 23-2. Concentrations of commonly employed local anesthetics

Drug	Group	Available concentrations (%)
Propoxycaine	Ester	0.4 (available with procaine)
Procaine	Ester	2 (available with propoxycaine)
Lidocaine	Amide	2
Mepivacaine	Amide	2 (with vasoconstrictor)
		3 (without vasoconstrictor)
Prilocaine	Amide	4
Bupivacaine	Amide	0.5
Etidocaine	Amide	1.5
Articaine	Amide	4

brane and absorption of solutions from multiple injection sites are other ways in which overdose may develop. Some forms of topical anesthetic are absorbed quite rapidly through the oral mucous membrane.

Rate of injection. The rate of injection is a very important factor in the cause or prevention of overdose reactions to all drugs. The intravenous injection of a local anesthetic drug may or may not produce signs and symptoms of overdose. Indeed, lidocaine is frequently administered intravenously in large doses (100 mg) in the management of several cardiac dysrhythmias. A major deciding factor in whether intravascular administration will prove clinically safe or hazardous is the rate at which the drug is administered. A 36 mg dose of lidocaine (one dental cartridge) administered rapidly intravenously (in less than 15 seconds) produces markedly elevated blood levels and virtually ensures an overdose reaction. On the other hand, 100 mg of lidocaine administered intravenously slowly (over several minutes), as in the management of cardiac dysrhythmias, produces a significantly lower blood level of the agent (greater distribution and biotransformation having occurred), with a lesser chance of overdose developing. Fig. 23-3 shows representative blood levels after administration of 30 mg of tetracaine via various routes. Many local-anesthetic overdose reactions result from the combination of inadvertent intravascular injection and too rapid a rate of injection. Both of these causes are virtually 100% preventable.

Vascularity of injection site. The greater the vascularity of the site of injection, the more rapid is the absorption of a drug away from that site and into the circulation. Although this is a desired situation with most parenterally administered drugs, it

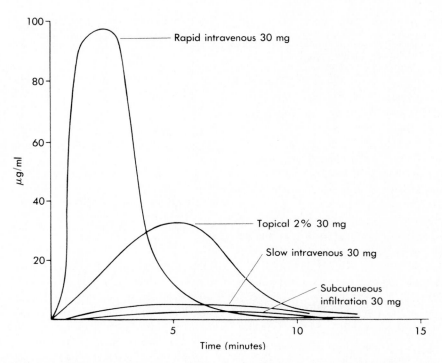

Fig. 23-3. Blood levels of local anesthetic (tetracaine) after administration by various routes. Note particularly the blood levels following rapid and slow intravenous administration. (From Adriani, J., and Campbell, B.: JAMA **162:**1527, 1956.)

is a decided disadvantage in the use of local anesthetics. These agents must remain in the area of injection to produce clinical pain control. Unfortunately for the dental profession (at least as far as local-anesthetic administration is concerned), the oral cavity is one of the more highly vascular areas of the entire body. A drug injected into the oral cavity can be expected to be absorbed into the blood more rapidly than the same drug injected elsewhere in the body. This factor, plus the inherent vasodilating properties of most local anesthetics, is the major reason for the addition of vasoconstrictors to most local anesthetics.

Presence of vasoconstrictors. As is discussed later in this chapter, the addition of a vasoconstrictor into a local-anesthetic solution produces a decrease in the rate of systemic absorption of the drug. The use of these agents, along with proper injection technique, has greatly reduced the clinical toxicity of local anesthetics. The box at left summarizes risk factors for local-anesthetic overdose.

Prevention

Virtually all overdose reactions to local anesthetics are preventable. Careful evaluation of the pa-

tient before dental treatment and equal care with drug administration technique eliminate this dangerous situation in all but a very few cases. Two sets of predisposing factors were presented in the previous section. The first set, patient factors, are those that cannot be eliminated but which, when present, require specific modification of dental management to prevent drug-related problems from developing. The second set of factors is related to the drugs themselves or to their administration. These factors are usually avoidable through proper drug selection and local-anesthetic injection technique.

Medical history questionnaire and dialogue history

The only questions directly related to the use of local anesthetics are included in the general drug use questions (Fig. 2-2). The doctor should carefully examine any adverse reaction to a local anesthetic and seek to determine its precise nature. The detailed dialogue history for this type of questioning is presented in Chapter 24.

In the absence of a previous history of adverse reaction to local anesthetics, the patient should be questioned concerning past experiences with den-

---

CAUSES OF HIGH BLOOD LEVELS OF LOCAL ANESTHETICS

1. Biotransformation of the drug is unusually slow
2. Drug is slowly eliminated from the body through the kidneys
3. Total dose administered of local anesthetic is too large
4. Absorption of the local anesthetic agent from the site of injection is unusually rapid
5. Local anesthetic agent is inadvertently administered intravascularly

From Moore, D.C.: Complications of regional anesthesia, Springfield, IL, 1955, Charles C. Thomas, Publisher.

OVERDOSE—PREDISPOSING FACTORS

Patient factors

Age (under the age of 6; over the age of 65)
Body weight (lower body weight increases risk)
Presence of pathology (for example, liver disease, congestive heart failure, pulmonary disease)
Genetics (for example, atypical plasma cholinesterase)
Mental attitude (anxiety decreases seizure threshold)
Sex (very slight increase in risk during pregnancy)

Drug factors

Vasoactivity of drug (vasodilator increases risk)
Dose of drug (higher dose increases risk)
Route of administration (intravascular route increases risk)
Rate of injection (rapid injection increases risk)
Vascularity of injection site (increased vascularity increases risk)
Presence of vasoconstrictor (decreases risk)

---

tal injections. Questions 2 and 3 may provide some relevant information in this area. The information gathered from this response is useful in an evaluation of the psychologic status of this patient. An adequate medical history enables the doctor to eliminate two potential causes of local anesthetic overdose: unusually slow biotransformation of the local anesthetic agent and unusually slow elimination of the agent from the body.

Etiology of overdose reactions

Before discussing the methods of prevention of local-anesthetic overdose, it is relevant to consider various ways in which high blood levels of local anesthetics may arise. Moore (1955) has stated that high blood levels of local anesthetics may occur in one or more of the ways listed in the box above. With these factors in mind, we can discuss the methods through which overdose reactions to local anesthetics may be avoided. As with the prevention of most other life-threatening situations in the dental office, the medical history questionnaire completed by the patient, as mentioned on this page, is important.

Biotransformation and elimination. Ester type local anesthetics (Table 22-3) undergo rapid biotransformation in the blood and liver. The major portion of this inactivation process occurs within the blood through hydrolysis to para-aminobenzoic acid by the enzyme pseudocholinesterase. Patients with a familial history of atypical pseudocholines-

terase are unable to detoxify ester type agents at a normal rate with the subsequent increased possibility that local anesthetic blood levels will reach overdose levels. Atypical pseudocholinesterase is thought to occur in 1 out of 2820 individuals. The patient with a questionable history should be referred to a physician for diagnostic tests, which may confirm or deny its existence. If atypical pseudocholinesterase is present, administration of ester type local anesthetics is relatively contraindicated.

Amide type anesthetics may be employed without an increased risk of overdose in these individuals. Amide type local anesthetics undergo biotransformation in the liver by microsomal enzymes. A history of liver disease (previous hepatitis or cirrhosis) does not absolutely contraindicate the use of these agents; however, prior liver disease is an indication that there may be some residual liver dysfunction and that the ability of the liver to biotransform the amide local anesthetics may be altered to some degree. In an ambulatory patient with a history of liver disease, amide type local anesthetics may still be given to the patient; however, they should be used judiciously (in other words, there is a relative contraindication to their administration). Minimal volumes should be employed for local anesthesia, keeping in mind that one cartridge may be capable of producing an overdose in this patient if liver function is compromised to a great enough degree. In my experience, however, such degrees of compromised liver function are more commonly observed in hospitalized patients than in ambulatory patients. Whenever doubt exists, medical consultation before injection of a local anesthetic agent may be indicated. In individuals with a greater degree of liver dysfunction, the use of ester type local anesthetics is also relatively contraindicated because the hydrolytic enzyme cholinesterase is produced in the liver, and liver dysfunction may disturb their biotransformation as well.

A small percentage of a local-anesthetic dose is eliminated from the blood in its active form through the kidneys (procaine 2%, lidocaine 10%, mepivacaine 1% to 15%). Renal dysfunction, however, does not usually lead to excessive blood levels of local anesthetics. As with liver dysfunction, however, it may be prudent to limit the dose of agent administered to the absolute minimum required for clinically effective pain control.

The patient undergoing renal dialysis also represents a relative contraindication to the administration of large local-anesthetic doses. This patient remains ambulatory between dialysis appointments and may come to the dental office for treatment. Undetoxified local anesthetic may accumulate in the blood of this patient, producing signs and symptoms of local anesthetic overdose.

The three remaining ways in which local-anesthetic overdose may develop are (1) too large a total dose, (2) rapid absorption of the local anesthetic into the circulation, and (3) inadvertent intravascular injection. Prevention of these is best accomplished through adherence to proper technique of local-anesthetic administration, which is reviewed following the discussion of each of these three factors.

Too large a total dose. If given to excess, all drugs are capable of producing signs and symptoms of overdose. The precise milligram dosage at which this occurs is impossible to predict consistently for all people. The principle of biologic variability greatly influences the manner in which individuals respond to drugs. Most drugs administered parenterally (such as local anesthetics) are commonly administered in a dosage form that has been calculated after consideration of a number of factors, including the age and physical status of the patient. A third consideration in the calculation of the maximum drug dosage is the weight of the patient receiving the drug. This factor is especially important in lighter patients. As mentioned previously, the larger the individual receiving the drug (within limits), the greater the drug distribution will be; therefore the blood level of the drug will be lower and the milligram dosage that may safely be administered will be larger.*

The manufacturers of local-anesthetic cartridges for dental use in the past did not indicate maximal dosages based on a dose per weight basis. Instead, generations of dentists were taught, for example, that the maximal dosage of lidocaine was 300 mg (without epinephrine) or 500 mg (with epinephrine), and so forth. Unfortunately, there have been cases in which these "maximal dosages" proved to be well in excess of an individual patient's "maximal tolerance," leading in some instances to morbidity or mortality. Such arbitrary doses for adult patients are meaningless when it is considered that one adult may weigh 200 pounds and another, 100 pounds. According to the "old" way of thinking, both of these persons were assumed to be capable of tolerating the same dosage of local anesthetic agent without adverse reaction. It becomes obvious that such thinking is erroneous. Distribution of the local anesthetic throughout the circulatory system of a muscular 200-pound adult results in a lower blood concentration than the same drug in a 100-pound adult. With all other potential factors being equal, the small adult has a greater chance of an overdose reaction than the larger adult does when exposed to the same drug dose. The overdose develops because the rate of absorption of the local anesthetic into the cardiovascular system exceeds the rate at which the liver is able to detoxify the agent (Fig. 23-4). Maximal dosages of local anesthetic drugs should therefore be calculated on a milligram per weight basis (kilogram or pound). Table 23-3 is a compilation of available information on maximal suggested dosages based on the patient's weight for several of the more commonly used dental local anesthetics.

---

*Although generally valid, there are always exceptions to this rule. Biologic variability and pathologic states can dramatically alter responsiveness to drugs; therefore care must always be exhibited when administering any drug.

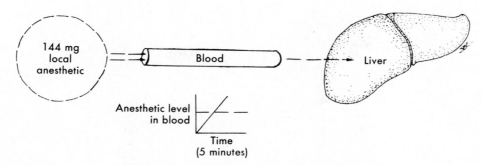

Fig. 23-4. Even in a patient with normal liver function, a large dose of local anesthetic may still be absorbed into the cardiovascular system more rapidly than the liver can remove it. This produces a rather rapid elevation of local anesthetic level. (From Malamed, S.F.: Handbook of local anesthesia, ed. 2, St. Louis, 1986, The C.V. Mosby Co.)

Table 23-3. Maximal recommended doses of commonly used local anesthetics*

Patient weight (lb)	Lidocaine 2%, with/without vasoconstrictor; 2.0 mg/lb up to 300 mg max		Mepivacaine 2% or 3%, 2.0 mg/lb up to 300 mg max			Prilocaine 4%, with/without vasoconstrictor; 2.7 mg/lb up to 400 mg max		Articaine (for adults) 4%, with vasoconstrictor; 3.2 mg/lb up to 500 mg max		Articaine (for children) 4%, with vasoconstrictor; 2.3 mg/lb up to 500 mg max	
	Mg	No. of cartridges	Mg	No. of cartridges		Mg	No. of cartridges	Mg	No. of cartridges	Mg	No. of cartridges
				2%	3%						
20	40	1.1	40	1.1	0.8	54	0.75	64	0.9	46	0.6
40	80	2.2	80	2.2	1.5	108	1.5	128	1.8	92	1.3
60	120	3.3	120	3.3	2.0	162	2.25	192	2.7	138	1.9
80	160	4.4	160	4.4	3.0	216	3.0	256	3.6	184	2.5
100	200	5.5†	200	5.5	3.5	270	3.75	320	4.4	230	3.0
120	240	6.5	240	6.5	4.0	324	4.5	384	5.33		
140	280	7.5	280	7.5	5.0	378	5.0	448	6.2		
160	300	8.0	300	8.0	5.5	400	5.5	500	7.0		
180	300	8.0	300	8.0	5.5	400	5.5	500	7.0		
200	300	8.0	300	8.0	5.5	400	5.5	500	7.0		

From Malamed, S.F.: Handbook of local anesthesia, ed. 2, St. Louis, 1986, The C.V. Mosby Co.
*Doses indicated are for normal healthy patients. Drug doses should be decreased for debilitated or elderly patients.
†0.2 mg epinephrine dose is limiting factor for 1:50,000 epinephrine.

It is highly unlikely that the dosages indicated in Table 23-3 will be reached. Rarely is there an indication for the administration of more than four or five cartridges during a dental appointment. Indeed, it is possible to achieve full mouth anesthesia (palatal, maxillary, and mandibular) with fewer than six cartridges of local anesthetic.

It is suggested that the doctor begin to think in terms of milligrams of local anesthetic injected instead of number of cartridges. It is therefore necessary to review the relationship between percent solution and the number of milligrams contained in that solution. A 1% solution of a local anesthetic contains 10 mg/ml of solution; a 2% solution contains 20 mg/ml, and so on. Table 23-4 summarizes the commonly used percentages in dental practice and the total number of milligrams found in the 1.8 ml dental cartridge.

Rapid absorption of drug into circulation. The addition of various vasoconstricting drugs to local anesthetic solutions has proved to be of great benefit. Not only do these agents increase the duration of action of the local anesthetic drugs by allowing them to remain in the area of injection for a greater

Table 23-4. Milligrams of local anesthetic per cartridge (1.8 ml) commonly used in dentistry

% concentration	=	mg/ml	× 1.8 ml	=	Total mg/cartridge
0.4		4			7.2
0.5		5			9
1		10			18
1.5		15			27
2		20			36
3		30			54
4		40			72

Table 23-5. Effect of vasoconstrictor (epinephrine 1:200,000) on peak local anesthetic level in blood

Local anesthetic	Dose (mg)	Peak level (µg/ml)	
		Without vasoconstrictor	With vasoconstrictor
Mepivacaine	500	4.7	3.0
Lidocaine	400	4.3	3.0
Prilocaine	400	2.8	2.6
Etidocaine	300	1.4	1.3

From Malamed, S.F.: Handbook of local anesthesia, ed. 2, St. Louis, 1986, The C.V. Mosby Co.

length of time in adequate concentration to produce conduction blockade, but vasoconstrictors also reduce the systemic toxicity of these drugs by retarding their absorption into the cardiovascular system (Table 23-5). Vasoconstricting drugs are considered an integral component of all local anesthetics whenever depth and duration of anesthesia are important. There are only a few indications in dentistry for using a local anesthetic solution without a vasoconstrictor.

The addition of vasoconstrictors to local anesthetic solutions has brought with it a different potential problem, however. Overdose of vasoconstricting agents has been reported. Because in most instances the vasoconstrictor in question is epinephrine, the potential reaction must not be taken lightly. Overdose of vasoconstrictors is discussed more fully later in this chapter.

Clinical experience with vasoconstrictors has led to the use of more and more dilute solutions with equally effective clinical application. Early local anesthetics contained epinephrine concentrations of 1:50,000. Later combinations were produced with 1:80,000 and 1:100,000 concentrations. Re-

search reports indicate that the optimal concentration of epinephrine for prolonging the duration of anesthesia with lidocaine may be as little as 1:250,000. Safety of a drug is increased with the use of the minimal effective concentration of both the local anesthetic and the vasoconstrictor.

Rapid uptake of local anesthetic agents may also occur following their application to the oral mucous membranes. As indicated in Fig. 23-3, absorption of some local anesthetics into the circulation following topical application is quite rapid, being exceeded only by direct intravenous injection. Another factor of importance in increasing the overdose potential of topically applied local anesthetics is the need to use them in a greatly increased concentration. This increase in concentration is necessary to produce adequate anesthesia of the mucous membranes. Injectable lidocaine is effective as a 2% solution, whereas lidocaine for topical application is used in a 5% or 10% concentration. It is readily apparent that the injudicious use of topical anesthetics may readily produce signs and symptoms of local anesthetic overdose. Other local anesthetics commonly employed as topical anesthetics include benzocaine and tetracaine. Both of these agents are ester type drugs and as such are rapidly detoxified by plasma pseudocholinesterase. Tetracaine is rather rapidly absorbed from mucous membranes, whereas benzocaine is poorly absorbed. Overdose reactions to benzocaine are virtually unknown. Tetracaine, on the other hand, has a significant toxicity and must therefore be employed judiciously. In addition, as esters, both of these agents are more likely to produce allergic reactions and localized tissue reaction (irritation) than are the amides.

Topical anesthetics are important agents for managing pain and anxiety. In spite of their potential for adverse reactions, it is common practice to apply topical anesthetics to the site of needle penetration before any intraoral injection. When used in small localized areas, there is little chance of significant blood levels developing; however, it is not uncommon to find topical anesthetics applied over large areas (quadrants or whole arches) before soft tissue procedures such as scaling and curettage. When used in this manner, significant blood levels are likely to be reached with a greater likelihood of overdose, particularly if this is later followed by injection of local anesthetics.

The preceding comments must not be taken as a recommendation against the use of topical anesthetics. Indeed, it is my feeling that topical anesthetics form an important part of every local-anesthetic procedure. However, the dentist must be aware of the potential complications so that they may be avoided. The following suggestions are offered for the use of topical anesthetics.

1. Amide type topical anesthetics should be employed whenever possible.

   COMMENT. Although overdose potential exists for all local anesthetics, other adverse reactions (local tissue reaction and allergy) are more frequently observed with the ester type agents.

2. Area of application should be small.

   COMMENT. There are only rare cases in which application of topical anesthetics to a full quadrant is indicated. Application of topical anesthetics to areas this size requires large quantities of the agent and results in a significant increase in the likelihood of overdose. It is my feeling that whenever larger areas (three or more teeth) require soft tissue anesthesia, injection of a local anesthetic should be considered.

3. Measured dosage forms of topical anesthetics should be used.

   COMMENT. Local anesthetics in the form of ointments and especially sprays are difficult to monitor as they are being applied. Overdose may be produced inadvertently with these devices. A spray form of an amide type anesthetic (lidocaine 10%) is available that delivers a metered dose of 10 mg with each application (Fig. 23-5).

Intravascular injection. Intravascular injection may occur with any type of intraoral injection but is much more likely to occur in certain anatomic areas. Table 23-6 lists the percentage of positive aspiration for various injections. Nerve block techniques usually possess the greatest potential for intravascular injection: 11% of aspiration tests in inferior alveolar nerve blocks, 5% of mental nerve blocks, and 3% of posterior-superior alveolar nerve blocks were positive, indicating that the needle bevel was lying within the lumen of a blood vessel (vein or artery).

Both intravenous and intraarterial injection may produce overdose reactions. It had previously been thought that only intravenous injection of a local anesthetic was capable of producing an overdose reaction and that intraarterial injection would not lead to elevated blood levels, since arterial blood travels distally from the heart, not toward the heart

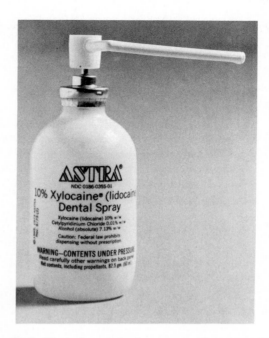

Fig. 23-5. Topical anesthetic spray with metered applicator. Depression of nozzle releases a 10 mg dosage of lidocaine.

Table 23-6. Percentage of positive aspiration for various intraoral injections

Injection	*% positive aspiration*
Inferior alveolar block	11.7
Mental block	5.7
Posterior superior alveolar block	3.1
Anterior superior alveolar block	0.7
(Long) buccal block	0.5

From Barlett, S.Z.: Clinical observations on the effects of injections of local anesthetics preceded by aspiration, Oral Surg. **33:**520, 1972.

as does venous blood. Aldrete (1977) has demonstrated, however, that intraarterial administration of local anesthetics may produce an overdose as rapidly as, or more rapidly than, an intravenous injection does. The mechanism of this reaction is a reversal of blood flow in the artery as the local anesthetic is rapidly injected. Such a mechanism during an inferior alveolar nerve block would entail the blood flowing in a retrograde fashion from the inferior alveolar artery to the internal maxillary artery, back to the external carotid, then to the common carotid, and finally to the internal carotid and the brain, a distance of only several inches (Fig. 23-6).

Intravascular injection of local anesthetics in the practice of dentistry should never occur. With care in injection technique and a knowledge of the anatomy of the area to be anesthetized, the incidence of overdose reaction from inadvertent intravascular injection may be minimized. Procedures necessary to prevent this complication include use of an aspirating syringe, use of a needle no smaller than 25 gauge, aspiration in at least two planes before injection, and slow injection of local anesthetic solution.

Recommending the use of an aspirating syringe for all injections would appear to be unnecessary because all dental schools teach its use to their students. However, in a survey on the injection techniques of practicing dentists, 21% of those surveyed stated that they employ nonaspirating syringes (Malamed, 1980). There can be no justification for the use of such devices for any injection procedure, because it is impossible to determine the location of the needle bevel with these instruments.

Needle size is an important factor in determining whether a needle is within a vessel before injection. The needles most commonly available are the 25, 27, and 30 gauge, the 27 gauge being the most frequently used. Needle gauge is of importance in several respects during local-anesthetic injection. Accuracy in injection technique is one critical point. For a local anesthetic to control pain, it must be deposited near the nerve. As a needle is passed through tissue toward the target nerve, it is deflected to varying degrees. The extent of deflection has been tested and is related to the caliber (gauge) of the needle. Needles with greater rigidity (larger

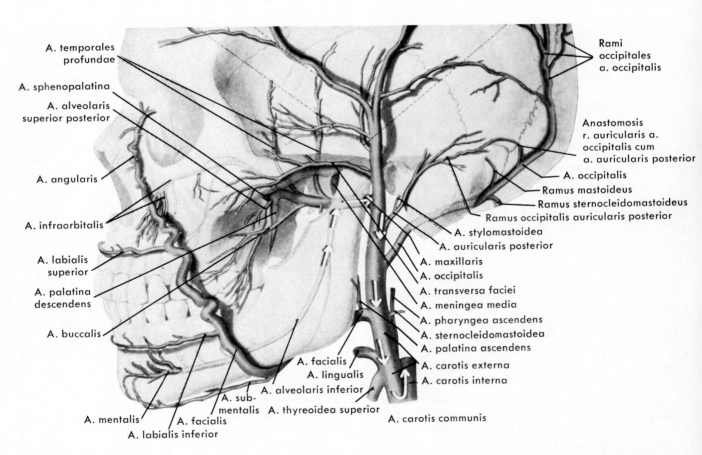

Fig. 23-6. Reverse carotid blood flow. Rapid intraarterial deposition of local anesthetic solution into the inferior alveolar artery produces an overdose reaction. Blood in the arteries reverses direction of flow because of the high pressure produced by the rate of injection. Arrows indicate the path of the solution into the cerebral circulation. (From Malamed, S.F.: Handbook of local anesthesia, ed. 2, St. Louis, 1986, The C.V. Mosby Co.)

gauge) were shown to deflect less when passed through tissues to the depth required for an inferior alveolar nerve block. The second critical point relating to needle gauge concerns reliability of aspiration. In other words, if a needle is in the lumen of a vessel, will aspiration tests always prove positive? Several studies have demonstrated conclusively that it is not possible to aspirate consistently with a needle gauge smaller than 25. Small-gauge needles are occluded more readily with tissue plugs or with the wall of the vessel than are larger needles, leading to false-negative aspirations. For injection techniques which have a greater likelihood of positive aspiration, a 23- or 25-gauge needle should always be employed. These techniques include all block injections, especially the inferior alveolar and posterior superior alveolar nerve blocks. Unfortunately, the majority of practicing dentists surveyed use the 27-gauge needle for inferior alveolar nerve blocks (64% use the 27-gauge needle; 34%, the 25-gauge needle).

The method by which aspiration is carried out is yet another factor of importance in preventing intravascular injection. All local-anesthetic needles have a bevel at the needle tip (Fig. 23-7, A). It is entirely possible (and indeed quite probable) for the bevel of a needle to be lying against the inner wall of a vessel. When negative pressure is created by pulling back on the thumb ring of the aspirating syringe, the wall of the vessel may be sucked up against the bevel of the needle, preventing entry of blood into the needle and cartridge (Fig. 23-7, B). Clinically this is interpreted as a negative aspiration, and injection of the local anesthetic follows. Injection of the local anesthetic requires positive pressure on the thumb ring to force the local anesthetic from the cartridge into the needle and out into the tissues. In this case, however, the positive pressure of the anesthetic solution pushes the vessel wall away from the needle bevel, and the local anesthetic solution is then deposited intravascularly (Fig. 23-7, C). A single aspiration test may therefore be inadequate to prevent intravascular injection. It is recommended that two or even three aspiration tests be made before injection. Each of these aspiration tests should be made with the bevel of the needle in a different position. To accomplish this, the hand holding the syringe must be turned approximately 45 degrees to reorient the bevel of the needle relative to the wall of the vessel. Return of blood into the dental cartridge is considered a positive aspiration and requires repositioning of the needle and reaspiration (with a negative result) before administration of the local-anesthetic solution. Only 60% of the dentists surveyed indicated they "always" aspirate before mandibular block;

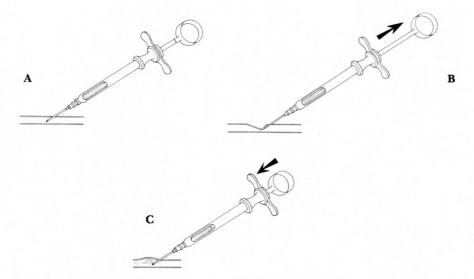

Fig. 23-7. Intravascular injection of local anesthetic. **A,** Needle is inserted in lumen of blood vessel. **B,** Aspiration test is performed. Negative pressure pulls vessel wall against bevel of needle; therefore no blood enters syringe (negative aspiration). **C,** Drug is injected. Positive pressure on plunger of syringe forces local anesthetic solution out through needle. Wall of vessel is forced away from bevel, and anesthetic solution is deposited directly into lumen of blood vessel.

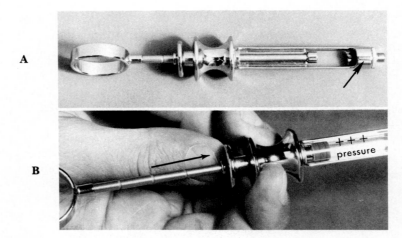

Fig. 23-8. A, Metal projection within the barrel depresses the cartridge diaphragm (*arrow*). **B,** Pressure on thumb disk (*arrow*) produces increased pressure within the cartridge. Release of pressure is all that is required for an aspiration test. (From Malamed, S.F.: Handbook of local anesthesia, ed. 2, St. Louis, 1986, The C.V. Mosby Co.)

25% said they "rarely" aspirate, and 15% said they "never" do. Recently, a self-aspirating syringe has become available for use in dentistry (Fig. 23-8). Its use makes aspiration much easier to perform.

The last factor related to prevention of overdose from intravascular injection concerns the rate of injection of the local-anesthetic solution. Rapid intravascular injection of a dental cartridge (1.8 ml) of a 2% local-anesthetic solution (36 mg) produces blood levels of anesthetic greatly in excess of those required for overdose (Fig. 23-9). In addition, the blood level elevation occurs rapidly so that the onset of the reaction is immediate. Rapid injection may be defined as administration of the contents of a dental cartridge in 30 seconds or less. The same quantity of solution injected slowly (60 seconds minimum) intravascularly produces blood levels below the minimum for overdose (see slow intravenous, Fig. 23-3). In the event that the blood level does exceed this minimal level, the onset of the reaction is slower, with signs and symptoms less severe than those observed following rapid injection.

Slow injection of drugs is perhaps the most important factor in prevention of all adverse drug reactions. It is difficult to inject a drug too slowly, but it is quite easy to inject too rapidly. It is recommended that the administration of one full 1.8 ml cartridge of local anesthetic take a *minimum of 60 seconds.* Such efforts significantly reduce the chance of an overdose reaction from intravascular injection. Of doctors surveyed, 46% administered a full cartridge of

solution for the inferior alveolar nerve block in fewer than 30 seconds. Only 15% responded that they took 60 seconds or longer for the same injection.

Technique of local anesthetic administration

Overdose reactions (and indeed all ADRs related to local anesthesia) may be minimized through the proper administration of local anesthetics, described as follows:

1. Preliminary medical evaluation should be completed before local-anesthetic administration.
2. Anxiety, fear, and apprehension should be managed before injection of a local anesthetic.
3. All dental injections should be administered with the patient in a supine or semisupine position. Patients should not receive local-anesthetic injections in the upright position unless absolutely necessary (as in severe cardiorespiratory disease).
4. Topical anesthetics should be applied to the site of injection before all injections.
5. The weakest effective concentration of local anesthetic solution should be injected in the smallest volume compatible with successful anesthesia.
6. The anesthetic solution selected should be appropriate for the patient and the dental treatment contemplated (duration of effect).
7. Vasoconstrictors should be included in all

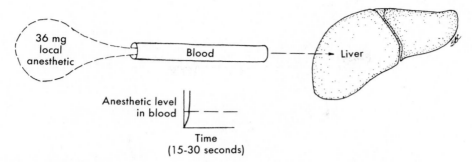

Fig. 23-9. Direct intravenous administration of one cartridge of local anesthetic produces marked elevation of local anesthetic level in the blood in a very short time. (From Malamed, S.F.: Handbook of local anesthesia, ed. 2, St. Louis, 1986, The C.V. Mosby Co.)

local anesthetics if not specifically contraindicated.

8. Aspirating syringes must always be employed for all injections.

9. Needles should be disposable, sharp, rigid, capable of reliable aspiration, and of adequate length for the contemplated injection techniques. All block techniques require use of long (1⅝-inch) 25-gauge needles. Short 27-gauge needles may be used for other injection techniques.*

10. Aspiration should be carried out in at least two planes before injection.

11. Injection should be made slowly, a minimum of 60 seconds being spent for each 1.8 ml dental cartridge.

12. *The patient should remain under observation following all local-anesthetic injections.* A member of the dental office staff who is capable of recognizing life-threatening situations should remain with the patient following administration of the local anesthetic. Not all local-anesthetic overdose reactions occur immediately following injection; many occur 5 or more minutes later. All too often, incidents are reported in which the doctor returns to the dental operatory to find the patient in the throes of a life-threatening drug reaction. Continuous observation of the patient permits prompt recognition and management of the situation with a greater probability of complete recovery.

---

*Variations may exist in needle selection for some regional nerve blocks. Local-anesthesia textbooks should be consulted for specific information.

Clinical Manifestations

Signs and symptoms of local-anesthetic overdose appear clinically in an individual whenever the blood level in an organ (such as the brain) rises to the critical level. The brain reacts to the concentration of local anesthetic delivered to it by the circulatory system regardless of the manner in which the local anesthetic entered the blood. The blood or plasma level of local anesthetic dictates the degree of severity and duration of the episode. The rate of onset of these manifestations corresponds to this blood level. There is a considerable difference in the rate of onset noted among the various causes of local-anesthetic overdose.

Onset, intensity, and duration

Rapid intravascular injection produces clinical signs and symptoms within seconds. The intensity of the reaction is normally greater with intravascular injection, and unconsciousness and seizures appear almost immediately. Duration of this form of overdose reaction is usually shorter than with other forms (Table 23-7) because of redistribution and continued biotransformation of the local anesthetic by the liver or serum cholinesterase while the reaction continues. This form of anesthetic overdose reaction is usually self-limiting and may occur with all types of local anesthetics.

Signs and symptoms of local-anesthetic overdose from too large a total dose or from unusually rapid absorption of the agent into the cardiovascular system do not occur as rapidly as those from intravascular injection. In these situations, clinical manifestations usually appear after 3 to 5 minutes and are initially mild. These may appear as a noticeable agitation of the patient, with an increase in

Table 23-7. Comparison of forms of local-anesthetic overdose

	Rapid intravascular	*Too large a total dose*	*Rapid absorption*	*Slow biotrans-formation*	*Slow elimination*
Likelihood of occurrence	Common	Most common	Likely with "high normal" dosages if no vasoconstrictors are used	Uncommon	Least common
Onset of signs and symptoms	Most rapid (seconds); intraarterial faster than intravenous	3-5 minutes	3-5 minutes	10-30 minutes	10 minutes to several hours
Intensity of signs and symptoms	Usually most intense	Gradual onset with increased intensity; may prove quite severe		Gradual onset with slow increase in intensity of symptoms	
Duration of signs and symptoms	2-3 minutes	Usually 5 to 30 minutes; depends on dose and ability to metabolize or excrete		Potentially longest duration because of inability to metabolize or excrete agents	
Primary prevention	Aspirate, slow injection	Administer minimal doses	Use vasoconstrictor; limit topical anesthetic use or use nonabsorbed type (base)	Adequate pretreatment physical evaluation of patient	
Drug groups	Amides and esters	Amides; esters only rarely	Amides; esters only rarely	Amides and esters	Amides and esters

intensity and a progression of symptoms over the next few minutes or longer if the blood level continues to rise. Clinically, the severity of these reactions may be as great as those witnessed in direct intravascular injection or they may not progress beyond a mild reaction. These reactions are also self-limiting because of the continued redistribution and biotransformation of the local anesthetic, but they tend to last significantly longer than the intravascular variety.

Unusually slow biotransformation or elimination of local anesthetics produces an even slower onset of clinical signs and symptoms. In two cases I have witnessed, the patients obtained adequate mandibular anesthesia and were undergoing restorative procedures for a period of time (15 and 25 minutes, respectively) before any clinical manifestations were noted. These manifestations included mild tremor, which progressed slowly to a mild convulsion over the next half hour. Because of patient inability to rid the body of the active form of the local anesthetic, these forms of overdose have the potential to persist for long periods of time.

Signs and symptoms

Local anesthetics produce depression of excitable membranes. The cardiovascular and, in particular, the central nervous systems are especially susceptible to these agents. The usual clinical expression of local-anesthetic overdose is one of apparent stimulation followed by a period of depression.

Minimal to moderate blood levels. The initial signs of central nervous system overdose are usually excitatory. At low overdose blood levels the patient usually becomes confused, talkative, apprehensive, and excited, and speech may be slurred. A generalized stuttering follows, which may lead to muscular twitching and tremor, commonly observed in the muscles of the face and in the distal parts of the extremities. Nystagmus may also be present. Blood pressure, heart rate, and respiratory rate are elevated.

Symptoms of overdose may include headache. In addition, a generalized feeling of lightheadedness and dizziness is usually reported first (the lightheadedness described as being different from that produced by alcohol), leading to visual and auditory disturbances (difficulty in focusing, blurred vision, and ringing in the ears). Numbness of the tongue and perioral tissues commonly develops, as does a feeling of either being flushed or chilled. As the reaction progresses and if the anesthetic blood level rises, drowsiness and disorientation occur, which may culminate in the loss of consciousness. The signs and symptoms of mild local-anesthetic

Table 23-8. Clinical manifestations of local-anesthetic overdose

Signs	Symptoms
Low to moderate overdose levels	
Confusion	Headache
Talkativeness	Lightheadedness
Apprehension	Dizziness
Excitedness	Blurred vision, unable to focus
Slurred speech	Ringing in ears
Generalized stutter	Numbness of tongue and perioral tissues
Muscular twitching and tremor of face and extremities	Flushed or chilled feeling
Nystagmus	Drowsiness
Elevated blood pressure	Disorientation
Elevated heart rate	Loss of consciousness
Elevated respiratory rate	
Moderate to high blood levels	
Generalized tonic-clonic seizure, followed by:	
Generalized CNS depression	
Depressed blood pressure, heart rate, and respiratory rate	

overdose resemble psychomotor or temporal lobe epilepsy (Chapter 21).

Moderate to high blood levels. As the blood level continues to rise, the clinical manifestations of the overdose reaction progress to a generalized convulsive state with tonic-clonic seizures. Following this phase of stimulation, there is an ensuing period of generalized central nervous system depression, characteristically of a degree of severity related to the degree of stimulation that preceded it. Therefore, if the patient underwent intensive tonic-clonic seizures, the period of depression will be more profound, with probable unconsciousness, respiratory depression, and possible respiratory arrest. If the stimulatory phase was mild (talkativeness, agitation), the depressant phase will be milder, with perhaps a period of disorientation and lethargy as the only clinically observable signs. Blood pressure, heart rate, and respiratory rate are usually depressed during this phase of the local-anesthetic overdose reaction—again to a degree proportionate to the degree of stimulation noted earlier. Table 23-8 summarizes clinical signs and symptoms.

Although the sequence just described is the usual sequence of clinical manifestations of local-anesthetic overdose, it is also possible that the excitatory phase of the reaction may be extremely brief or may not occur at all. This is true especially with lidocaine and mepivacaine. With these agents, patients exhibit drowsiness and nystagmus, which lead directly to generalized tonic-clonic seizure activity. Etidocaine and bupivacaine do not cause

drowsiness before seizures. Progression from the preseizure state of alertness to seizures is much more abrupt. The overdose reaction continues until the blood level of the local anesthetic falls below the minimal overdose level or until the reaction is terminated through appropriate drug therapy.

Pathophysiology

Local-anesthetic overdose is produced by an abnormally high blood level of the agent in various organs and tissues. In instances in which the entry of the local anesthetic into the blood exceeds its rate of removal, overdose levels may be reached, and the period of time required to do so varies with the causative element.

As stated previously, drugs do not merely affect a single organ or tissue, and all drugs have many actions. Local anesthetics are typical drugs in this regard. In the following discussion, both desirable and undesirable systemic actions of local anesthetics are discussed individually.

The term blood or plasma level refers to the amount of a drug that, following its administration, is absorbed into the circulatory system and transported in the blood plasma throughout the body. A sample of blood withdrawn from the patient may be analyzed to determine the amount of local anesthetic present per milliliter of blood. This is commonly referred to as the "blood level" or "plasma level" of a local anesthetic. Blood levels of drugs are measured in micrograms (μg) per milliliter (1000 μg = 1 mg).

Table 23-9. Overdose thresholds

Agent	Usual threshold for CNS signs and symptoms
Bupivacaine, etidocaine	1-2 μg/ml
Prilocaine	4 μg/ml
Lidocaine, mepivacaine	5 μg/ml

An additional factor to consider when discussing blood levels is that, although ranges are mentioned for various systemic effects, all individuals respond differently to drugs. Even though seizure activity may occur at a blood level of 7.5 μg/ml of lidocaine for most individuals, others may exhibit seizures at much lower levels, and still others may be able to tolerate blood levels greatly in excess of those listed without adverse response. A second factor is that different agents have different threshold levels at which signs and symptoms of overdose begin to appear (Table 23-9). It is not true that agents associated with higher plasma levels are less toxic, because these agents are usually less potent as local anesthetics and must be injected at higher concentrations (for example, bupivacaine 0.5% versus lidocaine 2%).

Local-anesthetic blood levels

Following the intraoral injection of local-anesthetic agents in the recommended manner, the solution gradually enters the blood. Circulating blood levels of lidocaine have been recorded following these injections and form the basis of the following discussion. Blood levels of other anesthetic agents vary from those reported for lidocaine (Fig. 23-10). In studies published by Cannell and coworkers (1975) it was demonstrated that, following the administration of 40 to 160 mg of lidocaine by intraoral injection, the blood level rose to a maximum of approximately 1.0 μg/ml. No adverse reactions were reported at those levels.

As the blood level of lidocaine increases, systemic actions are noted, some of which have considerable therapeutic value. When a blood level of 4.5 to 7.0 μg/ml is reached, definite signs of CNS irritability are noted. With an increase to 7.5 μg/ml or greater, seizure activity is present, whereas above a level of 10 μg/ml marked CNS depression is noted. Also occurring at overdose levels are adverse effects on the cardiovascular system; however, most adverse effects on the cardiovascular system do not develop until high overdose levels (for the CNS) have been

reached. Fig. 23-3 shows the effect of the various routes of administration on the blood level of the anesthetic.

Systemic activity of local anesthetics

Local anesthetic agents can exert a depressant effect on any excitable membrane. In the practice of dentistry these agents are normally applied to a specific region of the body where they produce their primary function: reversible blockade (depression) of peripheral nerve conduction. Other actions of local anesthetics are related to the absorption of the drugs into the circulation and their systemic activities on various excitable membranes including smooth muscle, the myocardium, and the central nervous system. Although high blood levels of local anesthetics produce undesirable systemic responses, at nonoverdose levels some desirable actions may be observed.

Cardiovascular action. Local anesthetics, particularly lidocaine, are frequently employed in the management of ventricular dysrhythmias, especially ventricular extrasystoles and ventricular tachycardia. Considerable data are available today that illustrate the alterations occurring in the myocardium with increasing blood levels of lidocaine.

It is generally considered that the minimal effective blood level of lidocaine for antidysrhythmic activity is 1.8 μg/ml. In the range from approximately 2 to 5 μg/ml, the actions of lidocaine on the myocardium include electrophysiologic changes only. These are a prolongation or abolition of the phase of slow depolarization during diastole in Purkinje fibers and a shortening of the action potential duration and of the effective refractory period. At this therapeutic level no alterations in myocardial contractility, diastolic volume, intraventricular pressure, or cardiac output are observed. The healthy, as well as the diseased, myocardium is well able to tolerate mildly elevated blood levels of local anesthetic without deleterious effect. When used to correct dysrhythmias, lidocaine is administered intravenously in a 50 to 100 mg bolus. Overdose reactions are a potential problem in these situations, but the benefit-risk ratio allows for judicious use. Increase of the lidocaine blood level to higher dose levels (5 to 10 μg/ml) produces a prolongation of conduction time through various portions of the heart, as well as an increase in diastolic threshold. This may be noted on the electrocardiogram as an increased P-R interval and QRS duration, and sinus bradycardia.

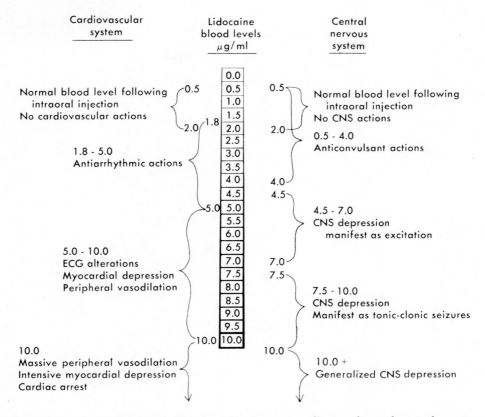

Fig. 23-10. Local-anesthetic blood levels and actions on cardiovascular and central nervous systems.

Along with this are noted decreased myocardial contractility, increased diastolic volume, decreased intraventricular pressure, and decreased cardiac output. Peripheral vascular effects observed at this level include vasodilation, which produces a fall in the blood pressure. This occurs as a result of the direct relaxant effect of the agent on the peripheral vascular smooth muscle.

Further increase in blood levels (>10 μg/ml of lidocaine) leads to an accentuation of the electrophysiologic and hemodynamic effects observed above, particularly a massive peripheral vasodilation, marked reduction in myocardial contractility, and a slowed heart rate, which may ultimately result in cardiac arrest.

Central nervous system actions. The central nervous system is extremely sensitive to the actions of local anesthetics. As cerebral blood levels of local anesthetics increase, clinical signs and symptoms develop. Local anesthetics cross the blood-brain barrier quite readily, producing a depressant effect on central nervous system function. At nonover-

dose levels of lidocaine (<5 μg/ml) there are no clinical signs of adverse effects on the CNS; however, a CNS-depressant action that has certain therapeutic usefulness is observed. When blood levels of lidocaine are between 0.5 and 4.0 μg/ml, this agent is capable of preventing various forms of seizure. Most clinically useful local anesthetic agents possess this anticonvulsant property (both procaine and lidocaine have been used to terminate or to decrease the duration of grand mal or petit mal seizures). The mechanism of this anticonvulsant action is thought to be a depression of hyperexcitable cortical neurons present in epileptic patients.

With an increase in the blood level above 4.5 μg/ml, initial signs and symptoms of CNS alteration appear. As discussed earlier, these are usually related to increased cortical irritability (agitation, talkativeness, and tremor). The symptom of numbness of the tongue and perioral tissues is thought to result from the rich blood supply to these tissues, allowing the drugs to produce blockade of the nerve endings. With a further increase in the blood level to 7.5 μg/ml or greater of lidocaine, generalized tonic-clonic seizures occur. Following this period of CNS stimulation, a further increase in the blood level of the local anesthetic results in termination of seizure activity and an electroencephalographic pattern consistent with generalized CNS depression. Respiratory depression and arrest are manifestations of this further depression.

It seems contradictory to state that local anesthetics are central nervous system depressants on the one hand, and then to claim that the first clinical manifestation of this CNS depression is CNS stimulation. This may be explained as follows: The stimulation and subsequent depression produced by high blood levels of local anesthetics result solely from depression of neuronal activity. The cerebral cortex receives both inhibitory and facilitory (stimulatory) impulses. If it is considered that these two groups of neurons are selectively depressed by different blood levels of local anesthetics, this seeming contradiction is explained. At blood levels of anesthetic capable of producing seizures, the inhibitory pathways in the cerebral cortex are depressed, but the facilitory pathways are not. This depression of the inhibitory pathways permits the facilitory neurons to function unopposed, leading to an increased excitation of the CNS and ultimately to seizures. With a further increase in local-anesthetic blood level, the facilitory neurons are depressed along with the inhibitory neurons, producing a state of generalized CNS depression. It must be noted here that the duration of the seizure, although primarily dependent on local-anesthetic blood level, can be further modified by the acid-base status of the patient. The higher the arterial carbon dioxide tension ($Paco_2$), the lower the local-anesthetic blood level required to precipitate generalized seizures. In contrast, the lower the $Paco_2$, the greater the drug blood level required to produce seizures. Lowering a patient's $Paco_2$ through hyperventilation raises the cortical seizure threshold to local anesthetics and lessens the chance that a drug will cause seizures.

Drug-induced seizures, in and of themselves, are not necessarily fatal. However, the mortality rate in untreated animals is over 60%. It appears that the duration of the seizure is an important factor in determining the degree of morbidity. The convulsing brain requires greatly elevated oxygen and glucose levels to continue functioning. To a degree, the body's own mechanisms can compensate for this; however, respiratory and circulatory support can greatly enhance the chances of survival. As cardiovascular depression is produced by even more elevated blood levels of the agent and respirations are further impaired by uncoordinated muscle spasm during the seizure, brain function will be affected even more through reduced cerebral blood flow and hypoxia. Fig. 23-10 summarizes the clinical effects of local anesthetics seen with increasing blood levels.

Management

Management of a local-anesthetic overdose is based on the severity of the reaction encountered. In most cases the reaction is mild and transitory, requiring little or no specific treatment. However, when the reaction is more severe and perhaps of longer duration, prompt therapy is required. As noted in the previous section, most local-anesthetic overdoses are self-limiting. The blood level of the local anesthetic decreases as the reaction progresses because of redistribution and biotransformation of the drug. It is a rare occasion indeed that drugs other than oxygen need to be administered to terminate a local-anesthetic overdose. Overtreatment of local-anesthetic overdose is a potential problem. In the rush of excitement that follows this unexpected reaction, drugs may be administered too freely. All anticonvulsants are CNS depressants and can delay recovery of consciousness.

The time for vigorous intravenous management is when the simpler measures have failed. However, by ending the seizure, these agents may give the rescuer a false sense of accomplishment; none of these drugs is wholly innocuous.

Before discussing management of the various degrees of local-anesthetic overdose, it must be repeated that *during and after administration of any local anesthetic, the patient must be observed continuously.* Careful observation of any change in the patient's behavior following administration of a local anesthetic permits the reaction to be managed at an earlier stage, with less potential hazard for the patient.

Mild overdose reaction with rapid onset

An overdose reaction that develops within 3 to 5 minutes following drug administration is considered rapid in onset. Possible causes of this reaction include intravascular injection, unusually rapid absorption, and too large a total dose of the local anesthetic. If the clinical manifestations do not progress beyond a mild degree of CNS excitation (talkativeness, increased anxiety, muscular twitching, perioral numbness, increased heart rate, blood pressure, and respiratory rate) with retention of consciousness, no definitive therapy is necessary. The local anesthetic will undergo redistribution and biotransformation, and the blood level will fall below the overdose level in a short time.

Step 1. Reassure patient.

Step 2. Administer oxygen. At this point, advantage may be taken of the fact that a lowered $Paco_2$ level will increase the seizure threshold to local anesthetics. Instruct the patient to hyperventilate on room air or, if oxygen is readily available, use either a full face mask or nasal hood and ask the patient to breathe deeply. This will usually suffice to prevent seizure activity in this situation.

Step 3. Initiate basic life support. Assess airway, breathing, and circulation, and implement as needed.

Step 4. Monitor vital signs. Postexcitation depression is mild in this form of reaction, and little or no therapy is required in its management. Oxygen may be administered and vital signs recorded.

Step 5. Administer anticonvulsant drug, if needed. The use of an anticonvulsant such as diazepam is not indicated in situations such as that described above. However, if the doctor is trained in venipuncture and has little difficulty in securing a vein, diazepam may be administered *slowly intravenously* and titrated at a rate of 2 mg per minute until the reaction ceases. Intravenous agents should always be titrated to clinical effect. Small doses of IV diazepam may prove effective. Doses as low as 2.5 to 5 mg have terminated seizures in humans. It must be reemphasized that for a mild reaction to a local anesthetic agent, as described, anticonvulsant drug therapy is normally *not indicated*.

Step 6. Recovery. The patient should be permitted to recover for as long as necessary. Dental treatment may or may not be continued following evaluation of the patient's physical and emotional status. Medical evaluation, preferably by an emergency room physician, should be seriously considered before discharge of the patient. If any anticonvulsant drug was administered, the patient must not be permitted to leave unescorted and should receive medical evaluation.

Mild overdose reaction with slow onset (>5 minutes)

If the patient exhibits signs and symptoms of local-anesthetic overdose after the local anesthetic has been administered in the recommended manner, if pain control has been achieved, and if dental treatment has begun, the most likely causes are ab-

normally slow biotransformation and excretion. Another possible cause is too large a total dose of the agent.

Step 1. Reassure patient.

Step 2. Administer oxygen and instruct patient to hyperventilate.

Step 3. Initiate basic life support.

Step 4. Monitor vital signs.

Step 5. Administer anticonvulsant if needed. Management of this situation entails terminating dental therapy, reassuring the patient, administering oxygen, controlled hyperventilation, and monitoring of vital signs. Reactions resulting from biotransformation or excretory dysfunction usually progress in intensity and are of longer duration than those caused by other types of overdose. If venipuncture can be performed, an intravenous infusion may be established and diazepam administered, 2 mg per minute, titrating until clinical manifestations subside.

Step 6. Summon medical assistance (optional). When venipuncture is not practical, medical assistance should be procured as early as possible.

The phase of postexcitement depression is relatively mild following a mild excitement phase. Use of diazepam to terminate the reaction may add to the level of depression but to a minor extent. Monitoring of the patient and adherence to the steps of basic life support are normally entirely adequate for this situation. Oxygen should be administered to the patient.

Step 7. Medical consultation. Following successful termination of a reaction of this nature, the patient should undergo evaluation by a physician to determine the possible causes of the reaction. This examination might include blood tests and renal and liver function tests to determine the ability of the patient to break down and excrete these agents. The doctor should make the initial consultation with the physician while the patient is still in the office.

Step 8. Recovery. Allow the patient to recover for as long as necessary, and make arrangements for the patient to be escorted to the local hospital or physician's office by an adult companion. Before further dental therapy requiring local anesthetics, a full medical evaluation should be sought.

Severe overdose reaction with rapid onset

If the signs and symptoms of overdose appear while the anesthetic syringe is still in the patient's mouth and the drug is being rapidly injected, intravascular injection is the most likely cause of this reaction. Because of the rapid elevation of blood level, the clinical manifestations are likely to be severe. Unconsciousness with or without convulsive seizures may be the initial clinical sign of the reaction.

Step 1. Position patient. Remove the syringe (if still present) from the victim's mouth and place the patient in the supine position. Management is based on the presence or absence of seizures.

Step 2. Protect patient from injury. Should seizures occur (which is common), management follows that described in Chapter 21 for all convulsive seizures. Such management includes prevention of injury to the patient by protecting the arms, legs, and head from hitting any hard objects. If possible (and only if easily possible), a soft object such as a handkerchief or cloth towel should be placed between the teeth of the patient to prevent possible injury to the tongue and lips. Extreme care must be exercised by the rescuer in this effort. Never place fingers between the teeth of a convulsing individual. Tight, binding articles of clothing such as ties, collars, and belts should be loosened. Prevention of injury is the primary aim of management.

Step 3. Basic life support. Basic life support procedures are instituted and oxygen is administered. Oxygen will assist in lowering the $Paco_2$ and will elevate the seizure threshold.

Step 4. Administer anticonvulsant. Additional assistance includes administration of oxygen during the tonic-clonic stage of the seizure, airway maintenance, and the monitoring of vital signs.

The blood level of the anesthetic agent continues to fall as it undergoes redistribution, biotransformation, and excretion. Within 1 to 2 minutes the blood level falls below the minimal overdose level, and the seizure ceases unless the patient has become acidotic during the seizure due to inadequate ventilation. In most cases, therefore, definitive drug therapy to terminate a seizure caused by overdose of local anesthetic is unnecessary. Intravenous administration of an anticonvulsant is not considered until the seizure has lasted longer than 4 to 5 minutes with little or no indication of subsiding. If possible, diazepam should be titrated slowly (2 mg per minute) until the seizure ends. In some situations, however, it may prove difficult to secure a vein on a patient in seizure. In this case, the patient should be maintained and medical assistance summoned.

Following the seizure, there is a period of generalized CNS depression that equals the excitation phase in intensity. During this phase the patient may be drowsy or unconscious, breathing may be shallow or absent, the airway may be partially or totally obstructed, and blood pressure and heart rate may be depressed or even absent. The use of anticonvulsants to terminate a seizure only adds to this state of depression. Barbiturates have a greater depressant effect than diazepam, although both are equally effective as anticonvulsants—thus the choice of diazepam for management of seizures.

Management of the postseizure phase requires adherence to the steps of basic life support. A patent airway may be maintained and oxygen or artificial ventilation administered, if indicated. Vital signs must be monitored and CPR begun (see Chapter 30) if blood pressure or heart beat is lost. More commonly, the blood pressure and heart rate are low, with a consistent return toward baseline levels with recovery.

Step 5. Additional management. Should the blood pressure remain depressed for extended periods (30 minutes), administration of a vasopressor such as 20 mg of methoxamine IM should be considered. This agent produces a mild elevation in blood pressure, the effect lasting for 1 hour or longer.

Step 6. Recovery. The patient should be allowed to rest until recovery is sufficient to permit discharge. Recovery includes a return of vital signs to approximately the baseline level and a loss of the disorientation and confusion present in the depression phase. Do not permit this patient to leave the dental office unescorted. Arrangements must be made to have the patient taken to a hospital emergency room where neurologic examination can be performed.

It was mentioned earlier that with the rapid rise in blood level following intravascular administration the first clinical sign may be unconsciousness. In this case, management follows that outlined in Chapter 5. Follow-up therapy is identical to that indicated for the postseizure patient.

Severe overdose reaction with slow onset

Overdose reactions that develop slowly (over a period of 15 to 30 minutes) are unlikely to progress to severe clinical signs and symptoms if the patient is being continuously observed and management is started promptly on recognition of the situation. Clinical manifestations most often progress from mild to tonic-clonic seizures over a relatively short period of time (5 minutes), or the progression may be much less pronounced. In either case, dental therapy must be stopped as soon as signs and symptoms are noted.

Step 1. Terminate dental therapy.

Step 2. Provide basic life support and administer oxygen.

Step 3. Administer anticonvulsant. If symptoms are mild at the onset but progress in severity, definitive drug therapy with an anticonvulsant is indicated.

Step 4. Summon medical assistance. Whether or not the anticonvulsant is administered, medical assistance should be summoned.

Step 5. Additional management. The postseizure state of depression once again requires strict adherence to the steps of basic life support to minimize significant morbidity and mortality. A mild vasopressor may be necessary if the blood pressure remains depressed for prolonged periods of time.

Step 6. Recovery. Patients should be allowed to recover for as long as necessary before being discharged to a hospital in the custody of an adult. Complete evaluation of these patients should be undertaken before readministration of a local anesthetic. Initial medical consultation should occur while they are in the dental office.

Management of local-anesthetic overdose is summarized in the box at right.

Local-anesthetic seizures should not lead to morbidity or death if appropriate resuscitation equipment is available, the patient is properly prepared, and the person administering the injection is well trained in the treatment of seizures. Local-anesthetic injections of any type should not be performed without these precautions.

EPINEPHRINE OVERDOSE REACTION
Precipitating Factors and Prevention

With the increasing use of vasoconstrictors in local-anesthetic solutions, a potentially new ADR has been introduced—overdose from the vasoconstrictor. Although a variety of vasoconstrictors is currently used in dentistry (Table 23-10), the most effective and the most widely employed is epinephrine. Overdose reactions are uncommon when agents other than epinephrine are employed because of the decreased potency of these agents. These reactions are also more likely to occur when greater concentrations of epinephrine are used. Table 23-11 outlines the concentrations (mg/ml) of the various epinephrine dilutions currently in use.

MANAGEMENT OF LOCAL-ANESTHETIC OVERDOSE

Mild overdose reaction (rapid onset)

   No formal therapy
Step 1 Reassure patient
  2 Administer oxygen
  3 Initiate basic life support
  4 Monitor vital signs
  5 Administer anticonvulsant (optional)
  6 Recovery

Mild overdose reaction (slow onset)

Step 1 Reassure patient
  2 Administer oxygen and instruct patient to hyperventilate
  3 Initiate basic life support
  4 Monitor vital signs
  5 Venipuncture if available (diazepam 2 mg/min until reaction stops)
  6 Summon medical assistance
  7 Medical consultation
  8 Recovery

Severe overdose reaction (rapid onset)

Step 1 Position patient (supine)
  2 Manage seizures
    Prevent injury
    Loosen tight garments
  3 Basic life support
    Ensure patent airway
    Administer oxygen
    Monitor vital signs
  4 Anticonvulsant after 4 to 5 minutes (diazepam 2 mg/min IV if possible)
    Manage postseizure depression
    Airway maintenance
    Oxygen, artificial ventilation
  5 Additional management
    Summon medical assistance
    Monitor vital signs
      CPR if indicated
      Methoxamine, 20 mg IM for low blood pressure
  6 Permit patient to recover before discharge to hospital

Severe overdose reaction (slow onset)

Step 1 Terminate dental therapy
  2 Basic life support and oxygen
  3 Anticonvulsant, if symptoms progress
  4 Summon medical assistance
  5 Manage postseizure depression
    Basic life support
    Vasopressor, if necessary
  6 Permit patient to recover before discharge to hospital

Table 23-10. Vasoconstrictors commonly employed in dentistry

Agent	Available concentrations	Maximal dose	Local anesthetic agents used with
Epinephrine	1:50,000	Healthy adult: 0.2 mg	Lidocaine 2%
	1:100,000	Cardiac patient: 0.04 mg	Articaine 4%
			Lidocaine 2%
	1:200,000		Articaine 4%
			Prilocaine 4%
Levonordefrin (Neo-Cobefrin)	1:20,000	Healthy adult: 1.00 mg	Mepivacaine 2%
		Cardiac patient: 0.2 mg	Procaine 2% with propoxycaine 0.4%
Levarterenol (Levophed)	1:30,000	Healthy adult: 0.34 mg	Procaine 2% with
		Cardiac patient: 0.14 mg	propoxycaine 0.4%

Table 23-11. Dilutions of vasoconstrictors used in dentistry

Dilution	Drug available	Mg/ml	Mg per cartridge (1.8 ml)	Maximum no. of cartridges used for healthy patient (H) and cardiac patient (C)
1:1000	Epinephrine (emergency kit)	1.0	Not applicable	Not available in local-anesthetic cartridge
1:10,000	Epinephrine (emergency kit)	0.1	Not applicable	Not available in local-anesthetic cartridge
1:20,000	Levonordefrin	0.5	0.09	10 (H), 2 (C)
1:30,000	Levarterenol	0.034	0.06	5 (H), 2 (C)
1:50,000	Epinephrine	0.02	0.036	5 (H), 1 (C)
1:100,000	Epinephrine	0.01	0.018	10 (H), 2 (C)
1:200,000	Epinephrine	0.005	0.009	20 (H), 4 (C)

The optimal concentration of epinephrine for prolongation of anesthesia with lidocaine is a 1:250,000 dilution. There is no rational reason for the use of the 1:50,000 dilution so frequently employed today for pain control. It contains twice the epinephrine per milliliter as a 1:100,000 dilution and four times that contained in a 1:200,000 dilution, while not adding any positive attributes to the solution. The only benefit of the 1:50,000 concentration of epinephrine over other concentrations appears to be in the control of bleeding (hemostasis). However, for its use as a hemostatic agent, epinephrine must be applied directly to the area where the bleeding is occurring or will occur. Only small quantities of the solution are necessary, and in many surgical areas only small quantities are feasible, because larger volumes actually interfere with the surgical procedure. Overdose reactions from this use of 1:50,000 epinephrine are rare.

There is yet another form in which epinephrine is used in dentistry that is even more likely to produce an overdose reaction or precipitate other life-threatening situations. This is the racemic epinephrine gingival retraction cord commonly used before taking impressions in crown and bridge procedures. The currently available epinephrine-impregnated cord contains from 310 to 1000 μg of racemic epinephrine per inch of cord. Racemic epinephrine is a combination of the levorotatory and dextrorotatory forms of epinephrine; the dextro form is about one twelfth to one eighteenth as potent as the levo form. However, because of the high concentration of epinephrine, these retraction cords are a potential source of danger to all patients, especially cardiac-risk patients. Epinephrine in an epinephrine-soaked cord is absorbed rapidly through gingival epithelium that has been disturbed (that is, abraded) by dental procedures (cavity preparation), whereas little absorption into the systemic circulation occurs through intact oral epithelium. Studies have demonstrated that from 24% to 92% of the applied epinephrine is absorbed into the circulation; the extreme variability is thought to result from the degree of vascular exposure (bleeding) and the length of time of the exposure.

When gingival retraction is necessary, it is recommended that other retraction materials be utilized. Effective agents that do not possess the adverse systemic actions of epinephrine are available and should be used. Such commercial preparations include Hemodent (containing aluminum chloride, hydroxyquinoline sulfate, phenocainium chloride, and ethyl aminobenzoate), and Alum (a saturated alum solution). The American Dental Association (1984) states the following in *Accepted Dental Therapeutics:* "Since effective agents which are devoid of systemic effects are available, it is not advisable to use epinephrine for gingival retraction, and its use is contraindicated in individuals with a history of cardiovascular disease."

Clinical Manifestations and Pathophysiology

The clinical manifestations of an overdose reaction to epinephrine appear in many ways to be quite similar to an acute anxiety response. Indeed, in the acute anxiety response most of the signs and symptoms are produced by the large increase in endogenous catecholamine release (epinephrine and norepinephrine) by the adrenal medulla. As with all drug overdose reactions, clinical manifestations relate to the usual pharmacology of the drug. Symptoms of an epinephrine overdose are listed in Table 23-12. The patient may make complaints such as "My heart is pounding" or "I feel nervous."

Signs of epinephrine overdose reaction include a sharp rise in both blood pressure (especially systolic) and heart rate. The rise in blood pressure is potentially hazardous, especially following inadvertent intravascular injection. Cerebral hemorrhage and cardiac dysrhythmias may be produced by an overdose of epinephrine. Subarachnoid hemorrhage has even been recorded following the subcutaneous administration of 0.5 mg of epinephrine. Blood pressures in excess of 400/300 torr have been recorded for a short time following this occurrence. In addition, epinephrine, a powerful cardiac stimulant, may predispose the heart toward ventricular dysrhythmias. The heart rate increases (140 to 160 beats per minute is common), and the rhythm may be altered. Ventricular premature contractions occur first, followed by ventricular tachycardia. Ventricular fibrillation may follow and is usually fatal unless immediately recognized and managed (Chapter 30).

Patients with preexisting cardiovascular disease are quite susceptible to these adverse actions of epinephrine. Increased workload on an already impaired cardiovascular system is likely to precipitate an acute exacerbation of a preexisting disorder such as anginal pain, acute myocardial infarction, heart failure, or cerebrovascular accident.

Overdose reaction from epinephrine is transitory, rarely lasting for more than a few minutes; however, the patient may feel tired and depressed for a prolonged period following the episode. The normally short duration of the epinephrine overdose reaction is related to the rapid biotransformation of epinephrine into inactive products in the body. The liver produces the enzymes necessary for the breakdown of epinephrine. These enzymes are monoamine oxidase (MAO) and catecholamine O-methyltransferase (COMT). Patients receiving monoamine oxidase inhibitors (MAO-I) in the management of depression are unable to break down epinephrine at a normal rate and are therefore more susceptible to overdose reactions from epinephrine.

Management

Most instances of epinephrine overdose are of such short duration that little or no formal management is required. On occasion, however, the reaction may appear prolonged, and some management will be desired.

Step 1. Terminate dental procedure. As soon as clinical manifestations of the overdose reaction appear, terminate the dental procedure and, if possible, remove the source of epinephrine from the patient. Following administration of a local anesthetic this is obviously impossible; however, a gingival retraction cord should be removed immediately.

Table 23-12. Clinical manifestations of epinephrine overdose

Symptoms	Signs
Fear	Elevated blood pressure
Anxiety	Elevated heart rate
Tenseness	
Restlessness	
Throbbing headache	
Tremor	
Perspiration	
Weakness	
Dizziness	
Pallor	
Respiratory difficulty	
Palpitation	

Step 2. Position patient. The conscious patient should be placed in a comfortable position (patient may determine position). The supine position is not recommended because of the accentuation of the cardiovascular effects (particularly the increased cerebrovascular blood flow) noted in that position. The semisitting or erect position minimizes to a small degree this elevation in cerebral blood pressure.

Step 3. Reassure patient. Increased anxiety and restlessness are usually noted in this reaction, along with other signs and symptoms such as palpitation and respiratory difficulty. These further increase the patient's apprehension and lead to an accentuation of the clinical problem. The doctor should reassure the patient that "everything will be all right in a moment."

Step 4. Initiate basic life support. Assess airway, breathing, and circulation and implement as needed.

Step 5. Monitor vital signs and administer oxygen. Blood pressure and heart rate should be monitored and recorded every 5 minutes during the episode. Rather striking elevations may be noted in both of these parameters, which gradually decline toward baseline over a period of time. Oxygen may be administered to the patient if necessary. If the patient complains of difficulty in breathing, oxygen should be administered by means of a nasal cannula, nasal hood, or full face mask.

Step 6. Allow patient to recover. Permit the patient to remain seated in the dental chair as long as necessary following the episode. Patients feel fatigued and depressed for variable lengths of time following this reaction. Do not discharge this patient if doubt remains as to the patient's ability for self-care (driving a car or walking unsupported). Should doubt remain, arrangements should be made for the patient to be escorted home from the dental office.

The proper steps for management of epinephrine overdose are summarized in the boxed material at right.

CENTRAL NERVOUS SYSTEM DEPRESSANT OVERDOSE REACTIONS

Whenever CNS depressant drugs are administered to a patient, there is always a possibility that an exaggerated degree of CNS depression may develop. Clinically this might simply be noted as slight oversedation, or it might result in an unconscious patient who has ceased breathing.

In the opinion of many, the group of drugs most likely to produce an overdose reaction is the barbiturate group. These drugs represented the first major breakthrough in the pharmacologic management of anxiety, and because of this, adverse reactions, such as allergy, addiction, and overdose potential, were tolerated. With the introduction of newer antianxiety drugs (for example, the benzodiazepines) that do not possess the same degree of abuse and overdose potential, the use of barbiturates has declined. The barbiturates still remain a very useful group in the dentist's and physician's armamentarium for management of anxiety.

Although the barbiturates present the greatest potential for adverse reaction, the narcotic analgesics are probably responsible for the greatest number of clinically significant episodes of overdose and respiratory depression. This is simply because the narcotics are used to a much greater degree than the barbiturates. The administration of narcotics is popular in the management of pediatric patients. In addition, narcotics are often employed intravenously, in addition to antianxiety drugs, to aid in achieving sedation and pain control in the adult patient. Goodson and Moore (1983) reported on 14 cases in pediatric dentistry in which the administration of narcotics (and other drugs) led to seven deaths and three cases of brain damage. Several narcotics were implicated in these reactions: alphaprodine (7 cases), meperidine (6 cases), and pentazocine (1 case).

Predisposing Factors and Prevention

Because the barbiturates and narcotics are commonly used for the preoperative management of anxiety, they are most often administered orally or intramuscularly. The clinical efficacy of a drug depends in large part on its absorption into the cardiovascular system and its subsequent blood level in different organs of the body. Only the inhalation and IV routes of drug administration permit titra-

---

**MANAGEMENT OF
EPINEPHRINE OVERDOSE**

Step 1 Terminate dental procedure
   2 Position patient—not supine
   3 Reassure patient
   4 Initiate basic life support
   5 Monitor vital signs, administer oxygen
   6 Allow patient to recover

tion. With oral and intramuscular administration, drug absorption is erratic, as demonstrated by the wide range of variability in clinical effectiveness. The normal distribution curve becomes important when drugs are administered by those routes in which titration is not possible. "Average" drug doses are based on this curve; therefore secobarbital, 100 mg or diazepam, 5 mg orally, produce a desired effect (mild sedation) in the majority of patients who receive them. For some patients, however, these doses are ineffective, and these persons will require a larger dose to attain the same clinical level of sedation. These persons are not risking potential overdose with the average dose, because a lack of adequate sedation is the clinical result.

The potential danger in the use of drugs lies with patients for whom an average dose of secobarbital or diazepam is too great. These are persons who are quite sensitive (not allergic) to the drug and require smaller than usual doses to obtain clinically effective sedation. It is normally not possible to predict in advance which patients will react in this manner. Only a previous history of an ADR can provide a clue to this occurrence. The medical history questionnaire should be carefully examined in relation to all drug reactions. When a history of drug sensitivity is obtained, great care must be exercised when barbiturates and narcotic analgesics are to be used. Lower than usual doses should be employed or different drug categories substituted. Nonbarbiturate sedative-hypnotic drugs, the benzodiazepines, and the narcotic agonist/antagonists may be used in place of these drugs.

Although the nature of the overdose cannot be easily predicted in advance, there is another way in which these drugs can produce an overdose reaction, a way that is preventable. It relates entirely to the goal being sought by the doctor when these drugs are administered. Some clinicians use the barbiturates or narcotics to achieve deep levels of sedation on apprehensive patients. When used in this manner by means of the oral or IM routes of drug administration, the potential for an overdose reaction is greatly increased. Most doctors who employ barbiturates for sedation in their practices have encountered patients who became uncooperative (less inhibited) after receiving these drugs. The procedure could not be completed because of the difficulty in managing an individual who has received a small overdose. Larger doses of this drug given to an anxious patient in an attempt to produce deeper levels of sedation may produce greater degrees of CNS depression, with possible loss of consciousness and respiratory depression.

Employing any CNS depressant drug to obtain deeper levels of sedation by routes of administration in which titration is not possible is, therefore, not advised and is an invitation to overdose. It cannot be recommended. Only those techniques that permit titration can safely be employed to achieve deeper levels of sedation, and then only in cases in which the doctor is thoroughly familiar with both the technique and the drugs to be administered and is able to manage all possible complications associated with the procedure.

The inhalation and IV routes are the only ones that permit titration. A factor that must be remembered regarding inhalation and IV sedation is that absorption of the drug(s) into the systemic circulation occurs rapidly so that drug responses (both therapeutic and adverse) may occur quite suddenly. Titration must always be employed when these techniques are used. Titration remains the greatest safety feature these techniques possess.

Table 23-13 summarizes recommendations for the various routes of drug administration.

Table 23-13. Summary of routes of drug administration

Route of administration	Control		Recommended safe sedative levels
	Titrate	*Rapid reversal*	
Oral	No	No	Light only
Rectal	No	No	Light only
IM	No	No	Adults: light, moderate
			Children: light, moderate, profound
IV	Yes	No (most drugs); yes (narcotics)	Adults and children*: light, moderate, profound
Inhalation	Yes	Yes	Any sedation level

*There is usually little need for IV sedation in normal healthy children. Most children who will permit a venipuncture will also permit a local anesthetic to be administered intraorally. IV sedation is of great benefit in managing handicapped children and adults.

Clinical Manifestations
Barbiturate and nonbarbiturate sedative-hypnotics

Barbiturates produce depression of a number of physiologic properties, including nerve tissue; respiration; and skeletal, smooth, and cardiac muscle. The mechanism of action (sedation and hypnosis) is depression at the level of the hypothalamus and the ascending reticular activating system, which produces a decrease in the transmission of impulses to the cerebral cortex. Further increases in the blood level of barbiturates produce depression at other levels of the central nervous system, such as profound cortical depression, depression of motor function, and finally depression of the medulla. This may be represented diagrammatically as follows:

Sedation (calming) → Hypnosis (sleep) → General anesthesia (unconsciousness with progressive respiratory and cardiovascular depression) → Respiratory arrest

Sedation and oversedation. At low (therapeutic) blood levels, the patient will appear calm and cooperative (sedated). As the barbiturate level in the blood increases, the patient will begin to fall into a rousable sleep (hypnosis). The doctor will notice the patient's inability to keep the mouth open in spite of constant reminders to do so. In addition, patients at this level of barbiturate-induced CNS depression have a tendency to overrespond to stimulation, especially that of a noxious nature. The unsedated adult patient may grimace in response to pain; the oversedated adult given barbiturates has an exaggerated response—perhaps yelling or jumping. This reflects the loss of self-control over emotion that is produced by the CNS-depressant action of the barbiturate.

Hypnosis. With continued elevation of the barbiturate level in the blood, hypnosis (sleep) ensues, with a minor degree of depression of respiratory function (decreased depth and increased rate of ventilation). At this level there is virtually no adverse action on the cardiovascular system, only a slight decrease in blood pressure and heart rate similar to that occurring in normal sleep. Dental treatment cannot be continued at this level of CNS depression, because the patient is unable to cooperate with the doctor by keeping the mouth open and may well require assistance in maintaining a patent airway (head tilt). The patient will still respond to noxious stimulation but in a sluggish manner.

General anesthesia. With a further increase in the barbiturate level in the blood, the degree of CNS depression broadens so that the patient is now unconscious (incapable of response to sensory stimulation, loss of protective reflexes, with attendant inability to maintain a patent airway). Respiratory movements are still present; however, with further increase in barbiturate blood levels, medullary depression occurs and is clinically evident as respiratory and cardiovascular depression. Respiratory depression is seen as shallow breathing movements at a slow or rapid rate. Ventilatory movements of the chest do not indicate that air is entering or leaving the lungs but only that the body is attempting to bring air into the lungs. Cardiovascular depression is evident as a continued decrease in blood pressure (caused by medullary depression and direct depression of the myocardium and vascular smooth muscle) and an increased heart rate. The patient develops a shocklike appearance, with a weak and rapid pulse and cold, moist skin.

Respiratory arrest. As the barbiturate blood level continues to increase or if the patient does not receive adequate therapy in the previous stage, respiratory arrest may occur. Respiratory arrest may readily be managed. If not managed adequately, it will soon progress to cardiac arrest.

Other nonbarbiturate sedative-hypnotic drugs, such as hydroxyzine, chloral hydrate, and promethazine, also possess the potential to produce overdose, although this is not as likely to occur as with the barbiturates. The potential for overdose varies significantly from drug to drug, but all sedative-hypnotic drugs have this potential to some degree.

Narcotic agonists

Meperidine, alphaprodine, morphine, and fentanyl are the most frequently used parenteral narcotics, with meperidine and alphaprodine the most popular in dentistry.

Meperidine, like most narcotic agonists, exerts its chief pharmacologic actions on the central nervous system. Therapeutic doses of meperidine produce analgesia, sedation, euphoria, and a degree of respiratory depression. Of principle concern, of course, is the respiratory depressant effect of the narcotic agonists. They are direct depressants of the medullary respiratory center. In human subjects, respiratory depression from narcotic agonists is evident even at doses that do not disturb the level of consciousness. The degree of respiratory depression produced by narcotics is dose dependent: the greater the dose of the drug, the more significant the level of depression of respiration. The newer narcotic agonist/antagonists, nalbuphine and butorphanol, offer the prospect of analgesia and sedation with minimal respiratory depression.

Death from narcotic overdose almost always is the result of respiratory arrest. All phases of respiration are depressed—rate, minute volume, and tidal volume. The respiratory rate may fall below 10 per minute. Rates of 5 to 6 per minute are not uncommon. The cause of the decreased respiratory activity is a reduction in the responsiveness of the medullary respiratory centers to increases in carbon dioxide tension (Pco_2) and also a depression of the pontine and medullary centers that are responsible for respiratory rhythm.

The cardiovascular effects of meperidine are not clinically significant when the drug is administered within the usual therapeutic dose range. Following the IV administration of meperidine, however, there is normally an increase in the rate of the heart, produced by atropine-like vagolytic properties of meperidine. At overdose levels the blood pressure remains quite stable until late in the course of the reaction, when it falls—primarily as a result of hypoxia. The administration of O_2 at this time will produce an increase in blood pressure despite continued medullary depression. Overly high blood levels of narcotic agonists can lead to the loss of consciousness.

Overdose reactions to both the sedative-hypnotic drugs and narcotic agonists are produced by a progressive depression of the central nervous system that is manifested by alterations in the level of consciousness and as respiratory depression that ultimately results in respiratory arrest. The loss of consciousness produced by barbiturates or narcotic agonists is not always "overdose"; in other words, loss of consciousness is sometimes desirable. For example, these drugs are very commonly administered as the primary agents in general anesthesia. However, when sedation is the goal, the loss of consciousness and respiratory depression must be considered to be serious complications of drug administration.

The duration and the degree of this clinical reaction will vary according to the route of administration, the dose of the drug administered, and the patient's individual sensitivity to the drug. In most situations, oral and rectal administration result in less CNS depression but with a longer duration; IM and submucosal administration result in a more profound level of depression that is relatively long acting, whereas IV administration produces the most profound level of depression that is of a shorter duration than that seen with the other techniques. The onset of respiratory depression following IV administration may be quite rapid; that following oral or rectal administration is considerably slower. Onset is intermediate in IM and subcutaneous administration.

Management
Sedative-hypnotic drugs

Management of the overdose reaction to sedative-hypnotic drug administration is concerned with correction of the clinical effects of CNS depression. Of primary importance is the management of respiratory depression through the administration of BLS (basic life support). Unfortunately, there is no effective antagonist that can reverse the CNS-depressant properties of the sedative-hypnotic drugs.

Step 1. Position patient. The patient is placed in the supine position with the feet elevated slightly

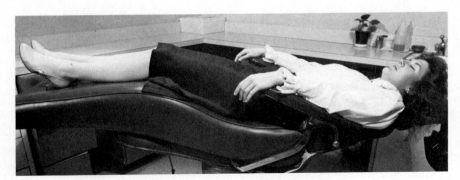

Fig. 23-11. Unconscious patient is placed in supine position with feet elevated slightly.

(Fig. 23-11). The goal in this situation, regardless of the level of consciousness (or unconsciousness) of the patient, is to ensure an adequate cerebral blood flow.

Step 2. Initiate basic life support. A patent airway must be ensured and the adequacy of breathing checked. Head tilt or head tilt–chin lift techniques may be used at this time (Fig. 23-12). The presence or adequacy of the patient's ventilatory efforts is next assessed by the rescuer, who places his or her ear 1 inch from the patient's mouth and nose and listens and feels for exhaled air while looking at the patient's chest to see if the patient is attempting to breathe spontaneously.

The maintenance of a patent airway is the most important step in management of the patient. The next step, adequate oxygenation, is contingent on successfully maintaining a patent airway.

Step 3. Administer oxygen. The patient may exhibit many different degrees of breathing. The patient may be conscious but overly sedated—responding, but slowly, to painful stimulation. In this situation the patient will probably be able to maintain his own airway and will be breathing spontaneously and rather effectively. The rescuer need only monitor the patient and, if desired, administer oxygen through a demand valve.

The patient may also be more deeply sedated and barely responsive to stimulation, with the airway partially or totally obstructed. In this situation airway maintenance will be necessary in addition to assisted ventilation. With patency of the airway ensured, the patient should receive oxygen through a full face mask. If spontaneous breathing is present but shallow, assisted positive pressure ventilation is indicated. This is accomplished with the full face mask sealed on the patient's face and oxygen forced into the lungs as the patient begins each breathing movement. When the positive pressure mask is used, this is accomplished by depressing the button on top of the mask until the patient's chest rises and then releasing the button. With the self-inflating bag-valve-mask device, the bellows bag is squeezed at the start of each inhalation. Head tilt must be maintained at all times.

If respiratory arrest has occurred, controlled artificial ventilation must be started immediately. The recommended rate for the adult is one breath every 5 seconds (12 per minute), one breath every 4 seconds for the child aged 1 year through 8 years (15 per minute), and one breath every 3 seconds for the infant under 1 year of age (20 per minute). Successful ventilation is indicated by elevation of the patient's chest. Overinflation is to be avoided because this will lead to abdominal distention and may result in inadequate ventilation and regurgitation.

Step 4. Monitor vital signs. The patient's vital signs must be monitored throughout the episode. Blood pressure, heart rate and rhythm, and respiratory rate should be recorded every 5 minutes, and a written record should be maintained. A second member of the emergency team is responsible for this task. If the blood level of the sedative-hypnotic drug increases significantly, the blood

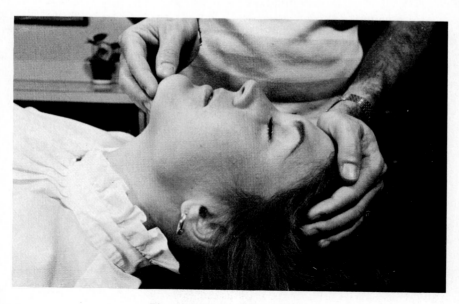

Fig. 23-12. Head tilt–chin lift.

pressure will decrease progressively while the heart rate increases. Should blood pressure and the pulse disappear, cardiopulmonary resuscitation must be instituted immediately.

In most cases of barbiturate or other sedative-hypnotic drug overdose, the patient is maintained in this manner until the blood level of the drug decreases and the patient demonstrates clinical recovery. In most cases, this apparent recovery is the result of redistribution of the drug, not biotransformation. However, the patient will appear more conscious (be more alert and responsive), breathing will improve (become deeper), and if depressed, the blood pressure will return to approximately baseline levels. The length of time this process will require depends on the drug administered and its route of administration.

Step 5. Summon medical assistance. In some situations, it may be prudent to summon medical assistance. The need for this will, of course, vary with the training of the doctor and staff, the nature of the incident, and the availability of medical assistance. This step must be considered when judged necessary by the doctor.

Step 6. Start intravenous infusion. If an IV infusion has not previously been established, it is prudent to establish one at this time. Although there are no effective antidotal drugs for sedative-hypnotic drug overdosage, hypotension may be treated most effectively through intravenously administered solutions or medications. As the blood pressure decreases, however, veins will become progressively more difficult to locate and cannulate. Establishing an IV line at the earliest possible time may prove invaluable later.

The venipuncture should be attempted only if the doctor is trained in this technique and has the necessary equipment and if the patient is receiving adequate care (BLS) from other personnel. A patent airway is more important that a patent vein.

Step 7. Definitive management. Definitive management of this situation is based primarily on the maintenance of an adequate airway and ventilation until the patient recovers.

Signs and symptoms of hypotension are checked by monitoring vital signs and determining adequacy of tissue perfusion.*

---

*Adequacy of tissue perfusion may be determined by pressing on nail bed or skin and releasing pressure. Adequate perfusion is present if color returns in not more than 3 seconds. If 4 or more seconds are required, tissue perfusion is inadequate and consideration must be given to the immediate infusion of intravenous fluids.

Step 8. Recovery and discharge. In the event that the overdose is profound and requires the assistance of outside medical personnel, the patient may require transportation to a hospital for observation and full recovery. Should this be necessary, the doctor should always accompany the patient to the hospital.

In most cases, however, the overdose is less severe, with diminished responsiveness and slight respiratory depression noted clinically. Management consists of positioning, airway maintenance, and assisted ventilation until recovery. Before discharge (in the custody of a responsible adult) the patient must be capable of standing and walking without assistance. Under no circumstances should the patient be discharged alone or if not adequately recovered.

The box below summarizes the management of sedative-hypnotic overdose.

Narcotic analgesics

Oversedation and respiratory depression are the primary clinical manifestations of narcotic overdose. Cardiovascular depression normally does not develop until quite late in the overdose reaction. Management of the patient who has received an absolute or relative overdose of a narcotic is the same as that described for the sedative-hypnotic

---

**MANAGEMENT OF
SEDATIVE-HYPNOTIC OVERDOSE**

Step 1 Position the patient—supine
  2 Initiate basic life support
    Obtain patent airway and check effectiveness of breathing
  3 Start artificial ventilation and administer O$_2$ as needed
  4 Monitor and record vital signs
  5 Summon medical assistance, if necessary
  6 Start IV infusion, if available and practical
  7 Start definitive management (as required): methoxamine 20 mg intramuscularly for prolonged hypotension
  8 Permit recovery for at least 1 hour; discharge patient home (with responsible adult) or hospital (doctor accompanies), as indicated

drugs with one major addition: specific antagonist drugs are available that rapidly reverse some of the clinical effects of the narcotics. Steps in the management of this patient follow.

Step 1. Position patient. The patient is placed in the supine position with feet elevated slightly.

Step 2. Initiate basic life support. The presence of a patent airway is ensured, and breathing is monitored.

Step 3. Administer oxygen. O_2 or artificial ventilation is administered if necessary. The administration of O_2 is especially important in the early management of a narcotic overdose. Little cardiovascular depression is normally observed, and in most cases it occurs as a result of hypoxia secondary to respiratory depression. The administration of O_2 to a patient with a patent airway will prevent or reverse any cardiovascular depression that is evident.

Step 4. Monitor vital signs. Vital signs are monitored every 5 minutes and entered on the record sheet. Should pulse and blood pressure be absent, cardiopulmonary resuscitation is initiated immediately.

Step 5. Definitive management. Definitive management is called for in cases in which a narcotic has been administered to the patient. Even when what is normally considered to be a small dose of a narcotic has been given, a narcotic antagonist should be administered to the patient if excessive respiratory depression has developed.

Nothing is administered to the patient until after a patent airway and adequate ventilation have been ensured and vital signs are monitored. At this point a narcotic antagonist is administered. The agent of choice, naloxone, should be administered intravenously if possible to take advantage of the more rapid onset of clinical activity with this route. If the IV route is unavailable, IM administration will suffice. The onset of action is slower, but the drug will prove effective if a narcotic has produced the respiratory depression. Regardless of the route of administration of naloxone, the doctor should continue to provide BLS as indicated from the time of naloxone administration until its onset of action, as determined by increased patient responsiveness and more adequate and rapid ventilatory efforts. Following IV administration, naloxone will demonstrate its actions within 1 to 2 minutes, and within 10 minutes following IM administration.

Naloxone is available in a 1 ml ampule containing 0.4 mg of the drug. The drug is loaded into a plastic disposable syringe, and if the IV route is available,

3 ml of diluent (any IV fluid) is added to the syringe, producing a final concentration of 0.1 mg of naloxone per milliliter. The drug is then administered to the patient at a rate of 0.1 mg (1 ml) per minute until the patient's ventilatory rate increases. If administered IM, a dose of 0.4 mg is administered into a suitable muscle mass, such as the mid-deltoid region of the upper arm, anterior-lateral thigh, or sublingually.

A potential problem with naloxone is the fact that its duration of clinical activity may be shorter than that of the narcotic it is being used to reverse. This is especially true in cases in which morphine is being used; it is less likely to occur with meperidine and still less likely with alphaprodine and fentanyl. Should this occur, the doctor and staff would notice an improvement of the patient's clinical picture as the naloxone began to act, and then see a recurrence of CNS depression approximately 30 or more minutes later. Because the narcotic producing the overdose continually undergoes redistribution and biotransformation during this time, in the event that such a reaction does recur, it would quite likely be of a much milder nature than the initial response. In cases in which longer-acting narcotics have been administered intramuscularly or submucosally, it may be prudent to follow the original IV dose of naloxone with a second IM dose (0.4 mg). In this manner, as the effect of the original naloxone dose is diminishing, the level of naloxone from the IM dose will be reaching a peak, thus preventing a relapse reaction. The availability in the near future of naltrexone, a longer-acting narcotic antagonist, will minimize this risk.

The administration of naloxone in cases of narcotic overdose is a very important step in overall patient management (see the following).

Step 6. Permit recovery. The patient is observed following the administration of naloxone and apparent clinical recovery. The patient may be transported to the recovery area but should remain there under constant supervision for at least 1 hour; on the other hand, if the doctor considers it prudent, treatment may continue. Vital signs should be recorded every 5 minutes, oxygen and suction must be available, and trained personnel should be present.

Step 7. Summon medical assistance. The summoning of medical assistance will be at the discretion of the doctor. If respiratory arrest (the cessation of breathing) has occurred, I recommend that medical assistance be summoned so that a postoperative evaluation of the patient can be obtained before discharge. If only a slight degree of depression is observed, the doctor may elect not to seek additional medical assistance.

Step 8. Discharge. Patient discharge may require the transport of the patient to a hospital facility for observation or follow-up treatment. Regardless of the indication for hospitalization, the doctor responsible for treating this patient should accompany the patient to the hospital or physician's office.

In most cases, this will prove unnecessary. Following a period of recovery in the dental or medical office, the patient can be discharged in the custody of a responsible adult companion, using the same criteria as established for IV and IM sedation. The patient must be able to stand and walk without aid from another person.

The box at right summarizes the management of narcotic overdose.

SUMMARY

The previous discussions dealt with overdose reactions of varying severity that occur following the administration of a single drug. Although single-drug overdose is not uncommon, especially following intramuscular or submucosal administration, most overdose reactions that are reported involve the administration of more than one medication. In many of these cases, drugs such as an antianxiety drug are combined with a narcotic analgesic to provide a level of sedation and some analgesia. To these will usually be added a local anesthetic for the control of operative pain.

When CNS-depressant drugs are being used together, the dosages of both agents *must* be reduced from their usual dosage to prevent an exaggerated, undesirable clinical response. As is demonstrated in Table 23-14 in most of the cases reported by Goodson and Moore, this was not done.

MANAGEMENT OF NARCOTIC OVERDOSE

Step 1 Position the patient—supine, feet elevated

2 Initiate basic life support
   Ensure patent airway, check for breathing

3 Start artificial ventilation; administer O_2, as indicated

4 Monitor and record vital signs

5 Start definitive management: naloxone 0.4 mg IM or IV (titrate 0.1 mg/ml)

6 Observe patient recovery for at least 1 hour

7 Summon medical assistance, if necessary

8 Discharge patient with responsible adult

Table 23-14. Dose administered relative to recommended maximum dose

Case	Narcotic analgesics (percentage)*	Antiemetic sedatives (percentage)*	Local anesthetics		
			(percentage)*	N₂O-O₂	Result
1	216	36	172	−	Fatality
2	173	145	237	−	Fatality
3	336	0	342	−	Fatality
4	127	27	267	+	Fatality
5	309	372	230	+	Brain damage
6	436	?	?	−	Fatality
7	100	136	107	−	Fatality
8	167	300	219	+	Brain damage
9	66	0	60	−	Recovery
10	66	92	?	+	Recovery
11	183	0	?	−	Recovery
12	200	558	0	−	Recovery
13	250	136	127	−	Brain damage
14	50	0	370	+	Fatality

From Goodson, J.M., and Moore, P.A.: J. Am. Dent. Assoc. **107:**239, 1983. Copyright by the American Dental Association. Reprinted by permission.
*Expressed as percentage of maximal recommended dose for that patient.

Another factor must be considered, one that most do not, as a rule, give much thought to when using sedative techniques. That is the fact that local anesthetics themselves are CNS depressants and can produce additive actions when administered in conjunction with the agents commonly employed for sedation. The maximal dosage of local anesthetic to be administered to any patient, but especially to a child or lighter-weight adult, should be based on the patient's body weight in kilograms or pounds. When no other CNS depressants are being administered, this maximal dose could be reached without adverse reaction if the patient is an ASA I and falls within the normal range on the bell-shaped curve. Maximal recommended doses of the most commonly used local anesthetics are presented in Table 23-15. When used in conjunction with other CNS depressants, the dosage of the local anesthetic should be minimized.

A primary goal of sedation is to produce a cooperative patient who still maintains protective reflexes. When possible, this goal should be achieved using the simplest technique available, as well as the fewest number of drugs possible. Polypharmacy, the combination of several drugs, may be necessary in some patients to achieve the desired level of sedation; however, if this same level can be produced with one drug, the combination ought not be employed. The use of drug combinations simply increases the opportunity for ADRs, as well as making it less obvious which drug has produced the problem and making management of the situation somewhat more difficult.

Within the individual techniques of sedation, it is recommended that single-drug regimens are preferable to combinations of drugs. Rational drug combinations are available for use in cases in which they are specifically indicated. With IV drug administration, the problem of severe ADRs should not occur if the technique of titration is adhered to

at all times. With intramuscular and oral drug administration, however, where titration is not available, the doctor must adjust drug dosages before their administration to the patient. Serious ADRs are more likely to occur with these techniques.

Consideration must also be given to the use of multiple techniques of sedation in a patient. It will not be uncommon for a patient who presents a management problem to receive an oral antianxiety drug before arrival in the office, followed by either IM, submucosal, IV, or inhalation sedation in addition to local anesthesia during the treatment. Wherever oral premedication with CNS depressants have been used, the dosages of all other CNS depressants should be decreased. This is critical when the IM or submucosal routes are used, since titration is unavailable. With inhalation and IV sedation, careful titration of drugs to the patient who has been orally premedicated will usually produce the desired sedation level with a lower dose of the drug being used.

How, then, may overdose reactions best be prevented?

Goodson and Moore (1983) made the following recommendations concerning the use of sedative techniques in which narcotics are being administered.

1. Be prepared for emergencies

Continuous monitoring of the cardiovascular and respiratory systems should be employed. An emergency kit containing drugs such as adrenaline, O_2, and naloxone should be readily available, in addition to equipment and trained personnel. In their article, Goodson and Moore state that "because multiple sedative drug techniques can easily induce unconsciousness, respiratory arrest, and convulsions, practitioners should be prepared and trained to recognize and control these occurrences."

2. Individualize drug dosage

When drugs are used in combination, the dosage of each drug must be carefully selected. The toxic effects of drug combinations appear to be additive. Drug selection must be based on the patient's general health history. The presence of systemic disease usually indicates the need for a reduction of dosage.

Because most sedative drugs are available in quite concentrated form, and because children will require very small dosages, extreme care must be

Table 23-15. Maximal recommended local-anesthetic doses

Drug	Dose		Absolute maximal dose
	Mg/kg	*Mg/lb*	
Lidocaine	4.4	2.0	300
Mepivacaine	4.4	2.0	300
Prilocaine	6.0	2.7	400
Bupivacaine	2.0	0.9	90

taken when these drugs are being prepared for administration.

Fixed-dose administration of drugs based on a range of ages (for example, 4 to 6 years: 50 mg) should not be employed. Dosages based on body weight or surface area of the patient or titration are preferred, if possible.

Should the selected drug dosage prove to be inadequate, it is prudent to consider a change in the technique of sedation or in the drugs being used (at a subsequent appointment), rather than increasing the drug dosage to a higher and potentially more dangerous level.

3. Recognize and expect adverse drug effects

When combinations of CNS-depressant drugs have been administered, the potential for excessive CNS and respiration depression is increased and should be expected.

• • •

The Dentists Insurance Company (TDIC), in a retrospective study of deaths and morbidity in dental practice over a 3-year period, concluded that in most of those incidents that were related to the administration of drugs there were three common factors:

1. Improper preoperative evaluation of the patient
2. Lack of knowledge of drug pharmacology by the doctor
3. Lack of adequate monitoring during the procedure

These three factors greatly increased the risk of serious ADRs developing, with a negative outcome.

An overdose reaction to the administration of CNS-depressant drugs may not always be a preventable complication; however, with care on the part of the doctor, the incidence of these events should be extremely low, and a successful outcome should occur virtually every time. With techniques such as IV and inhalation sedation, in which titration is possible, overdosage should rarely develop at all. With oral, IM, and SM drug administration, in which the doctor has no control over the drug effect because of the inability to titrate, greater care must be expended by the doctor in preoperative evaluation of the patient, determination of the appropriate drug dosage, and monitoring throughout the procedure so that excessive CNS or respiratory depression may be observed and treated immediately. When the oral, SM, and IM routes of administration are employed, the onset of adverse reactions may be delayed. The adverse reaction may not develop until after the rubber dam is in place and the dental procedure started. Monitoring during the procedure therefore becomes extremely important to patient safety.

BIBLIOGRAPHY

Adatia, A.K.: Intravascular injection of local anesthetics, Br. Dent. J. **138**:328, 1975.

Adjepon-Yamoah, K.K., Nimmo, J., and Prescott, L.F.: Gross impairment of hepatic drug metabolism in a patient with chronic liver disease, Br. Med. J. **4**:387, 1974.

Adriani, J., and Campbell, B.: Fatalities following topical application of local anesthetics to mucous membranes, JAMA **162**:1527, 1956.

Aldrete, J.A., and Daniel, W.: Evaluation of premedicants as protective agents against convulsive (LD_{50}) doses of local anesthetic agents in rats, Anesth. Analg. **50**:127, 1971.

Aldrete, J.A., and others: Effects of hepatectomy on the disappearance rate of lidocaine from blood in man and dog, Anesth. Analg. **49**:687, 1970.

Aldrete, J.A., Narang, R., and Sada, T.: Untoward reactions to local anesthetics via reverse intracarotid flow, J. Dent. Res. **54**:145, 1975.

Aldrete, J.A., and others: Reverse carotid blood flow—a possible explanation for some reactions to local anesthetics, J. Am. Dent. Assoc. **94**:1142, 1977.

Alexander, R.E.: Epinephrine is safe for heart patients, Med. Times **99**:132, 1971.

American Dental Association: Accepted dental therapeutics, ed. 40, Chicago, 1984, American Dental Association.

American Medical Association: AMA drug evaluations, ed. 4, Littleton, Mass., 1980, Publishing Sciences Group, Inc.

Ausinsch, B., Malagod, M.H., and Munson, E.S.: Diazepam in the prophylaxis of lignocaine seizures, Br. J. Anaesth. **48**:309, 1976.

Bartlett, S.Z.: Clinical observations on the effects of injections of local anesthetics preceded by aspiration, Oral Surg. **33**:520, 1972.

Bigger, J.T., Jr., and Mandel, W.J.: Effect of lidocaine on the electrophysiological properties of ventricular muscle and Purkinje fibers, J. Clin. Invest. **49**:63, 1970.

Boynes, R.N., and others: Pharmacokinetics of lidocaine in man, Clin. Pharmacol. Ther. **12**:105, 1970.

Braid, D.P., and Scott, D.B.: The systemic absorption of local analgesic drugs, Br. J. Anaesth. **37**:394, 1965.

Cannell, H., and others: Circulating levels of lignocaine after peri-oral injections, Br. Dent. J. **138**:87, 1975.

Cohen, M.B., Gravitz, L.A., and Knappe, T.A.: Twenty-five versus twenty-seven gauge needles, J. Am. Dent. Assoc. **78**:1312, 1969.

Covino, B.G.: Comparative clinical pharmacology of local anesthetic agents, Anesthesiology **35**:158, 1971.

Covino, B.G., and Vassallo, H.G.: Local anesthetics: mechanisms of action and clinical use, New York, 1976, Grune & Stratton, Inc.

Crottu, J.J.: The epidemiology of salicylate poisoning, Clin. Toxicol. **1**:381, 1968.

deJong, R.H., and Heavner, J.E.: Diazepam prevents local anesthetic seizures, Anesthesiology **34**:523, 1971.

deJong, R.H., and Heavner, J.E.: Local anesthetic seizure prevention: diazepam versus pentobarbital, Anesthesiology **36**:449, 1972.

deJong, R.H., Heavner, J.E., and Oliveira, L.F.: Effects of nitrous oxide on the lidocaine seizure threshold and diazepam protection, Anesthesiology **37**:299, 1972.

deJong, R.H., and Heavner, J.E.: Convulsions induced by local anaesthetic: time course of diazepam prophylaxis, Can. Anaesth. Soc. J. **21**:153, 1974.

deJong, R.H.: Toxic effects of local anesthetics, JAMA **239**:1166, 1978.

Dhuner, K.G.: Frequency of general side reactions after regional anaesthesia with mepivacaine with and without vasoconstrictors, Acta Anaesthesiol. Scand. **48**(suppl):23, 1972.

Downs, J.R.: Atypical cholinesterase activity: its importance in dentistry, J. Oral Surg. **24**:256, 1966.

Englesson, S.: The influence of acid-base changes on central nervous system toxicity of local anaesthetic agents, Acta Anaesthesiol. Scand. **18**:79, 1974.

Englesson, S., and Matousek, M.: Central nervous system effects of local anesthetic agents, Br. J. Anaesth. **47**:241, 1975.

Fein, B.T.: Aspirin shock associated with asthma and nasal polyps, Ann. Allergy **29**:598, 1971.

Feinstein, M.B., Lenard, W., and Mathias, J.: The antagonism of local anesthetic induced convulsions by the benzodiazepine derivative diazepam, Arch. Int. Pharmacodyn. Ther. **187**:144, 1970.

Freeman, D.W., and Arnold, N.I.: Paracervical block with low doses of chloroprocaine, JAMA **231**:56, 1975.

Goodson, J.M., and Moore, P.A.: Life-threatening reactions after pedodontic sedation: an assessment of narcotic, local-anesthetic, and antiemetic drug interaction, J. Am. Dent. Assoc. **107**:239, 1983.

Greenblatt, D.J., and others: Pharmacokinetic approach to the clinical use of lidocaine intravenously, JAMA **236**:273, 1976.

Harrison, D.C., and Alderman, E.L.: Relation of blood levels to clinical effectiveness of lidocaine. In Scott, D.B., and Julian, D.C., editors: Lidocaine in the treatment of ventricular arrhythmias, Edinburgh, 1971, E & S Livingstone.

Hine, C.H., and Pasi, A.: Fatality after use of alphaprodine in analgesia for dental surgery. Report of a case, J. Am. Dent. Assoc. **84**:858, 1972.

Holroyd, S.V.: Clinical pharmacology in dental practice, ed. 2, St. Louis, 1978, The C.V. Mosby Co.

Jebson, P.R.: Intramuscular lignocaine 2% and 10%, Br. Med. J. **3**:566, 1971.

Kramer, H.S., Jr., and Mitton, V.A.: Complications of local anesthesia, Dent. Clin. North Am. **17**:443, 1973.

LaGruta, V., Amato, G., and Zagami, M.T.: The importance of the caudate nucleus in the control of convulsive activity, Electroencephalogr. Clin. Neurophysiol. **31**:57, 1971.

Lear, E., and others: Atypical pseudocholinesterase: a clinical report, Anesth. Analg. **55**:243, 1976.

Lindorf, H.H., Ganssen, A., and Mayer, P.: Thermographic representation of the vascular effects of local anesthetics, Electromedica **4**:106, 1974.

Malamed, S.F.: Local anesthetic survey, Unpublished data, 1980.

Malamed, S.F.: Handbook of local anesthesia, ed. 2, St. Louis, 1986, The C.V. Mosby Co.

Moore, D.C.: Complications of regional anesthesia, Springfield, IL, 1955, Charles C. Thomas, Publisher.

Moore, D.C., and others: Arterial and venous plasma levels of bupivacaine (Marcaine) following epidural and intercostal nerve blocks, Anesthesiology **45**:39, 1976.

Morgan, D.J., and others: Disposition and placental transfer of etidocaine in pregnancy, Eur. J. Clin. Pharmacol. **12**:359, 1977.

Morikawa, K.I., and others: Effect of acute hypovolaemia on lignocaine absorption and cardiovascular response following epidural block in dogs, Br. J. Anaesth. **46**:631, 1974.

Munson, E.S.: Diazepam treatment of local anesthetic induced seizures, Anesthesiology **37**:523, 1972.

Munson, E.S.: Mepivacaine overdose in a child, Anesth. Analg. **52**:422, 1973.

Munson, E.S., and others: Etidocaine, bupivacaine and lidocaine seizure thresholds in monkeys, Anesthesiology **42**:471, 1975.

Munson, E.S., Gutnick, M.J., and Wagman, I.H.: Local anesthetic induced seizures in rhesus monkeys, Anesth. Analg. **49**:986, 1970.

Nation, R.L., Triggs, E.J., and Selig, M.: Lignocaine kinetics in cardiac patients and aged subjects, Br. J. Clin. Pharmacol. **4**:439, 1977.

Parnell, A.G.: Intravascular injection of local anaesthetics, Br. Dent. J. **139**:162, 1976.

Reidenber, M.M., James, M., and Dring, L.G.: The rate of procaine hydrolysis in serum of normal subjects and diseased patients, Clin. Pharmacol. Ther. **13**:279, 1972.

Rood, J.P.: Circulating levels of lignocaine after peri-oral injections, Br. Dent. J. **138**:206, 1975.

Sakabe, T., and others: The effects of lidocaine on canine cerebral metabolism and circulation related to the electroencephalogram, Anesthesiology **40**:433, 1974.

Schallek, W., Scholosser, W., and Randall, L.C.: Recent developments in the pharmacology of the benzodiazepines, Adv. Pharmacol. Chemother. **10**:119, 1972.

Scott, D.B., and others: Factors affecting plasma levels of lignocaine and prilocaine, Br. J. Anaesth. **44**:1040, 1972.

Scott, D.B.: Evaluation of clinical tolerance of local anaesthetic agents, Br. J. Anaesth. **47**:328, 1975.

Scott, D.B.: Evaluation of the toxicity of local anesthetic agents in man, Br. J. Anaesth. **47**:56, 1975.

Spear, P.W., and Protass, L.M.: Barbiturate poisoning—an endemic disease, Med. Clin. North Am. **57**:1471, 1973.

Thomson, P.: Lidocaine pharmacokinetics in advanced heart failure, liver disease, and renal failure in humans, Ann. Intern. Med. **78**:499, 1973.

Tucker, G.T., and others: Systemic absorption of mepivacaine in commonly used regional block procedures, Anesthesiology **37**:277, 1972.

Verrill, P.J.: Adverse reactions to local anesthetics and vasoconstrictor drugs, Practitioner **214**:380, 1975.

Wesseling, H., Bovenhurst, G.H., and Wiers, J.W.: Effects of diazepam and pentobarbitone on convulsions induced by local anesthetics in mice, Eur. J. Pharmacol. **13**:150, 1971.

Zinman, E.J.: Toxicity and mepivacaine, J. Am. Dent. Assoc. **92**:858, 1976.

Zsigmond, E.K., and Eilderton, T.E.: Survey of local anesthetic toxicity in the families of patients with atypical plasma cholinesterase, J. Oral Surg. **33**:833, 1975.

24 *Allergy*

Allergy has previously been defined as a hypersensitive state acquired through exposure to a particular allergen, reexposure to which produces a heightened capacity to react. Allergic reactions cover a broad range of clinical manifestations, from mild, delayed reactions occurring as long as 48 hours after exposure to the antigen to immediate and life-threatening reactions developing within seconds of exposure. A classification of allergic reactions is presented in Table 24-1. Although all allergic phenomena are important, two forms are of particular consequence in the practice of dentistry. The type IV, or delayed, reaction, seen clinically as contact dermatitis, is particularly relevant because of the significant number of dental personnel who develop this form of allergic response. The type I, or anaphylactic (immediate), reaction, may present the dental office staff with the most acutely life-threatening emergency situation of any discussed in this textbook.

Contact dermatitis, although a non–life-threatening situation, is of special interest and is discussed briefly at the conclusion of this chapter. The immediate-onset allergic reactions are of primary importance and receive major emphasis in the following discussion. The type I reaction may be subdivided into several forms of response, including generalized and localized anaphylaxis. A list of type I allergic reactions follows:*

Type I immediate hypersensitivity:
    Generalized (systemic) anaphylaxis
    Localized anaphylaxis
        Urticaria (in the skin)
        Bronchial asthma (in the respiratory tract)
        Food allergy (in the gastrointestinal tract and other organs)

---

*From Gell, P.G.H., and Coombs, R.R.A.: Clinical aspects of immunology, ed. 3, Oxford and London, 1975, Blackwell Scientific Publications.

The major forms of type I reaction are discussed following a presentation of several terms relevant to this chapter.

allergen An antigen that can elicit allergic symptoms

anaphylactoid Anaphylactoid reactions, which mimic true IgE-mediated anaphylaxis, are idiosyncratic reactions that occur generally when the patient is first exposed to a particular drug or agent. Although not immunologically mediated, their emergency management is the same as that of immunologically mediated reactions.

angioedema (angioneurotic edema) Noninflammatory edema involving the skin, subcutaneous tissue, underlying muscle, and mucous membranes, especially those of the gastrointestinal and upper respiratory tract; occurs in response to an allergen; the most critical area of involvement is the larynx (laryngeal edema)

antibody Those substances found in the blood or tissues that respond to the administration of, or react with, an antigen. They differ in structure (for example, IgE and IgG) and are capable of eliciting a distinct response (anaphylaxis or serum sickness)

antigen Any substance foreign to the host that is capable of activating an immune (allergic) response by stimulating the development of a specific antibody

atopy A "strange disease"; a clinical hypersensitivity state subject to hereditary influences; examples include asthma, hay fever, and eczema

pruritus Itching

urticaria A vascular reaction of the skin marked by the transient appearance of smooth, slightly elevated patches, which are redder or paler than the surrounding skin and often attended by severe itching

All allergic reactions are mediated through immunologic mechanisms that are similar, regardless of the specific antigen responsible for precipitating the response. Therefore an allergic reaction to the venom of a stinging insect may be identical to that seen following aspirin or penicillin administration to a previously sensitized individual. This must be

301

Table 24-1. Classification of allergic diseases (after Gell and Coombs)

Type	Mechanism	Principal antibody or cell	Time of reactions	Clinical examples
I	Anaphylactic (immediate, homocytotropic, antigen-induced, antibody-mediated)	IgE	Seconds to minutes	Anaphylaxis (drugs, insect venom, antisera) Atopic bronchial asthma Allergic rhinitis Urticaria Angioedema Hay fever
II	Cytotoxic (antimembrane)	IgG IgM (activate complement)	—	Transfusion reactions Goodpasture's syndrome Autoimmune hemolysis Hemolytic anemia Certain drug reactions Membranous glomerulonephrosis
III	Immune complex (serum sickness-like)	IgG (form complexes with complement)	6-8 hours	Serum sickness Lupus nephritis Occupational allergic alveolitis Acute viral hepatitis
IV	Cell-mediated (delayed) or tuberculin-type response	—	48 hours	Allergic contact dermatitis Infectious granulomas (tuberculosis, mycoses) Tissue graft rejection Chronic hepatitis

Adapted from Krupp, M.A., and Chatton, M.J.: Current medical diagnosis and treatment, Los Altos, CA, 1984, Lange Medical Publications.

differentiated from the overdose or toxic drug reaction that is a direct extension of the normal pharmacologic properties of the drug involved. Overdose reactions are much more frequently encountered than are allergic drug reactions,* even though to the nonmedical individual any adverse drug reaction is usually considered to be an "allergy." It is hoped that following the discussions in this section the reader will be able to fully evaluate any "allergic" history to determine what really occurred and will be able to differentiate between these two important ADRs. Chapter 25 presents a differential diagnosis of the several ADRs and other clinically similar reactions.

Allergy is a frightening word to those health professionals responsible for primary care of patients. In the dental profession, many drugs that have a significant potential for allergenicity are administered or prescribed to patients. Although the concept of prevention has been stressed repeatedly

throughout this book, in no other situation is this concept of greater importance than in allergy. Although allergy is not the most common adverse drug reaction seen, it is frequently involved with the more serious of these reactions. Emphasis is placed on the more immediate forms of allergic reactions and on those specific drugs and chemicals in common use in dental practice.

PREDISPOSING FACTORS

The number of persons with significant allergy is not small. Of the population in the U.S., 15% have allergic conditions severe enough to require medical management. Thirty-three percent of all chronic disease in children is allergic in nature. Individuals with allergy problems represent a potentially serious risk when receiving dental treatment. Although never without risk, drug utilization is normally accomplished without significant occurrence of adverse effects (indeed, if ADRs occurred more frequently, we would avoid using any drugs in dentistry). However, in an individual with a genetic predisposition to allergy (the atopic patient),

---

*85% of adverse drug reactions result from the pharmacologic actions of the drug; 15% are immunologic reactions.

great care must be taken before use of any drug. The patient with multiple allergies (for example, hay fever, asthma, or allergy to numerous foods) is much more likely to elicit an allergic response to the drugs used in dentistry than a patient with no prior history of allergy.

Although the patient's prior history is the major factor in determining a risk of allergy, the specific drug to be employed is also of extreme importance. In allergy, as opposed to overdose, prior drug contact (sensitizing dose) is almost always necessary for the reaction to develop (such is not the case in anaphylactoid reactions). Signs and symptoms of allergy appear only after a subsequent (challenge) dose is administered to the patient. Without the sensitizing and challenge doses, allergy will not occur.

Various drug groups are more highly allergenic than are others. In one survey, the barbiturates, the penicillins, meprobamate, codeine, and the thiazide diuretics were responsible for over 70% of the allergic reactions encountered. Other substances implicated with fatal systemic anaphylaxis include venom of the hymenoptera (honeybees, yellow jackets, hornets, and wasps), stings of fire ants (solenopsis), iodines (radiopaque contrast media and the iodine in disclosing solutions), vaccines, biologic extracts (insulin, heparin), salicylates, sulfonamides, opiates, and local anesthetics. Listed below are the major drugs used in dental practice that possess significant allergic potential.

Antibiotics
  Penicillins
  Sulfonamides
  Ampicillin
Analgesics
  Acetylsalicylic acid (ASA—aspirin)
  Narcotics
    Morphine
    Meperidine
    Codeine
Antianxiety drugs
  Barbiturates
Local anesthetics
  Esters
    Procaine
    Propoxycaine
    Benzocaine
    Tetracaine
All local anesthetics with paraben preservatives
  or bisulfites
Other agents
  Acrylic monomer (methyl methacrylate)

The hymenoptera, penicillin, and aspirin are the three most common causes of anaphylaxis.

Antibiotics

Probably the most significant ADR associated with antibiotics is the ability of some agents to produce allergic reactions. Some antibiotics such as erythromycin are associated with a very low incidence of allergy; others, particularly the sulfonamides and penicillins, frequently produce allergic responses. In virtually all cases, the allergic reactions associated with antibiotic therapy are not life threatening. The penicillins, the most commonly used antibiotics in dentistry, are the major exceptions.

It has been estimated that the incidence of allergy to penicillin ranges anywhere from 5% to 10% of those receiving the drug. Approximately 2.5 million persons in the United States are allergic to penicillin. Of patients receiving penicillin, 0.004% to 0.04% will develop anaphylaxis, and 10% of these persons will die. This accounts for from 100 to 300 deaths per year.

In a survey on the nature and extent of penicillin side reactions, 150 cases of anaphylaxis were studied. Of the patients observed, 14% had a history of other allergies, 70% had previously received penicillin, and over 33% had experienced a prior immediate allergic reaction to the drug. When death occurred, it normally occurred within 15 minutes.

Allergy to penicillin may be induced by any mode of administration. The topical route is probably the most likely to sensitize an individual (5% to 12% sensitized), the oral route the least likely (0.1% sensitized). However, it is also possible to be sensitized to penicillin without knowledge of prior exposure, since penicillin is a natural contaminant of our environment. The penicillin mold is airborne and may be found in bread, cheese, milk, and fruit.

Analgesics

Allergy to any of the pain-relieving drugs employed in dentistry may occur. This is true regarding the narcotic analgesics such as codeine and meperidine, but the incidence of true allergy to these agents is quite low, even though "allergic to codeine" is listed frequently on medical history questionnaires. A thorough dialogue history (p. 306) is required to determine the exact nature of the ADR that occurred. In most instances, the "allergy" to codeine turns out to be merely annoying side effects of the agent such as nausea, vomiting, drowsiness, dysphoria (restlessness), or constipation.

The incidence of allergy to aspirin is relatively high, with symptoms ranging from mild urticaria to anaphylaxis. Previous ingestion of aspirin without ill effect is no guarantee against a subsequent allergic reaction to the drug. Allergic reactions to aspirin also take the form of angioedema and asthma (bronchospasm). Asthma is the chief allergic manifestation in most persons sensitive to aspirin but especially in the middle-aged female who also has nasal polyps. Death may result. The overall incidence of allergy to aspirin is estimated to be from 0.2% to 0.9%.

Antianxiety Drugs

Of the many agents employed for anxiety reduction in dentistry, the barbiturates probably possess the greatest potential for sensitization of patients. Although not as common as allergy to penicillin or aspirin, allergy to these agents usually manifests itself in the form of skin lesions such as hives and urticaria or, less frequently, in the form of blood dyscrasias such as agranulocytosis or thrombocytopenia. Allergy to barbiturates occurs much more frequently in persons with a history of asthma, urticaria, and angioedema. A history of allergy to any of the barbiturates is an *absolute contraindication* to the use of any of these agents.

Local Anesthetics

Local anesthetics are the most commonly employed drugs in dentistry and probably the most important. Without the availability of these agents, the practice of dentistry would revert to the days when all dental procedures were associated with pain. Allergy to local anesthetics does occur; however, the incidence of such reactions has dramatically decreased since the introduction of amide type local anesthetics in the 1940s. Allergic manifestations of local anesthetics may range from an allergic dermatitis (commonly occurring in dental office personnel) to a typical asthmatic attack to fatal systemic anaphylaxis. Hypersensitivity to local anesthetics occurs much more frequently in response to the ester type local anesthetics such as procaine, propoxycaine, benzocaine, tetracaine, and compounds related to them such as procaine penicillin G, and procainamide (an antidysrhythmic drug). Local anesthetics of the amide type are essentially free of this problem, yet the frequency

of reports of allergy to amide type drugs in the dental and medical literature and on medical history questionnaires seems to be increasing. This apparent contradiction may be cleared up with careful evaluation of these alleged local-anesthetic allergies. Several investigators, most notably Aldrete and Johnson (1970), have investigated these reports and performed extensive evaluations of each case, seeking to determine the true nature of the reaction. In most cases, the reactions were the result of psychogenic factors or drug overdose (Chapter 23); in other cases, the reactions demonstrated were of an allergic nature. When an ester type local anesthetic is employed, a true allergic reaction is frequently elicited; however, with use of the amide type local anesthetics, a purported allergic reaction is frequently shown to be another type of response (overdose, idiosyncrasy, or psychogenic).

Although true allergy to the amide type local anesthetics is extremely rare, patients *have* demonstrated true allergic reactions to the contents of the dental cartridge. The dental cartridge contains a number of ingredients besides the local-anesthetic solution (Table 24-2). Of special interest with respect to allergy is the presence of a preservative, methylparaben, in dental cartridges. Parabens—methyl, ethyl, and propyl—are included in many drugs, foods, and cosmetics. It is difficult if not im-

Table 24-2. Contents of local-anesthetic cartridge

Ingredient	Function
Local anesthetic agent	Conduction blockade
Vasoconstrictor	Decrease absorption of local anesthetic into blood, thus increasing duration of anesthesia and decreasing toxicity of anesthetic
Sodium metabisulfite	Preservative for vasoconstrictor
Methylparaben*	Preservative to increase shelf life; bacteriostatic
Sodium chloride	Isotonicity of solution
Sterile water	Diluent

*Methylparaben has been excluded from all local-anesthetic cartridges manufactured in the United States since January, 1984. It is still found in multiple-dose vials of medications and in many local anesthetic solutions manufactured in other countries.

possible to avoid contact with these agents. Because of the increasing use of the parabens, the frequency of sensitization to them has greatly increased. Parabens are used increasingly in nondrug items such as skin creams, hair lotions, suntan preparations, face powder, soaps, lipsticks, toothpastes, syrups, soft drinks, and candies. In response to the increasing incidence of allergic reactions to these products, certain products have been marked as "hypoallergenic" and do not contain any parabens.

Patients with a history of allergy to an amide type local anesthetic were tested (Aldrete and Johnson, 1970), using the anesthetic agent without methylparaben and with the preservative alone. In every instance, the patient exhibited a positive response to the preservative but a negative response to the amide anesthetic without the preservative. Paraben allergy is almost exclusively limited to a dermatologic type response. In 1984 the Food and Drug Administration (FDA) ordered the removal of paraben preservatives from all local anesthetic cartridges manufactured in the United States.

Allergy to sodium bisulfite or metabisulfite is being reported with increasing frequency. Bisulfites are antioxidants and are commonly used in restaurants where they are sprayed on fruits and vegetables to keep them appearing "fresh." For example, sliced apples sprayed with bisulfite do not turn brown (become oxidized). Persons with bisulfite allergy frequently respond to contact with bisulfite with severe respiratory allergy, such as bronchospasm. Bisulfite allergy should alert the doctor to the possibility of this same type of response if sodium bisulfite or metabisulfite are included in the dental cartridge. Bisulfites are present in all cartridges of local anesthetic which contain a vasoconstrictor.

Topical anesthetic agents are also potentially allergenic. Many of the topical anesthetics are esters—benzocaine and tetracaine being the most commonly employed. Many topical anesthetics, even the amide types, contain preservatives such as the parabens (methyl, ethyl, propyl), so that allergy is always possible when these agents are used.

Clinical manifestations of allergy related to topical-anesthetic application may span the entire spectrum of allergic responses; however, the most common response is allergic contact stomatitis, which may include mild erythema, edema, and ulcerations. If widespread and severe, the edema may lead to difficulty in swallowing and breathing.

Other Agents

"Denture sore mouth" is the name commonly given to inflammatory changes of the mucous membranes developing beneath dentures. Most frequently the oral mucosa of the palate and maxillary ridges are involved, with the tissue appearing bright red and edematous and the patient complaining of soreness, rawness, dryness, and burning.

The acrylic resins used in most dentures today are capable of producing allergic responses. This is much more likely to be seen when self-cured acrylics are used than with heat-cured acrylics. In addition, dental personnel and laboratory technicians may develop contact dermatitis to these materials. These reactions occur most frequently on the fingers and hands and are almost always caused by the acrylic monomer (the liquid), methyl methacrylate.

Heat-cured acrylics are less frequently associated with allergy because the monomer is more completely utilized in the polymerization process. In cold-cured or self-cured acrylics, it is likely that small amounts of monomer remain unpolymerized, and it is this that produces the allergic response in sensitized individuals. Cold-curing or self-curing acrylics are employed in denture repair and relining procedures, as well as in the fabrication of temporary crowns, bridges, and splints.

PREVENTION
Medical History Questionnaire

The medical history questionnaire contains several questions relating to allergy.

QUESTION 7. Are you allergic to (that is, itching, rash, swelling of hands, feet, or eyes) or made sick by penicillin, aspirin, codeine, or any drugs or medications?
QUESTION 9. Circle any of the following which you have had or have at present:
- **Asthma**
- **Hay fever**
- **Sinus trouble**
- **Allergies or hives**

COMMENT. These questions seek to determine if ADRs have occurred. ADRs are not uncommon; the most frequently reported reactions are usually labeled "allergy." Any positive response to these questions by a patient must be thoroughly evaluated by means of the dialogue history.

In all instances, it is prudent to assume that the allergy does exist until the exact type of reaction can be determined. The dialogue history is a vital part of this evaluation, as is medical consultation with an allergy specialist in the event that any doubt remains concerning allergy. The drug or drugs in question, as well as any related drugs, should not be used until the alleged allergy has been disproved.

Substitute drugs may be employed in place of most of the drugs that commonly cause allergic reactions. These agents possess many of the same desirable clinical effects as the primary drugs without their allergic potential. The only drug group in which the substitute agents are not as clinically effective as the primary agents is the local anesthetic group. Because these are also the most important drugs employed in dental practice, much of the following discussion is related to the problem of local-anesthetic allergy.

Dialogue History

Following an affirmative response to the question about a previous adverse drug reaction, the doctor should seek as much information as possible from the patient directly. The following questions should be asked (with slight modification where indicated) in evaluation of an alleged drug "allergy."

QUESTION. *What drug was used?*

COMMENT. A patient who is truly allergic to a drug should be told the exact (generic) name of the substance. Many persons with documented allergic histories wear a Medic Alert tag, which lists the items to which they are sensitive. However, the most common responses to this question are, "I'm allergic to local anesthetics" or "I'm allergic to Novocain" or "I'm allergic to all '-caine' drugs." Novocain (procaine), an ester, is rarely used today as a local anesthetic in dentistry, the amides having virtually replaced the esters. Yet patients routinely refer to the local anesthetics they receive as "shots of Novocain." There are two reasons for this: first, the name Novocain has become virtually synonymous with dental injections. Second, in spite of the fact that most doctors do not use procaine or procaine-propoxycaine, many doctors themselves still refer to local anesthetics as "Novocain" although they use amide type local anesthetics almost exclusively. Therefore the usual response to the question remains "I'm allergic to Novocain." This response, if received from a patient who has been

managed properly in the past following an adverse reaction, indicates that the patient was sensitive to the ester type local anesthetics but not to the amide local anesthetics. However, the answers usually received are too general and too vague to permit any conclusions to be drawn.

QUESTION. *What amount of drug was administered?*

COMMENT. This question seeks to determine whether there was a definite dose-response relationship, as might be seen in an overdose reaction. The problem is that the patient rarely knows these clinical details and can provide little or no assistance.

QUESTION. *Did the solution contain vasoconstrictors or preservatives?*

COMMENT. The reaction may have been an overdose reaction to the vasoconstrictors in the solution. If an allergic reaction did occur, perhaps it was related to the preservative and not to the local anesthetic. Unfortunately, however, most patients are unable to furnish this information.

QUESTION. *Were you taking any other medication at the time?*

COMMENT. This question seeks to determine the possibility that drug interaction or another drug was responsible for the reported adverse reaction.

QUESTION. *What was the time sequence of events?*

COMMENT. When, in relation to the administration of the drug, did the reaction occur? Most of the ADRs associated with local-anesthetic administration occur during or immediately following the injection. Syncope, hyperventilation, overdose, and anaphylaxis are most likely to develop at the time of injection, although any of these reactions may occur later during dental therapy, too. Also, seek to determine how long the episode lasted. How long was it until the patient was discharged from the office? Was dental therapy continued following the episode? Dental therapy that continued following the episode indicates that the reaction was probably not an allergic response.

QUESTION. *What position were you in when the reaction took place?*

COMMENT. Injection of local anesthetics into a patient in the upright position is most likely to produce a psychogenic reaction (vasodepressor syncope). This does not exclude the possibility of other reactions having occurred; however, if the patient was in the supine position during injection, vasodepressor syncope seems less likely to be the cause of the reaction, even though loss of consciousness may occur on occasion in these circumstances.

QUESTION. How did the reaction manifest itself? What happened?

COMMENT. This is an important question in that it allows the patient to describe what actually occurred. The "allergy" in many instances is explained by the answer to this question. The signs and symptoms the patient describes should be recorded and evaluated to make a tentative diagnosis of the ADR. See the chapters on overdose reaction (Chapter 23), vasodepressor syncope (Chapter 6), allergy (Chapter 24), and the differential diagnosis of drug reactions (Chapter 25) for complete listings of clinical signs and symptoms of each of these responses. Did the patient lose consciousness? Did seizures occur? Was there a skin reaction or respiratory distress?

Allergic reactions involve one or more of the following "systems": the skin (itching, swelling, rash), the gastrointestinal system (diarrhea, nausea and vomiting, cramping), the exocrine glands (running nose, watery eyes), the respiratory system (wheezing, laryngeal edema), and the cardiovascular and/or genitourinary system. Most often, patients describe their "allergic" reaction as one in which they suffered palpitations, severe headache, sweating, and mild shaking (tremor). Such reactions are usually of psychogenic origin or are related to the administration of overly large doses of vasoconstrictors (such as epinephrine) and are not allergenic in nature. Hyperventilation, an anxiety-induced reaction in which the patient loses control of his breathing—breathing rapidly and deeply—leads to signs and symptoms of dizziness, light-headedness, and peripheral (fingers, toes, lips) paresthesias.

QUESTION. What therapy was given?

COMMENT. When the patient is able to describe the management of the reaction, the doctor can usually determine its cause. Were drugs administered? If so, what drugs? Epinephrine, anticonvulsants, aromatic ammonia? Knowledge of specific management of these situations can lead to an accurate diagnosis.

Drugs employed in the management of allergic reactions include three drug types or categories: epinephrine (Adrenalin); antihistamines, including diphenhydramine (Benadryl) and chlorpheniramine (Chlor-Trimeton); and corticosteroids, including hydrocortisone sodium succinate (Solu-Cortef). The use of one or more of these agents increases the possibility that an allergic response did occur. Anticonvulsants such as diazepam (Valium) and the injectable barbiturates, including pentobarbital (Nembutal), are administered to manage seizures induced by overdose of local anesthetics, whereas aromatic ammonia is frequently employed in the treatment of syncopal episodes. Oxygen may be administered in any or all of these reactions.

QUESTION. Were the services of a physician or paramedical personnel required? Were you hospitalized?

COMMENT. An affirmative response indicates that a more serious reaction occurred. Most psychogenic responses are ruled out in this instance.

QUESTION. What is the name and address of the doctor (or dentist, physician, or hospital) who was treating you at the time the adverse reaction took place?

COMMENT. If possible, it is usually valuable to speak to the doctor who managed the previous episode. He is in most instances able to locate the records and describe in detail what actually occurred. Direct discussion with the dentist or physician normally provides a wealth of information with which the knowledgeable practitioner can determine the precise nature of the previous reaction.

Medical Consultation

If doubt remains in the doctor's mind following the dialogue history, it must still be assumed that the patient is allergic to the drug(s) in question, and they should not be used. At this point, the doctor should consider referral of the patient to a doctor who will be able to more fully evaluate the nature of the previous reaction. This doctor will also be able to perform certain tests that will prove more reliable in assessing the patient's local-anesthetic "allergy." Among the more commonly used tests are skin testing, passive transfer methods, and blood tests, such as the basophil degranulation test.

Skin testing is still the primary mode of testing for local-anesthetic allergy. Although several varieties of skin tests are used, the intracutaneous test is considered to be among the most reliable. Intracutaneous testing involves the injection of 0.1 ml of the test solution and is thought to be 100 times more sensitive than the cutaneous test. It is, however, more unpleasant because it requires multiple needle punctures. Other problems associated with its use involve "false positives" produced by the local release of histamine. However, intracutaneous testing is clinically useful, since a negative response probably means that the patient can safely receive the local anesthetic tested. No instance of an immediate allergic reaction has ever been reported in a patient with a previously negative intracutaneous response for a given agent.

In all instances where skin testing is employed, the anesthetic solutions should not contain any preservatives. Tests for allergy to methylparaben should be done separately. If a positive response occurs from this ingredient, local anesthetics to which the patient is not allergic should be used provided they do not contain any preservative. All dental cartridges manufactured in the United States since January, 1984 do not contain methylparaben.

The protocol for intracutaneous testing for allergy to local anesthetics that is currently in use at the University of Southern California School of Dentistry is summarized as follows: After an extensive dialogue history and review of the patient's medical history, 0.1 ml of each of the following is deposited intracutaneously: 0.9% normal saline, 1% or 2% lidocaine, 3% mepivacaine, and 4% prilocaine, all without methylparaben, followed by 0.1 ml of bacteriostatic water and one or more local anesthetics containing methylparaben. Following successful completion of this phase of the testing (60 minutes), 1 ml of one of the preceding local-anesthetic solutions that tested negative is administered intraorally by means of supraperiosteal (infiltration) injection, atraumatically (but without use of topical anesthetic), above a maxillary anterior tooth. This is termed a challenge test, and it frequently provokes the so-called allergic reaction, that is, signs and symptoms of a psychogenic response.

After having completed more than 100 local-anesthetic allergy test procedures, I have encountered four allergic responses to the paraben preservative and none to the local anesthetic agent itself. Numerous psychogenic responses have developed during either the intracutaneous or intraoral test-

ing procedures. Skin testing is not without risk, however. Severe, immediate allergic reactions may be precipitated by the administration of as little as 0.1 ml of a drug to a sensitized patient. Emergency drugs and equipment for resuscitation must always be readily available when allergy testing is contemplated.

Allergy Testing in the Dental Office

It is occasionally suggested that, in an emergency situation (toothache, infection), the doctor should carry out skin testing in the dental office. It is my firm conviction that dental-office allergy testing not be considered for several reasons. First, skin testing, although potentially valuable, is not foolproof. Localized histamine release (false-positives) may result from the trauma of the needle insertion. A negative reaction, although commonly taken to indicate that a drug may safely be injected, may also prove unreliable. In some cases, the drug itself is not the agent to which the patient is sensitive. Instead, a metabolite resulting from the biotransformation of the drug may be the causative agent. The skin·test would be negative or delayed many hours under these circumstances. A second and even more compelling factor for not using skin testing in the dental office is the possibility that even the minute quantity of drug being employed (0.1 ml) might precipitate an immediate and acute systemic anaphylactic response in the truly allergic patient. Drugs and equipment needed in the management of anaphylaxis and cardiopulmonary arrest must always be available when these tests are performed.

Dental Therapy Modification
Allergy to drugs other than local anesthetics

When a patient is proved to be truly allergic, precautions must be taken to prevent the patient from receiving that agent. The dental chart should be marked with an easily visible sign that the patient "has a drug sensitivity to _____." For all of the more highly allergenic drugs prescribed in dentistry, other drugs are available that are usually equipotent in therapeutic effect but that possess a much lower allergenicity.

Penicillin allergy may be circumvented through the use of erythromycin; it is a drug possessing virtually the same clinical spectrum of effectiveness as penicillin G with a lesser incidence of allergy. Sensitization reactions including skin lesions, fever, and anaphylaxis have been reported to erythromycin but are much less frequent than penicillin allergy. Erythromycin remains the classic substitute drug for penicillin G.

Acetaminophen is the drug employed in cases of allergy to aspirin. Although as effective an analgesic as aspirin, acetaminophen is not as effective as an antipyretic. However, it is not cross-allergenic with aspirin and may be administered to the salicylate-sensitive patient.

Allergy to the narcotic analgesics is rarely encountered; the unpleasant side effects of nausea and vomiting are the most commonly encountered reactions. However, in the presence of a true narcotic allergy, none of the narcotics may be used because they are all cross-allergenic. Nonnarcotic analgesics will be of some value in this situation.

Barbiturate allergy is an absolute contraindication to use of *any* barbiturate, because cross-allergenicity exists among all group members. However, the chemical structures of the nonbarbiturate sedative-hypnotics are sufficiently different so that cross-allergenicity does not occur. These drugs may safely be employed in patients with barbiturate allergy. Included in this group of drugs are flurazepam, diazepam, triazolam, chloral hydrate, and hydroxyzine.

Allergy to methyl methacrylate monomer is most readily avoided by not employing acrylic resins. If, however, acrylic resins must be used, heat-cured acrylic is much less allergenic than cold-cured or self-cured acrylic.

Table 24-3 summarizes the substitute drugs discussed above. In all cases, it is still possible for a patient to be allergic to one of the substitute drugs. Therefore the doctor must specifically question the patient about any drug before it is administered.

When considering the use of these or any other drugs, several additional factors must be kept in mind. The likelihood of an allergic reaction to a drug increases with duration and the number of courses of therapy. One remarkable example is a patient who had received 16 courses of penicillin therapy without adverse reaction over many years but developed anaphylactic shock with the seventeenth. Although long-term therapy is rarely necessary in dentistry, one must remember that acute allergic reactions may occur even in the absence of a previous history of allergy.

The route of administration of a drug is also of importance. It must be understood that allergic symptoms can arise following any route of administration. The site of administration is frequently the main target area for the allergic symptoms, especially following topical application of drugs. Of significance, however, is the finding that anaphylactic reactions occur much less commonly following enteral rather than parenteral administration of drugs. The frequency of other types of allergic drug reaction may also be decreased by using the oral route. It is important therefore to consider the method of administration of a drug and, when possible, to administer the drug orally rather than parenterally. Penicillin is an example of a highly allergenic drug. There are extremely few indica-

Table 24-3. Allergenic drugs and possible substitutes

| Category | Drug | Usual substitute | |
		Generic	Proprietary
Antibiotics	Penicillin	Erythromycin	Ilosone Erythrocin
Analgesics	Acetylsalicylic acid (aspirin)	Acetaminophen	Tylenol Tempra Datril
	Narcotic	No equally effective substitute presently available	
Sedative-hypnotics	Barbiturates	Flurazepam	Dalmane
		Diazepam	Valium
		Triazolam	Halcion
		Chloral hydrate	Noctec
		Hydroxyzine	Atarax, Vistaril
Acrylic	Methyl methacrylate	Avoid use if possible, otherwise heat-cured acrylic	

tions for the parenteral administration of this agent in the dental office, since oral administration has been shown to result in adequate blood levels of penicillin in a relatively short time. Antianxiety agents may require parenteral administration when employed in an acutely apprehensive patient. The risk of allergy must be weighed against the potential benefit to be accrued from the use of the drug in this manner. Local anesthetics, however, are a drug group that must be administered parenterally to be effective. Allergic reactions observed following this mode of administration tend to be more severe.

Management
Alleged allergy to local anesthetics

Routine dental care. When there is a doubtful history of allergy to any local anesthetic drug, these drugs should not be administered to the patient. Routine dental therapy requiring any local anesthetic (topical, injectable) may need to be delayed until a thorough evaluation of the patient is completed by an allergist. Dental therapy not requiring local or topical anesthesia might be carried out during this period.

Emergency dental care

The patient in pain or with an oral infection presents a more difficult situation. In most instances, the patient is a new patient in the office, has a tooth requiring extraction or pulpal extirpation, and has a normal medical history except for an alleged "allergy to Novocain." Following questioning of this patient, the "allergy" seems most likely to have been a psychogenic reaction (vasodepressor syncope), but some doubt remains. How might this patient be managed?

Option 1. Probably the most practical approach to this patient is an immediate medical consultation (personal physician or allergist) and arranging an appointment for the patient with the allergist. Dental therapy should *not* be carried out. Pain may be managed orally with various analgesics, and infection may be controlled with antibiotics. These are temporary measures only. Following evaluation of the patient by the physician as to whether allergy exists, definitive dental therapy may be carried out.

Option 2. A second approach might be to use a general anesthetic in place of a local anesthetic for the management of the dental emergency. Although a highly useful and relatively safe technique when properly performed, there are complications and problems associated with the use of general anesthesia, not the least of which is the fact that it is unavailable in most dental offices. However, general anesthesia remains a viable alternative to local anesthesia in the management of the allergic patient, provided adequate facilities and well-trained personnel are available.

Option 3. A third option to consider when emergency treatment is necessary and general anesthesia is not available is to use an antihistamine (for example, diphenhydramine) as a local anesthetic for the management of pain during therapy. Most injectable antihistamines possess local anesthetic properties. Several are more potent local anesthetics than procaine. Diphenhydramine (Benadryl) has been the most commonly used of the antihistamines in this regard. Used as a 1% solution with 1:100,000 epinephrine, diphenhydramine has produced pulpal anesthesia of up to 30 minutes' duration. An unwanted side effect frequently noted during its injection is a burning or stinging sensation. The use of nitrous oxide and oxygen along with this agent minimizes discomfort.

Another possible unwanted result of the use of an antihistamine as a local anesthetic is postoperative tissue swelling and soreness. These unpleasant actions must be considered before the use of these agents. For these reasons, the use of diphenhydramine as a local anesthetic is limited to those instances in which there is a questionable history of local-anesthetic allergy, the patient has a dental emergency requiring immediate physical intervention, and general anesthesia is not a reasonable alternative. It must again be kept in mind that allergy may develop to any drug, including the antihistamines. The patient should be questioned concerning prior exposure to antihistamines or other drugs before they are used.

It is important to remember that there are almost no dental emergency situations in which physical intervention is absolutely necessary. Appropriate drug therapy with immediate medical consultation (option 1) probably remains the most reasonable mode of action in these cases of alleged "local-anesthetic allergy" coupled with a dental emergency.

Confirmed Allergy to Local Anesthetics

Management of the patient with documented allergy to local anesthetics varies according to the nature of the allergy. If the local-anesthetic allergy is limited to the ester type agents (procaine, propoxycaine, benzocaine, or tetracaine), the amide type solutions (lidocaine, mepivacaine, or prilocaine) may be used. If the local-anesthetic "allergy" is actually an allergy to the paraben preservative, the amide type agents may be injected if they do not contain any preservative. On occasion, however, it is reported that a patient is allergic to all "-caine" drugs. I recommend that this report undergo careful scrutiny and that the method by which this conclusion was reached be reexamined (what tests were carried out and by whom; were pure solutions used, or were preservatives present?). All too often patients are labeled "allergic" to all local anesthetics when in reality they are not. These patients often have their dental treatment carried out in a hospital setting, usually under general anesthesia, when a proper evaluation might prevent this, saving the patient much time and money and decreasing the risk.

In concluding this important section on the prevention of allergy, I offer the following from a report on local-anesthetic allergy by Aldrete and Johnson (1970):

A strong plea is made for a thorough evaluation of the circumstances surrounding an adverse reaction to a local anesthetic before the label of "allergic to procaine," "allergic to lidocaine," or "allergic to all -caine drugs" is entered on the front of the patient's chart. We believe that untoward reactions observed during the use of local anesthetic agents are quite frequently the result of overdosage. . . . The benefits obtained from the use of local anesthetic agents should not be denied to a patient just because of an untoward response during a previous exposure to one of them. Instead, details of the circumstances surrounding the incident, such as sequence of events, other drugs administered, and the type of procedure, must be evaluated.

CLINICAL MANIFESTATIONS

The various forms that allergic reactions may take are listed in Table 24-1. In addition to these classifications, it is also possible to list reactions according to the length of time elapsed between contact with the antigen and the appearance of clinical manifestations. The two categories in this grouping are *immediate* and *delayed* reactions. Immediate reactions are those that occur within seconds to hours of exposure and include types I, II, and III of the Gell and Coombs classification system (Table 24-1). Delayed allergic reactions occur hours to days following antigenic exposure. The type IV reaction is an example of delayed response.

Of great significance to the dental practitioner are the immediate reactions, in particular the type I, or anaphylactic, reaction. Most allergic drug reactions are immediate. A number of organs and tissues are affected during immediate allergic reactions, particularly the skin, cardiovascular system, respiratory system, and gastrointestinal tract. *Generalized (systemic) anaphylaxis* by definition affects all the systems mentioned above. When hypotension occurs, resulting in loss of consciousness, the term *anaphylactic shock* may be employed.

Immediate allergic reactions may also manifest themselves through any number of combinations involving these systems. Reactions involving one organ system are referred to as *localized anaphylaxis*. Examples include bronchial asthma, in which the respiratory system is the "target," and urticaria, in which the skin is the target organ. The skin and respiratory reactions are discussed individually, followed by a description of generalized anaphylaxis.

Onset

The period elapsing between the exposure of the patient to the antigen and the development of clinical symptoms is of great importance. In general, the more rapidly signs and symptoms occur following exposure, the more intense is the ultimate reaction. Conversely, the greater the time elapsing between exposure and onset, the less intense the reaction. However, cases have been reported of systemic anaphylaxis arising many hours following exposure. Of importance too is the rate of progression of the signs and symptoms once they appear. If they appear and rapidly increase in intensity, the reaction is more likely to be life threatening than is one that progresses slowly or not at all once initial signs and symptoms appear. These time factors have a bearing on the management of allergic reactions.

Skin Reaction

Allergic skin reactions are the most common sensitization reaction to drug administration. Many types of allergic skin reactions may occur; the three most important types are localized anaphylaxis, contact dermatitis, and drug eruption. Drug eruption constitutes the most common group of skin manifestations of drug allergy. Included in this category are urticaria, erythema (rash), and angioedema (localized swelling measuring several centimeters in diameter).

Urticaria is associated with wheals (smooth,

slightly elevated patches of skin) and frequently with intense itching (pruritis). Angioedema is a process in which localized swelling occurs in response to an allergen. Several forms of angioedema exist, but they are clinically similar. The skin is usually of normal temperature and color (unless accompanied by urticaria and/or erythema) and pain and itching are uncommon. The areas most frequently involved include the face, hands, feet, and genitalia. Of special interest in dentistry is the potential involvement of the lips, tongue, pharynx, and larynx, leading to obstruction of the airway. (This is discussed further in the following section on respiratory reactions.) Angioedema is observed most frequently following administration of topical anesthetics (ester type local anesthetics or methylparaben) to oral mucous membranes. Within 30 to 60 minutes, the tissue in contact with the allergen appears quite swollen and erythematous.

Allergic skin reactions, if they are the sole manifestation of an allergic response, are normally not considered life threatening. Yet a skin reaction that occurs rapidly following drug administration may be only the first indication of the generalized reaction to follow.

Contact dermatitis is the allergic reaction most often observed in members of the dental profession. The sensitization process may require years of constant exposure before clinical symptoms occur. These include erythema, induration (hardness), edema, and vesicle formation. Chronic reexposure to the specific antigen results in dry, scaly lesions resembling eczema.

Respiratory Reactions

Clinical signs and symptoms of allergy may be related entirely to the respiratory tract, or signs and symptoms of respiratory tract involvement may occur along with other systemic responses. In a slowly developing generalized allergic reaction, respiratory reactions normally follow the skin, exocrine, and gastrointestinal responses but precede cardiovascular signs and symptoms. Asthma is the classic respiratory manifestation of allergy. It represents the clinical result of constriction of bronchial smooth muscle and is often termed bronchospasm. Signs and symptoms of an allergic asthmatic attack are identical to the nonallergic asthmatic attack. They include respiratory distress, dyspnea, wheezing, flushing, possible cyanosis, perspiration, tachycardia, greatly increased anxiety, and the use of accessory muscles of respiration. Asthma is described fully in Chapter 13.

A second respiratory manifestation of acute allergy may be the extension of angioedema to the larynx, which produces swelling of the vocal apparatus with subsequent obstruction of the airway. Clinical manifestations of this include little or no exchange of air from the lungs (*look* to see if chest is moving; *feel* that there is little or no air; *listen* for wheezing, indicating partial obstruction, or no sound, indicating total obstruction). The occurrence of significant angioedema represents one of the most ominous clinical signs. Acute airway obstruction leads rapidly to death of the patient unless immediately corrected.

Laryngeal edema represents the effects of allergy on the upper airway. Asthma represents the actions of allergy on the lower airway.

Generalized Anaphylaxis

Generalized anaphylaxis is a most dramatic and acutely life-threatening allergic reaction and may cause death within a few minutes. It may develop following the administration of an antigen by any route but is most likely to occur following parenteral administration. The time from antigenic challenge to the onset of reaction is quite variable, but typically the reaction develops rapidly, reaching a maximal intensity within 5 to 30 minutes. Delayed responses of an hour or more have also been reported. It is thought that this is a result of the rate at which the antigen enters the circulatory system.

The signs and symptoms of generalized anaphylaxis are highly variable. Four major clinical syndromes are recognized: skin reactions, smooth muscle spasm (gastrointestinal and genitourinary tracts and respiratory smooth muscle), respiratory difficulty, and cardiovascular collapse. In typical generalized anaphylaxis, the symptoms progressively move through these four areas; however, in cases of fatal anaphylaxis, respiratory and cardiovascular disturbances predominate and are evident early in the reaction.

In a "typical" generalized anaphylactic reaction, patients may begin to complain that they feel "sick" and may develop intense itching (pruritus), flushing (erythema), and giant hives (urticaria) over the face and upper chest. Nausea, possibly followed by vomiting, may also occur. These early symptoms are primarily related to the skin. Other reactions that are noted during the early phase of the reaction include conjunctivitis, vasomotor rhinitis (inflammation of the mucous membranes of the nose, marked by increased mucous secretion), and pilomotor erection (the feeling of "hair standing on end").

Associated with the development of skin symptoms are various gastrointestinal and genitourinary disturbances related to spasm of smooth muscle. Severe abdominal cramps, nausea and vomiting, diarrhea, and fecal and urinary incontinence may occur.

Respiratory symptoms normally follow the skin reactions. Keep in mind, however, that in a rapidly developing reaction, all symptoms may occur within a very short time with considerable overlap. In particularly severe reactions, respiratory and cardiovascular symptoms may be the only signs present.

Respiratory symptoms begin with a feeling of substernal tightness or a pain in the chest. A cough may develop, as well as wheezing and dyspnea. If the respiratory disturbances are severe, cyanosis may ensue, noticed initially in mucous membranes and the nailbeds. Laryngeal edema may also develop, producing acute airway obstruction.

Signs and symptoms of cardiovascular disturbance occur next and include pallor, lightheadedness, palpitation, tachycardia, hypotension, and cardiac dysrhythmias followed by the loss of consciousness and cardiac arrest. With the loss of consciousness the anaphylactic reaction may more properly be called anaphylactic shock.

The duration of the reaction or any part of it may vary from minutes to a day or more. With prompt and appropriate therapy the entire reaction may be terminated rapidly; however, the two most serious sequelae, hypotension and laryngeal edema, may persist for hours or days in spite of therapy. Death may occur at any time, the usual cause (from autopsy reports) being upper airway obstruction produced by laryngeal edema. Table 24-4 summarizes the signs and symptoms of allergic responses.

PATHOPHYSIOLOGY

The clinical manifestations of allergy are the result of an antigen-antibody reaction. Such reactions form a part of the body's defense mechanisms (immune system), which are described in the following material to provide a better understanding of the processes involved in allergy.

Antigens, Haptens, and Allergens

An *antigen* is any substance capable of inducing the formation of an antibody. Antigens are foreign to the species into which they are injected or ingested and may be harmful or harmless. Most anti-

Table 24-4. Clinical manifestations of allergy

Area affected	Manifestation
Skin	Urticaria—wheal and flare
	Pruritis
	Angioedema
	Erythema
Respiratory	Dyspnea
	Wheezing
	Flushing
	Cyanosis
	Perspiration
	Tachycardia
	Increased anxiety
	Use of accessory muscles of respiration

Generalized anaphylaxis—usual progression

Phase I: Skin	Patient "feels sick"
	Intense itching, flushing, and giant hives over chest and face
	Nausea and vomiting
	Conjunctivitis and vasomotor rhinitis (increased mucous secretion)
	"Hair standing on end" (piloerection)
Phase I: Gastrointestinal and genitourinary	Abdominal cramps
	Nausea and vomiting
	Diarrhea
	Fecal and urinary incontinence
Phase II: Respiratory	Feeling of substernal tightness
	Cough, wheezing
	Dyspnea
	Cyanosis, if severe
	Laryngeal edema
Phase III: Cardiovascular	Pallor
	Lightheadedness
	Palpitation
	Tachycardia
	Hypotension
	Cardiac dysrhythmia
	Loss of consciousness
	Cardiac arrest

gens are proteins with a molecular weight between 5000 and 40,000. Materials under a molecular weight of 5000 are usually not allergenic or antigenic. Virtually all proteins, whether of animal, plant, or microbial origin, possess antigenic potential.

Drugs, however, are not proteins and commonly possess a very low molecular weight (500 to 1000), which makes them unlikely antigens. The hapten theory of drug allergy explains the mechanism through which drugs may act as antigens. A *hapten* is a specific, protein-free substance that can combine to form a complex with a "carrier" protein. The hapten itself is not antigenic; however, when coupled with the carrier protein, it may provoke an immune response. The hapten may combine with the carrier protein outside the body and then be injected into the individual, or the hapten may combine with tissue proteins of the host after administration into the body. The latter mechanism is the one by which most drugs become antigens and thus capable of inducing antibody formation and causing an allergic reaction. Penicillin, aspirin, and barbiturates are examples of haptens. Haptens are also termed incomplete antigens. An *allergen* is an antigen capable of eliciting allergic symptoms. It is obvious that not every antigen is an allergen. An antigen or allergen may stimulate the production of several classes of immunoglobulins, each of which possesses different functions.

Antibodies (Immunoglobulins)

An antibody is a substance found in the blood or tissues that responds to the administration of an antigen or reacts with it. The molecular weights of these substances may range from 150,000 (IgG = immunoglobulin G) to 900,000 (IgM). The basic structure of an antibody molecule consists of two heavy and two light polypeptide chains linked in a Y configuration by covalent disulfide bonds. The base of the heavy chain (termed F_c for crystallizable unit) binds the antibody to the surface of a cell, while the arms of the antibody bind with the receptor sites on the antigen. Immunoglobulins are classified as IgA, IgD, IgE, IgG, and IgM according to structural differences in the heavy chains. Each immunoglobulin differs in its biologic functions and in the type of allergic response it may produce (Tables 24-1 and 24-5).

IgA is found principally in the serum and in external secretions such as saliva and sputum. It represents 5% to 10% of all immunoglobulins. It plays a role in the defense mechanisms of the external surfaces of the body, including the mucous membranes. The fetus begins to produce IgA during the last 6 months in utero, and adult levels are reached by 5 years of age.

IgD has been identified; however, its biologic functions remain unknown at this time.

IgE, the antibody responsible for immediate hypersensitivity, is synthesized by plasma cells in the nasal mucosa, respiratory tract, gastrointestinal tract, and lymphoid tissues. The half-life of IgE is approximately 2 days, serum levels normally being quite low—0.03 mg/100 ml.

IgG represents approximately 80% of antibodies in normal serum, and its chief biologic functions are the binding to and enhancement of the phagocytosis of bacteria and neutralization of bacterial toxins. IgG also crosses the placenta and imparts immune protection to the fetus, which remains for the first 6 months after birth. Shortly after birth the infant begins to synthesize IgG, and by the age of 4 to 5 years IgG levels approach adult levels.

IgM, the heaviest of the antibodies, is active in both agglutinating and in cytolytic reactions and accounts for 5% to 10% of all immunoglobulins. The fetus begins production of IgM during the final 6 months of fetal life, and adult levels are reached by 1 year of age.

Antibodies possess the ability to bind with the specific antigen that induces their production. This immunologic specificity is based on similarities in the structures of the antigen and antibody. Antibodies possess at least two specific antigen-binding sites per molecule (the F_{ab} fragments). IgM possesses five, and IgA probably has more than two. Antibodies are not entirely specific, and cross-sensitivity is possible between chemically similar substances.

Table 24-5. Properties of human immunoglobulins

	IgA	IgD	IgE	IgG	IgM
Molecular weight	180,000	150,000	200,000	150,000	900,000
Normal serum concentration (mg/100 ml)	275	5	0.03	1200	120
Primary function	Local or mucosal reactions and infections	Unknown	Type I hypersensitivity	Infection Type III hypersensitivity	Possible role in particular antigens

Defense Mechanisms of the Body

When a person is exposed to a foreign substance, the body attempts to protect itself through a number of mechanisms. These include the anatomic barriers, which attempt to exclude the antigen from the body. Examples of these barriers include the epithelium of the gastrointestinal tract, the sneeze and cough mechanisms, and the mucociliary blanket of the tracheobronchial tree. Once foreign substances are inside the body, two other nonspecific defense mechanisms are brought into play. These include mobilization of phagocytic blood cells such as leukocytes, histiocytes, and macrophages, and the production of nonspecific chemical substances such as lysozymes and proteolytic enzymes, which assist in removal of the foreign substance. A more specific defense mechanism is also employed. IgA antibody is produced by plasma cells in response to the antigen, and IgA then acts to aid in the removal or the detoxification of the antigen from the host.

Through these processes of anatomic localization, phagocytosis, and destruction, the antigen is usually eliminated, resulting in little or no damage to the host. If, however, the antigen remains (because of genetic defects in the patient such as atopy or the nature of the antigen itself), additional defense mechanisms may be called into play that may ultimately prove harmful to the host. These include reactions that result in formation of antibodies that, on subsequent exposure to the antigen, may result in the formation of precipitates of antigen-antibody complexes within cells or blood vessels (type III response), or may result in the subsequent release of the chemical mediators of the type I allergic response (see Table 24-1).

There are at least three possible results of an antigen-antibody reaction: (1) the production of antibodies that combine with the antigen to neutralize it or change it so that it becomes innocuous; (2) the antigen-antibody combination occurring within blood vessels in magnitude great enough to produce actual precipitates with small blood vessels, which results in occlusions with subsequent ischemic necrosis (for example, the Arthus reaction—type III); and (3) the antigen-antibody union, activating proteolytic enzymes that release certain chemicals from cells, which in turn act to produce the anaphylactic response. The first response is of benefit to the host, leading to elimination of the foreign material; the two other reactions are capable of producing injury and death.

Type I Allergic Reaction—Anaphylaxis

The type I (anaphylactic or immediate) allergic reaction is of great concern to the doctor. For any true allergic reaction to occur, the patient must have previously been exposed to the antigen. This is termed the sensitizing dose, and the subsequent exposure to the antigen is termed the challenge dose.

Sensitizing dose

During the sensitization phase the patient receives the initial exposure to the antigen. In response to the antigen, plasma cells produce immunoglobulins specific for that antigen. When a susceptible (atopic) individual is exposed, antigen-specific immunoglobulin E (IgE) antibodies are formed, which interact only with that particular antigen (or very closely related antigens, that is, cross-sensitivity). IgE antibodies are cytophilic and selectively attach themselves to the cell membranes of circulating basophils and tissue mast cells.

A latent period of variable duration (days to months) ensues, during which time IgE antibody continues to be produced (attaching to basophils and mast cells) while the level of antigen progressively decreases. Following this latent period, there is no antigen present, but high levels of IgE-sensitized basophils and mast cells remain. The patient is then "sensitized" to the specific antigen.

Challenge (allergic) dose

Subsequent exposure to the antigen results in an antigen-antibody interaction thought to be initiated by the bridging of two adjacent IgE molecules on the membranes of the sensitized mast cells or basophils. In the presence of the cations calcium and magnesium, this bridging begins a complex series of intramembrane and intracellular events that culminates in the release of pharmacologically active substances from the cells, which are termed the chemical mediators of allergy. The major chemical mediators are thought to be histamine and slow-reacting substance of anaphylaxis (SRS-A). These mediators in turn may directly produce local and systemic pharmacologic effects, cause the release of other mediators, or activate reflexes that ultimately produce the clinical picture of anaphylaxis. Other chemical mediators implicated in the type I allergic reaction include various kinins, especially bradykinin; eosinophilic chemotactic factor of anaphylaxis (ECF-A); serotonin (5-hydroxytryptamine); and possibly prostaglandins.

Chemical mediators of anaphylaxis

The endogenous chemicals released from tissue mast cells or circulating basophils are ultimately responsible for the clinical manifestations of allergy. These chemicals explain the similarity in allergic reactions regardless of the antigen that induces the response (penicillin, aspirin, procaine, and so on). The level of intensity of an allergic reaction may vary greatly (anaphylaxis, mild urticaria) from patient to patient. Factors involved in determining the variability of magnitude of an allergic response include (1) the amount of antigen or antibody present, (2) the affinity of antibody for the antigen, (3) the concentration of chemical mediators, (4) the concentration of receptors for mediators, and (5) the affinity of mediators for receptors. All of these factors, except for the antigen, are endogenous, which explains the wide variation in individual susceptibility. The major chemical mediators of allergy are briefly described with their primary biologic functions.

Histamine. Histamine is a widely distributed normal constituent of many tissues of the body, including the skin, lungs, nervous system, and gastrointestinal tract. In many tissues it is stored within the mast cell (a fixed-tissue cell) or in the circulating blood in basophils. It is stored in these sites in a physiologically inactive form and is electrostatically bound to heparin in granule form. When an IgE-induced antigen-antibody reaction occurs, these granules undergo a process in which they are activated and released from the basophils and mast cells without damage to the cell.

Particularly important pharmacologic actions of histamine include those on the cardiovascular system, smooth muscle, and glands. Cardiovascular actions of histamine include capillary dilation and increased capillary permeability. The action of capillary dilation is probably the most important action effected by histamine. All capillaries are involved following parenteral administration. This effect is most obvious in the skin of the face and upper chest, the so-called blushing area, which becomes hot and flushed. The increase in capillary permeability leads to an outward passage of plasma protein and fluid into extracellular spaces and to the formation of edema.

Other cardiovascular responses to histamine include the "triple response." When administered subcutaneously or released in the skin, histamine produces (1) a localized red spot extending a few millimeters around the site of injection, (2) a brighter red flush or "flare" that is irregular in outline and extends for about 1 cm beyond the original red spot, and (3) localized edema fluid, which forms a wheal that is noted in about 1.5 minutes and occupies the same area as the original red spot. Histamine is also the chemical mediator of pain and itch.

Because of the cardiovascular actions of histamine, there is a decrease in venous return and a significant reduction in the systemic blood pressure and cardiac output. The hypotension that results is normally of short duration because of the rapid inactivation of histamine and other compensatory reflexes that are activated in response to histamine release (such as increased catecholamine release from the adrenal medulla).

Histamine relaxes vascular smooth muscle in humans; however, most nonvascular smooth muscle undergoes stimulation (constriction). Smooth muscle constriction is most prominent in the uterus and bronchi. Bronchiolar smooth muscle constriction leads to the clinical syndrome of asthma (bronchospasm). Smooth muscle of the gastrointestinal tract is moderately constricted, whereas that of the urinary bladder and gallbladder is only slightly constricted.

Actions of histamine on exocrine glands involve the stimulation of secretions. Stimulated glands include the gastric, salivary, lacrimal, pancreatic, and intestinal glands. Increased secretion from mucous glands leads to the clinical syndrome of rhinitis, which is prominent in many allergic reactions.

Histamine is considered to be the major chemical mediator of anaphylaxis. The physiologic responses to histamine may be moderated or blocked by the administration of pharmacologic doses of antihistamines *before* the release of histamine.

Slow-reacting substance of anaphylaxis. Slow-reacting substance of anaphylaxis (SRS-A) is thought to be released from previously sensitized (IgE) mast cells and basophils and is found in rich abundance in the lungs. SRS-A was recently identified as the leukotrienes C and D_5. Its only known pharmacologic action is that of a marked and prolonged bronchial smooth muscle contraction. This bronchoconstrictive action is slower and longer lasting than that of histamine. The actions of SRS-A are not diminished or reversed by antihistaminic drugs.

Other mediators. Several other chemicals are thought to be involved in the allergic response. These include bradykinin, eosinophilic chemotactic factor of anaphylaxis, serotonin, and prostaglandins.

Bradykinin is thought to be involved in producing the inflammatory response and smooth muscle contraction seen in asthma. Other pharmacologic actions of importance include vasodilation, increased permeability of blood vessels, and the production of pain. Blood levels of bradykinin are significantly increased during anaphylaxis.

Eosinophylic chemotactic factor of anaphylaxis (ECF-A) may be produced in the lungs when challenged by a specific antigen. It is thought to be responsible for the attraction of eosinophils to the site of the allergic reaction.

Serotonin, or 5-hydroxytryptamine, is a vasoactive chemical that is of undetermined importance as a mediator in human anaphylaxis. Serotonin increases capillary permeability and produces smooth muscle constriction.

Prostaglandins have been thought to play a possible role in allergy because of the bronchoconstrictive properties of one fraction (prostaglandin fraction F_2). Other prostaglandin fractions, however, exert bronchodilating properties.

MANAGEMENT

The clinical expression of allergy may be quite varied. Of concern to the doctor are the signs and symptoms of immediate allergy, which range from mild skin lesions to angioedema to generalized anaphylaxis. The speed with which symptoms of allergy appear and the rate at which they progress have some determining effect on the mode of management of the reaction.

Skin Reactions

Skin lesions may range from localized angioedema to diffuse erythema, urticaria, and pruritis. Management of these reactions is based on the speed at which they appear following antigenic challenge (drug administration).

Delayed reactions

Skin reactions that appear after a considerable lapse of time following antigenic exposure (60 minutes or more) and do not progress may be considered non–life threatening. These include a mild skin reaction or a localized mucous membrane reaction following application of topical anesthetics.

Step 1. Initiate basic life support. Assess airway, breathing, and circulation and implement as needed.

Step 2. Administer antihistamine. Management of the patient consists of the immediate intramus-

cular administration of an antihistamine such as diphenhydramine (50 mg) or chlorpheniramine (10 mg). The patient is then given a prescription for diphenhydramine, 50 mg, to be taken orally every 4 to 6 hours for 2 to 3 days.

Step 3. Medical consultation. A consultation with the patient's physician or an allergist should follow, and evaluation of the patient should be completed before further dental therapy. A complete list of all drugs and chemicals administered to the patient should be compiled for use by the allergist.

If the skin reaction is mild but the patient has left the dental office, the patient should be requested to return to the office where the therapy just described will be employed. Should the reaction occur at a time when the patient is unable to return to the dental office, the patient should be advised to arrange to see a physician or to report to the emergency room of a hospital. The doctor should accompany the patient to the hospital.

Antihistamines reverse the actions of histamine by occupying the receptor sites on the effector cell (competitive antagonism). Antihistamines thereby prevent the agonist molecules (histamine) from occupying these sites without initiating a response themselves. The protective responses of antihistamine include control of edema formation and itch. Other allergic responses such as hypotension and bronchoconstriction are influenced little, if at all, by antihistamines. It can be seen therefore that antihistamines are only of value in mild allergic responses in which small quantities of histamine have been released or in the prevention of reactions in allergic individuals.

Immediate reactions

Allergic skin reactions that arise in less than 60 minutes should be managed more aggressively. Other allergic symptoms of a relatively minor nature included in this section are conjunctivitis, rhinitis, urticaria, pruritus, and erythema.

Step 1. Initiate basic life support. Assess airway, breathing, and circulation and implement as needed.

Step 2. Administer epinephrine. Recommended management of these reactions involves the immediate intramuscular or subcutaneous administration of 0.3 to 0.5 mg of a 1:1000 epinephrine solution (adult), 0.25 mg (child), or 0.125 mg (infant).

Step 3. Administer antihistamine. Following epinephrine, an antihistamine (diphenhydramine, 50 mg, or chlorpheniramine, 10 mg) should be administered IM. The pediatric dose of diphenhydramine is 25 mg.

Step 4. Medical consultation. Consultation with a physician, allergist, or hospital emergency room before discharge of the patient is essential in any situation in which epinephrine has been administered. It may be necessary to transfer the patient to the physician's office or hospital for observation.

Step 5. Observe patient. In most cases, the clinical signs and symptoms disappear following this management. After the patient has been observed in the dental office for a period of time (1 hour, approximately) for signs of a recurrence, the patient may be discharged in the company of an adult.

Step 6. Prescribe oral antihistamine. An antihistamine should be prescribed for oral administration following consultation with the physician. Further evaluation of this patient must occur before subsequent dental treatment.

Respiratory Reactions
Bronchial constriction (bronchospasm)

Bronchial smooth muscle constriction results in asthma. Management of the acute asthmatic episode is described in depth in Chapter 13 and includes the following:

Step 1. Terminate dental therapy.

Step 2. Position patient in the semierect position.

Step 3. Initiate basic life support, implement as needed.

Step 4. Administer oxygen through cannula, nose piece, or face mask.

Step 5. Administer a bronchodilator. Epinephrine may be administered by means of an aerosol inhaler (Medi-haler Epi) (Fig. 24-1) or by intramuscular or subcutaneous injection (0.3 ml of a 1:1000 dilution for adults). The potent bronchodilating actions of epinephrine usually terminate bronchospasm within a few minutes of administration. Epinephrine is the drug of choice because it effectively reverses the actions of both of the causative agents of bronchospasm—histamine and SRS-A. Antihistamines do not relieve bronchospasm produced by SRS-A. Other bronchodilators, such as metaproterenol, may be used in the management of bronchospasm.

Step 6. Observe patient. The patient should remain in the dental office for observation, because a recurrence of bronchospasm is possible as the epinephrine undergoes rapid biotransformation. Should symptoms reappear, epinephrine is readministered intramuscularly, subcutaneously, or by inhalation (aerosol).

Step 7. Administer antihistamine. The IM administration of an antihistamine minimizes recurrence of bronchospasm because the antihistamine occupies the histamine receptor site, preventing a relapse. Diphenhydramine, 50 mg IM for adults or 2 mg/kg IM or IV for children, is recommended.

Step 8. Medical consultation and discharge. Following medical consultation and observation (60 minutes, approximately), the patient may be discharged to return home or transferred to a hospital.

Step 9. Prescribe oral antihistamine. Oral antihistamines should be prescribed and a thorough allergy evaluation concluded before subsequent dental therapy.

Diphenhydramine, 50 mg every 4 to 6 hours, is recommended for the adult, whereas 25 mg every 4 to 6 hours for 2 to 3 days is suggested for the child.

Laryngeal edema

The second and probably more life-threatening respiratory allergic manifestation is the development of laryngeal edema. It may be diagnosed when no air movement can be heard or felt through the mouth and nose despite vigorous spontaneous respiratory movements or when a patent airway cannot be obtained. A partially obstructed larynx in the presence of spontaneous respiratory movements produces a characteristically high-pitched crowing sound (in contrast to the wheezing of bronchospasm), whereas total obstruction is accompanied by silence. The patient soon loses consciousness from lack of oxygen (hypoxia or anoxia).

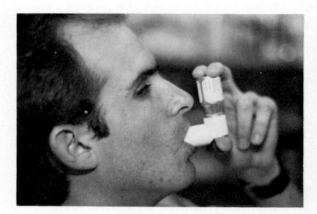

Fig. 24-1. Aerosol spray of bronchodilator for management of bronchial spasms.

Step 1. Position patient and initiate basic life support. Immediate management of acute laryngeal edema involves placing the patient in the supine position and initiating basic life support, as required.

Step 2. Administer epinephrine. Immediately administer 0.3 ml of 1:1000 epinephrine IM or IV if possible (0.125 to 0.25 ml for infant or child).

Step 3. Maintain airway. In the presence of a partially obstructed airway, epinephrine administration may halt or even reverse the progress of the laryngeal edema.

Step 4. Summon medical assistance. Oxygen must be administered and medical assistance summoned.

Step 5. Additional drug management. An antihistamine (diphenhydramine, 50 mg, adult; 25 mg, pediatrics) and corticosteroids (hydrocortisone, 100 mg) should be administered IM or IV. Corticosteroids inhibit edema and capillary dilation. They are of little immediate value, however, because of their slow onset of action, even when administered intravenously. The function of corticosteroids is the prevention of a relapse, whereas that of epinephrine, a more rapidly acting drug employed during the acute phase, is to halt or reverse the deleterious actions of histamine and SRS-A. These procedures are normally adequate to maintain the patient. With the arrival of medical assistance the patient is transferred to a hospital for further therapy and observation.

Step 6. Cricothyrotomy. A totally obstructed airway may not be cleared by epinephrine and other drug administration. In this case, it is necessary to create an emergency airway to maintain the life of the patient. Time is of the essence, and it is not possible to delay action until medical assistance arrives. A cricothyrotomy is the procedure of choice for the establishment of an airway in this situation. (The technique is described in Chapter 11.) Once an airway is obtained, oxygen must be administered, artificial ventilation employed if needed, and vital signs monitored. Before the arrival of medical assistance, the agents previously administered can halt the progression of the reaction and might even reverse it. The patient will require hospitalization following transfer from the dental office by the paramedics.

Epinephrine and Allergy

Epinephrine is the most important drug in the initial management of all immediate allergic reactions. Its actions effectively counteract the effects of histamine and the other chemical mediators of allergy. Although antihistamines reverse several allergic symptoms, especially edema and itch, they are of little value with others such as bronchospasm and hypotension. Epinephrine possesses properties to reverse all of these actions and has a more rapid onset of action than do antihistamines.

The actions of epinephrine are classified as beta-adrenergic and alpha-adrenergic effects. The beta-adrenergic effects of epinephrine mimic those produced by efferent sympathetic (adrenergic) nerve activity on the heart ($beta_1$) and lungs ($beta_2$), whereas alpha-adrenergic properties mimic those of the nerves on the peripheral vasculature. Useful beta-adrenergic actions of epinephrine include bronchodilation, increased myocardial contractility, increased heart rate, and constriction of arterioles with a redistribution of blood to the systemic circulation. Useful alpha-adrenergic actions include cutaneous, mucosal, and splanchnic vasoconstriction, with a total increase in systemic vascular resistance. This action, in addition to the $beta_1$-adrenergic actions (increased heart rate and myocardial contractility), leads to increased cardiac output. Increased cardiac output, in addition to the increased systemic vascular resistance, produces an increased systemic blood pressure. Through as yet unknown mechanisms, epinephrine also reverses rhinitis and urticaria.

Although epinephrine is rapid acting, it is also a short-acting drug (owing to its rapid biotransformation). Therefore whenever epinephrine is used in an emergency situation, the patient should be observed long enough to ensure that symptoms do not recur. In addition, care must be taken when considering the reinjection of epinephrine. Administration of epinephrine produces dramatic increases in heart rate and blood pressure (epinephrine injection has produced cerebrovascular hemorrhage) and increases the risk of the development of irregularities in the heart's rhythm. Before reinjection of epinephrine (0.3 ml of 1:1000 in the adult, 0.125 to 0.25 ml in infants and children), the cardiovascular status of the patient must be evaluated and the risk of reinjection carefully weighed against the benefits. In the presence of rapid heart rate (arbitrarily defined as 144 beats per minute or higher in the adult) or cardiac dysrhythmias, it may be prudent to delay the readministration of epinephrine and administer antihistamine and corticosteroid instead. However, if the patient's condition continues to deteriorate, epinephrine must be readministered.

Generalized Anaphylaxis

In generalized anaphylaxis a wide range of clinical manifestations may occur; however, the cardiovascular system is involved in virtually all reactions. In a rapidly progressing anaphylactic reaction, cardiovascular collapse may occur within minutes of the onset of symptoms. Immediate and aggressive management of the situation is imperative if a successful result is to be achieved. In the dental office, this reaction most probably occurs during or immediately following administration to a previously sensitized patient of oral penicillin or aspirin. A much more remote possibility might be the injection of an ester-type local anesthetic. Two other life-threatening situations may also develop in this latter situation that may occasionally mimic anaphylaxis: vasodepressor syncope and an overdose reaction to the local anesthetic. In the immediate management of this situation, there must be an attempt to diagnose the actual cause.

Signs of allergy present

Should any clinical signs such as urticaria, erythema, pruritus, or wheezing be noted before the patient's collapse, the diagnosis of the problem is obviously allergy, and management proceeds accordingly.

Step 1. Position patient. The patient is placed in the supine position.

Step 2. Basic life support. The airway is opened (head tilt), and the steps of basic life support are carried out as needed.

Step 3. Administer epinephrine. The doctor should have previously summoned the emergency

---

MANAGEMENT OF ALLERGIC REACTIONS

Skin reactions (delayed)

Step 1 Initiate basic life support, as needed
2 Antihistamine IM (diphenhydramine 50 mg, chlorpheniramine 10 mg, and oral antihistamine)
3 Medical consultation

Skin reactions (immediate)

Step 1 Initiate basic life support, as needed
2 Epinephrine, 0.125-0.3 ml of 1:1000 IM, SC
3 Antihistamine IM
4 Consult with physician
5 Observe patient
6 Oral antihistamine

Respiratory reactions — bronchial constriction

Step 1 Terminate dental therapy
2 Position patient (semierect)
3 Initiate basic life support, as needed
4 Administer oxygen
5 Epinephrine via aerosol inhaler or 0.125-0.3 ml of 1:1000 IM, SC
6 Observe patient
7 Antihistamine IM or IV
8 Medical consultation
9 Oral antihistamine

Respiratory reactions — laryngeal edema (partial obstruction)

Step 1 Position patient (supine)
2 Epinephrine, 0.125-0.3 ml of 1:1000 IM, SC

3 Airway maintenance (head tilt)
4 Summon medical assistance
5 Additional drug therapy antihistamine and corticosteroid IM or IV

Laryngeal edema (total obstruction)

Step 1 Position patient (supine)
2 Epinephrine, 0.125-0.3 ml of 1:1000 IM, SC
3 Oxygen
4 Summon medical assistance
5 Antihistamine and corticosteroid IM or IV
6 Cricothyrotomy (if needed)
7 Transfer to hospital

Generalized anaphylaxis (if allergy symptoms appear)

Step 1 Position patient (supine)
2 Initiate basic life support
3 Epinephrine, 0.125-0.3 ml of 1:1000 IM, SC
4 Summon medical assistance
5 Monitor vital signs every 5 minutes
6 Additional drug therapy Antihistamine and corticosteroid IM or IV
7 Transfer to hospital

Generalized anaphylaxis (no signs of allergy present)

Step 1 Position patient (supine)
2 Initiate basic life support
3 Monitor vital signs
4 Summon medical assistance

team. Epinephrine from the emergency kit (0.3 ml of 1 : 1000 for adults, 0.25 ml for children, and 0.125 ml for infants) is administered IM or SC as quickly as possible. Because of the immediate need for epinephrine in this situation, a preloaded syringe of epinephrine is kept in the emergency kit. Epinephrine is the only injectable agent that is kept in a preloaded form to prevent confusion when looking for the drug.

Epinephrine usually produces a clinical improvement in the patient. The respiratory and cardiovascular signs and symptoms should decrease in severity, breath sounds improve as bronchospasm decreases, and blood pressure increases. Should the clinical picture fail to improve or continue to deteriorate (increased severity of symptoms) within 3 to 5 minutes of the first epinephrine dose, a second appropriate dose may be administered. Subsequent doses (0.125 to 0.3 ml of 1 : 1000 solution) may be administered as needed, if the potential risk of epinephrine administration (excessive cardiovascular stimulation) is kept in mind.

Step 4. Summon medical assistance. Airway maintenance and artificial ventilation (oxygen, if available) must be provided as needed throughout the management phase. Medical assistance should be sought at the earliest convenience.

Step 5. Monitor vital signs. Cardiovascular status must be monitored continuously. Blood pressure and heart rate (carotid artery) should be recorded at least every 5 minutes, and closed chest compression should be started if cardiac arrest occurs.

During this acute, life-threatening phase of the obvious anaphylactic reaction, management consists of the administration of oxygen and epinephrine, with continual monitoring of vital signs. Until an improvement in the patient's status is noted, no additional therapy is indicated.

Step 6. Additional drug therapy. Once clinical improvement is noted (increased blood pressure, decreased bronchospasm), additional therapy may be started. This includes administration of an antihistamine and a corticosteroid (both IM or IV). Their function is to prevent a possible recurrence of symptoms and to obviate the need to continue the administration of epinephrine. They are not administered during the acute phase of the reaction because they are too slow in onset of action and they do not do enough immediate good to justify their use initially. Epinephrine and oxygen are the only drugs to administer during the acute phase of the anaphylactic reaction.

Throughout this text, it has been stressed that definitive therapy with drugs is of secondary importance to the ABCs of basic life support. Drugs need not be administered in all emergency situations. Unfortunately, the anaphylactic reaction is different. Once diagnosis of an acute, generalized allergic reaction has been made, it is imperative that drug therapy (epinephrine) be initiated as soon as possible following the start of basic life support. Review of clinical reports demonstrates the effectiveness of immediate drug therapy in anaphylaxis. Recovery from anaphylaxis is related to the rapidity with which effective treatment is instituted. Delay in treatment increases the mortality rate. Eighty-seven percent of those experiencing anaphylaxis provoked by bee stings survived if treated within the first hour, but only 67% of dying patients were treated in this first hour.

No signs of allergy

A second clinical picture might well be one in which the patient receiving a potential allergen loses consciousness without any obvious signs of allergy being observed.

Step 1. Position patient. Management of this situation, which might prove to result from any of a number of causes, will require immediate positioning of the patient in the supine position.

Step 2. Basic life support. Victims of vasodepressor syncope rapidly recover consciousness once they are properly positioned with an ensured airway. Patients who do not recover at this point should continue to have the elements of basic life support applied (breathing, circulation).

Step 3. Monitor vital signs. Blood pressure and heart rate should be monitored every 5 minutes, and cardiopulmonary resuscitation should be begun if needed.

Step 4. Summon medical assistance. If vital signs are present but the patient does not regain consciousness, continue to support the patient and call for medical assistance as soon as possible. In the absence of definitive signs and symptoms of allergy, epinephrine and other drug therapy are not indicated. Any of a number of other situations may be the cause of the unconsciousness: for example, overdose reaction, hypoglycemia, cerebrovascular accident, and acute adrenal insufficiency may be causative factors. Continuation of the steps of basic life support until medical assistance arrives is the most rational mode of management in this situation.

Laryngeal edema

Laryngeal edema is yet another possible development during the generalized anaphylactic reaction. Should airway maintenance become difficult in spite of adequate head tilt and a clear pharynx (obtained by suctioning), it may become necessary to perform a cricothyrotomy to obtain an airway. Laryngeal edema is a serious manifestation of allergy. Once airway patency has been ensured (cricothyrotomy), epinephrine may be administered (0.125 to 0.3 ml of 1:1000 solution), followed by an antihistamine and corticosteroid. Once stabilized, the patient should be transferred to a hospital for definitive management and observation.

The management of allergic reactions is summarized in the box on p. 320.

BIBLIOGRAPHY

Adriani, J.: Reactions to local anesthetics, JAMA **196:**405, 1966.

Aldrete, J.A., and Johnson, D.A.: Evaluation of intracutaneous testing for investigation of allergy to local anesthetic agents, Anesth. Analg. **49:**173, 1970.

Beaven, M.A.: Histamine, N. Engl. J. Med. **294:**30, 320, 1976.

Booth, B.H., and Patterson, R.: Electrocardiographic changes during human anaphylaxis, JAMA **211:**627, 1970.

Braham, R.L.: Angioneurotic edema with idiopathic pigmentation of the lips: a case report, J. Dent. Child. **38:**60, 1971.

Buisseret, P.D.: Allergy, Sci. Am. **247:**86, 1982.

Campbell, K.B.: Neurologic manifestations of allergic disease, Ann. Allergy **31:**485, 1973.

Capurro, N., and Levi, R.: The heart as a target organ in systemic allergic reactions, Circ. Res. **36:**520, 1975.

Chue, P.W.Y.: Emergency management of anaphylactic reactions, Dent. Surv. **51:**32, July, 1975.

Chue, P.W.Y.: Acute angioneurotic edema of the lips and tongue due to emotional stress, Oral Surg. **41:**734, 1976.

David, J.R.: Lymphocyte mediators and cellular hypersensitivity, N. Engl. J. Med. **288:**143, 1973.

deShazo, R.D., and Salvaggio, J.E.: Anaphylactic emergencies: update on changing picture, Mod. Med. **50:**112, 1982.

Eggleston, D.J.: Anaphylaxis, Aust. Dent. J. **20:**263, 1975.

Ellis, E.F.: Allergic emergencies, Pediatr. Clin. North Am. **26:**903, 1949.

Epstein, W.L.: Contact dermatitis, Clin. Pharmacol. Ther. **16:**892, 1974.

Foreman, J.C.: The pharmacological control of immediate hypersensitivity, Annu. Rev. Pharmacol. Toxicol. **21:**63, 1981.

Foreman, J.C., and Lichtenstein, L.M.: Clinical pharmacology of acute allergic disorders, Annu. Rev. Med. **31:**181, 1980.

Foucard, T.: Acute anaphylaxis in children, Pediatrics **7:**176, 1978.

Gell, P.G.H., and Coombs, R.R.A.: Clinical aspects of immunology, ed. 3, Oxford and London, 1975, Blackwell Scientific Publications.

Glauda, N.M., Henerfer, E.O., and Super, S.: Nonfatal anaphylaxis caused by oral penicillin: report of case, J. Am. Dent. Assoc. **90:**159, 1975.

Harris, R.J., and Harris, R.L.: Multiple antibiotic allergies, J. Am. Dent. Assoc. **97:**994, 1978.

Houwerzijil, J., deFast, G.C., and Nater, J.P.: Tests for drug allergies, Lancet **1:**655, 1975.

Kaliner, M.: Immunologic mechanisms for release of chemical mediators of anaphylaxis from human living tissue, Can. Med. Assoc. J. **110:**431, 1974.

Kelly, J.F., and Patterson, R.: Anaphylaxis, JAMA **227:**1431, 1974.

Krupp, M.A., and Chatton, M.J.: Current medical diagnosis and treatment, Los Altos, CA, 1984, Lange Medical Publications.

Levine, M.I.: Chronic urticaria, J. Allergy Clin. Immunol. **55:**276, 1975.

Lichtenstein, L.M.: Control of IgE—mediated histamine release. In Austen, K.F., and Lichtenstein, L.M., editors: Asthma, physiology, immunopharmacology and treatment, New York, 1973, Academic Press, Inc.

Little, J.W., and Falace, D.A.: Dental management of the medically compromised patient, ed. 2, St. Louis, 1984, The C.V. Mosby Co.

Lowell, F.C.: "Asthma," "rhinitis," and "atopy" reconsidered (editorial), N. Engl. J. Med. **300:**669, 1979.

Maddison, S.E.: Delayed hypersensitivity and cell mediated immunity, Clin. Pediatr. **12:**529, 1973.

Malamed, S.F.: The use of diphenhydramine HCl as a local anesthetic in dentistry, Anesth. Prog. **20:**76, 1973.

Michel, R.G., Hudson, W.R., and Pope, T.H.: Angioneurotic edema, Arch. Orolaryngol. **101:**544, 1975.

Murrow, D.H., and Luther, R.R.: Anaphylaxis: etiology and guidelines for management, Anesthesiol. Analg. **55:**493, 1976.

Norman, P.S.: Allergic rhinitis and sinusitis, Postgrad. Med. **54:**94, 1973.

Norman, P.S.: Specific therapy in allergy: pro (with reservations), Med. Clin. North Am. **58:**111, 1974.

Pallasch, T.J.: Clinical drug therapy in dental practice, Philadelphia, 1973, Lea & Febiger.

Parker, C.W.: Drug allergy, N. Engl. J. Med. **292:**511, 1975.

Pascoe, D.J.: Anaphylaxis. In Pascoe, D.J., and Grossman, M., editors: Quick reference to pediatric emergencies, ed. 3, Philadelphia, 1984, J.B. Lippincott Co.

Patterson, R., and Anderson, J.: Allergic reactions to drugs and biologic agents, JAMA **248:**2637, 1982.

Patterson, R., and Valentine, M.: Anaphylaxis and related allergic emergencies including reactions to insect stings, JAMA **248:**2632, 1982.

Patterson, R., Zeiss, C.R., and Kelly, J.F.: Classification of hypersensitivity reactions, N. Engl. J. Med. **295:**277, 1976.

Peters, G.A., Karnes, W.E., and Bastron, J.A.: Near fatal and fatal reactions to insect sting, Ann. Allergy **41:**268, 1978.

Ravindranathan, N.: Allergic reaction to lignocaine, Br. Dent. J. **138:**101, 1975.

Roth, M., Schreier, L., and Cutler, R.: Adrenalin treatment for hereditary angioneurotic edema, Ann. Allergy **35:**175, 1975.

Schwartz, H.C.: Local anesthesia, J. Am. Dent. Assoc. **89:**157, 1974.

Sidon, M.A., and Aldrete, J.A.: A patient with multiple allergies—what anesthetic to use? J. Am. Dent. Assoc. **82:**366, 1971.

Slavin, R.G.: Skin tests in the diagnosis of allergies of the immediate type, Med. Clin. North Am. **58:**65, 1974.

Spark, R.P.: Fatal anaphylaxis to oral penicillin, Am. J. Clin. Pathol. **56:**407, 1971.

Speer, F.: Aspirin allergy: a clinical study. South. Med. J. **68:**314, 1975.

Treatment of anaphylactic shock (editorial), Br. Med. J. **282:**1011, 1981.

25 Drug-related Emergencies: Differential Diagnosis

The use of drugs is not without risk. In this section, several adverse drug reactions (ADRs) are described that are potentially life threatening. These reactions are compared so that the doctor called on to manage them may be better able to rapidly diagnose the precise cause of the reaction and initiate appropriate therapy. Included in the differential diagnosis is vasodepressor syncope, because it is a common drug-related reaction.

PAST MEDICAL HISTORY

Past medical history is of great importance in the prevention of ADRs. Careful evaluation of a patient's prior drug response is a major factor in prevention of these reactions. "Allergy" must be documented; however, the drug or drugs producing the reaction *must* be avoided until the patient undergoes more definitive evaluation. When allergy exists, alternative drugs may be used.

Drug overdose reactions are more difficult to evaluate from the medical history. Patients commonly record all adverse drug reactions as "allergy." Only a careful dialogue history and knowledge of the pharmacology of the drug in question can lead to a diagnosis of prior overdose reaction.

Vasodepressor syncope is commonly associated with parenteral drug administration, particularly the administration of local anesthetics. A history of "blacking out" whenever an injection is administered should lead the doctor to suspect vasodepressor syncope and take measures to prevent its recurrence.

AGE OF PATIENT

Allergic and overdose reactions may occur at any age. Children appear to have a greater potential to develop allergy than do adults; however, many children "outgrow" their childhood allergies (especially food allergies).

Drug overdose reactions may also develop in any patient, but children represent a greater risk, especially with CNS-depressant drugs such as sedative-hypnotics, narcotic analgesics, and local anesthetics. Adult dosages of these agents must *never* be administered to children.

Vasodepressor syncope, on the other hand, is only rarely observed in younger patients or in patients after the age of 40. The age span from late teens to late 30s, primarily in males, represents the "high risk" category for vasodepressor syncope.

SEX OF PATIENT

Drug overdose and allergic reactions are not found more often in one sex than the other. However, vasodepressor syncope is much more common in males. The most likely candidate for vasodepressor syncope is the male under the age of 35 years.

POSITION OF PATIENT

The patient's position when clinical signs and symptoms appear is relevant primarily in the administration of local anesthetics. Patient position has no bearing on the development of the allergic or the overdose reaction. Both may develop with the patient in the upright or supine position. Vasodepressor syncope, however, is rarely observed if local anesthetics are administered to a patient placed in the supine position. Injection of local anesthetics into a patient seated upright is much more likely to lead to vasodepressor syncope. Positioning of the patient once clinical symptoms develop also aids in diagnosing the cause of the reaction if unconsciousness is a clinical sign. Placement of the unconscious patient in the supine position leads to rapid improvement in the case of vasodepressor syncope but produces no significant improvement in drug overdose or allergy.

ONSET OF SYMPTOMS

Vasodepressor syncope, drug overdose, and allergy may develop immediately following drug administration, or they may develop more slowly. Vasodepressor syncope most often occurs immediately *before* the actual administration of the drug but may also develop during or after its administration. Syncope occurring just before drug administration is caused by neither allergy nor drug overdose and is most often related to fear.

Clinical symptoms developing *during* drug administration may be related to any of these reactions; however, in this situation the dose of drug injected is of great importance (see below).

Signs and symptoms that appear *following* the administration of a drug most probably represent drug overdose or allergy. Vasodepressor syncope may also occur at this time, but in this situation the acute precipitating factor is most probably related to different factors, such as the sight of blood or dental instruments.

PRIOR EXPOSURE TO DRUG

Prior exposure to a specific drug or to a closely related agent is essential for an allergic response to occur. Vasodepressor syncope is not truly a drug-related situation except in the sense that the psychologic aspect of receiving a drug may precipitate the reaction. (Injection of sterile water might just as readily precipitate vasodepressor syncope. The important factor in the reaction is *injection*.) Drug overdose is not related to prior exposure to a drug. It may occur with the first exposure to the agent or with the twentieth exposure.

DOSE OF DRUG ADMINISTERED

Vasodepressor syncope is unrelated to the dose of drug administered. Drug overdose reactions are in most instances related to the quantity of the drug administered. Overdose represents an extension of the normal pharmacologic actions of a drug beyond its desirable therapeutic effect and is related to elevated blood levels of a drug. Relative overdose may develop in patients for whom "normal" therapeutic doses produce adverse effects, illustrating the phenomenon of biologic variability as represented by the normal distribution curve. Allergy is not normally related to absolute dosage of drug administered. Allergy testing using 0.1 ml of an agent may produce fatal systemic anaphylaxis in a previously sensitized patient.

OVERALL INCIDENCE OF OCCURRENCE

Vasodepressor syncope is the most commonly occurring adverse reaction. Of true adverse drug reactions, minor side effects (nonlethal, undesirable drug actions that develop at therapeutic levels, for example, nausea or sedation) are encountered most frequently. Drug overdose represents the most common of the life-threatening situations that occur, whereas only 15% of ADRs are truly allergic in nature.

SIGNS AND SYMPTOMS
Duration of Reaction

Overdose reactions to local anesthetics are normally self-limiting. Inadvertent intravascular injection of one cartridge of local anesthetic may lead to acute clinical symptoms for 1 to 2 minutes before the blood level falls below overdose levels. Overdose reaction to epinephrine is of extremely short duration because of the rapid biotransformation of the agent into inactive forms. Vasodepressor syncope is commonly self-limiting, because patients regain consciousness once they are placed in the supine position.

Allergy, on the other hand, may persist for extended periods. As long as any antigen exists within the patient's body, the allergic response will continue. It is not uncommon for acute reactions to persist for hours or days in spite of vigorous treatment.

Changes in Appearance of Skin

Allergy is frequently seen clinically as a skin reaction. Flushing (erythema) may occur in other emergency situations, as well as in allergy; however, when flushing is accompanied by urticaria, pruritus (itching), or both, the clinical diagnosis of allergy is appropriate.

Epinephrine overdose may also produce erythema, yet other clinical signs allow for ready differentiation of this reaction from allergy. These signs of epinephrine overdose include intense headache, tremor, increased anxiety, tachycardia, and greatly elevated blood pressure.

Pallor and cold, clammy skin are observed in vasodepressor syncope and possibly in local-anesthetic overdose as hypotension develops. Pallor may also be noted in epinephrine overdose reaction. Edema is noted only in allergic reactions.

Appearance of Nervousness

An increase in outward nervousness (described as fear, apprehension, or agitation) may be observed in the local-anesthetic overdose reaction and in the epinephrine overdose reaction. The patient with vasodepressor syncope is nervous before and during the administration of the drug but does not normally become progressively more nervous in the postinjection period. This patient's major complaint is one of "feeling bad" or "feeling faint." Allergic patients do not develop marked nervousness; most of these patients complain of "feeling terrible."

Loss of Consciousness

Local-anesthetic overdose, acute systemic anaphylaxis, and vasodepressor syncope may all lead to the loss of consciousness. All may also produce milder reactions that do not develop to this degree. Epinephrine overdose seldom produces unconsciousness unless serious cardiovascular complications develop.

Presence of Seizures

Local-anesthetic overdose is most likely to produce generalized seizures of a tonic-clonic variety. Milder seizure movement (individual muscles such as a finger or facial muscle twitching) may occur in vasodepressor syncope. Mild tremor of the extremities is normally observed in overdose to epinephrine. Seizures do not usually occur with allergy unless hypoxia is present.

Respiratory Symptoms

Dyspnea (difficulty in breathing) may be present in any of these situations. Respiratory symptoms are most marked in the allergic reaction. Wheezing produced by bronchial smooth muscle constriction leads to a definitive diagnosis of asthma or allergy. Because management of both of these clinical entities is identical, precise diagnosis is not immediately required.

A high-pitched crowing sound should lead the doctor to consider laryngeal obstruction. This may be produced by a foreign object in the posterior pharynx or by laryngeal edema resulting from an allergic reaction.

In the absence of other signs of allergy (such as a skin reaction) the airway should be suctioned to remove any possible foreign material before further management.

Total airway obstruction is most probably produced by the tongue in an unconscious patient. If, following airway maneuvers and suctioning, the obstruction persists, lower airway obstruction should be considered. Regardless of the cause (edema or foreign object), an airway must be established rapidly (manual thrust or cricothyrotomy).

Cardiovascular Symptoms
Heart rate

Heart rate increases during the presyncopal phase of vasodepressor syncope, but it decreases dramatically to approximately 50 to 60 beats per minute once consciousness is lost and remains low during the postsyncopal period. Local-anesthetic overdose and allergic reactions are also associated with increases in heart rate, but the rate does not decrease to lower levels if consciousness is lost. A "shock reaction" develops that is characterized by rapid heart rate and low blood pressure, producing a weak, thready pulse. Epinephrine overdose, on the other hand, produces a dramatic increase in heart rate (and blood pressure), leading to a "full and bounding" pulse. In addition, the heart rate may become irregular during the epinephrine reaction owing to the effects of the drug on the myocardium.

Blood pressure

Blood pressure remains at the baseline level or is only slightly depressed during the presyncopal phase of vasodepressor syncope. With loss of consciousness, however, blood pressure drops significantly. In acute allergic reactions, blood pressure falls precipitously because of the massive vasodilation that occurs. Indeed, this reaction (acute systemic anaphylaxis) is one of the most likely of all the ADRs to lead to cardiovascular collapse (cardiac arrest).

During the early phase of a local-anesthetic overdose reaction, blood pressure is usually slightly

Table 25-1. Comparison of drug-related emergencies (by common factors)

Related (common) factors	Vasodepressor syncope	Overdose: local-anesthetic or epinephrine	Drug allergy
Age of patient	18-40 years most common	Any age; more likely in children than in adults	Any age
Sex of patient	More common in males	No sexual difference in occurrence	No sexual difference in occurrence
Position of patient	Unlikely in supine position	Not related to position	Not related to position
Onset of symptoms	Before, during, or immediately following administration	During or following administration	During or following administration
Prior exposure to drug	Not related	May occur with any drug, any administration	Prior exposure; "sensitizing dose" required
Dose of drug administered	Not related	Dose-related	Not dose-related
Overall incidence of occurrence	Most common drug-related emergency	Overdose is the most common *true* drug-related emergency (85% of all ADRs)	Rare; represents 15% of all ADRs

Table 25-2. Comparison of drug-related emergencies (by signs and symptoms)

Signs and symptoms	Vasodepressor syncope	Overdose		Drug allergy
		Local anesthetic	Epinephrine	
Duration of acute symptoms	Brief, following positioning	Self-limiting (2-30 minutes)	Extremely brief (usually seconds)	Long; hours to days
Appearance of skin	Pale, cold, and moist	Not relevant	Erythematous	Erythematous, presence of urticaria, itching, edema
Appearance of nervousness	No drastic increase	Increased anxiety, agitation	Fear, anxiety present	Not present
Loss of consciousness	Yes—vasodepressor syncope is most common cause of loss of consciousness	Yes—in severe reaction	No—rarely, if ever	Yes—in severe reaction
Presence of seizures	Rare—limited to mild, localized	Yes; tonic-clonic seizure	Mild tremor	No—unless hypoxia present
Respiratory symptoms	Not diagnostic	Not diagnostic	Not diagnostic	Wheezing, laryngeal edema
Cardiovascular symptoms				
Heart rate (pulse)	Initial elevation (presyncope), then depression (syncope)	Increased Weak and thready	Dramatic increase in palpitations Full and bounding	Increased Weak and thready
Blood pressure	Initially normal (presyncope); then depression	Initial increase, then depression	Dramatic increase	Significant depression
Most significant diagnostic criteria	Presyncopal manifestations; rapid recovery following positioning	CNS "stimulation" following drug administration	Palpitations; intense headache; brief duration	Erythema, urticaria, and pruritis; bronchospasm

elevated. As the reaction progresses, the blood pressure returns to baseline or falls below this level. Blood pressure during an epinephrine overdose reaction is dramatically increased. Pressures greatly in excess of 200 torr systolic and 120 torr diastolic may be observed during this reaction.

SUMMARY

Each of these clinical syndromes is presented with several outstanding features:

Vasodepressor syncope has a presyncopal phase of relatively long duration. The patient feels faint and lightheaded, the skin loses color, and perspiration is evident. Consciousness is regained rapidly following supine positioning of patient. This reaction commonly results from fear and is the most frequent emergency.

Local-anesthetic overdose is related to high blood levels of local anesthetic. It is commonly produced by rapid intravascular injection or administration of too large a dose. Signs and symptoms of stimulation (agitation, increased heart rate and blood pressure, and possible seizures) are followed by depression (lethargy, cardiovascular depression, respiratory depression, and loss of consciousness).

Epinephrine overdose is most frequently produced by the use of excessive concentrations of epinephrine in gingival retraction cord and less commonly in local anesthetics. The most prominent clinical signs include greatly increased nervousness, mild tremor, intense throbbing headache, and greatly increased blood pressure and heart rate. Epinephrine reactions are usually brief. The patient seldom loses consciousness.

Allergy may manifest itself in a variety of ways. However, obvious clinical signs of allergy include the skin reactions of flushing, urticaria, and itching. Edema may also occur. The presence of wheezing with respiratory efforts also signifies allergy. Allergy is the least common ADR but is usually the most dangerous of these reactions.

Tables 25-1 and 25-2 compare the different types of adverse drug reactions.

26 Chest Pain: General Considerations

There are a great many specific causes for the clinical symptom of chest pain that are entirely noncardiac in origin. Yet the sudden onset of chest pain is invariably a frightening experience, because it immediately invokes thoughts of "heart attack" in the mind of the victim. Because cardiovascular disease *is* the major cause of death in the United States today, this concern is not entirely unfounded. The almost universal presence of signs of cardiovascular disease in adults means that we are all potential victims of one or more of the clinical manifestations of cardiovascular disease. If we add to this the additional stresses involved in dental therapy, it becomes evident that many dental patients represent an increased risk during treatment. Recognition of these potentially high-risk patients and specific modifications in dental therapy diminish the chances of life-threatening situations developing.

Although chest pain is one of the major clinical clues to the presence of significant heart disease, the underlying disease process has normally been present for a considerable time before the appearance of clinical symptoms. Indeed, chest pain need not be the presenting symptom of this disease process. Previous chapters have discussed two clinical expressions of cardiovascular disease: heart failure, presenting as respiratory difficulty (Chapter 14), and cerebrovascular ischemia and infarction (Chapter 19), presenting as altered consciousness. In this section, three additional clinical manifestations of heart disease are discussed. Two of these, angina pectoris (Chapter 27) and myocardial infarction (Chapter 28), most commonly present as chest pain. Another clinical syndrome of cardiovascular disease, cardiac arrest, is discussed in Chapter 30. Cardiac arrest is a possible acute complication of all forms of cardiovascular disease, or it may be the initial indication of the presence of cardiovascular disease.

Table 26-1 lists three possible causes of the symptom of chest pain which may be encountered in dental situations.

The major factor underlying all forms of cardiovascular disease is atherosclerosis. Atherosclerosis is a special type of thickening and hardening of medium-sized and large arteries that accounts for a large proportion of heart attacks and cases of ischemic heart disease. It also accounts for many strokes (those caused by cerebral ischemia and infarction), numerous instances of peripheral vascular disease, and most aneurysms of the lower abdominal aorta, which can rupture and cause sudden fatal hemorrhage. Atherosclerosis is present in approximately 90% of patients with significant noncongenital heart disease. When present in arteries that supply blood to the myocardium, the disease state is termed coronary artery disease (CAD). Other common names for CAD are: coronary heart disease, ischemic heart disease, and atherosclerotic coronary artery disease. We may define CAD as a narrowing or occlusion of the coronary arteries, usually by atherosclerosis, which results in an imbalance between the requirement for and the supply of oxygen to the myocardium. An understanding of CAD and atherosclerosis leads to a greater knowledge of their clinical expressions. The remainder of this chapter concerns the important factors of cardiovascular disease, responsible for approximately 50% of all deaths in this country.

Table 26-1. Causes of chest pain

Cause	Frequency	Where discussed
Angina pectoris	Most common	Chest pain (Section VII)
Hyperventilation syndrome	Common	Respiratory difficulty (Section III)
Acute myocardial infarction	Less common	Chest pain (Section VII)

The following are definitions of terms to be used in this section:

hypoxia Reduced oxygen supply to tissue despite adequate perfusion

anoxia Absence of oxygen supply to tissue despite adequate perfusion

ischemia Oxygen deprivation accompanied by inadequate removal of metabolites consequent to inadequate perfusion

infarction Area of coagulation necrosis in a tissue caused by local ischemia, resulting from obstruction of circulation to the area

PREDISPOSING FACTORS

In 1981, cardiovascular disease was responsible for an estimated 989,610 deaths in the United States. Of this figure, 559,000 died from myocardial infarction, and the remainder succumbed to cerebrovascular accidents, rheumatic heart disease, and other causes such as aneurysms and pulmonary emboli (Table 26-2).

The number of deaths per year from cardiovascular disease has declined each year since 1950. More than 40% of this decrease has occurred since 1979. Still, the death rate from cardiovascular disease is disturbing.

An even more disturbing figure, however, is the overall incidence of cardiovascular disease in the United States. According to information from the American Heart Association, more than 42 million persons have clinical evidence of one or more forms of cardiovascular disease. These persons represent a great potential risk to the dental practitioner. Most of these persons are ambulatory, and a significant number may be asymptomatic, perhaps even unaware of their disease state, when appearing in the dental office for routine dental therapy. As is evident in the following discussion, any procedure or incident that results in an increase in the workload of this individual's cardiovascular system is potentially dangerous.

Coronary artery disease occurs more frequently in males. Its overall incidence shows a 4:1 male to female rate of occurrence. Of all deaths in men

Table 26-2. Number of deaths in the United States from cardiovascular disease, cancer, and accidents, 1981

Cause of death	Number (estimated)
Cardiovascular diseases	989,610
Acute myocardial infarction (heart attack)	559,000
Cerebrovascular accident (stroke)	164,300
Rheumatic fever, rheumatic heart disease	7,700
Congenital heart defects	6,500
Cancer	422,720
Accidents	102,130

Data from 1984 Heart Fact Reference Sheet, American Heart Association.

between the ages of 55 and 64, 40% are from coronary artery disease. In whites between the ages of 35 and 44 years there is a 5.2:1 male to female ratio for CAD, which progressively falls until, between the ages of 65 and 74, the male to female ratio for whites with CAD is 2.3:1. For nonwhites, these male to female ratios are 2.5:1 and 1.5:1, respectively. In general, the female rate lags behind the male rate by about 10 years in whites and about 7 years in nonwhites.

Data show that 2% of clinical CAD occurs before the age of 30 years. The incidence increases with age; 80% of CAD occurs between the sixth and eighth decades of life, with the peak incidence in men occurring between 50 and 60 years of age and in women, between 60 and 70 years of age.

The widespread occurrence and increasing incidence of coronary artery disease has prompted much research into its causes. In addition, possible methods are being researched to prevent CAD from progressing to the point of clinical morbidity and mortality. To date, this research has identified a number of factors that, when present, can increase the probability of an individual's developing clinical manifestations of CAD. Major risk factors for heart disease are listed in the box below. Although the evidence relating these factors to a significant increase in morbidity and mortality from CAD is clear-cut, much controversy remains within the medical profession concerning the effects of removing or managing these factors.

Major Modifiable Risk Factors

The following are major risk factors of heart disease that can be modified with a resulting decrease in risk.

Smoking

Cigarette smoking is a major risk factor for acute myocardial infarction and death from CAD. Results of several studies demonstrate that total mortality (all causes), total cardiovascular morbidity and mortality, and the incidence of CAD are about 1.6 times higher in male smokers than in male nonsmokers. There is also a direct relationship between these events and the number of cigarettes smoked daily.

Fortunately, the excessive risk factor for CAD declines in ex-smokers within a year or two of their discontinuation of smoking, but it does remain slightly greater than the risk associated with nonsmokers.

Several reasons for the increased risk caused by smoking have been postulated, including the effects of nicotine and carbon monoxide on the heart, coronary arteries, and blood. Nicotine increases the myocardial demand for oxygen, increases adhesiveness of platelets, and lowers the threshold for ventricular fibrillation. Carbon mon-

oxide prevents oxygen from forming oxyhemoglobin, thereby decreasing oxygen availability to tissues. Blood carbon monoxide levels in smokers range from 1 to 20%, compared with normal levels of 0.5% to 1.0% (blood levels of from 20% to 80% occur in carbon monoxide poisoning). When a person stops smoking, the carbon monoxide blood level falls, and the increased risk of CAD falls to approximately that of the nonsmoker. This factor also explains the increased incidence of cardiovascular abnormalities noted in automobile passengers on crowded Los Angeles freeways (Aronow, 1973). These subjects were exposed to a significantly higher level of gasoline engine exhausts, of which carbon monoxide is a major part. Carbon monoxide levels in their blood reached 1.4% to 3.0%.

Blood lipids

Among the recognized risk factors for the development of atherosclerosis, one of the most well documented is the relationship between blood lipid levels and CAD. The evidence associating increased serum cholesterol levels with increased incidence of CAD is extensive and unequivocal. Stated quite simply, persons with the highest cholesterol levels are at greatest risk to develop CAD, but even those with lower serum cholesterol levels are not completely risk-free.

Several types of lipoproteins have been identified. Low density lipoprotein (LDL) is known to be atherogenic and is the lipoprotein most directly associated with coronary artery disease. High density lipoprotein (HDL) demonstrates an inverse association with risk of CAD (higher HDL levels equate with lower risk of development of CAD). There is, however, no cut-off point in serum cholesterol levels below which there is no risk. Persons with blood cholesterol levels in excess of 300 mg% have a risk of developing CAD four times greater than do those with blood cholesterol levels less than 200 mg%. Mean levels for total plasma cholesterol (mg/dl) in white men are 200 between ages 35 and 39, 213 between ages 45 and 49, and 221 between ages 65 and 69, whereas plasma LDL cholesterol levels in these same groups are 133, 143, and 150, respectively.

Blood pressure

The risk of morbidity and mortality from CAD, as well as the risk of other diseases produced or exacerbated by atherosclerosis, show a smooth, direct relationship to blood pressure levels over the

---

**MAJOR RISK FACTORS
OF HEART DISEASE**

Factors that CANNOT be changed

Heredity
Sex
Race
Age

Factors that CAN be changed

Cigarette smoking
High blood pressure
High blood cholesterol levels
Diabetes

entire range of values. As with blood lipids, there is no cut-off point at which risk suddenly changes from low to high.

Management of high blood pressure through the administration of antihypertensive medications can decrease the risk to the patient. Damage that has developed within arteries over the years from high blood pressure cannot be undone (see Pathophysiology section, p. 334); however, the atherosclerotic process will be slowed if the patient's blood pressure is lowered.

Abnormal glucose tolerance

Hyperglycemia and glucose intolerance are associated with an increased risk of developing CAD. Overt diabetes mellitus has long been recognized as a precursor of vascular disease. Males with glucose intolerance have a 50% greater chance of developing CAD than do those with normal values, whereas in females the risk is doubled. In non-insulin-dependent diabetes the major cause of mortality is CAD. Both non-insulin-dependent and insulin-dependent adult onset diabetics are at in-

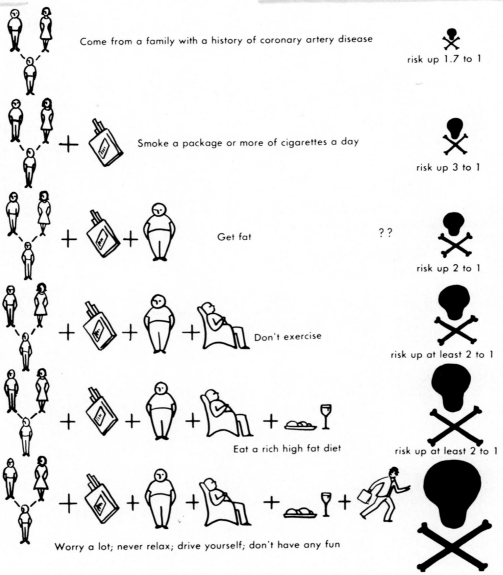

Fig. 26-1. How to die from coronary heart disease. The total increase in risk of death from coronary disease from all factors is at least 10 to 1, and may be more like 30 to 1. (From Phibbs, B.: The human heart: a guide to heart disease, ed. 4, St. Louis, 1979, The C.V. Mosby Co.)

Table 26-3. Death and major nonfatal events in untreated and treated hypertensive patients

	Initial diastolic blood pressure			
	115-129 torr*		90-114 torr*	
	70 untreated men‡	*73 actively treated men*	*194 untreated men*	*186 actively treated men*
Cardiovascular deaths	4	0	19	8
Major nonfatal events†	23	2	57	14

From Veterans Administration Cooperative Study Group on Antihypertensive Agents (1970). II. Results in patients with diastolic blood pressure averaging 90-114 mm Hg, JAMA **213:**1143, 1970.

*Average period of observation for men with diastolic blood pressure of 115-129 was 18 months; for men with diastolic blood pressure of 90-114, it was 40 months.

†Includes congestive heart failure, CV thrombosis, cerebral hemorrhage, MI, grade 3 or 4 retinopathy, and azotemia.

‡Includes 20 patients whose diastolic blood pressure exceeded 124 torr at three separate clinic visits.

creased risk for developing CAD. Mortality in juvenile onset insulin-dependent diabetes is primarily associated with renal disease.

Major Unmodifiable Risk Factors

Several other major risk factors of heart disease are unable to be modified at this time. These include heredity, sex, race, and age.

Heredity: Persons with either parents or siblings who are affected by CAD before the age of 50 years have a significantly greater risk of developing the disease themselves at a younger age than those who do not have such a history. This risk may be as great as 5:1.

Sex: As was previously discussed, CAD remains predominantly a male disease. The premenopausal female is relatively unaffected by CAD. Following menopause, the incidence of CAD in females increases, but it never reaches that of males.

Race: Blacks have an almost 45% greater chance of developing high blood pressure than do whites.

Age: The incidence of CAD increases with age.

Minor Risk Factors

Other factors related to an increased risk of significant CAD that are less well supported by clinical evidence include gout, menopause and oral contraceptives, obesity, physical activity, and type of personality and behavior. In addition, it is known that individuals with certain noncardiac diseases demonstrate a higher incidence of significant CAD. Hypercholesterolemia, high blood pressure, and diabetes mellitus have been mentioned previously. Another disease with significant CAD rates includes uncontrolled hypothyroidism. Fig. 26-1 shows the increased risk of death that is presented by some of these factors.

Table 26-4. Effectiveness of antihypertensive treatment in reducing death and major nonfatal events

	Percentage of patients with events		Effectiveness of treatment (%)*
Initial diastolic blood pressure	*Control*	*Treated*	
90-114 torr	33.3	11.8	70
115-129 torr	33.6	2.7	93

From Veterans Administration Cooperative Study Group on Antihypertensive Agents (1970). II. Results in patients with diastolic blood pressure averaging 90-114 mm Hg, JAMA **213:**1143, 1970.

*Effectiveness of treatment is the difference between percentages of incidence of events in control and treated groups, divided by percentage of incidence in control group.

PREVENTION

Unfortunately, primary prevention (prevention of initial development) of atherosclerosis and coronary artery disease has not yet been effectively demonstrated. Research into the known risk factors may ultimately demonstrate the feasibility of prevention of clinical CAD. To date, however, secondary prevention (prevention of death after clinical symptoms have developed) is the norm, but in too many cases this effort proves to be too late to prevent the occurrence of mortality or significant morbidity.

Emphasis is currently being placed on the elimination of any known risk factors that may be present. Smoking is discouraged, optimal weight and physical fitness are encouraged, and special diets and medications are recommended for those with elevated cholesterol levels in the blood. Uncontrolled hyperthyroidism or diabetes mellitus is

Table 26-5. Mortality from all causes for stepped care (SC) and referred care (RC) participants* during 5-year followup, by diastolic blood pressure (DBP) at entry

DBP at entry (torr)	Sample size		Deaths		Life table death rate per 100 (SE)†		95% confidence limits for difference in RC and SC rates	Percentage of reduction in mortality for SC group‡
	SC	RC	SC	RC	SC	RC		
TOTAL	5,485	5,455	349	419	6.4 (0.3)	7.7 (0.4)§	0.37-2.29	16.9
90-104	3,903	3,922	231	291	5.9 (0.4)	7.4 (0.4)§	0.40-2.62	20.3
105-114	1,048	1,004	70	77	6.7 (0.8)	7.7 (0.8)	−1.25-3.21	13.0
115+	534	529	48	51	9.0 (1.2)	9.7 (1.3)	−2.84-4.18	7.2

From Hypertension Detection and Follow-up Program Cooperative Group. Five year findings of the hypertension detection and follow-up program. I. Reduction in mortality of persons with high blood pressure, including mild hypertension, JAMA **242**:2562, 1979.

*Stepped care (SC) patients received rigorous antihypertensive drug therapy from time of diagnosis of their elevated blood pressure; referred care (RC) patients were managed in a manner consistent with usually accepted techniques, which might not include immediate use of antihypertensive drugs.

†SE indicates standard error.

‡(RC rate − SC rate)/(RC rate) × 100.

§$P < 0.1$.

Table 26-6. Clinical manifestations of atherosclerosis

	Manifestation	Mechanism
Noncardiac		
Diabetes mellitus	Diabetic retinopathy and blindness	Atherosclerosis of retinal vessels
	Increased infection and poor healing of lower limb, with possible amputation of toes or feet	Atherosclerosis of arteries to legs
Cerebral arteries	Transient ischemic attack	Transient occlusion of vessels
	Cerebrovascular infarction	Prolonged occlusion of vessels
Cardiac		
Coronary artery disease	Angina pectoris	Transient, localized myocardial ischemia
	Myocardial infarction	Prolonged arterial occlusion
	Intermediate coronary syndrome (unstable angina)	Prolonged myocardial ischemia, with or without myocardial necrosis
	Heart failure	Gradual fibrosis of myocardium; occurs commonly following MI
	Dysrhythmias	Gradual fibrosis of myocardium; occurs commonly following MI
	Sudden death (cardiopulmonary arrest)	Any of the above and/or ventricular dysrhythmias

brought under control, and elevations in blood pressure are corrected. However, the evidence being gathered concerning the effectiveness of many of these therapies in preventing morbidity and mortality is conflicting. Management of elevated blood pressure *has* been effectively demonstrated to produce a significant decrease in the morbidity and mortality rate from CAD. The Veterans Administration studies (Tables 26-3 and 26-4) proved conclusively that reduction of elevated blood pressure leads to a highly significant decrease in the incidence of fatal and nonfatal cardiovascular events. More recently, the Hypertension Detection and Follow-up Program Cooperative Group has demonstrated that vigorous drug management of even mild elevations in blood pressure (diastolic blood pressure 90-104 torr) leads to significant reductions (a decline of 20.3%) of cardiovascular morbidity and mortality (Table 26-5). Therefore the recording of blood pressure on all dental patients before dental therapy might prove to be a life-saving procedure. A suggested protocol for dental management of patients with elevated blood pressure is presented in Chapter 2.

Another significant factor that may be applied to the dental office setting is the reduction of stress related to dental treatment. Physical and psychologic stress increases the work of the myocardium and therefore its oxygen requirement. In the patient with impaired coronary blood flow, this additional requirement for oxygen may not be met and may lead to an acute exacerbation of some form of heart disease. The Stress Reduction Protocol (Chapter 2) is invaluable in the management of most patients with CAD. Of particular importance will be the administration of supplemental oxygen through a nasal cannula or nasal hood during the dental treatment.

CLINICAL MANIFESTATIONS

Atherosclerosis does not produce clinical manifestations of disease. It is only when the degree of atherosclerosis becomes great enough to produce a deficit in blood supply to an area of the body that symptoms become apparent. The nature of the clinical syndrome depends on these factors:

1. The size and location of the tissue inadequately supplied with blood
2. The severity of the deficiency
3. The rate of development of the deficiency
4. The duration of the deficiency

For example, cerebrovascular ischemia is a manifestation of atherosclerosis that occurs in the brain. If the oxygen deficiency is mild, transient ischemic attacks (TIA) may be the sole clinical manifestation,

whereas a true CVA develops with infarction of neuronal tissues if the oxygen deprivation is more complete. TIA is normally of short duration, usually resolving without residual neuronal deficiency; CVA produces permanent neuronal damage. The clinical manifestations of atherosclerosis in the coronary vessels (angina pectoris, myocardial infarction, heart failure, cardiac dysrhythmias, and sudden death) are summarized in Table 26-6.

Angina pectoris (see Chapter 27) is a transient, localized ischemia of the myocardium, whereas a myocardial infarction (Chapter 28) results from arterial occlusion. Heart failure and cardiac dysrhythmias quite frequently develop following myocardial infarction (as chronic complications), but they may also occur through a process of gradual fibrosis of the myocardium and the conduction system of the heart in the absence of myocardial infarction. Sudden death (cardiopulmonary arrest) may develop following any of the above-mentioned mechanisms or through the occurrence of ventricular fibrillation. (See Chapter 30.)

PATHOPHYSIOLOGY
Atherosclerosis

Atherosclerosis is an ongoing process that starts *in utero* as soon as blood begins to flow in rudimen-

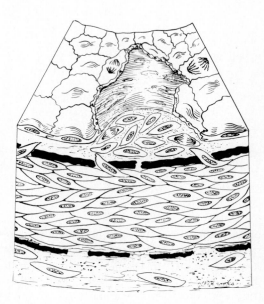

Fig. 26-3. Development of atherosclerosis. Smooth muscle cells migrate from media into the intimal layer through fenestrae in internal elastic lamina. (From Ross, R., and Glomset, J.A.: N. Engl. J. Med. **295:**369-377, 420-425, 1976.)

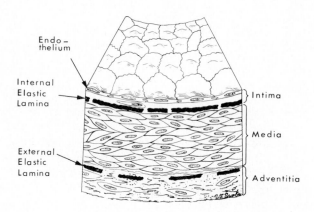

Fig. 26-2. Structure of normal muscular artery. (From Ross, R., and Glomset, J.A.: N. Engl. J. Med. **295:**369-377, 420-425, 1976.)

tary blood vessels. It is found in all individuals at certain sites of predilection. Atherosclerosis may therefore be considered a reactive biologic response of arteries to the forces being generated by the flow of blood. Texon (1974) has described atherosclerosis as "the price we pay for blood flow as a requirement of life."

The basic factor in the development of the atherosclerotic lesion (termed an atheroma) is a multiplication of the smooth muscle cells of the intimal layer of the blood vessel in response to pressure changes within the vessel (Figs. 26-2 and 26-3). In a normal blood vessel, there is constant movement of lipids into and out of the intimal layer. However, when proliferative changes occur within the intimal smooth muscle cells, the ability of these cells to maintain a steady level of lipids is altered, and the influx of lipids into the intima becomes predominant. This influx is initially made up of cholesterol, triglycerides, and phospholipids and appears as a yellowish streak or plaque that is visible within the lumen of the artery (Fig. 26-4). As the lesion progresses, cholesterol becomes the predominant lipid. Fibrous tissue next grows into and around the atheroma, and finally calcium is deposited into the lesion. The atheroma, which began as a soft fatty lesion, becomes a larger, harder lesion.

With the increase in size, the lesion may cause obstruction of blood flow through the vessel at the point of the lesion, leading to chronic ischemia (heart failure, dysrhythmias), acute ischemia (angina pectoris, TIA), or infarction (myocardial or cerebrovascular infarction). If the endothelial layer of the blood vessel breaks down, the atheromatous material is exposed to circulating blood platelets, which then clump and initiate thrombus formation with subsequent acute clinical manifestations (myocardial infarction, CVA, or cardiac arrest).

Location

Sites of predilection of atherosclerosis are illustrated in Fig. 26-5. Atherosclerosis of the coronary vessels occurs predominantly in the proximal segments of medium-sized coronary arteries, especially at branching points. Interestingly, only those vessels that run over the surface of the myocardium are susceptible to the development of atheroma-

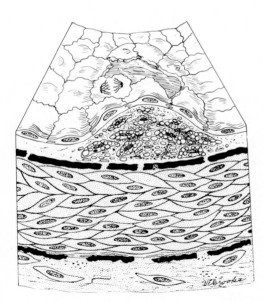

Fig. 26-4. Development of atherosclerosis. Lipid deposition within intimal cells and their surrounding connective tissue matrix. Lumen of vessel progressively narrows. (From Ross, R., and Glomset, J.A.: N. Engl. J. Med. **295:**369-377, 420-425, 1976.)

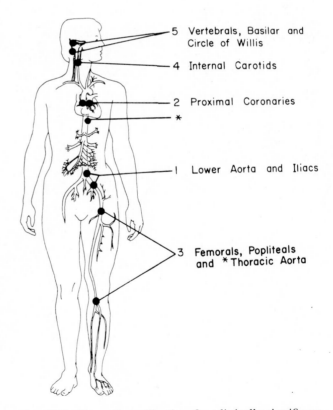

Fig. 26-5. Sites of predilection for clinically significant atherosclerosis, ranked in usual order of occurrence. Substantial exceptions can occur, often without an obvious reason. (From Braunwald, E., editor: Heart disease, Philadelphia, 1980, W.B. Saunders Co.)

tous lesions. Vessels that enter the myocardium (the penetrating or muscular branches) do not demonstrate atheromata. The explanation for this is not yet known. The most common site in which clinically significant atherosclerosis develops in the heart, leading to major morbidity and mortality, is the anterior descending branch of the left coronary artery. Occlusion of this vessel leads to infarction of the anterior portion of the left ventricle. The blood supply to the myocardium is shown in Fig. 26-6.

Chest Pain

The basic mechanism of cardiac pain is a decrease or cessation of blood flow to the myocardium. Episodes of cardiac pain occur when critical myocardial ischemia is produced by an absolute decrease of the coronary blood flow or by oxygen demand of the myocardium that is greater than the available blood supply.

The precise mechanism of cardiac pain production is unknown. Current theories suggest that cardiac pain results from an accumulation of metabolites within the ischemic portion of the myocardium. This rapid accumulation of metabolites within the heart muscle, occurring with transient ischemia (angina pectoris) or prolonged ischemia (myocardial infarction), is responsible for triggering pain impulses. Other theories on the genesis of cardiac pain include those suggesting that vasomotor reflexes or vasospasms produce paroxysms of cardiac pain (the pain arising from the coronary vessels themselves) or that cardiac pain is provoked by distention of the walls of coronary vessels proximal to the site of an occlusion. Sudden obstruction of a major coronary vessel (primarily by thrombosis) and the occurrence of myocardial infarction are often associated with violent pain, yet if the vessel occlusion develops gradually there may be no clinically evident signs. This is primarily because of the gradual development of an effective collateral circulation between the left and right coronary arteries. In the presence of an adequate collateral circulation, an occlusion of the right coronary artery may not lead to infarction of that part of the tissue that is also supplied by the left coronary artery (Fig. 26-6). Unfortunately, in the normal heart there is usually a minimally developed collateral circulation, which in part explains the greater incidence of acute episodes of cardiac disease.

MANAGEMENT

Management of the acute clinical manifestations of coronary artery disease is directed toward the specific clinical entity that develops. In the patient with congestive heart failure, primary management of the acute episode is directed at alleviation of re-

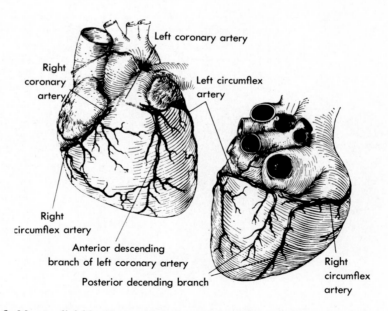

Fig. 26-6. Myocardial blood supply. *Left,* anterior heart. *Right,* posterior heart. (From Goldman, M.J.: Principles of clinical electrocardiography, ed. 9, Los Altos, CA, 1976, Lange Medical Publications.)

spiratory distress, which presents as the major immediate symptom. Angina and acute myocardial infarction produce acute paroxysms of chest discomfort of varying intensity and duration. Immediate management of these clinical entities is directed at alleviation of this discomfort. In all instances of clinical CAD, goals of management include decreasing the workload of the myocardium (thereby decreasing the myocardial oxygen requirement) and providing the victim with an increased supply of oxygen. When sudden death is imminent (as in cardiopulmonary arrest), the goal of immediate therapy is of course the prevention of biologic death. The principles of basic life support must be applied as rapidly and as effectively as possible. Cardiac arrest is a possible complication of all forms of coronary artery disease.

BIBLIOGRAPHY

Agnew, T.M., and others: Coronary artery disease: recent developments, N.Z. Med. J. **84**:52, 1976.

Altschule, M.D.: Foreword to Symposium on atherosclerosis, Med. Clin. North Am. **58**:243, 1974.

Altschule, M.D.: The etiology of atherosclerosis, Med. Clin. North Am. **58**:397, 1974.

American Heart Association: Heart facts 1984, Dallas, 1984, The Association.

Aronow, W.S.: Smoking, carbon monoxide and coronary heart disease, Circulation **48**:1169, 1973.

Astrup, P., and Kjeldsen, K.: Carbon monoxide, smoking, and atherosclerosis, Med. Clin. North Am. **58**:323, 1973.

Ball, K., and Turner, R.: Smoking and the heart: the basis for action, Lancet **2**:822, 1974.

Barnes, B.O.: On the genesis of atherosclerosis, J. Am. Geriatr. Soc. **21**:350, 1973.

Baroldi, G.: Coronary thrombosis: facts and beliefs, Am. Heart J. **91**:683, 1976.

Bellet, S., DeGuzmas, N.T., and Kostis, J.B.: The effect of inhalation of cigarette smoke on ventricular fibrillation threshold in normal dogs and dogs with acute myocardial infarction, Am. Heart J. **83**:67, 1972.

Blackburn, H.: Concepts and controversies about the prevention of coronary heart disease, Postgrad. Med. J. **52**:417, 1976.

Braunwald, E., and Sobel, B.E.: Coronary blood flow and myocardial ischemia. In Braunwald, E., editor: Heart disease: a textbook of cardiovascular medicine, Philadelphia, 1980, W.B. Saunders Co.

Buell, J.C., and Eliot, R.S.: Stress and cardiovascular disease, Mod. Concepts Cardiovasc. Med. **47**:19, 1979.

Dimsdale, J.E.: Emotional causes of sudden death, Am. J. Psychiatry **134**:1361, 1977.

Driscoll, D.J., Glicklich, L.B., and Gallen, W.J.: Chest pain in children: a prospective study, Pediatrics **57**:648, 1976.

Eleventh Bethesda Conference: Prevention of coronary heart disease, Am. J. Cardiol. **47**:713, 1981.

Eliot, R.S., and others: Influence of environmental stress on the pathogenesis of sudden cardiac death, Fed. Proc. **36**:1719, 1971.

Eliot, R.S.: Stress and cardiovascular disease, Eur. J. Cardiol. **5**:97, 1977.

Eliot, R.S., and Forker, A.D.: Emotional stress and cardiac disease, JAMA **236**:2325, 1976.

Engel, H.J., Page, H.L., Jr., and Campbell, W.B.: Coronary artery disease in young women, JAMA **230**:1531, 1974.

Epstein, S.E., Gerber, L.H., and Borer, J.S.: Chest wall syndrome: a common cause of unexplained cardiac pain, JAMA **241**:2793, 1979.

Friedman, G.D., Siegelaub, A.B., and Dales, L.G.: Cigarette smoking and chest pain, Ann. Intern. Med. **83**:1, 1975.

Friedman, M., and Rosenman, R.H.: Type A: your behavior and your heart, New York, 1974, Alfred A. Knopf, Inc.

Goldman, M.J.: Principles of clinical electrocardiography, ed. 9, Los Altos, CA, 1976, Lange Medical Publications.

Hammond, E.C., Garfinkel, L., and Seidman, H.: Longevity of parents and grandparents in relation to coronary heart disease and associated variables, Circulation **43**:31, 1971.

Hennekens, C.H., and others: Coffee drinking and death due to coronary heart disease, N. Engl. J. Med. **294**:633, 1976.

Hypertension Detection and Follow-up Program Cooperative Group. Five year findings of the hypertension detection and follow-up program. I. Reduction in mortality of persons with high blood pressure, including mild hypertension, JAMA **242**:2562, 1979.

Intersociety Commission for Heart Disease Resources Report: Primary prevention of the atherosclerotic diseases, Circulation **62**:A, 1970.

Jenkins, C.D.: Recent evidence supporting psychologic and social risk factors for coronary disease, N. Engl. J. Med. **294**:1033, 1976.

Kannel, W.B.: Some lessons in cardiovascular epidemiology from Framingham, Am. J. Cardiol. **37**:269, 1976.

Kannel, W.B., Castell, W.P., and Gordon, T.: Cholesterol in the prediction of atherosclerotic disease. New perspectives based on the Framingham study, Ann. Intern. Med. **90**:85, 1979.

Kannel, W.B., and others: Precursors of sudden coronary death, Circulation **51**:606, 1975.

Keys, A.: Coronary heart disease—the global picture, Atherosclerosis **22**:149, 1975.

Kuo, P.T.: Hyperlipidemia and coronary artery disease, Med. Clin. North Am. **58**:351, 1974.

Lefkowitz, R.J.: Smoking, catecholamines and the heart, N. Engl. J. Med. **295**:615, 1976.

Levy, R.I.: Declining mortality in coronary heart disease, Atherosclerosis **1**:312, 1981.

Levy, R.I., and Feinleib, M.: Risk factors for coronary artery disease and their management. In Braunwald, E., editor: Heart disease: a textbook of cardiovascular medicine, Philadelphia, 1980, W.B. Saunders Co.

Lynch, J.J., and others: Psychological aspects of cardiac arrhythmias, Am. Heart J. **93**:645, 1977.

McNamara, J.J., and others: Coronary artery disease in combat casualties in Viet Nam, JAMA **216**:1185, 1971.

Miller, N.E., and others: The Tromso heart study. High density lipoprotein and coronary heart disease. A prospective case control study, Lancet **1**:965, 1977.

Nye, E.R.: Epidemiology of ischemic heart disease, N.Z. Med. J. **80**:288, 1974.

Oslo Study Group: Effect of diet and smoking intervention on the incidence of coronary heart disease: report from the Oslo Study Group of a randomised trial in healthy man, Lancet **2**:1301, 1981.

Rosenman, R.H., and others: Multivariate prediction of coronary heart disease during 8.5 year follow up in the Western Collaborative Group study, Am. J. Cardiol. **37:**903, 1976.

Ross, R., and Glamset, J.A.: The pathogenesis of atherosclerosis, N. Engl. J. Med. **295:**369 and 420, 1976.

Russek, H.I., and Russek, L.G.: Etiologic factors in ischemic heart disease: the illusive role of emotional stress, Geriatrics **27:**81, 1972.

Sampson, J.J., and Cheitlin, M.D.: Pathophysiology and differential diagnosis of chest pain, Prog. Cardiovasc. Dis. **13:**507, 1971.

Stamler, J.: Lifestyles, major risk factors, proof, and public policy, Circulation **58:**3, 1978.

Steinbaugh, M., and Strong, W.B.: Primary prevention of atherosclerosis: nutritional aspects, South. Med. J. **68:**328, 1975.

Sugiura, M., and others: A clinicopathological study on the heart diseases in the aged, Jpn. Heart J. **16:**526, 1975.

Texon, M.: Atherosclerosis, its hemodynamic basis and implications, Med. Clin. North Am. **58:**257, 1974.

Veterans Administration Cooperative Study Group on Antihypertensive Agents (1970). II. Results in patients with diastolic blood pressure averaging 90-114 mm Hg, JAMA **213:**1143, 1970.

Warren, J.V.: A revolution in coronary artery disease, J. Chronic Dis. **26:**547, 1973.

Wissler, R.W.: Principles of the pathogenesis of atherosclerosis. In Braunwald, E., editor: Heart disease: a textbook of cardiovascular medicine, Philadelphia, 1980, W.B. Saunders Co.

Workshop Four: Emotional stress in coronary artery disease, J. S.C. Med. Assoc. **72**(suppl):88, 1976.

Wright, I.S.: Cardiovascular diseases: role of psychogenic and behavior patterns in development and aggravation, N.Y. State J. Med. **75:**2128, 1975.

Wright, I.S.: Problems which inhibit the prevention of cardiovascular diseases, Bull. N.Y. Acad. Med. **51:**104, 1975.

27 *Angina Pectoris*

Angina is a Latin word describing a spasmodic choking or suffocating pain; *pectoris* is the Latin word for chest. These words describe the basic clinical manifestations of angina pectoris, also called simply angina, the classic expression of chronic coronary artery disease (CAD). A working definition of angina is that it is a characteristic thoracic pain, usually substernal; precipitated chiefly by exercise, emotion, or a heavy meal; relieved by vasodilator drugs and a few minutes' rest; and a result of a moderate inadequacy of the coronary circulation. The major clinical characteristic of angina is chest "pain." However, the pain is seldom described by a victim as such. Much more commonly, the sensation is described as a dull, aching discomfort.

Angina is clinically important to the dental practitioner because it is usually a sign of significant coronary artery disease. Its onset indicates that the victim's coronary arteries are not providing the myocardium with an adequate oxygen supply. If this inadequacy is prolonged excessively, actual infarction of the myocardial tissues may occur. The patient with a history of angina therefore represents a significant risk during dental therapy. Any factor that produces an increase in myocardial oxygen requirements may precipitate an acute episode of chest pain, which is usually readily managed through vasodilator drug therapy but may ultimately lead to myocardial infarction, acute dysrhythmias, or cardiac arrest. Therefore prevention of the acute episode proves ultimately more satisfactory than management of the episode.

PREDISPOSING FACTORS

The factors that lead to the initial development of angina are those previously discussed in Chapter 26 on chest pain (see box on p. 330). Acute clinical episodes of angina of effort (i.e., precipitated by effort) are usually precipitated by factors that produce a relative inability of the coronary arteries to supply adequate oxygenated blood to the myocardium. Commonly observed precipitating factors are listed in the box on p. 340.

There is another form of angina that is more likely to occur at rest than with effort, may develop at odd times during the day or night (even awakening patients from sleep), and is often associated with dysrhythmias or conduction defects. It is termed *coronary artery spasm* or *Prinzmetal's variant angina.* Variant angina is more common in women under the age of 50 years, whereas the typical angina of effort is uncommon in women of this age in the absence of severe hypercholesterolemia, high blood pressure, or diabetes mellitus. Another syndrome, termed *unstable angina,* also exists. Other names for this syndrome are preinfarction angina, intermediate coronary syndrome, premature or impending myocardial infarction, or coronary insufficiency. This syndrome is an intermediate between angina of effort and acute myocardial infarction; it is important because of the adverse prognosis and the unpredictability of sudden onset of acute myocardial infarction in some of the patients experiencing it. Patients with unstable angina should be managed in the dental office as if they had recently had an acute myocardial infarction. This syndrome will be discussed in depth in this chapter.

Angina may develop with the patient at rest or even during apparently restful sleep. Clinical study has demonstrated that in most of the instances in which an acute anginal episode develops during sleep, it is preceded by a dream in which the patient is emotionally stimulated or is exercising. There are striking elevations in the respiratory rate, blood pressure, and heart rate. Within the dental office, factors such as fear, anxiety, and pain are more likely causes of anginal episodes. Each of these factors results in elevated blood levels of the catecholamines epinephrine and norepinephrine, which act to produce an increase in the heart rate, increased strength of myocardial contraction, and an increase in blood pressure. The oxygen requirement of the myocardium increases, and if the coronary arteries are unable to provide for this added requirement, the pain of angina results.

PREVENTION

As has been stressed previously, the prevention of life-threatening situations is much preferred to their management after they occur. In no other category is this more true than that of chest pain, because the outcome frequently is the death of the patient. With the multitude of stresses placed on the doctor and the dental patient, it is probable that most persons experience an increase in cardiac workload during dental appointments. Determination of the high-risk patient permits modification of dental therapy and in most instances prevents the occurrence of chest pain. Because stress is the major element precipitating anginal pain, the elimination of stress is the chief preventive measure.

Medical History Questionnaire

QUESTION 9. Circle any of the following which you have had or have at present:
- **Heart disease**
- **Angina pectoris**
- **Heart surgery**

COMMENT. An affirmative answer to any part of this question should be followed with the dialogue history to determine the nature of the cardiac problem and its severity. Coronary bypass surgery is frequently indicated in patients with intolerable angina pectoris.

QUESTION 10. When you walk up stairs or take a walk, do you ever have to stop because of pain in your chest or shortness of breath, or because you are very tired?

COMMENT. "Pain" occurring in the chest during exertion (such as walking or climbing a flight of stairs) is an indication of classic angina pectoris.

QUESTION 6. Have you taken any medicine or drugs during the past 2 years?

COMMENT. Patients with angina pectoris normally have with them a supply of sublingual nitroglycerin tablets that are used to terminate an acute anginal episode. Since its introduction in January of 1986

> **PRECIPITATING FACTORS IN ANGINA PECTORIS**
>
> Physical activity
> Hot, humid environment
> Cold weather
> Large meals
> Emotional stress (argument, anxiety, or sexual excitement)
> Caffeine ingestion
> Fever, anemia, or thyrotoxicosis
> Cigarette smoking
> Smog
> High altitudes
> Smoke from *another* person's cigarettes

---

more and more anginal patients have started to use the more stable oral spray form of nitroglycerin in place of sublingual tablets. Many patients with a history of angina are also receiving other medications, such as long-acting nitrates, to prevent the occurrence of acute anginal episodes. Although the frequency of anginal episodes may be decreased with the long-acting nitrates, there is no convincing evidence that these agents prolong life. More recently, beta-blocking agents and calcium entry–blocking agents have been employed to prevent acute anginal episodes. Calcium entry–blockers are especially useful when coronary artery spasm is present, although they may relieve pain in the absence of spasm because they produce vasodilation. Additionally, nitroglycerin ointment and transdermal nitroglycerin have recently been added to the treatment armamentarium. Nitroglycerin ointment provides relief for 4 to 6 hours, whereas transdermal nitroglycerin provides slow, continuous release of the drug over a 24-hour period. Table 27-1 lists those agents used in the prevention of anginal episodes.

Dialogue History

For patients with a possible history of angina, the dialogue history should be used to determine the following information concerning "anginal pains":

QUESTION. What precipitates your anginal episode?

COMMENT. Most commonly, anginal pain occurs during exertion. The amount of exertion required to precipitate angina varies from patient to patient but is usually relatively constant for each patient. Can the patient walk two level city blocks or climb one flight of stairs without developing chest pain? is a question that will provide helpful information. Of particular importance for the doctor is the relationship of emotional factors to anginal episodes and the patient's attitude toward dentistry.

QUESTION. How frequently do you suffer anginal attacks?

COMMENT. The frequency of anginal episodes varies from patient to patient. Attacks may occur infrequently, perhaps once a week or once a month, or the patient may experience acute episodes several times a day. On average the patient with a history of angina experiences one or two epi-

Table 27-1. Agents used to prevent anginal episodes

Generic name	Proprietary name	Usual dosage	Route of administration	Side effects
Long-acting nitrates				
Isosorbide dinitrate	Isordil Sorbitrate	5-10 mg every 3 hours 5-30 mg four times daily or 40 mg twice daily	Sublingual Oral	Headache Flushing Tachycardia Dizziness
Pentaerythritol tetranitrate	Peritrate	10-20 mg four times daily or 80 mg twice daily	Oral	Postural hypotension
Erythrityl tetranitrate	Cardilate	5-15 mg four times daily	Sublingual and oral	Tachyphylaxis to nitroglycerin with prolonged use
Beta-blocking agents				
Propranolol	Inderal	10-80 mg twice daily or four times daily	Oral	For all beta blockers: development of asthma, severe bradycardia, atrioventricular conduction defects, and left ventricular failure
Metoprolol	Lopressor	50 mg twice daily	Oral	
Nadolol	Corgard	40 mg once daily	Oral	
Atenolol	Tenormin	50-100 mg once daily	Oral	
Pindolol	Visken	5-10 mg twice daily	Oral	
Timolol	Blocadren	10-20 mg twice daily	Oral	
Calcium entry–blocking agents				
Verapamil	Calan, Isoptin	240-480 mg daily in 3-4 divided doses	Oral	For all calcium channel blockers: peripheral edema, hypotension, dizziness, lightheadedness, headache, weakness, nausea, constipation
Diltiazem	Cardizem	180-240 mg daily in 3-4 divided doses	Oral	
Nifedipine	Procardia	10-20 mg three times daily	Oral	
Nitroglycerin				
	Nitrostat	1 tablet sublingual q 5 min at onset of acute angina	Sublingual tablet or spray, just before activity	For all forms: headache, hypotension
	Nitrobid Nitrol Nitrong Nitrostat	1-2 inches q 8 hours	Ointment, every 4-8 hours	
	Nitrodisc Nitro-dur Transderm-Nitro	Appropriate-size pad every day	Transdermal patch, every 24 hours	

sodes per week. The risk of an episode being precipitated in the dental office is obviously increased in a patient with a greater frequency of episodes under other conditions.

QUESTION. *How long do your anginal episodes last?*

COMMENT. Angina is by definition of short duration. If the episode is precipitated by exertion and the patient stops and rests, the discomfort normally ceases within 2 to 10 minutes. Chest pain lasting less than 30 seconds is usually not anginal. This brief duration commonly points to a problem of noncardiac origin, such as musculoskeletal pain, hiatal hernia, or functional pain. Chest pain lasting for hours suggests acute myocardial infarction, pericarditis, dissecting aortic aneurysm, musculoskeletal disease, herpes zoster, or anxiety. Anginal episodes developing after a large meal tend to be longer lasting and more difficult to treat.

QUESTION. *How does nitroglycerin affect the anginal episode?*

COMMENT. Nitroglycerin in tablet, spray, or ointment form greatly shortens the duration of the anginal episode. In most cases, nitroglycerin terminates the anginal attack within 2 to 4 minutes. The clinical management of chest pain in the dental patient is initiated by the administration of nitroglycerin, and subsequent treatment is based on the patient's response or lack of response to this agent. Chest pain lasting 10 minutes or more may prove to be acute myocardial infarction or unstable angina. Pain of esophageal spasm or esophagitis may also be relieved by nitroglycerin; however, pain of esophagitis (and peptic ulcer) is also relieved by ingestion of food and antacids, whereas anginal pain is not.

QUESTION. *Describe a typical anginal episode.*

COMMENT. Anginal episodes for each patient are usually consistent in frequency, intensity, radiation, and duration. An increase in severity of any of these parameters is a clinical sign of unstable angina and should be evaluated further (by means of medical consultation).

The diagnosis of angina pectoris depends almost entirely on the dialogue history, and it is quite important to permit the patient sufficient time to describe the symptoms without interruption. Patients frequently use gestures to describe the location and quality of the symptom (Fig. 27-1), such as placing

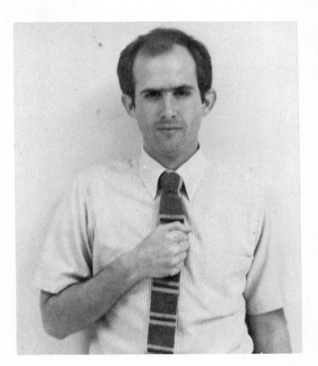

Fig. 27-1. The Levine sign, an indicator of angina pectoris.

their closed fist against their sternum—the "Levine sign."

Physical Examination

Physical examination of a patient with a history of angina will yield essentially normal findings during a period between episodes. Physical findings during the acute episode are described on p. 345.

Unstable Angina

Unstable angina represents a syndrome that lies between angina pectoris and acute myocardial infarction in the spectrum of clinical manifestations of coronary heart disease. Synonyms for unstable angina include intermediate coronary syndrome, preinfarction angina, premature or impending myocardial infarction, and coronary insufficiency. Unstable angina is extremely significant because of the increased risk of acute MI, as well as the unpredictability of the occurrence of MI. Patients developing unstable angina should be managed in the dental office as would patients having recently (within the past 6 months) suffered a myocardial infarction. They represent an ASA IV risk and ought not to be considered for elective dental treatment. In fact, it is considered prudent medical management to hospitalize these patients with monitoring in a coronary care unit to minimize the risk of fatal dysrhythmias and death.

Unstable angina will be recognized from the dialogue history obtained from the anginal patient (see section on dialogue history). As mentioned previously, the characteristics of an acute anginal episode for a given patient are fairly consistent from episode to episode. Unstable angina is a syndrome in which the pain differs in character, duration, radiation, and severity—in which the pain, over a period of hours or days, demonstrates a crescendo (increasing) quality or occurs at rest or during the night.

Not all patients with unstable angina will develop signs of myocardial infarction. However, they are considered to be in a precarious balance for myocardial oxygen supply and demand and must be treated as if they had a minor myocardial infarction.

Clinical reports on the prognosis following medical treatment of unstable angina indicate a low mortality rate during the period of hospitalization—approximately 5%. However, the mortality rate over the next 1 to 2 years is about 15%. Medical management of unstable angina includes bed rest; the administration of nitrates (including intravenous nitroglycerin), beta-blocking agents (Table 27-1), and calcium channel blockers (Table 27-1); and psychologic rest and reassurance. Nitroglycerin ointment or transdermal nitroglycerin are frequently employed.

When medical treatment has not improved or eliminated the patient's symptoms, or if they become worse, surgical intervention may be indicated (that is, aortocoronary bypass).

Evidence shows that patients who are admitted to a coronary care unit because of unstable angina suggestive of myocardial infarction, but in whom infarction is never demonstrated, have a higher death rate over the next 1 to 2 years than ordinary anginal patients.

Only emergency dental treatment should be considered for patients with unstable angina, and then only after consultation with their physician and preferably within a hospital environment.

Dental Therapy Considerations

Prevention of acute episodes of angina during dental therapy is predicated on minimizing stress so that the amount of oxygen delivered through the coronary arteries is adequate to meet the requirements of the myocardium.

The Stress Reduction Protocols are particularly important to the anginal patient. Specific consideration must be given to the intraoperative aspects of the protocol, in particular the length of the appointment, pain control during therapy, and the use of psychosedation. The average patient with angina pectoris is an ASA physical status III (Table 27-2).

Length of appointment

An important factor in preventing the occurrence of anginal episodes during dental treatment is to avoid overstressing the patient. No time limit can be stated, because patient tolerance varies considerably. However, dental treatment should be halted when a patient demonstrates signs or symptoms of fatigue such as sweating, fidgety movements, or increased anxiety. Permit the patient to rest before permitting discharge.

Supplemental oxygen

Anginal patients are excellent candidates to routinely receive supplemental oxygen through a nasal cannula or nasal hood during dental treatment. A flow of 3 to 5 liters per minute will minimize the possibility of inadequate oxygenation of the myocardium.

Pain control during therapy

Pain is stressful; therefore its control in the anginal patient is extremely important. The prevention of pain during dental therapy can best be ensured by the appropriate use of local-anesthetic drugs. The question that arises all too frequently concerns the advisability of using a vasoconstrictor in conjunction with the local anesthetic in the patient with cardiac risk.

A wealth of clinical evidence has accumulated that supports the statement that, for most cardiac patients, local-anesthetic solutions containing a vasoconstrictor (epinephrine) are indicated during dental therapy. The American Dental Association in conjunction with the American Heart Association published the findings of a joint committee that researched this potential problem (see *Journal of the American Dental Association,* May 1964).

To summarize the available clinical data concerning this question, it may be stated that, if pain control proves inadequate, cardiac patients are potentially at greater risk from the effects of endogenously released catecholamines (epinephrine and norepinephrine) than they are from a properly

Table 27-2. Dental therapy considerations in angina pectoris

Frequency of angina	Patient's abilities	ASA physical status	Considerations
0-1 per month	Patient can walk two level city blocks or climb one flight of stairs	II	Usual ASA II considerations and supplemental oxygen
2-4 per month	Patient can walk two level city blocks or climb one flight of stairs	II	Usual ASA II considerations to include possible premedication with nitroglycerin 5 minutes before therapy and supplemental oxygen
2-3 per week	Pain develops before patient walks two level city blocks or climbs one flight of stairs	III	Usual ASA III considerations to include possible premedication with nitroglycerin 5 minutes before therapy and supplemental oxygen
Daily episodes *or* recent (within past 2-3 weeks) changes in character of episode: Increased frequency, duration, or severity Radiation to new site Precipitated by less activity Decreased pain relief with usual nitroglycerin dose	Patient unable to walk two level city blocks or climb one flight of stairs	IV	Usual ASA IV considerations

administered (aspiration negative, slowly injected) local anesthetic containing epinephrine. Under the stress of pain or anxiety the adrenal medulla releases extremely high levels of epinephrine (approximately 280 μg per minute) and norepinephrine (approximately 56 μg per minute) into the circulation, whereas with proper injection technique of a local anesthetic containing 1:50,000 epinephrine, less than 1 μg per minute of epinephrine is added to the circulatory system. Table 27-3 summarizes these clinical findings.

Adequate depth of anesthesia to permit tooth manipulation (extraction, cavity preparation) without the patient experiencing pain is the major factor determining the ultimate blood level of catecholamines. Local-anesthetic solutions that contain no vasoconstrictor (for example, plain lidocaine, prilocaine, and mepivacaine) are less likely to provide pulpal anesthesia of sufficient duration to permit completion of dental therapy before the patient experiences pain. The addition of minimal concentrations of epinephrine (1:200,000 and 1:100,000) prolongs the duration of pulpal anesthesia in most cases well beyond the time required for treatment, so that the patient does not experience any pain and the release of endogenous catecholamines is thus minimized.

Table 27-3. Catecholamine blood levels

	Epinephrine (μg/min)	Norepinephrine (μg/min)
Resting adrenal medullary secretion	7.0	1.5
Stress	280.0	56.0
Local anesthesia (1:50,000 epinephrine in 1.8 ml)	<1.0	—

The maximal dose of epinephrine recommended for administration to the cardiac-risk patient at one appointment is 0.04 mg. To put this figure in terms of commonly used epinephrine concentrations, we may employ one cartridge (1.8 ml) of a local anesthetic containing a 1:50,000 concentration of epinephrine (0.02 mg/ml), two cartridges with 1:100,000 epinephrine (0.01 mg/ml), or four cartridges with 1:200,000 epinephrine (0.005 mg/ml).

If the doctor is confronted with a patient who states that he cannot receive epinephrine, consultation with the patient's physician should be completed before initiating dental therapy. If considerable doubt persists concerning a particular patient after medical consultation about the proper use of epinephrine in local anesthetics, it is recommended that a second opinion be obtained or that a local anesthetic with a different vasoconstrictor or an agent that provides sufficient duration of pulpal anesthesia without a vasoconstrictor be employed. Examples of these are mepivacaine containing levonordefrin, the combination of procaine and propoxycaine with levophed, and prilocaine without vasoconstrictor (when used for block anesthesia only). A textbook on local anesthesia and the drug package insert should be consulted before selecting the local anesthetic. One definite contraindication to the use of vasoconstrictors in local anesthetics is the presence of cardiac dysrhythmias that persist in spite of antidysrhythmic therapy.

One additional factor must be mentioned regarding the use of epinephrine in the cardiac patient: 8% racemic epinephrine, a combination of the dextrorotatory and levorotatory forms commonly used in gingival retraction cord before the taking of impressions in many dental procedures, contains approximately 4% (40 mg/ml) of the pharmacologically active levo form of epinephrine, which is 40 times the epinephrine concentration used in acute emergency situations (anaphylaxis). Absorption of epinephrine through the mucous membrane into the cardiovascular system is normally rapid and is even more so with active bleeding such as that occurring after subgingival tooth preparation. Blood levels of epinephrine rise rapidly in this situation, leading to cardiovascular manifestations of epinephrine overdose (Chapter 23). Tachycardia, palpitation, sweating, tremor, and headache are the usual clinical symptoms. In the patient with preexisting, clinically evident or subclinical cardiovascular disease, this increase in cardiovascular activity may prove to be life threatening. The American Dental Association recommends that racemic epinephrine cord not be used for any patient with a history of or suspicion of cardiovascular disease. Indeed, there are very few indications for the use of racemic epinephrine in any dental procedure in any patient.

Psychosedation

The use of psychosedation during the dental appointment may be indicated for the patient who experiences acute anginal episodes once a week or more often or the anginal patient who is fearful of dental therapy. Of the various techniques currently in use, inhalation sedation with nitrous oxide and oxygen is my primary technique for all cardiac patients. My reasons for preferring this technique include (1) the increased percentage of oxygen that the patient is always receiving along with the nitrous oxide (most sedation units available in the United States do not deliver less than 27% to 30% oxygen), (2) the anxiolytic properties of nitrous oxide, which successfully reduce the stress of dental therapy (thereby minimizing endogenous catecholamine release), and (3) the minor but potentially highly significant analgesic properties of nitrous oxide. As discussed in Chapter 28, nitrous oxide and oxygen are commonly employed in the immediate management of acute myocardial infarction in many countries and more recently in the United States.

Additional considerations

Vital signs. Patients with a history of angina should have their vital signs recorded before each dental visit. Minimally, these recordings should include the blood pressure, pulse rate, and respiratory rate. It is also suggested that measurements be taken after the dental therapy is completed.

Nitroglycerin. It has been suggested by some authorities that nitroglycerin be administered prophylactically to anginal patients before each dental appointment. Nitroglycerin exerts a clinical effect within 2 to 4 minutes, with a duration of action of approximately 30 minutes. It is my feeling that prophylactic premedication with nitroglycerin should be reserved for the anginal patient who experiences episodes of anginal pain more than once a week and who exhibits fear of dentistry. However, I do feel that before beginning dental therapy on the higher risk anginal patient, the doctor should request the patient's supply of nitroglycerin spray or tablets, which should be placed where it will be readily available for immediate use if needed. Although this medication is also present in the dental emergency kit, the patient's own medication should be used preferentially.

CLINICAL MANIFESTATIONS

The primary clinical manifestation of angina is chest pain. The doctor managing this patient usually has been forewarned about this medical situation through the patient's medical history questionnaire and is prepared to manage it. Although most instances of anginal pain are terminated easily, it is always possible that a supposed anginal attack is actually a more severe manifestation of coronary artery disease—unstable angina or acute myocardial infarction. The initial clinical manifestations of all of these coronary syndromes are quite similar; therefore immediate management is based on the response of the patient to certain initial steps in treatment.

Signs and Symptoms
Pain

The patient becomes acutely aware of the sudden onset of chest pain and stops any activities. In the dental chair, the patient normally sits upright and presses a fist to the chest. If questioned about the pain, the patient commonly describes it as a sensation of squeezing, burning, pressing, choking, aching, bursting, tightness, or "gas." In fact, on many occasions episodes of cardiac pain are mistaken for indigestion—not infrequently with a fatal outcome (see Chapter 28). The patient may state that it feels as if there is a heavy weight on the chest. In describing this sensation, many anginal victims hold a clenched fist to their chest as they describe their attacks. Sharp pains are not typical of angina pectoris. In addition, respiratory movements (inspiration) do not exaggerate the discomfort. The sensation is more a dull, aching, heavy pain than a searing hot or knifelike pain. The pain is located substernally, most commonly in the middle of the sternum, but it may appear just to the left of the sternum. Finally, pain of cardiac origin tends to be more generalized than non-cardiac pain which can often be localized to one specific site (see radiation of pain below).

Radiation of pain

Chest pain normally spreads or radiates to other locations in the body that are distant from the chest. Fig. 27-2 shows the more common pathways of radiation. Typically, the sensation radiates to the left shoulder and distally down the medial surface of the arm, occasionally as far as the hand and fingers, following the distribution of the ulnar nerve. The sensation felt is that of an ache, numbness, or tingling discomfort. Less commonly the pain may radiate to the right shoulder only or to both shoulders. Other sites of radiation include the left side of the neck (usually described as a constricting sensation), with continuation up into the left side of the face and mandible. Mandibular pain, for which the victim sought dental care, has been reported as the sole clinical manifestation of chest pain in one case of angina. Another possible yet relatively uncommon area of radiation is the upper epigastrium (Table 27-4).

Patient reaction to anginal pain varies. In some individuals, the discomfort of angina subsides with-

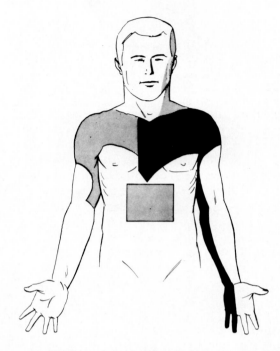

■ Substernal pain projected to left shoulder and arm (ulanar nerve distribution)

▨ Less frequent referred sites including right shoulder and arm, left jaw, neck, and epigastrium

Fig. 27-2. Radiation patterns of chest pain. (From Jastak, J.T., and Cowan, F.F., Jr.: Dent. Clin. North Am. **17:**363, 1973.)

out their having to stop activities. Other individuals experience moderate pain that persists but does not become more intense. The victim is able to tolerate this level of discomfort and is not forced to stop activities. In most anginal patients, however, the clinical progression is of a different nature. In these persons the pain becomes progressively more intense, eventually forcing the victim to seek relief by terminating activities, taking medication, or both.

It must always be kept in mind that the clinical characteristics of acute anginal episodes are reasonably consistent for each patient from episode to episode. The intensity, frequency, radiation, and duration of the episodes demonstrate little or no variation. Changes in the normal pattern of the disease, with an increase in frequency, duration, or intensity, are ominous signs and should be reported immediately to the patient's physician. This is termed unstable, or preinfarction, angina and is a syndrome of accelerating or worsening anginal episodes. It is commonly associated with recent obstructive dis-

Table 27-4. Clinical manifestations of angina pectoris

Sudden onset with exertion
Characteristics of "pain":
    Squeezing, choking, burning, pressing, tightness, "gas"
    "Heavy weight" on chest
    Respiratory movements do not intensify pain
    Substernal
    Generalized, not localized
Radiation (see Fig. 27-2)
    To left shoulder, medial aspect of left arm
    Right shoulder
    Left side of face, left mandible
    Upper epigastrium
Subsidence of pain with nitroglycerin or rest

ease of the coronary arteries and frequently precedes acute myocardial infarction or sudden death.

Physical Examination

During acute anginal episodes, the following signs and symptoms may be noted: The patient is apprehensive and usually sweating and may press the fist to the sternum and appear anxious to take nitroglycerin. The heart rate is markedly elevated, as is the blood pressure (blood pressures of 200 torr/150 torr having been recorded in normotensive patients during acute anginal episodes). Respiratory difficulty (dyspnea) and a feeling of faintness may also be noted during the episode.

Complications

Although most anginal episodes resolve without residual complications, it is possible for acute emergency situations to develop. Acute cardiac dysrhythmias occurring during the episode are most common. Although these are normally not life threatening, ventricular dysrhythmias may occur with a possibility of ventricular fibrillation and sudden death. A second potential complication of angina is acute myocardial infarction.

Prognosis

The prognosis for the anginal patient depends largely on the severity of the underlying disorder (CAD) and the presence or absence of additional risk factors. In men with angina the annual mortality rate is 1.4% if they have no history of myocardial infarction, a normal ECG, and normal blood pressure. This rate increases to 7.4% annually if they have elevated blood pressure, to 8.4% if they have an abnormal ECG, and to 12% annually if both the

blood pressure is elevated and the ECG is abnormal. Other factors, such as the presence of diabetes mellitus, heart failure, cardiac dysrhythmias, and cardiac hypertrophy, tend to decrease life expectancy even further. Fifty percent of all anginal patients die suddenly (cardiac arrest). Thirty-three percent die following myocardial infarction, and most of the remainder succumb to heart failure.

PATHOPHYSIOLOGY

Angina is caused by the temporary inability of the coronary arteries to supply adequate oxygenated blood to the myocardium. The patient with coronary artery disease may be asymptomatic at rest or during moderate exertion because the coronary arteries may be able to deliver an adequate supply of oxygen to the myocardium under these circumstances. Any further increase in the oxygen requirement of the myocardium above this critical level (which varies from patient to patient) results in a relative oxygen deficiency and the development of myocardial ischemia, with the subsequent appearance of clinical manifestations of anginal pains. As mentioned previously, the pain of angina is most probably related to the metabolic changes produced in the myocardium by ischemia. The actual source of the pain is not known. The myocardium has no true pain fibers (some pain fibers do accompany the coronary blood vessels), so it is difficult to imagine the mechanism of pain production. It is thought that the metabolic byproducts of ischemia stimulate the nerve fibers of the sympathetic nervous system to initiate nerve impulses, which are carried to the ganglia of the neck and from there are relayed to the deep intercostal and transverse thoracic muscles of the anterior chest. This produces the characteristic squeezing sensation of angina. Clinical confirmation of this theory is obtained from the fact that an intercostal nerve block usually relieves the pain of angina.

Further evidence for the validity of this theory comes from patients with spontaneous angina (onset of anginal pain while the patient is at rest). The increases in blood pressure and heart rate seen during acute anginal episodes are consistently observed *before* the onset of pain. Changes in the electrocardiogram also occur from 1 to 3 minutes *before* the pain. These factors indicate that a buildup of the metabolic products of ischemia occurs before stimulation of pain fibers.

Some of the most dangerous occurrences observed during the anginal episode include continuing elevation in blood pressure and tachycardia. Both of these produce a potentially dangerous feedback system. Myocardial oxygen requirements continue to increase as the workload of the heart continues to rise (with increasing blood pressure and rapid heart rate). If the coronary arteries are unable to deliver the oxygen required, the degree of myocardial ischemia increases, which in turn increases the chances of acute, possibly lethal, dysrhythmias and myocardial infarction. Rapid management of the anginal episode therefore becomes quite important.

Coronary artery spasm (Prinzmetal's variant angina) has been demonstrated to occur either spontaneously or by exposure to cold, by exposure to ergot-derivative drugs used to treat migraine headaches, or by mechanical irritation from a cardiac catheter. Spasm has been observed in the large coronary arteries, whether healthy or atherosclerotic, resulting in decreased coronary blood flow. Prolonged spasm of the coronary arteries in angina may result in documented episodes of myocardial infarction—even in the absence of visible coronary artery disease.

MANAGEMENT

The primary goal in the management of the acute anginal episode is to decrease the myocardial oxygen requirement.

Step 1. Terminate dental therapy. Immediately on the patient experiencing chest pain, all dental procedures should be terminated. In many instances, the precipitating factor is a part of the dental treatment (such as a local-anesthetic syringe, scalpel, or hand piece) and merely terminating the procedure proves beneficial.

Step 2. Position patient. The anginal patient is conscious and usually apprehensive. Permit the patient to be positioned in the most comfortable manner. Most commonly this is sitting or standing upright. The supine position is rarely preferred by the patient and in fact commonly makes the pain appear subjectively to be more intense.

Step 3. Administer vasodilator. A member of the emergency team should immediately get the emergency kit and oxygen. As soon as possible, nitroglycerin should be administered orally (spray) or sublingually (tablet). The patient's own supply is preferred because the dosage will be correct for the patient. The number of sprays or tablets administered is determined by the patient's requirement (0.3 to 0.6 mg is the usual dosage).

Effects and side effects of nitroglycerin. Nitroglycerin normally reduces or eliminates anginal discomfort dramatically within 2 to 4 minutes. Commonly observed side effects of nitroglycerin administration include a fullness or pounding in the head, flushing, tachycardia, and possible hypotension (if the patient is sitting upright).

Action of nitroglycerin. Nitroglycerin is the single most effective agent available for the management of acute anginal episodes. In normal individuals, the administration of nitroglycerin decreases coronary artery resistance and increases coronary blood flow. This mechanism is probably of little consequence in patients with significant CAD, however. The probable mechanism of action of nitroglycerin in anginal patients is its ability to produce a decrease in the systemic vascular resistance through arterial and venous dilation. This leads to a decrease in venous return of blood to the heart and a decrease in cardiac output, which results in a lessened cardiac workload. A decrease in cardiac work produces a lesser oxygen requirement of the myocardium and a reversal of the oxygen insufficiency that existed during the episode.

Step 4. If necessary, administer alternative vasodilator medications. If the patient's nitroglycerin tablets are ineffective in terminating the anginal pains, a second dose may be administered either from the patient's drug supply or from the emergency kit supply, which may be fresher than the patient's. Nitroglycerin tablets lose potency unless they are stored in tightly sealed glass containers. This is one possible explanation for the failure of the patient's nitroglycerin to act to relieve anginal pains. Nitroglycerin spray is more stable than the sublingual tablets and is preferred in this situation. A test for nitroglycerin potency is to place a tablet on the tongue; the drug is still potent if a tingling sensation is felt as the tablet dissolves, with a feeling of coolness throughout the mouth similar to mint candy but without the taste. A second explanation for nitroglycerin's failure to provide relief is that the episode is not angina at all but is an acute myocardial infarction. Administration of nitroglycerin and the patient's subsequent response to it is a major factor in the differential diagnosis of these two important cardiovascular syndromes.

The American Heart Association recommends that in a patient with known angina pectoris emergency medical care be sought if chest pain is not relieved by three nitroglycerin tablets or spray doses over a 10-minute period. In a person with previously unrecognized coronary disease, the persistence of chest pain for 2 minutes or longer is an indication for emergency medical assistance.

If nitroglycerin is unavailable or ineffective in terminating an episode, the use of amyl nitrite should be considered. Amyl nitrite is available in 0.3 ml ampules, which are crushed and then inhaled. The patient should be in the recumbent position when this agent is administered. Amyl nitrite is not recommended for use unless the anginal episode is severe and unrelieved by nitroglycerin and unless the patient has high blood pressure with a markedly elevated diastolic pressure.

Effects and side effects of amyl nitrite. Once inhaled, amyl nitrite normally produces relief of anginal discomfort within 10 seconds. Because of its extreme potency, there are uncomfortable side effects that invariably occur with its use. These include a flushing of the face, pounding of the pulse, dizziness, and a pounding headache. (The person administering amyl nitrite may also experience the clinical effects of the drug if vapors are inadvertently inhaled.)

Action of amyl nitrite. Amyl nitrite causes profound peripheral arterial vasodilation. With the administration of one ampule, the blood pressure falls precipitously. Amyl nitrite has a negligible effect on the veins; therefore little venous pooling occurs. Amyl nitrite markedly decreases cardiac output.

Effects and side effects of calcium slow-channel blockers. Patients known to have coronary artery spasm as a component of their anginal episodes will respond to the administration of nifedipine (10 to 20 mg) sublingually. Nifedipine, verapamil, and diltiazem are calcium entry-blocking agents.

Verapamil has been the most extensively studied agent in this relatively new group of drugs for emergency cardiac care. Its actions are representative of the other agents in the group. The therapeutic usefulness of verapamil is based on its slow-channel blocking properties, particularly the inward flow of calcium ions in cardiac and vascular smooth muscle. By blocking calcium influx and supply to the myocardial contractile mechanism, verapamil exerts a direct depressant effect on the inotropic state and therefore on the myocardial oxygen requirement. Verapamil also reduces contractile tone in vascular smooth muscle, which results in coronary and peripheral vasodilation, which in turn reduces systemic vascular resistance. Additionally, the calcium slow-channel blockers

---

MANAGEMENT OF ANGINA

Step 1 Terminate dental therapy
2 Position patient (upright position most comfortable)
3 Administer vasodilator
Nitroglycerin preferred
4 Amyl nitrite, if needed
Nifedipine, if needed
5 Other medications
Oxygen, if needed
Narcotics contraindicated in angina
6 Modify further dental therapy to prevent recurrence

---

exhibit antidysrhythmic effects, specifically by slowing conduction and prolonging refractoriness in the AV (atrioventricular) node. The current primary use of verapamil and other calcium slow-channel blockers is as an antidysrhythmic agent. (It is highly effective in the management of PSVT [paroxysmal supraventricular tachycardia]). Its hemodynamic properties account for its beneficial actions in managing angina induced by coronary artery spasm.

Step 5. If necessary, administer other medications. Oxygen may be administered to the patient during an anginal episode. However, in the absence of vasodilator drugs the pain of angina may not be decreased by the administration of oxygen. Oxygen should be administered as a supplement to the vasodilating agents, not in lieu of them.

Pain-relieving narcotics such as morphine and meperidine (Demerol) should not be used because they do not treat the cause of pain (inadequate oxygen supply). The only indication for narcotic administration is acute myocardial infarction (see Chapter 28).

Step 6. Modify further dental therapy. Following the anginal episode, it should be determined what factors have caused it to occur. Definite alteration of dental therapy should be considered for the future to prevent the episode from recurring. The patient may be treated or dismissed after being allowed to rest for a proper length of time (approximately 15 to 30 minutes). Vital signs should be recorded before discharge.

Dental treatment may resume at any time (same day, next day) following cessation of the acute anginal episode, unlike in the post-myocardial infarction patient (see Chapter 28) in which a six month waiting period is recommended.

The management of angina is summarized in the box on p. 349.

BIBLIOGRAPHY

Alderman, E.L., and others: Coronary artery syndromes after sudden propranolol withdrawal, Ann. Intern. Med. **81:**625, 1974.

Alpert, J.S., and Braunwald, E.: Pathological and clinical manifestations of acute myocardial infarction. In Braunwald, E., editor: Heart disease: a textbook of cardiovascular medicine, Philadelphia, 1980, W.B. Saunders Co.

American Dental Association Council on Dental Therapeutics: American Dental Association and American Heart Association joint report: Management of dental problems in patients with cardiovascular disease, J. Am. Dent. Assoc. **68:**533, 1964.

American Dental Association Council on Dental Therapeutics: Accepted dental therapeutics, Chicago, 1985, The Association.

American Heart Association: Heart attack: signals and actions for survival, Dallas, 1976, The Association.

Antman, E.M., Stone, P.H., and Muller, J.E.: Calcium channel blocking agents in the treatment of cardiovascular disorders, I: Basic and clinical electrophysiologic effects, Ann. Intern. Med. **93:**875, 1980.

Aronow, W.S., and Stemmer, E.A.: Two year follow up of angina pectoris: medical or surgical therapy, Ann. Intern. Med. **82:**208, 1975.

Aronow, W.S.: Effect of passive smoking on angina pectoris, N. Engl. J. Med. **299:**21, 1978.

Boakes, A.J., and others: Adverse reactions to local anaesthetic/vasoconstrictor preparations, Br. Dent. J. **133:**137, 1972.

Braunwald, E.: The history. In Braunwald, E., editor: Heart disease: a textbook of cardiovascular medicine, Philadelphia, 1980, W.B. Saunders Co.

Burggraf, G., and Parker, J.O.: Hemodynamic effects of amyl nitrite in coronary artery disease, Am. J. Cardiol. **32:**772, 1973.

Cairns, J.A., Fantus, I.G., and Klassen, G.A.: Unstable angina pectoris, Am. Heart J. **92:**373, 1976.

Capone, R., and others: A comparison of the action of short and long action nitrites on the peripheral circulation, Clin. Res. **20:**204, 1972.

Carleton, R.A., and Johnson, A.D.: Coronary arterial spasm: a clinical entity? Mod. Concepts Cardiovasc. Dis. **43:**87, 1974.

Chahine, R.A.: Unstable angina: the problem of definition, Br. Heart J. **37:**1246, 1975.

Chahine, R.A., and Luchi, R.J.: Coronary arterial spasm: culprit or bystander? Am. J. Cardiol. **37:**937, 1976.

Clausen, J.P., and Trap-Jensen, J.: Heart rate and arterial blood pressure during exercise in patients with angina pectoris: effect of training and of nitroglycerin, Circulation **53:**436, 1976.

Cohn, P.F., and Braunwald, E.: Chronic coronary artery disease. In Braunwald, E., editor: Heart disease: a textbook of cardiovascular medicine, Philadelphia, 1980, W.B. Saunders Co.

Conti, C.R., and others: Unstable angina pectoris: morbidity and mortality in 57 consecutive patients evaluated angiographically, Am. J. Cardiol. **32:**745, 1973.

Desai, D.C., and Alexander, S.: Treatment of severe angina pectoris, Dent. Clin. North Am. **56:**599, 1972.

Diamond, G.A., and Forrester, J.S.: Analysis of probability as an aid in the clinical diagnosis of coronary artery disease, N. Engl. J. Med. **300:**1350, 1979.

DiCarlo, F.J.: Nitroglycerin revisited: chemistry, biochemistry, interactions, Drug Metab. Rev. **4:**1, 1975.

Enos, W.F., Holmes, R.H., and Beger, J.: Coronary disease among United States soldiers killed in action in Korea, JAMA **152:**1090, 1953.

Frank, C.W., Weinblatt, E., and Shapiro, S.: Angina pectoris in men: prognostic significance of selected medical factors, Circulation **47:**509, 1973.

Friedman, G.D., Siegelaub, A.B., and Dales, L.G.: Cigarette smoking and chest pain, Ann. Intern. Med. **83:**1, 1975.

Fulton, M., and others: Natural history of unstable angina, Lancet **1:**860, 1972.

Gerstenblith, G., and others: Nifedipine in unstable angina: a double-blind, randomized trial, N. Engl. J. Med. **306:**885, 1982.

Glover, J.: Vasoconstrictors in dental anaesthetics contraindication—fact or fallacy, Aust. Dent. J. **13:**65, 1968.

Goldstein, R.E., and others: Alterations in the circulatory response to exercise following a meal and their relationship in postprandial angina pectoris, Circulation **44:**90, 1971.

Gordon, T., and Kannel, W.B.: Predisposition to atherosclerosis in the head, heart, and legs: the Framingham study, JAMA **221:**661, 1972.

Guthrie, R.B., and others: Pathology of stable and unstable angina pectoris, Circulation **51:**1059, 1975.

Harrison, J.D.: Effect of retraction materials on gingival sulcus epithelium, J. Prosthet. Dent. **11:**514, 1961.

Heberden, W.: Some account of a disorder of the breast, Med. Trans. Coll. Physicians (London) **2:**59, 1872.

Hillis, L.D., and Braunwald, E.: Coronary artery spasm, N. Engl. J. Med. **299:**695, 1978.

Holroyd, S.V., Watts, D.T., and Welch, J.T., Jr.: The use of epinephrine in local anesthetics for dental patients with cardiovascular disease: a review of the literature, J. Oral Surg. **18:**492, 1960.

Horowitz, L.D., Herman, M.V., and Gorlin, R.: Clinical response to nitroglycerin as a diagnostic test for coronary artery disease, Am. J. Cardiol. **29:**149, 1972.

Houston, J.B., and others: Effect of r-epinephrine impregnated retraction cord on the cardiovascular system, J. Prosthet. Dent. **24:**373, 1970.

Hurst, J.W., and King, S.B.: The problem of chest "pain," JAMA **236:**2100, 1976.

Jastak, J.T., and Cowan, F.F., Jr.: Patients at risk, Dent. Clin. North Am. **17:**363, 1973.

Judge, T.E.: Vasodilators, Practitioner **212:**2, 1974.

Kannel, W.B., and Feinleib, M.: Natural history of angina pectoris in the Framingham study: prognosis and survival, Am. J. Cardiol. **29:**154, 1972.

Kent, R.I.: Prognosis of symptomatic or mildly symptomatic patients with coronary artery disease, Am. J. Cardiol. **49:**1823, 1982.

Killip, T.: Prodromes in myocardial infarction and unstable angina, Postgrad. Med. **57:**10, 1975.

Klaus, A.P., and others: Comparative evaluation of sublingual long acting nitrates, Circulation **48:**519, 1973.

Kleiger, R.E.: Chest pain in patients seen in emergency clinics, JAMA **236:**595, 1976.

Maseri, A., and Chierchia, S.: Coronary artery spasm: Demonstration, definition, diagnosis, and consequences, Prog. Cardiovasc. Dis. **25:**169, 1982.

Maseri, A., Parodi, O., and Fox, K.M.: Rational approach to the medical therapy of angina pectoris: the role of calcium antagonists, Prog. Cardiovasc. Dis. **25:**269, 1983.

Mayer, G.A.: Instability of nitroglycerin tablets, Can. Med. Assoc. J. **110:**788, 1974.

Mulcahy, R., and others: Unstable angina: natural history and determinants of prognosis, Am. J. Cardiol. **48:**525, 1981.

Munoz, R.J.: The cardiovascular effects of anxiety and r-epinephrine retraction cord in routine fixed prosthodontic procedures, J. Calif. Dent. Assoc. **46:**10, 1970.

Nayler, W.G., and Szeto, J.: Effects of verapamil on contractility, oxygen utilization, and calcium exchangeability in mammalian heart muscle, Cardiovasc. Res. **6:**120, 1972.

New York Heart Association: Report of the special committee of the New York Heart Association, Inc., on the use of epinephrine in connection with procaine in dental procedures, J. Am. Dent. Assoc. **50:**108, 1955.

Nies, A.S., and Shand, D.G.: Clinical pharmacology of propranolol, Circulation **52:**6, 1975.

Pague, W.L., and Harrison, J.D.: Absorption of epinephrine during tissue retraction, J. Prosthet. Dent. **18:**242, 1967.

Palmer, E.D.: Serious heart disease simulated by hiatus hernia, U.S. Armed Forces Med. J. **8:**477, 1957.

Parker, J.O., and others: The influence of changes in blood volume on angina pectoris: a study of the effect of phlebotomy, Circulation **41:**593, 1976.

Parmley, W.W.: Beta blockers in coronary artery disease, Cardiovasc. Rev. Rep. **2:**655, 1981.

Parmley, W.W.: The combination of beta-adrenergic-blocking agents and nitrates in the treatment of stable angina pectoris, Cardiovasc. Rev. Rep. **3:**1425, 1982.

Phatak, N.M., and Lang, R.L.: Systemic hemodynamic effects of r-epinephrine gingival retraction cord in clinic patients, J. Oral Ther. Pharmacol. **2:**393, 1966.

Port, S., Cobb., F.R., and Jones, R.H.: Effects of propranolol on left ventricular function in normal man, Circulation **61:**358, 1980.

Proudfit, W.L., and Hodgman, J.R.: Physical signs during angina pectoris, Prog. Cardiovasc. Dis. **10:**283, 1968.

Reeves, T.J., and others: Natural history of angina pectoris, Am. J. Cardiol. **33:**423, 1974.

Robinson, B.F.: Relation of heart rate and systolic blood pressure to the onset of pain in angina pectoris, Circulation **35:**1073, 1967.

Sampson, J.J., and Cheitlin, M.D.: Pathophysiology and differential diagnosis of cardiac pain, Prog. Cardiovasc. Dis. **13:**507, 1971.

Sampson, J.J., and Hyatt, K.H.: Management of the patient with severe angina pectoris; an internist's point of view, Circulation **46:**1885, 1972.

Scanlon, P.J.: The intermediate coronary syndrome, Prog. Cardiovasc. Dis. **23:**351, 1981.

Scheidt, S., Wolk, M., and Killip, T.: Unstable angina pectoris; natural history, hemodynamics, uncertainties of treatment and the ethics of clinical study, Am. J. Med. **60:**409, 1976.

Singh, B.N.: The pharmacology of slow channel blocking drugs, Cardiovasc. Rev. Rep. **4:**179, 1983.

Singh, B.N., Collett, J.T., and Chew, C.Y.: New perspectives in the pharmacologic therapy of cardiac arrhythmias, Prog. Cardiovasc. Dis. **22:**243, 1980.

Stamler, J.: Epidemiology of coronary heart disease, Med. Clin. North Am. **57:**5, 1973.

Tempero, K.F.: Angina pectoris; diagnosis, evaluation and therapy, Geriatrics **28:**76, 1973.

Thompson, R.H.: The clinical use of transdermal delivery devices with nitroglycerin, Cardiovasc. Rev. Rep. **4:**91, 1983.

Timberlake, D.L.: Epinephrine in tissue retraction, Ariz. Dent. J. **17:**14, 1971.

Victor, M.F., and others: Unstable angina pectoris of new onset: a prospective clinical and arteriographic study of 75 patients, Am. J. Cardiol. **47:**228, 1981.

Warren, S.G., Bremer, D.L., and Orgain, E.S.: Long-term propranolol therapy for angina pectoris, Am. J. Cardiol. **37:**420, 1978.

Wehrmacher, W.H.: The painful anterior chest wall syndromes, Med. Clin. North Am. **42:**111, 1958.

Winsor, T., and Berger, H.J.: Oral nitroglycerin as a prophylactic antianginal drug; clinical, physiologic, and statistical evidence of efficacy based a three phase experimental design, Am. Heart J. **90:**611, 1975.

28 Acute Myocardial Infarction

Myocardial infarction may be defined as a clinical syndome resulting from a deficient coronary arterial blood supply to a region of myocardium; it results in cellular death and necrosis. The syndrome is usually characterized by severe and prolonged substernal pain similar to but more intense and of longer duration than that of angina pectoris. Common complications of myocardial infarction include shock, heart failure, and cardiac arrest. Synonyms for myocardial infarction include coronary occlusion, coronary thrombosis, and heart attack.

Each year more than 1.5 million Americans suffer acute myocardial infarction. It is the leading cause of death in the United States and is responsible for 35% of deaths occurring in men between the ages of 35 and 50 years. A male living in North America has a 1 in 3 chance of suffering a myocardial infarction or sudden death before the age of 65 years (for women, this risk is 1 out of 10). Although a relatively common clinical occurrence, myocardial infarction unfortunately still has a high mortality rate; approximately 60% of acute myocardial infarction victims do not survive long enough to reach an acute care facility's emergency room. In 1981, 1,500,000 persons in the United States suffered an acute myocardial infarction. Over 60% of deaths from acute myocardial infarction occur within 60 minutes of the onset of signs and symptoms. Most of these result from development of lethal dysrhythmias, usually ventricular fibrillation.

For the patient to have a greater chance of survival, the dental practitioner must be aware of ways to prevent this clinical entity, how to recognize its signs and symptoms, and how to manage it effectively. Killip (1975) has stated that, once admitted to a hospital, the patient has already survived a significant risk.

In addition to management of the acute myocardial infarction, the dental practitioner is asked to manage the needs of the patient who has survived a previous myocardial infarction. The American Heart Association estimates that there are 4,600,000 victims of myocardial infarction still living in the United States. As with post-CVA patients and patients with angina, there is always an increased risk when status post–myocardial infarction patients are treated. The mortality rate of these patients is three to four times that of normal persons even 10 years after the infarction.

In myocardial infarction, a portion of myocardium dies. Depending on the extent of myocardial damage and the presence or absence of acute complications such as dysrhythmias, heart failure, and cardiac arrest, the victim either survives or succumbs during the acute phase of the disease. After the acute phase, further complications such as heart failure may arise, which are related to the inability of the heart to carry out its primary function as a pump because of the size of the infarcted area of myocardium. Heart failure is commonly seen following myocardial infarction. Knowledge of the presence of a compromised myocardium enables the dental practitioner to modify dental therapy so as to decrease the medical risk presented by the patient.

PREDISPOSING FACTORS

The primary etiologic factor in acute myocardial infarction is coronary artery disease (atherosclerosis; CAD). CAD is a factor in more than 90% of all episodes. Other risk factors in myocardial infarction include obesity, being a male (especially during the fifth to seventh decades of life), and undue stress (see also Chapter 26). Friedman (1974) has described the cardiac risk patient as a "coronary prone" individual. This person is further characterized as having a type A behavior pattern (Elek, 1974), described as follows:

Foremost is a frightening and often obsessive sense of time urgency. He is determined to accomplish too much in too little time. He struggles both with his environment and with himself, but mainly with the latter. He is alert, very intense, and usually hostile. He is very competitive and ambitious; he wants recognition and seeks advancement. He tends to speed up his ordinary activities by looking at his watch often, by being on time, by hating to wait in line at the bank, movie, or restaurant. He is usually in occupations subject to deadlines. These patients themselves have labeled the type-A behavior pattern as the "hurry-up" disease.*

In addition, a strong family history of cardiovascular disease, an abnormal electrocardiogram, elevated blood pressure, enlarged heart size, and/or an elevated blood cholesterol level add to the risk of a person suffering acute myocardial infarction. Immediate predisposing factors in myocardial infarction include a significant decrease in blood flow through the coronary arteries (as in coronary thrombosis) or an increase in the level of cardiac work without a corresponding increase in the supply of oxygen to the myocardium (as seen in stress). This situation of decreased perfusion is termed myocardial ischemia.

Acute myocardial infarction is usually considered to be the direct result of a sudden obstruction of a major coronary artery. However, infarction may also occur in the absence of arterial occlusion, just as occlusion may be present without infarction (in the presence of an effective collateral circulation). Spasm of one or more diseased coronary arteries has also been implicated in the pathogenesis of myocardial infarction.

Location and Extent of Infarction

As described in Chapter 26, the anterior descending branch of the left coronary artery is the most common site of clinically significant atherosclerosis. Not surprisingly, this vessel is the most

*From Elek, S.R.: Psychological management of patients with coronary-prone type-A behavior pattern, JAMA **229**:1805, 1974. Copyright 1974 American Medical Association.

common site of thrombosis leading to myocardial infarction. With occlusion of this vessel, the anterior portion of the left ventricle becomes ischemic, and in the absence of adequate collateral circulation, infarction occurs with subsequent myocardial necrosis throughout the distribution of the occluded artery. Occlusion of the left circumflex artery produces anterolateral infarction. Thrombosis of the right coronary artery leads to infarction of the posteroinferior portion of the left ventricle and might also involve the right ventricular myocardium. The extent of infarction is therefore related to several factors, including the anatomic distribution of the occluded vessel, the adequacy of collateral circulation, the extent of existing coronary artery disease throughout the myocardium, and whether previous infarctions have occurred.

PREVENTION

Prevention of a first myocardial infarction in a high-risk patient (see CAD risk factors, p. 330), although a seemingly impossible task, may be attempted by the dental practitioner through strict adherence to the Stress Reduction Protocol. This protocol minimizes the potentially adverse effects of undue stress on the workload and oxygen requirement of the myocardium, thereby reducing the risk from one of the immediate predisposing factors of acute myocardial infarction (increased cardiac workload). The other immediate predisposing factors—thrombosis, occlusion, or spasm of a coronary blood vessel—obviously cannot be prevented by the doctor.

The dental patient with a previous history of myocardial infarction should be identified, and the doctor must attempt to gather as much information concerning the current physical status of this patient as possible so that an accurate determination of risk may be established before dental therapy. This necessitates use of the written medical history questionnaire, physical examination of the patient, and the dialogue history.

Medical History Questionnaire
QUESTION 9. Circle any of the following which you have had or have at present:
- **Heart disease**
- **Heart attack**

COMMENT. An affirmative reply must be followed by a detailed dialogue history to determine the degree of risk represented by this patient.

QUESTION 6. Have you taken any medicine or drugs during the past 2 years?

COMMENT. Survivors of myocardial infarction (termed status post–myocardial infarction) will be receiving medications according to the degree of residual myocardial damage and the presence of post-MI complications.

Post–myocardial infarction patients frequently receive one or more of the following drug groups: diuretics—for management of heart failure and high blood pressure; digitalis or dopamine—for heart failure; antidysrhythmics; nitrates (e.g., nitroglycerin)—if anginal pains are present in the post-MI periods; and possibly antiplatelet agents, such as sulfinpyrazone (Anturane) and aspirin. Beta-adrenergic blockers such as propranolol are also frequently prescribed. Table 28-1 summarizes the drugs used in the post-MI period.

Anticoagulants such as coumarin, heparin, and Dicumarol are only infrequently employed today in the management of the status post–myocardial infarction patient.

QUESTION 10. When you walk up stairs or take a walk, do you ever have to stop because of pain in your chest or shortness of breath, or because you are very tired?

COMMENT. The presence of one or more of these symptoms of poor cardiorespiratory reserve indicates a greater risk during management of this patient.

Dialogue History

In the presence of a positive history of cardiovascular disease (angina, myocardial infarction), the doctor should continue with the following dialogue history:

QUESTION. Has there been any alteration in the pattern of your episodes of angina in the last month?

COMMENT. As discussed in Chapter 27, anginal episodes are usually fairly constant for each patient. Any increase in rate of frequency, duration, or severity or decrease in level of precipitating factors

Table 28-1. Medications employed for patients with status post–myocardial infarction

Drug category	Example(s)	Rationale
Diuretics	Hydrochlorothiazide	High blood pressure Heart failure
Inotropic agents	Digitalis Dopamine Dobutamine Amrinone	Heart failure
Antidysrhythmics	Digitalis Lidocaine/tocainide Procainamide Quinidine sulfate Disopyramide (Norpace)	Atrial fibrillation with rapid ventricular rate Ventricular dysrhythmias
Nitrates	Nitroglycerin—ointment, transdermal, or sublingual tablet or spray forms Long-acting nitrates (Table 27-1)	Anginal pains
Antiplatelet agents	Sulfinpyrazone (Anturane)	Shown in two studies to reduce incidence of sudden death and recurrent myocardial infarction (for up to 7 months post-MI)
	Aspirin	Still prescribed, although a large, multicenter study found no reduction in deaths from recurrent myocardial infarction
Beta-adrenergic agents	Propranolol Timolol Alprenolol Metoprolol	Several studies have shown beta-blockers to decrease likelihood of sudden death and reinfarction in months following acute myocardial infarction

may well be an indication of preinfarction or unstable angina. Immediate consultation with the patient's physician is desirable in this instance.

QUESTION. When did you have your last myocardial infarction?

COMMENT. Length of time elapsed since the last myocardial infarction is significant in relation to the risk involved in dental therapy. Following a myocardial infarction, there is an increased risk of reinfarction. The patient represents an increased risk during dental therapy regardless of the amount of time elapsed since the initial episode. However, in the immediate postinfarction period there is a significantly higher risk of reinfarction. In a survey by Weinblatt and coworkers (1968), the reinfarction rate (noted during surgery or in the immediate postoperative period [24 hours]) was 37% if the surgical procedure occurred within 3 months of the initial episode. If performed within 4 to 6 months of the episode, the reinfarction rate dropped to 16%; if surgery was postponed for longer than 6 months following the episode, the reinfarction rate fell to 5%. These figures compare to an infarction rate of 0.1% in persons with no prior history of infarction. During the recovery period, collateral circulation to the infarcted area improves, thereby allowing the heart to "heal" and minimizing the size of the residual infarct. This process of healing normally requires approximately 6 months. The increased risk represented by the status post–myocardial infarction patient is illustrated by an overall mortality rate of 30% within the first month after the infarction. The majority of these deaths are related to the presence of significant dysrhythmias. Although this high mortality rate does decrease with time, after 10 years the postinfarction mortality rate is still four times that of a "normal group."

Physical Examination

Vital signs should be recorded before and immediately following dental appointments for all post–myocardial infarction patients. (See p. 16 [Table 2-1] for suggested management of patients according to their blood pressure.)

Additional examination of the patient may not provide any reliable indication of previous myocardial infarction. Many survivors of a mild myocardial infarction appear to be in extremely fine physical and mental condition. Much research has been carried out concerning the role of physical exercise in the rehabilitation of myocardial tissues following infarction. Findings have led to comprehensive physical training programs for many of these persons. Patients are permitted to resume normal activities (such as walking and sexual activity) in a graded manner during convalescence. Such programs result in both subjective and objective improvement, recorded as decreases in heart rate and blood pressure, as well as a return to normal or near normal life style and improved morale. Unfortunately, there is much less evidence for improvement in ventricular function and little convincing evidence that these programs, with exercise, decrease the recurrence of myocardial infarction or the mortality rate. It must always be remembered therefore that regardless of the *apparent* state of physical fitness of post–myocardial infarction patients, they must still be considered a high risk during all dental procedures.

Post–myocardial infarction patients who have a significant degree of ventricular damage may also have clinical signs and symptoms of congestive heart failure. (See Chapter 14 for a discussion of this clinical entity.) Visual examination of these patients may reveal a degree of peripheral cyanosis (nailbeds, mucous membranes), coolness of the extremities, peripheral edema (ankles), and possible orthopnea (difficulty in breathing that is relieved by sitting upright). These patients represent a considerable risk during dental treatment.

Dental Therapy Considerations

Dental therapy considerations for the post–myocardial infarction patient include reduction in stress that is related to dental therapy and possible alteration in drug therapy, dental therapy, or both (Table 28-2).

The status post–myocardial infarction patient represents an ASA III risk.

Stress reduction

The post–myocardial infarction patient is relatively stress intolerant; therefore, the Stress Reduction Protocol (see p. 40) should be adhered to rather strictly. Of special importance in this patient are intraoperative stress reduction and adequate pain control.

The administration of supplemental oxygen to the status post–myocardial infarction patient will minimize the risk of development of hypoxia and myocardial ischemia. A flow of 4 to 6 liters per minute of oxygen through a nasal cannula (humidified) or nasal hood is recommended.

Oxygen may also be delivered in conjunction with nitrous oxide. Nitrous oxide–oxygen inhala-

Table 28-2. Dental therapy considerations for status post–myocardial infarction patients

Number of episodes	ASA physical status	Considerations
One documented myocardial infarction at least 6 months previously; no residual cardiovascular complications	III	Usual ASA III considerations to include followup after therapy by telephone; supplemental oxygen during treatment
One documented episode at least 6 months previously; angina, CHF, or dysrhythmia present	III or IV	Use of dialogue history to determine level of risk; usual ASA III considerations include possible premedication with nitroglycerin 5 minutes preop (if angina); oxygen through nasal cannula or nasal hood; and followup after therapy by telephone
More than one documented episode, most recent one at least 6 months previously; no further cardiovascular complications	III	Usual ASA III considerations to include supplemental oxygen during treatment and followup after therapy by telephone
Documented episode less than 6 months previously, or severe post-MI complications	IV	Usual ASA IV considerations

tion sedation is the most highly recommended sedation technique for the cardiac risk patient. Its value in the management of acute episodes of myocardial infarction is discussed later in this chapter. Other sedation techniques may be used if deemed necessary by the doctor. In all sedation techniques, hypoxia must be avoided. The use of supplemental oxygen will minimize this risk.

Adequate pain control during the dental procedure must be ensured. As discussed in Chapter 27, endogenous catecholamine release is potentially more dangerous to the cardiac risk patient than is the 0.01 mg/ml of exogenous epinephrine introduced into the tissues with a properly administered local anesthetic containing epinephrine in a 1:100,000 concentration. However, vasoconstrictors are contraindicated in patients with intractable cardiac dysrhythmias.

The duration of an appointment for the status post–myocardial infarction patient is variable but should never exceed a patient's level of tolerance.

It is strongly recommended that no routine dental therapy, even procedures as seemingly innocuous as prophylaxis, be considered for a post–myocardial infarction patient for at least 6 months following the infarction. Emergency dental therapy, such as that for infection and pain, ought not to be managed within the dental office setting during this 6-month period. The clinical problem may be initially managed through the administration of oral medications (antibiotics and/or analgesics) alone, with any additional therapy being carried out in a hospital setting. It must be stressed that only emergency procedures should be considered on the post–myocardial infarction patient within 6 months of the episode, and then only if medications have been ineffective and a hospital setting is available for the contemplated therapy.

Medical consultation should be considered before the dental management of a post–myocardial infarction patient if any doubt remains in the doctor's mind after a full dental, medical, and psychological (anxiety) evaluation of the patient. If the doctor is contemplating emergency dental therapy for this patient within the 6-month waiting period, medical consultation is strongly recommended before treatment.

Anticoagulant or antiplatelet therapy

Medical consultation is also indicated before treatment that involves a degree of hemorrhage (periodontal surgery, oral surgery) if the patient is currently receiving anticoagulant or antiplatelet therapy. The post-MI use of anticoagulants is much less common today that it was in the recent past. Dental surgery is frequently performed in patients whose prothrombin time is 20% to 30% of normal without the development of bleeding problems. In most instances, therefore, the proposed dental procedure does not have to be postponed, and the patient's anticoagulant medication does not need alteration. The doctor, however, should take all possible precautions to prevent hemorrhage from occurring. Possible steps include a hemostatic dressing placed within the socket, multiple sutures in the surgical area, intraoral pressure packs, ice packs (extraoral), the avoidance of mouth rinses, and a soft diet for 48 hours following the procedure.

CLINICAL MANIFESTATIONS
Pain

The chief clinical manifestation of acute myocardial infarction is the sudden onset of severe pain of the anginal type. Acute myocardial infarction may occur without an obvious precipitating cause, often arising during a period of rest or sleep, or it may occur during or immediately following a period of unusually strong exercise (Table 28-3). There is considerable evidence that emotional stress is a precipitating factor. The pain builds rapidly to maximal intensity, lasting for prolonged periods of time (30 minutes to several hours) if unmanaged.

The pain is usually described as a pressing or crushing sensation, like a deep ache within the chest. The patient may state that "it feels like there is a heavy rock or someone sitting on my chest." Rarely is the pain described as sharp or stabbing. It is located over the middle to upper third of the sternum and, much less commonly, over the lower third of the epigastrium.

Rest does not reduce the pain, nor does the use of nitroglycerin. The pain of myocardial infarction is most effectively relieved through the administration of narcotics such as morphine. Radiation of pain occurs throughout the same pattern as that of angina (see Fig. 27-2).

In 5% to 15% of cases, pain is either absent or minor and is overshadowed by immediate complications such as acute pulmonary edema, CHF, profound weakness, shock, syncope, or cerebral thrombosis. This type of infarction is termed a "painless infarction."

Other Clinical Signs and Symptoms

The patient with acute myocardial infarction may appear to be in acute distress. A cold sweat is usually present, and the patient feels quite weak. The patient appears apprehensive and expresses an intense fear of impending doom. (Although "intense fear of impending doom" may appear to the reader to be an overly dramatic and thus silly statement, rest assured that many victims of acute myocardial infarction do indeed verbally report this "intense fear of impending doom!") In contrast to anginal patients who lie, sit, or stand still, realizing that all activity increases the discomfort, patients with acute myocardial infarction will often be restless, moving about in a futile attempt to find a comfortable position for themselves.

Dyspnea is usually present also, and the patient

Table 28-3. Patient activity at onset of myocardial infarction

Activity	Percentage of patients
At rest	51
Modest or usual exertion	18
Physical exertion	13
Sleep	8
During surgical procedure	6
Other	4

Data from Alpert, J.S., and Braunwald, E.: Pathological and clinical manifestations of acute myocardial infarction. In Braunwald, E., editor: Heart disease, a textbook of cardiovascular medicine, Philadelphia, 1980, W.B. Saunders Co.

complains that the crushing pressure on the chest prevents normal breathing. Respiratory movements do not intensify the painful sensation. Nausea and vomiting frequently occur, especially if the pain is severe.

Other clinical signs and symptoms may include a feeling of lightheadedness or faintness, coughing, wheezing, and abdominal bloating. This last symptom may lead victims to think that they are suffering from an upset stomach or indigestion, thereby delaying the initiation of proper treatment and increasing the chance of death.

The doctor should suspect an acute myocardial infarction in the following three situations:
1. New onset of chest pain suggestive of myocardial ischemia either at rest or with ordinary activity. Chest pain appearing for the first time usually indicates occlusion of a coronary artery. It is unlikely to be "simple" angina of effort.
2. A change in a previously stable pattern of anginal pain—either an increased frequency or severity, or the occurrence of rest angina for the first time
3. Chest pain suggestive of myocardial ischemia in a patient with known coronary artery disease if unrelieved by rest and/or nitroglycerin

Physical Findings

The patient appears restless and apprehensive and possibly in severe pain. Color may be poor, the face ashen gray, and nailbeds and other mucous membranes cyanotic. The skin is cool, pale, and moist. The heart rate (pulse) may be weak, thready, and rapid, although a slow rate (bradycardia) may occasionally be present. Significant dysrhythmias are often present (premature ventricular contractions [PVCs] are seen in 95% of patients with acute myocardial infarction). Blood pressure may be normal but more commonly is low, decreasing dramatically over the first few hours and possibly falling to shock levels. Respirations appear rapid and shallow. If the left ventricle is the major site of the infarction, left ventricular failure may become clinically evident with labored breathing, a frothy sputum, and other signs of congestive heart failure (dependent edema), or pulmonary edema may gradually develop (Table 28-4).

Acute Complications

The greatest risk of death from myocardial infarction is during the first 4 to 6 hours after the onset of signs and symptoms. Complications such as acute dysrhythmias and cardiac arrest can occur abruptly during this time. The majority of deaths occur in the first hour and are related to the presence of dysrhythmias, such as ventricular tachycardia and ventricular fibrillation. PVCs are very common. Their presence indicates increased irritability of damaged myocardium and may presage the development of ventricular tachycardia or ventricular fibrillation. Ventricular fibrillation is 15 times more likely to occur in the first hour after the onset of signs and symptoms than in the following 12 hours. Ventricular fibrillation develops in the first hour in approximately 36% of persons with acute myocardial infarction. The significant mortality rate from myocardial infarction is in part based on the average delay between the onset of signs and symptoms

Table 28-4. Clinical manifestations of acute myocardial infarction

Symptoms	Signs
Pain	Restlessness
Severe to intolerable	In acute distress
Prolonged, >30 min	Skin—cool, pale, moist
Crushing, choking, knifelike	Heart rate—bradycardia to tachycardia; PVCs common
Retrosternal	
Radiates: left arm, hand, epigastrium, shoulders, neck, jaw	
Nausea and vomiting	
Weakness	
Dizziness	
Palpitations	
Cold perspiration	
Sense of impending doom	

of myocardial infarction and entering the emergency medical system, which is 3 hours!

The doctor must prepare for acute complications. As mentioned, survival of a patient through the prehospitalization period is indeed a good omen. Once the patient is hospitalized in a specialized cardiac care unit (CCU), the chances for survival increase significantly. The most dangerous period is that time spent waiting for medical assistance to arrive. Adequate preparation by the dental office staff can improve the chances of a successful outcome of this situation.

PATHOPHYSIOLOGY

Acute myocardial infarction is usually the direct result of a sudden occlusion of a major coronary vessel. The obstruction may result from acute thrombosis, subintimal hemorrhage, or the rupture of an atheromatous plaque, which then initiates the formation of a clot. The artery most often involved in coronary occlusion is the anterior descending branch of the left coronary artery, which supplies the anterior left ventricle. There are two major types of myocardial infarction; the transmural infarct and the nontransmural infarct. In the *transmural infarct* the myocardial necrosis involves the full thickness of the ventricular wall. Necrosis in the *nontransmural infarct* involves subendocardium, the intramural myocardium, or both, without extension all the way through the ventricular wall to the epicardium.

An occlusion may occur rapidly, or it may develop over a prolonged period. In either case, it is possible that even total occlusion of a coronary vessel may not lead to ischemia and infarction. In the presence of an adequate collateral circulation, the myocardial tissue supplied by the occluded vessel still receives an adequate blood supply through collateral vessels. Collateral circulation in the normal heart is usually poorly developed; however, it has been demonstrated that, immediately following occlusion of a coronary artery, the collateral blood flow doubles. The enlargement of these vessels over the next 3 to 4 weeks is a major element in the finding that the size of the area of myocardial necrosis is usually smaller than would be expected.

Myocardial infarction may occur even though the vessel is not totally occluded. In an area dependent for its blood supply on collateral circulation (a previously infarcted area with adequate collateral circulation), a minimal change in blood supply through the vessel may lead to infarction. This may come about through a partial occlusion of the vessel or from a change in vascular resistance in the vessel.

Infarction of the myocardium produces alterations in the contractility of the heart. Because the left ventricle is most commonly involved, the blood supply to the periphery may become inadequate. This leads to many of the clinical signs and symptoms observed in myocardial infarction, such as a cool, moist skin, peripheral cyanosis, and tachycardia. The larger the infarct, the greater the degree of circulatory inadequacy (heart failure). Left ventricular filling pressures increase significantly even in the presence of a small infarct. If the infarction is larger, there is a greater increase in the left ventricular filling pressure and clinical evidence of left heart failure. Infarction of 35% or more of left ventricular mass leads to clinical evidence of hypotension, decreased cardiac output, and cardiogenic shock.

Cardiogenic shock occurs in approximately 10% of acute myocardial infarctions. Its presence is ominous because it is associated with a higher mortality rate. It normally develops approximately 10 hours following the onset of the infarction and may be produced by cardiac dysrhythmias, the continued presence of severe pain, the onset of acute pulmonary edema, or pulmonary embolism. Clinical evidence of cardiogenic shock includes hypotension (systolic blood pressure below 80 torr) and signs of an inadequate peripheral circulation (mental confusion, cool skin, peripheral cyanosis, tachycardia, and a decreased urinary output).

Probably the most threatening feature of the early postinfarction period (1 to 2 hours) is the presence of cardiac dysrhythmias. Most patients (95%) exhibit these abnormalities in heart rhythm. They are significant in that they may produce alterations in the normal sequence of atrial and ventricular contraction, thereby leading to inadequate blood flow, and/or they may produce an aberrant focus of electrical depolarization in the myocardium. They also may adversely affect the ventricular rate, producing bradycardia (slow rate), ventricular tachycardia (an extremely rapid contraction rate with insufficient time for ventricular filling), ventricular fibrillation (irregular, uncoordinated, ineffective contraction of individual muscle bundles), or asystole (complete absence of contractions). Commonly observed dysrhythmias are shown in Fig. 30-1. Death occurring in the early postinfarction period, although it may be produced by the infarction of a large mass of myocardium, is normally the result of an acute dysrhythmia.

Survival following myocardial infarction depends on many factors. Most important of these are the state of left ventricular function and the severity of obstructive lesions in the coronary vascular bed. Complete clinical recovery (no chronic complications) and a normal ECG are compatible with a 10- to 20-year period of survival. However, patients who exhibit residual congestive heart failure usually die within 1 to 5 years.

MANAGEMENT

Clinical management of acute myocardial infarction is based on recognizing it and applying the steps of basic life support. It may be difficult to differentiate immediately between the pain of angina and that of acute myocardial infarction. Although there are slight differences, the dental practitioner may find it difficult to determine which of these clinical entities is present.

Step 1. Diagnosis. The suspicion of acute myocardial infarction must be based on the patient's history. If the history (record of clinical signs and symptoms) is consistent with a diagnosis of acute myocardial infarction, the patient must be treated accordingly. Although the electrocardiogram (ECG) may confirm acute myocardial infarction, the ECG may also appear to be entirely normal. For this reason, a single, normal ECG tracing cannot reliably exclude the diagnosis of past acute myocardial infarction.

It is suggested that management of chest pain be approached as if it were angina unless it is obviously not of anginal origin. Therefore the initial steps in management of these patients include termination of dental therapy and allowing the patient to find a comfortable position. If patients have a history of angina, their nitroglycerin tablets or spray should be available and used at this time. Nitroglycerin from the emergency kit is used only if patients do not have their own supply. Before administering nitroglycerin, the patient's vital signs should be recorded. Nitroglycerin should *not* be administered if the systolic blood pressure is below 100 torr (because it can decrease the mean arterial pressure). Nitroglycerin normally acts within 2 to 4 minutes to dramatically reduce or terminate the discomfort of angina. Should the pain continue or increase in severity in spite of the administration of this agent, we must consider the very real possibility of an acute myocardial infarction.

Step 2. Initiate basic life support and implement as needed.

Step 3. Summon medical assistance. With the failure of nitroglycerin to ease the patient's discom-

---

MANAGEMENT OF
ACUTE MYOCARDIAL INFARCTION

Step 1 Diagnosis
Administer nitroglycerin

2 Initiate basic life support and implement as needed

3 Summon medical assistance

4 Administer oxygen and monitor vital signs

5 Relieve pain
SC or IV morphine or meperidine or a nitrous oxide–oxygen mixture by means of a nasal hood

6 Manage complications
Dysrhythmias: Do not administer antidysrhythmic agents unless electrocardioscope is present
Congestive heart failure: see Chapter 14
Cardiac arrest: see Chapter 30

7 Transport patient to hospital; doctor should accompany patient to hospital

---

fort, medical assistance should immediately be sought. It must always be remembered that mortality from myocardial infarction is greatest during the first few hours, the majority of deaths occurring before the patient is admitted to the hospital. Over 60% of all deaths from myocardial infarction occur within the first few hours after the onset of symptoms. Three quarters of all deaths occur within the first 24 hours. Most deaths occurring before hospitalization are the result of life-threatening dysrhythmias that frequently occur in the immediate postinfarction period, as well as the misinterpretation or denial of signs and symptoms by the patient or medical personnel. Early entry into the emergency medical services (EMS) system is often vital for patient survival. As mentioned previously, the average time from onset of symptoms to EMS entry is more than 3 hours.

The availability of trained paramedical personnel in mobile coronary care units has led to a significant decrease in the mortality rate from myocardial infarction. Definitive therapy (advanced cardiac life support) can be started at the scene or while en route to the hospital. (The cities of Seattle, Washington and Belfast, Ireland have demonstrated the value of such trained personnel.)

Step 4. Administer oxygen and monitor vital signs. Oxygen should be administered to the pa-

tient while awaiting medical assistance. Vital signs (blood pressure, pulse rate, and respirations) should be monitored on a regular basis (every 5 minutes) and recorded.

There is evidence suggesting that increased arterial oxygen tension (Pao_2) may decrease the size of the infarct. Oxygen should be delivered through a nasal cannula or nasal hood at a flow rate of 4 to 6 liters per minute.

Step 5. Relieve pain. Prolonged pain during myocardial infarction is a potentially life-threatening situation. It will lead to increased anxiety on the part of the patient, and it contributes to excessive activity of the autonomic nervous system, producing an increase in cardiovascular workload and oxygen requirement. In addition, prolonged, intense pain is one of the causative factors of cardiogenic shock, which has a high mortality rate.

Parenteral analgesics. The use of potent analgesics is recommended for relief of the pain of myocardial infarction. Intravenous administration of 2 to 5 mg of morphine sulfate repeated every 5 to 15 minutes provides adequate pain relief and allays apprehension. Morphine sulfate may be administered subcutaneously in a dose of 5 to 15 mg. Morphine should not be readministered if the respiratory rate is less than 12 respirations per minute. Meperidine (50 to 100 mg IM) may be administered in place of morphine. Intramuscular injection of these analgesic drugs provides adequate pain relief of long duration. Intravenous administration may also be considered, but the drugs require readministration in a shorter period of time.

Other analgesics. Another useful analgesic medication may already be present in the dental office. A mixture of nitrous oxide and oxygen, more commonly employed as an antianxiety agent in dental practice, has been employed in Great Britain and several other countries since 1967 in premixed cylinders containing 50% nitrous oxide (N_2O) and 50% oxygen (O_2) (Entonox). Recently, premixed cylinders of nitrous oxide (35%) and oxygen (65%) (Dolonox) have been used in the United States in the treatment of myocardial infarction. In Britain, the nitrous oxide–oxygen mixture is employed on emergency ambulances and serves as the primary agent for pain relief in acute cardiovascular emergency situations. The primary advantage of this agent is that it provides the patient with a gaseous analgesic agent that by itself has little effect on blood pressure. This contrasts with the use of parenteral analgesics, which are more likely to reduce blood pressure and produce adverse side effects (for example, respiratory depression, nausea, and vomiting). The use of this mixture also provides the patient with a source of enriched oxygen (50% to 65% versus 21% in atmospheric air).

Although premixed nitrous oxide and oxygen is available through medical suppliers in the United States, any available source of these gases may be employed in this situation. A 35% concentration of nitrous oxide is administered through the nasal hood or by means of a full face mask. When the patient is ready to be transported from the dental office to the hospital, the medical or paramedical personnel will administer a parenteral analgesic to provide continuing pain relief during the journey should portable sources of N_2O-O_2 be unavailable.

Step 6. Manage complications. The major complications of acute myocardial infarction likely to develop in the dental office while medical assistance is being awaited are acute dysrhythmias, congestive heart failure, and cardiac arrest. The management of *acute dysrhythmias* requires intravenous administration of various drugs. In addition, the presence of an electrocardioscope and a person knowledgeable in its interpretation are essential. Agents that may be employed to manage dysrhythmias include lidocaine and atropine. It is again emphasized that without an electrocardiographic monitor no antiarrhythmic drugs should be administered to a patient with dysrhythmias.

Left ventricular failure may develop if a significant portion of the myocardium has been infarcted. Respiratory symptoms are most prominent, with dyspnea and acute pulmonary edema occurring. (Management of this complication is discussed fully in Chapter 14.) Essentials of management include positioning the patient and reducing the circulating blood volume through the use of a bloodless phlebotomy. In addition, oxygen should be administered to this patient.

Cardiac arrest, indicative of acute cardiorespiratory collapse, needs immediate effective management. Chapter 30 covers this subject more fully.

Step 7. Transport to hospital. Once the patient's condition has been stabilized (relief of pain and stabilization of heart rhythm and blood pressure), transport to a primary care facility (emergency room) should be considered. It is desirable for the doctor to accompany the patient in the ambulance or by car from the dental office to the hospital and to remain with the patient until a physician is in attendance.

The management of acute myocardial infarction is summarized in the box on opposite page.

BIBLIOGRAPHY

Adgey, A.A.J., and others: Acute phase of myocardial infarction. Prehospital management of the coronary patient, Minn. Med. **59:**347, 1976.

Alderman, E.L.: Analgesics in the acute phase of myocardial infarction, JAMA **229:**12, 1974.

Alpert, J.S., and Braunwald, E.: Pathological and clinical manifestations of acute myocardial infarction. In Braunwald, E., editor: Heart disease: a textbook of cardiovascular medicine, Philadelphia, 1980, W.B. Saunders Co.

Altschule, M.D.: Physiology in acute myocardial infarction, Med. Clin. North Am. **58:**399, 1974.

American Heart Association: Heart Facts, Dallas, 1984, The Association.

Astvad, K., and others: Mortality from acute myocardial infarction before and after establishment of a coronary care unit, Br. Med. J. **1:**567, 1974.

Baroldi, G.: Coronary thrombosis: facts and beliefs, Am. Heart J. **91:**683, 1976.

Bassler, T., and Scaff, J.: Impending heart attacks, Lancet **1:**544, 1976.

Bigger, J.T., Jr., and others: Ventricular arrhythmias in ischemic heart disease: mechanism, prevalence, significance, and management, Prog. Cardiovas. Dis. **19:**255, 1977.

Bolooki, H., and others: Myocardial revascularization after acute infarction, Am. J. Cardiol. **36:**395, 1975.

Brest, A.N., and others: Myocardial infarction without obstructive coronary artery disease, Am. Heart J. **88:**219, 1974.

Buchanan, R.A., Jr., Russel, R.O., and Rackley, C.E.: Myocardial infarction in patients less than 45 years old, South. Med. J. **69:**691, 1976.

Cobb, L.A., and others: Resuscitation from out of hospital ventricular fibrillation: 4 years follow-up, Circulation **51-52** (suppl. III):223, 1975.

Cohen, B.S.: A program of rehabilitation after acute myocardial infarction, South. Med. J. **68:**145, 1975.

Cohen, L.S., and Ross, A.M.: Long term management of complicated myocardial infarction, Postgrad. Med. **57:**17, 1975.

Coronary Drug Project Research Group: Prognostic importance of premature beats following myocardial infarction, JAMA **223:**116, 1973.

Cosby, R.S., Giddings, J.A., and See, J.R.: Late complications of myocardial infarction, JAMA **236:**1717, 1976.

Dolder, M.A., and Oliver, M.F.: Myocardial infarction in young men: study of risk factors in nine countries, Br. Heart J. **37:**493, 1975.

Eisele, J.H., and others: Myocardial performance and N_2O analgesia in coronary artery disease, Anesthesiology **44:**16, 1976.

Elek, S.R.: Psychological management of patients with coronary-prone type-A behavior pattern, JAMA **229:**1805, 1974.

Epstein, S.E., and others: The early phase of acute myocardial infarction: pharmacologic aspects of therapy, Ann. Intern. Med. **78:**918, 1973.

Friedman, E.H.: Type A or B behavior, JAMA **228:**1369, 1974.

Friedman, M., and Rosenman, R.H.: Type A behavior and your heart, New York, 1974, Alfred A. Knopf, Inc.

Fulton, M., and others: Natural history of unstable angina, Lancet **1:**860, 1972.

Gelson, A.D.N., and others: Course of patients discharged early after myocardial infarction, Br. Med. J. **1:**1555, 1976.

Gillespie, T.A., and Sobel, B.E.: A rationale for therapy of acute myocardial infarction. Limitation of infarct size, Adv. Intern. Med. **22:**319, 1976.

Gillum, R., and others: Delay in the prehospital phase of acute myocardial infarction, Arch. Intern. Med. **136:**649, 1976.

Glasser, S.P.: The problems of patients with cardiovascular disease undergoing dental treatment, J. Am. Dent. Assoc. **94:**1158, 1977.

Graham, I., and others: Natural history of coronary heart disease. A study of 586 men surviving an initial acute attack, Am. Heart J. **105:**249, 1983.

Horgan, J.H.: Rehabilitation after myocardial infarction, J. Irish Med. Assoc. **66:**661, 1973.

Hutter, A.M., Jr.: Early hospital discharge after myocardial infarction, N. Engl. J. Med. **288:**1141, 1973.

Jenkins, C.D.: Recent evidence supporting psychologic and social risk factors for coronary disease, N. Engl. J. Med. **294:**987, 1976.

Kavanagh, T., Shephard, R.H., and Pandit, V.: Marathon running after myocardial infarction, JAMA **229:**1602, 1974.

Kerr, F., and others: A double blind trial of patient controlled nitrous oxide/oxygen analgesia in myocardial infarction, Lancet **1:**397, 1975.

Kerr, F., and Donald, D.W.: Analgesia in myocardial infarction, Br. Heart J. **36:**117, 1974.

Khan, A.H., and Haywood, L.J.: Myocardial infarction in nine patients with radiologically patent coronary arteries, N. Engl. J. Med. **291:**427, 1974.

Killip, T.: Management of arrhythmias in acute myocardial infarction, Hosp. Prac. **7:**121, 1971.

Killip, T.: Arrhythmias in myocardial infarction, Med. Clin. North Am. **60:**233, 1975.

Klatsky, A., Friedman, G.D., and Siegelaub, A.: Coffee drinking prior to acute myocardial infarction, JAMA **226:**540, 1973.

Kleiger, R.E.: Chest pain in patients seen in emergency clinics, JAMA **236:**595, 1976.

Lassers, B.W., and others: Left ventricular failure and acute myocardial infarction, Am. J. Cardiol. **25:**511, 1970.

Levenstein, J.H.: Emergency management of acute myocardial infarction by the general practitioner, S. Afr. Med. J. **50:**531, 1976.

Levy, R.I.: Progress in prevention of cardiovascular disease, Prev. Med. **7:**464, 1978.

Librach, G., and others: The initial manifestations of acute myocardial infarction, Geriatrics **31:**41, 1976.

Madias, J.E., and Hood, W.B., Jr.: Reduction of precordial ST-segment elevation in patients with anterior myocardial infarction by oxygen breathing, Circulation **53**(suppl. 1):198, 1976.

Manning, D.P.: First aid in acute myocardial infarction, Br. Med. J. **1:**711, 1976.

Maroko, P.R., and others: Reduction of infarct size by oxygen inhalation following acute coronary occlusion, Circulation **52:**360, 1975.

Maseri, A., and others: Coronary vasospasm as a possible cause of myocardial infarction. A conclusion derived from the study of "preinfarction" angina, N. Engl. J. Med. **299:**1271, 1978.

Morris, D.C., Hurst, J.W., and Logue, R.B.: Myocardial infarction in young women, Am. J. Cardiol. **38:**299, 1976.

Moss, A.J., editor: Symposium on the prehospital phase of acute myocardial infarction, Arch. Intern. Med. **129:**681, 1972.

Moss, A.J., and Goldstein, S.: The prehospital phase of acute myocardial infarction, Circulation **41:**737, 1970.

Nancekievill, D.: Apparatus for the administration of Entonox

(50% N_2O: 50% O_2 mixture) by intermittent positive pressure, Anaesthesia, **29:**736, 1974.

Neill, W.A., and Oxendine, J.M.: Exercise can promote coronary collateral development without improving perfusion of ischemic myocardium, Circulation **60:**1513, 1979.

Nemec, E.D., Manfield, L., and Kennedy, J.W.: Heart rate and blood pressure responses during sexual activity in normal males, Am. Heart J. **92:**274, 1976.

Norris, R.M., and Mercer, C.J.: Significance of idioventricular rhythms in acute myocardial infarction, Prog. Cardiovas. Dis. **16:**455, 1974.

Oliva, P.B., and Breckinridge, J.C.: Arteriographic evidence of coronary arterial spasm in acute myocardial infarction, Circulation **56:**366, 1977.

Pantridge, J.F., and Geddes, J.S.: A mobile intensive care unit in the management of myocardial infarction, Lancet **2:**271, 1967.

Pantridge, J.F., Webb, S.W., and Adgey, A.A.J.: Arrhythmias in the first hours of acute myocardial infarction, Prog. Cardiovasc. Dis. **23:**265, 1981.

Partridge, J.R., and Geddes, J.S.: Diseases of the cardiovascular system. Management of acute myocardial infarction, Br. Med. J. **2:**168, 1976.

Propper, R.H.: Prefatal cardiac arrhythmias, J. Oral Surg. **33:**929, 1975.

Rose, R.M., and others: Occurrence of arrhythmias during the first hour in acute myocardial infarction, Circulation **50** (suppl. 3):111, 1974.

Scanlon, P.J., and others: Accelerated angina pectoris: clinical, hemodynamic, arteriographic and therapeutic experience in 85 patients, Circulation **47:**19, 1973.

Schaffer, W.A., and Cobb, L.A.: Recurrent ventricular fibrillation and modes of death in survivors of out-of-hospital ventricular fibrillation, N. Engl. J. Med. **293:**259, 1975.

Shekelle, R.B., and Liu, S.C.: Public beliefs about causes and prevention of heart attacks, JAMA **240:**756, 1978.

Sobel, B.E.: Propranolol and threatened myocardial infarction, N. Engl. J. Med. **300:**191, 1979.

Sobel, B.E., and Braunwald, E.: Management of acute myocardial infarction. In Braunwald, E., editor: Heart disease: a textbook of cardiovascular medicine, Philadelphia, 1980, W.B. Saunders Co.

Stamler, J.: Major coronary risk factors before and after myocardial infarction, Postgrad. Med. **57:**25, 1975.

Staples, A.F.: Cardiopulmonary crises in the dental office, Dent. Clin. North Am. **17:**473, 1973.

Stern, M.S., and others: Nitrous oxide and oxygen in acute myocardial infarction, Circulation **58**(suppl. II):171, 1978.

Thompson, P.L., and Lown, B.: Nitrous oxide as an analgesic in acute myocardial infarction, JAMA **235:**924, 1976.

Wallace, W.A., Napodano, R.J., and Yu, P.N.: Early care of acute myocardial infarction, Arch. Intern. Med. **136:**974, 1976.

Walsh, M.J., and others: Mobile coronary care, Br. Heart J. **34:**701, 1972.

Weinblatt, E., and others: Prognosis of men after first myocardial infarction: mortality and first recurrence in relation to selected parameters, Am. J. Public Health **58:**1329, 1968.

Wolk, M.J., Scheidt, S., and Killip, T.: Heart failure complicating acute myocardial infarction, Circulation **45:**1125, 1972.

Wynne, J., and others: Beneficial effects of nitrous oxide in patients with ischemic heart disease, Circulation **55-56**(suppl. III):18, 1977.

29 *Chest Pain: Differential Diagnosis*

The two major clinical syndromes that confront the dental practitioner and that exhibit chest pain are angina pectoris and acute myocardial infarction. Yet there are occasions when the dental patient (or the doctor) may have other forms of chest pain. Indeed, everybody experiences various forms of chest pain at times. Fortunately, most of these pains are unrelated to cardiac disease and for the most part are innocuous. However, most of those experiencing chest pain have stopped and thought, "This pain I am feeling now is the real thing." With this in mind, we will first discuss the major differences between this common form of chest pain and the chest pain of cardiovascular disease. Following this discussion is a differential diagnosis of the two major forms of chest pain. Table 29-1 lists several of the possible causes of chest pain.

NONCARDIAC CHEST PAIN

Noncardiac chest pain can usually be differentiated from the pain of angina and myocardial infarction in the following manner: sharp (knifelike) chest pain that increases in intensity with inspiration and diminishes with exhalation is usually not related to cardiac syndromes. Chest pain that is aggravated by movement (twisting, turning, or stretching of the sore area) is most often related to muscle or nerve injuries, not to cardiac disease. It must be noted that I have used the word "usually" when describing the typical chest pains. Instances occur in which patients are aware of a sharp, knifelike pain that may in fact be related to cardiac disease. Variations from the "typical" are expected, and the practitioner of dentistry is well advised to take note of this.

Probably the most common cause of noncardiac chest pain is the *muscle strain* that occurs after exercise or physical exertion. This form of pain is normally localized (the patient can point to a specific site of discomfort), does not radiate, and is made worse by breathing and movement. A heating pad or mild analgesic medication may give relief.

Pericarditis is an inflammation of the outer membrane covering the heart and is most commonly caused by viral infection. The pain of pericarditis is similar to that of angina or myocardial infarction, occurs in the midsternum, and is described as "oppressive." Clues to its differential diagnosis include the aggravation of the pain of pericarditis on breathing and swallowing, the characteristic relief of the pain when the patient bends forward from the waist, and very often the presence of a fever before the onset of pain.

Esophagitis with or without *hiatal hernia* produces a substernal or epigastric burning pain that is precipitated by eating or lying down after a meal. The pain is relieved by antacids. There often is an acid reflux into the mouth.

Pulmonary embolism usually indicates the sudden occlusion of a blood vessel within the lungs by an embolus that has been "thrown" (broken loose) from the legs. The patient experiences a sudden severe chest pain that is commonly associated with the coughing up of blood-tinged sputum.

A less common cause of acute chest pain is the *dissecting aortic aneurysm*. The patient experiences sudden, acute, severe chest pain that is often greatest at onset. Typically it spreads up and down the chest and back over a period of hours. The dissecting aortic aneurysm may rapidly lead to death.

Two other very common causes of chest pain often make it difficult to differentiate between car-

Table 29-1. Causes of chest pain

Cardiac related	Non–cardiac related
Angina pectoris	Muscle strain
Myocardial infarction	Pericarditis
	Esophagitis
	Hiatal hernia
	Pulmonary embolism
	Dissecting aortic aneurysm
	Acute indigestion
	Intestinal "gas"

diac and noncardiac pain. These are the pains of *acute indigestion* and *"gas."* It has been mentioned previously that one of the major factors leading to the high initial mortality rate associated with myocardial infarction is the misinterpretation or denial of clinical symptoms by the patient or the attending physician. The symptoms are commonly written off as indigestion or gas pains and are later discovered to have been produced by acute myocardial infarction. The pain of gas is normally sharp and knifelike and increases in intensity on breathing. This fact should assist in differentiating gas pain from cardiac pain. Acute indigestion is similar to the pain of angina or myocardial infarction, and therefore all patients with this symptom should receive careful evaluation. Epigastric discomfort may be a manifestation of myocardial ischemia or infarction and should not be dismissed lightly. Unusual or prolonged indigestion should rouse suspicion, particularly in a high-risk individual.

CARDIAC CHEST PAIN

Angina and acute myocardial infarction are the two most common causes of cardiac-related chest pain in the dental office. Differential diagnosis is essential because these two syndromes represent quite different risks to the patient and are managed in dissimilar manners. The following discussion is offered to assist in this differential diagnosis.

Prior Medical History

The patient with angina is most commonly aware of the existence of the disease and is receiving medications to manage acute anginal episodes as they occur. It is possible but highly unlikely that a patient without a history of angina will suffer a first episode within the dental office setting. Most first episodes of chest pain for patients in the dental environment will prove to be either myocardial infarction or unstable angina.

A medical history of a prior myocardial infarc-

tion may also be available. Many patients who survive an acute myocardial infarction later develop episodes of angina and have medication for it.

Age of Patient

Coronary artery disease is present in all age groups. Clinical evidence may develop in young individuals, or it may never develop at all. There is no clinical difference between the age of patients developing either of these two coronary syndromes. Clinical evidence of CAD is most commonly noted in men between the ages of 50 and 60 years, whereas in women its greatest incidence is found between the ages of 60 and 70 years.

Sex of Patient

Coronary artery disease remains primarily a disease of males. The overall male-to-female ratio is 4:1. Before the age of 40 years, the ratio rises to 8:1.

Circumstances Associated with Onset of Symptoms

The clinical symptomatology of angina is usually associated with exertion, whether physical or mental. Myocardial infarction, on the other hand, may occur during or immediately following a period of exertion, but it also commonly occurs during periods of rest. Angina rarely occurs during rest, although coronary artery spasm may provoke anginal pain at any time.

Clinical Symptoms and Signs
Location of chest pain

Location of chest pain is not a reliable indicator of the nature of the pain. Both anginal pain and the pain of acute myocardial infarction occur substernally or just to the left of the midsternal region.

Description of chest pain

Chest pain associated with either of these two syndromes is usually not described as pain by the patient. More commonly the sensation is described as "squeezing," "pressing," or "crushing." The pain associated with myocardial infarction is more intense than that of angina and is more commonly described as pain or as being "intolerable."

Radiation of chest pain

Differentiation between the two syndromes is difficult to make using radiation of pain as a criterion. Radiation of chest pain commonly occurs to the left shoulder and medial side of the left arm, following the distribution of the ulnar nerve. Less frequently the pain may radiate to the right shoulder, the mandibular region, or the epigastrium. Both syndromes have similar radiation patterns.

Duration of chest pain

The pain associated with acute myocardial infarction is normally of long duration and lasts from 30 minutes to several hours if untreated. As mentioned in Chapter 28, untreated cardiac pain may produce cardiogenic shock. Pain associated with angina is almost always brief. Merely terminating the activity that induced the episode brings relief within 3 to 5 minutes. Anginal episodes that have been precipitated by eating a large meal or feeling anger are of a longer duration, perhaps lasting 30 minutes or more.

Response to medication

Probably the most reliable diagnostic tool is the response of the patient to the administration of medications. A vasodilator, preferably nitroglycerin but possibly amyl nitrite or nifedipine, is administered to the patient. The pain of angina will be relieved approximately 2 to 4 minutes following administration of nitroglycerin and within 1 minute following amyl nitrite administration. These agents may temporarily diminish the pain of myocardial infarction, but more commonly they will have no effect on the pain. The pain of myocardial infarction is commonly managed through administration of narcotic analgesics (such as morphine).

Administration of a vasodilator to the patient with presumed cardiac-related chest pain offers one of the most reliable methods of differentiating between the pain of angina and that of acute myocardial infarction. For this reason, this administration represents the first step in clinical management of chest pain in the dental office.

Physical Examination
Heart rate

The heart rate noted during episodes of angina is quite rapid and may feel "full" or "bounding." A rapid heart rate is also present during acute myocardial infarction; however, because the blood pressure is usually decreased, the pulse may feel weak or thready. The heart rate during acute myocardial infarction may also be slow.

Blood pressure

Episodes of angina are normally accompanied by marked elevations in blood pressure, whereas blood pressure in acute myocardial infarction may be normal but more commonly is decreased.

Respiration

Patients with either coronary syndrome may exhibit respiratory difficulty during the acute episode. The respiratory rate is more rapid, and the depth of each respiration may be more shallow than usual. In myocardial infarction the left ventricle may fail, producing clinical evidence of left heart failure.

Other signs and symptoms

Overall appearance. Patients with myocardial infarction or angina appear quite apprehensive and may be bathed in a cold sweat. The anginal patient can compare this episode with previous episodes, which may give a clue as to the seriousness of the present episode. Anginal episodes tend to be quite similar in an individual patient. Any change in severity, duration, or frequency may indicate the occurrence of unstable angina or myocardial infarction. Patients with acute myocardial infarction often have a great fear of impending doom.

Skin. In myocardial infarction, facial skin may appear ashen gray. The nailbeds and other mucous membranes of the victim may demonstrate varying degrees of cyanosis. These changes rarely occur during anginal episodes.

SUMMARY

As is evident, the clinical diagnosis of chest pain is difficult to make. However, management of cardiac-related chest pain invariably results in an accurate diagnosis. This depends primarily on the response of the patient to the administration of nitroglycerin.

One other important factor that bears repetition at this time is that anginal episodes for a given patient are usually similar from episode to episode. Any change in these attacks that produces a more severe episode may indicate the occurrence of acute myocardial infarction.

Noncardiac chest pain is usually easily differentiated from cardiac-related chest pain because of the nature of the pain itself. However, two common forms of discomfort, acute indigestion and "gas," are quite difficult to differentiate from cardiac-related chest pain. These symptoms must not be ignored. Careful evaluation is required, and medical consultation should be considered if doubt remains in the dental practitioner's mind.

30 *Cardiac Arrest and Cardiopulmonary Resuscitation*

Angina pectoris, myocardial infarction, and heart failure are three clinical manifestations of significant atherosclerosis of the coronary arteries. Associated with each of these clinical situations is the possible development of acute complications. Among these are cardiac dysrhythmias and cardiopulmonary collapse, which is also called cardiac arrest or sudden death. It must be noted that cardiac arrest may also occur as a clinical entity in the absence of other cardiovascular manifestations.

Of the victims of cardiac arrest, 25% have no clinical signs or symptoms before the onset of sudden death. Stated another way, the first clinical sign of significant atherosclerosis may be the death of the patient.

Sudden death is defined by the World Health Organization as clinical death that occurs within 24 hours after the onset of symptoms. Clinical death that occurs within 30 seconds of the onset of symptoms is termed instantaneous death. For the purposes of our discussion in this section, the term sudden death is defined as death occurring within 1 hour of the onset of signs and symptoms.

Death, as referred to in these definitions, is clinical death as opposed to biologic death. *Clinical death* occurs at the moment of cardiopulmonary arrest but may, on occasion, be reversed if promptly recognized and effectively managed. *Biologic death* ensues when permanent cellular damage has occurred, primarily from lack of an adequate oxygen supply. Biologic or cellular death of neuronal (brain) tissue takes place when delivery of oxygen is inadequate for approximately 4 to 6 minutes.

The magnitude of sudden death is apparent when it is noted that of the more than 540,000 deaths occurring in 1984 from ischemic heart disease, a majority of these occurred outside of the hospital—usually within 1 hour after the onset of symptoms. Sudden, unexpected death from myocardial infarction is therefore—in terms of absolute loss of life—the greatest single acute medical problem today.

With the introduction of closed chest cardiac massage by Kouwenhoven, Jude, and Knickerbocker in 1960, a new era in cardiac resuscitation began. Sudden death, previously a nonreversible situation, became reversible in many instances with the effective application of these new procedures.

The precipitating cause of death in most cases of sudden death is the lethal dysrhythmia ventricular fibrillation. It is estimated that ventricular fibrillation occurs in structurally sound hearts in excess of 900 times a day in the United States in victims outside of a hospital. Ventricular fibrillation therefore is the major cause of death from ischemic heart disease. Ventricular fibrillation most often occurs within the first 2 hours following the onset of clinical symptoms of coronary artery disease (most commonly acute myocardial infarction); however, it may also occur in the absence of any signs and symptoms of acute myocardial infarction or other ischemic heart disease.

Ventricular fibrillation is often reversible if adequate oxygenation of the myocardium is maintained until defibrillation is successfully carried out. Adequate circulation may be provided through the prompt and effective application of the steps of basic life support. The survival rate of victims of out-of-hospital cardiac arrest resulting from ventricular fibrillation (based on patients discharged from a hospital) is approximately 14% if the person initially finding the victim does not initiate basic life support (BLS) procedures. This compares to a survival rate of over 40% for those who receive basic life support immediately, followed closely in time by advanced cardiac life support (ACLS). If BLS is not begun immediately, the victim's brain is hypoxic for a longer period of time before circulation of oxygenated blood is restored. Permanent damage (biologic death) to neuronal tissues is more severe, and the victim's chance of having a level of neurologic activity close to the prearrest level is decreased. In some selected subgroups, resuscitation has been effective in 60% to 80% of cases (Lund and Skulber, 1976; Carveth, 1974). Table 30-1 demonstrates survival rates after cardiac arrest resulting from ventricular fibrillation.

Basic life support or cardiopulmonary resuscitation (CPR) is readily carried out without the use of any adjunctive equipment or drug therapy. As described in the following, basic life support consists of airway maintenance, artificial ventilation, and external chest compression of the victim so that a continuous supply of oxygenated blood is delivered to the brain and heart, thereby preventing nonreversible (biologic) death.

CARDIOPULMONARY ARREST

Although disease of the cardiovascular system is the most common cause of sudden death (cardiopulmonary arrest), many other life-threatening situations may also terminate in this clinical entity (Table 30-2). Regardless of the precise nature of the cause, it is imperative that cardiac arrest be recognized and managed in as short a time as possible, thereby minimizing the period of anoxia.

Cardiopulmonary arrest is comprised of two specific entities: pulmonary arrest and cardiac arrest. Pulmonary, or respiratory, arrest occurs with cessation of effective respiratory movements, whereas cardiac arrest refers to the cessation of circulation or the presence of circulation inadequate to sustain life.

Respiratory arrest may develop in the absence of cardiac arrest. However, if respiratory arrest is unmanaged or if it is managed ineffectively, cardiac function rapidly deteriorates with cardiac arrest supervening in a short period of time, depending in part on the degree of oxygen deprivation. Cardiac arrest can occur in the absence of respiratory arrest (for example, with electric shock); however, this is quite rare, and in such circumstances respiratory arrest inevitably follows within a few seconds. In most instances, respiratory arrest precedes cardiac arrest.

Table 30-1. Survival rate from cardiac arrest resulting from ventricular fibrillation, as related to promptness of initiation of CPR and ACLS*

Initiation of CPR (minutes)	Arrival of ACLS (minutes)	Survival rate (%)
0-4	0-8	43
0-4	16+	10
8-12	8-16	6
8-12	16+	0
12+	12+	0

From Eisenberg, M.S., Bergner, L., and Hallstrom, A.: JAMA **241:**1905, 1979.
*Data from Project Restart, King County, Washington.

Table 30-2. Possible causes of cardiac arrest*

Cause	Frequency	Where discussed in text
Myocardial infarction	Most common	Chest pain (Section VII)
Sudden death (no other symptoms)	Most common	Cardiac arrest (Chapter 30)
Airway obstruction	Common	Respiratory difficulty (Section III)
Drug overdose reaction	Common	Drug-related emergencies (Section VI)
Anaphylaxis	Less common	Drug-related emergencies (Section VI)
Seizure disorders	Less common	Seizure disorders (Section V)
Acute adrenal insufficiency	Less common	Unconsciousness (Section II)

*All medical emergency situations may ultimately lead to cardiac arrest. In most instances, prompt recognition and initiation of effective management of the specific situation prevents cardiac arrest from happening.

Pulmonary (Respiratory) Arrest

Recognition and management of respiratory arrest have previously been described. The reader is referred to Chapter 5 for a full discussion.

Cardiac Arrest

The term cardiac arrest must be defined to prevent possible confusion. At one time, cardiac arrest was used to indicate that the heart had stopped beating, a situation today referred to as ventricular standstill or *asystole*. The meaning of the term cardiac arrest has been expanded to include other clinical situations in which the circulation of blood is absent or, if present, is inadequate to maintain life. Cardiac arrest as defined today may therefore result from any of the following: electromechanical dissociation, ventricular fibrillation, or ventricular standstill (asystole) (Fig. 30-1).

In electromechanical dissociation, the heart is still beating but so weakly that effective circulation of blood throughout the cardiovascular system is not accomplished. This situation may be caused by drugs, including local anesthetics, barbiturates, and narcotics, all of which are used in dentistry (see Chapter 23). It may also result from severe hemorrhage and shock.

Ventricular fibrillation is a dysrhythmia in which the individual myocardial muscle bundles contract independently of each other as opposed to the normal regular, coordinated, and synchronized contraction of myocardial fibers. Although myocardial elements are still contracting, little or no effective circulation is present. Ventricular fibrillation is a common occurrence in the period immediately following myocardial infarction (within the first 2 to 4 hours) and is the leading cause of death from ischemic heart disease. In humans, ventricular fibrillation is 15 times more frequent during the first hour after the onset of signs and symptoms of acute myocardial infarction than during the following 12 hours.

Ventricular standstill or asystole refers to the absence of contractile movements of the myocardial fibers. Cardiac arrest in its strictest sense refers to ventricular standstill. A severe lack of oxygen to the myocardial muscle is the most common cause of this situation.

Although there are several forms of cardiac arrest (asystole, fibrillation, and electromechanical dissociation), in an emergency the precise nature of the arrest is not immediately relevant. The clinical picture of all three is the same: The victim loses consciousness, and respiration, blood pressure, and pulse are absent. Time is of the essence, because every second that passes without effective circulation adds to the degree of hypoxia or anoxia in the tissues of the body and to the development of respiratory and metabolic acidosis, all factors which make effective resuscitation less likely to occur.

Immediate clinical management of cardiopulmonary arrest is therefore based on the need to furnish the victim with a supply of well-oxygenated blood adequate to maintain life (prevent clinical death) until definitive management may be initiated.

CARDIOPULMONARY RESUSCITATION

The technique of cardiopulmonary resuscitation (CPR) has undergone intensive scrutiny by various segments of the medical community. Standardization of technique is being sought so that teaching of the procedures will not lead to confusion among those called on to use them.

In May 1973, the American Heart Association and the National Academy of Sciences National Research Council cosponsored a National Conference on Standards of Cardiopulmonary Resuscitation (CPR) and Emergency Cardiac Care (ECC), which for the first time presented standardized procedures for basic and advanced life support (American Heart Association, 1974). In the years since the first conference a significant body of research has added to our understanding of the phenomenon of cardiac arrest and cardiopulmonary resuscitation. In 1979 and 1985, a second and third conference, respectively, were called to update these standards. The techniques of basic life support described in the following material and elsewhere in this text are those recommended by the 1985 conference.*

Two broad areas of training in life support were established at these conferences. Basic life support and advanced cardiac life support represent differing degrees of training and responsibility in the management of the victim of cardiac arrest and implementation of cardiopulmonary resuscitation to maintain life until a victim recovers sufficiently to be transported to a hospital or until advanced life support is available. Basic life support includes the

---

*See "Standards and guidelines for cardiopulmonary resuscitation (CPR) and emergency cardiac care (ECC)," *Journal of the American Medical Association,* **255:**2905, 1986.

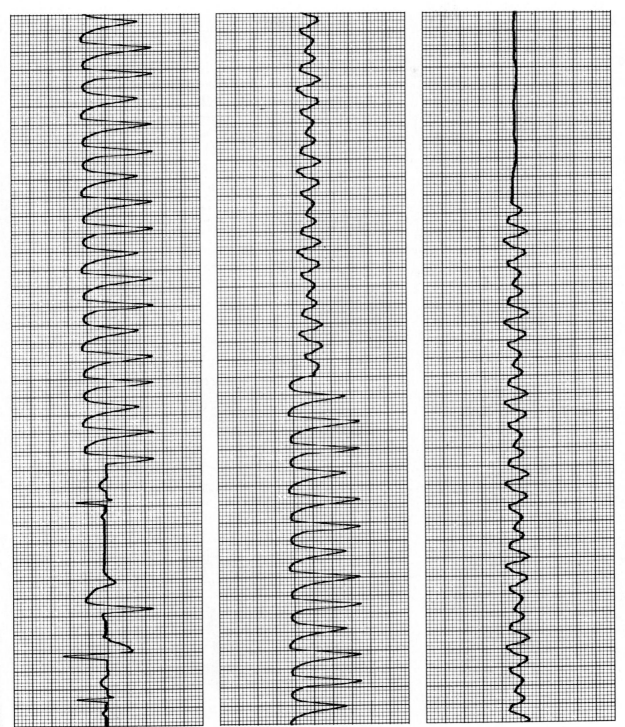

Fig. 30-1. Dysrhythmias leading to cardiac arrest. *Top,* premature ventricular contraction (PVC) leading to ventricular tachycardia (VT); *middle,* VT leading to ventricular fibrillation (VF); *bottom,* VF leading to asystole.

ABC steps of cardiopulmonary resuscitation (Fig. 30-2). Advanced life support consists of training in the following areas: basic life support; use of adjunctive equipment and techniques such as endotracheal intubation and open chest internal cardiac compression; cardiac monitoring (electrocardiography) for recognition of dysrhythmias; defibrillation technique; establishment of an intravenous infusion; stabilization of the victim's condition; and the employment and use of definitive therapy, including administration of drugs to correct acidosis and to assist in establishing and maintaining an effective cardiac rhythm and circulation.

The level of training in life support varies according to an individual's requirements. I recommend that all dental office personnel receive certification in *basic life support course C,* at the very least. More and more frequently today, dentists are receiving training and certification in advanced cardiac life support. Training at this level is valuable because of the potential complications associated with the administration of drugs in dental practice,

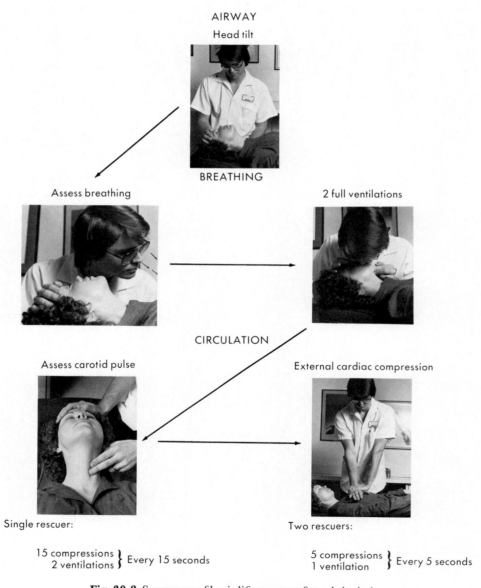

AIRWAY
Head tilt

BREATHING

Assess breathing

2 full ventilations

CIRCULATION

Assess carotid pulse

External cardiac compression

Single rescuer:

15 compressions ⎫
2 ventilations ⎬ Every 15 seconds

Two rescuers:

5 compressions ⎫
1 ventilation ⎬ Every 5 seconds

Fig. 30-2. Summary of basic life support for adult victim.

such as local anesthetics, antibiotics, analgesics, and sedatives. All other dental office personnel (dental hygienists, dental assistants, and nonchairside personnel) should be knowledgeable in, and capable of, proper application of the techniques of basic life support (at the BLS course C level).

Training in BLS should be repeated at least annually by all office personnel and if possible more frequently. Weaver and others (1979) demonstrated that retention of skills by trainees who do not perform CPR regularly is quite limited. Only 11.7% of 61 trainees were capable of properly performing one-person CPR on mannequins, compared to 85% of the same group 6 months earlier.

BLS courses are sponsored by many organizations, including the American Heart Association, American Red Cross, dental societies, and fire departments. The BLS level C program involves training in four areas:

1. Single-rescuer CPR
2. Two-rescuer (team) CPR
3. Obstructed airway
4. Pediatric basic life support

Table 30-3 lists the various levels of training provided by the American Heart Association.

Team Approach

In no other life-threatening situation is prompt recognition and management of greater importance than in cardiac arrest. Although it is possible for a single individual to effectively perform cardiopulmonary resuscitation, the procedure becomes even more efficient when a trained team of rescuers is available. The team approach to basic life support is described below (two-rescuer sequence). Dental office personnel should receive their training together so that they may interact effectively as a team when called on to do so.

Basic Life Support

As mentioned earlier, basic life support consists of the application (as needed) of the procedures of airway maintenance (A), breathing (B), and circulation by means of chest compression (C) to the victim of any medical emergency (including cardiac arrest) until recovery, or until the victim can be stabilized and transported to an emergency care facility or until advanced life support is available.

Two of the three components of cardiopulmonary resuscitation have previously been discussed. Airway maintenance and artificial ventilation in the unconscious patient are outlined in Chapter 5; lower airway obstruction is discussed in Chapter 11. Together these comprise the A and B parts of cardiopulmonary resuscitation. Fig. 30-2 summarizes the important steps of basic life support.

Witnessed and Unwitnessed Cardiac Arrest

In the management of cardiac arrest, two separate clinical situations are considered (see box below and on p. 389). In *unwitnessed cardiac arrest* the victim is unconscious when discovered by the rescuer. The rescuer has not seen the victim collapse and consequently has no knowledge as to the length of time since the cessation of breathing and

Table 30-3. Levels of certification, American Heart Association

Basic life support	Advanced cardiac life support
National faculty	
Affiliate faculty	
Instructor-trainer	Instructor-trainer
Instructor	Instructor
Provider	Provider

BLS course A: Heart-saver + adult obstructed airway

BLS course B: Heart-saver + adult and pediatric obstructed airways + pediatric BLS module (for lay-persons)

BLS course C: Heart-saver + adult and pediatric obstructed airways + pediatric one- and two-rescuer CPR (for health-care professionals)

BLS course D: Pediatric CPR + pediatric obstructed airway

BLS course E: For specially defined populations such as physically challenged

---

MANAGEMENT OF WITNESSED, MONITORED CARDIAC ARREST

Step 1 Recognize unconsciousness
  2 Call for help; position patient
  3 Deliver single precordial thump
  4 Open airway
  5 Check for breathing
  6 Ventilate four times
  7 Check carotid artery
  8 Begin external chest compression
     Single rescuer—15:2 ratio
     Team rescue—5:1 ratio

Text continued on p. 376.

CPR and ECC Performance Sheet
One-Rescuer CPR: Adult

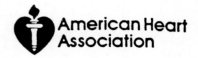
American Heart Association

Name _____   Date _____

Step	Activity	Critical Performance	S	U
1. Airway	Assessment: Determine unresponsiveness.	Tap or gently shake shoulder.		
		Shout "Are you OK?"		
	Call for help.	Call out "Help!"		
	Position the victim.	Turn on back as unit, if necessary, supporting head and neck (4–10 sec).		
	Open the airway.	Use head-tilt/chin-lift maneuver.		
2. Breathing	Assessment: Determine breathlessness.	Maintain open airway.		
		Ear over mouth, observe chest: look, listen, feel for breathing (3–5 sec).		
	Ventilate twice.	Maintain open airway.		
		Seal mouth and nose properly.		
		Ventilate 2 times at 1–1.5 sec/inspiration.		
		Observe chest rise (adequate ventilation volume.)		
		Allow deflation between breaths.		
3. Circulation	Assessment: Determine pulselessness.	Feel for carotid pulse on near side of victim (5–10 sec).		
		Maintain head-tilt with other hand.		
	Activate EMS system.	If someone responded to call for help, send him/her to activate EMS system.		
		Total time, Step 1—Activate EMS system: 15–35 sec.		
	Begin chest compressions.	Rescuer kneels by victim's shoulders.		
		Landmark check prior to hand placement.		
		Proper hand position throughout.		
		Rescuer's shoulders over victim's sternum.		
		Equal compression—relaxation.		
		Compress 1 1/2 to 2 inches.		
		Keep hands on sternum during upstroke.		
		Complete chest relaxation on upstroke.		
		Say any helpful mnemonic.		
		Compression rate: 80–100/min (15 per 9–11 sec).		
4. Compression/Ventilation Cycles	Do 4 cycles of 15 compressions and 2 ventilations.	Proper compression/ventilation ratio: 15 compressions to 2 ventilations per cycle.		
		Observe chest rise: 1–1.5 sec/inspiration; 4 cycles/52–73 sec.		
5. Reassessment*	Determine pulselessness. (If no pulse: Step 6.)†	Feel for carotid pulse (5 sec).		
6. Continue CPR	Ventilate twice.	Ventilate 2 times.		
		Observe chest rise; 1–1.5 sec/inspiration.		
	Resume compression/ventilation cycles.	Feel for carotid pulse every few minutes.		

* 2nd rescuer arrives to replace 1st rescuer: (a) 2nd rescuer identifies self by saying "I know CPR. Can I help?" (b) 2nd rescuer then does pulse check in Step 5 and continues with Step 6. (During practice and testing only one rescuer actually ventilates the manikin. The 2nd rescuer simulates ventilation.) (c) 1st rescuer assesses the adequacy of 2nd rescuer's CPR by observing chest rise during ventilations and by checking the pulse during chest compressions.

† If pulse is present, open airway and check for spontaneous breathing: (a) If breathing is present, maintain open airway and monitor pulse and breathing. (b) If breathing is absent, perform rescue breathing at 12 times/min and monitor pulse.

Instructor _____   Check: Satisfactory _____ Unsatisfactory _____
4/86

CPR and ECC Performance Sheet
Two-Rescuer CPR: Adult*

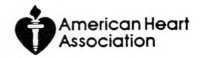
American Heart Association

Name _____ Date _____

Step	Activity	Critical Performance	S	U
1. Airway	One rescuer (ventilator): Assessment: Determines unresponsiveness.	Tap or gently shake shoulder.		
		Shout "Are you OK?"		
	Positions the victim.	Turn on back if necessary (4–10 sec).		
	Opens the airway.	Use a proper technique to open airway.		
2. Breathing	Assessment: Determines breathlessness.	Look, listen and feel (3–5 sec).		
	Ventilator ventilates twice.	Observe chest rise: 1–1.5 sec/inspiration.		
3. Circulation	Assessment: Determines pulselessness.	Palpate carotid pulse (5–10 sec).		
	States assessment results.	Say "No pulse."		
	Other rescuer (compressor): Gets into position for compressions.	Hands. shoulders in correct position.		
	Locates landmark notch.	Landmark check.		
4. Compression/Ventilation Cycles	Compressor begins chest compressions.	Correct ratio compressions/ventilations: 5/1.		
		Compression rate: 80–100/min (5 compressions/3–4 sec).		
		Say any helpful mnemonic.		
		Stop compressing for each ventilation.		
	Ventilator ventilates after every 5th compression and checks compression effectiveness.	Ventilate 1 time (1–1.5 sec). Check pulse to assess compressions.		
	(Minimum of 10 cycles.)	Time for 10 cycles: 40–53 sec.		
5. Call for Switch	Compressor calls for switch when fatigued.	Give clear signal to change.		
		Compressor completes 5th compression.		
		Ventilator completes ventilation after 5th compression.		
6. Switch	Simultaneously switch:			
	Ventilator moves to chest.	Move to chest.		
		Become compressor.		
		Get into position for compressions.		
		Locate landmark notch.		
	Compressor moves to head.	Move to head.		
		Become ventilator.		
		Check carotid pulse (5 sec).		
		Say "No pulse."		
		Ventilate once.†		
7. Continue CPR	Resume compression/ventilation cycles.	Resume Step 4.		

* (a) If CPR is in progress with one rescuer (lay person), the entrance of the two rescuers occurs after the completion of one rescuer's cycle of 15 compressions and 2 ventilations. The EMS should be activated first. The two new rescuers start with Step 6. (b) If CPR is in progress with one professional rescuer, the entrance of a second professional res- cuer is at the end of a cycle after check for pulse by first rescuer. The new cycle starts with one ventilation by the first rescuer, and the se- cond rescuer becomes the compressor.

† During practice and testing only one rescuer actually ventilates the manikin. The other rescuer simulates ventilation.

Instructor _____ Check: Satisfactory _____ Unsatisfactory _____

CPR and ECC Performance Sheet
One Rescuer CPR: Infant

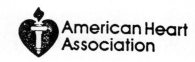
American Heart Association

Name _____ Date _____

Step	Activity	Critical Performance	S	U
1. Airway	Assessment: Determine unresponsiveness.	Tap or gently shake shoulder.		
	Call for help.	Call out "Help!"		
	Position the infant.	Turn on back as unit. supporting head and neck.		
		Place on firm, hard surface.		
	Open the airway.	Use head-tilt/chin-lift maneuver to sniffing or neutral position.		
		Do not overextend the head.		
2. Breathing	Assessment: Determine breathlessness.	Maintain open airway.		
		Ear over mouth, observe chest: look, listen, feel for breathing (3–5 sec).		
	Ventilate twice.	Maintain open airway.		
		Make tight seal on infant's mouth and nose with rescuer's mouth.		
		Ventilate 2 times, 1–1.5 sec/inspiration.		
		Observe chest rise.		
		Allow deflation between breaths.		
3. Circulation	Assessment: Determine pulselessness.	Feel for brachial pulse (5–10 sec).		
		Maintain head-tilt with other hand.		
	Activate EMS system.	If someone responded to call for help, send him/her to activate EMS system.		
		Total time, Step 1–Activate EMS system: 15–35 sec.		
	Begin chest compressions.	Draw imaginary line between nipples.		
		Place 2–3 fingers on sternum, 1 finger's width below imaginary line.		
		Equal compression-relaxation.		
		Compress vertically, 1/2 to 1 inches.		
		Keep fingers on sternum during upstroke.		
		Complete chest relaxation on upstroke.		
		Say any helpful mnemonic.		
		Compression rate: at least 100/min (5 in 3 sec or less).		
4. Compression/Ventilation Cycles	Do 10 cycles of 5 compressions and 1 ventilation.	Proper compression/ventilation ratio: 5 compressions to 1 slow ventilation per cycle.		
		Pause for ventilation.		
		Observe chest rise: 1–1.5 sec/inspiration; 10 cycles/45 sec or less.		
5. Reassessment	Determine pulselessness. (If no pulse: Step 6.)*	Feel for brachial pulse (5 sec).		
6. Continue CPR	Ventilate once.	Ventilate 1 time.		
		Observe chest rise; 1–1.5 sec/inspiration.		
	Resume compression/ventilation cycles.	Feel for brachial pulse every few minutes.		

* If pulse is present, open airway and check for spontaneous breathing. (a) If breathing is present, maintain open airway and monitor breathing and pulse. (b) If breathing is absent, perform rescue breathing at 20 times/min and monitor pulse.

Instructor _____ Check: Satisfactory _____ Unsatisfactory _____

4/86

CPR and ECC Performance Sheet
One-Rescuer CPR: Child*

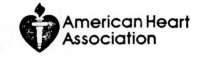 American Heart Association

Name _____ Date _____

Step	Activity	Critical Performance	S	U
1. Airway	Assessment: Determine unresponsiveness.	Tap or gently shake shoulder.		
		Shout "Are you OK?"		
	Call for help.	Call out "Help!"		
	Position the victim.	Turn on back as unit, if necessary, supporting head and neck (4–10 sec).		
	Open the airway.	Use head-tilt/chin-lift maneuver.		
2. Breathing	Assessment: Determine breathlessness.	Maintain open airway.		
		Ear over mouth, observe chest: look, listen, feel for breathing (3–5 sec).		
	Ventilate twice.	Maintain open airway.		
		Seal mouth and nose properly.		
		Ventilate 2 times at 1–1.5 sec/inspiration.		
		Observe chest rise.		
		Allow deflation between breaths.		
3. Circulation	Assessment: Determine pulselessness.	Feel for carotid pulse on near side of victim (5–10 sec).		
		Maintain head-tilt with other hand.		
	Activate EMS system.	If someone responded to call for help, send him/her to activate EMS system.		
		Total time, Step 1—Activate EMS system: 15–35 sec.		
	Begin chest compressions.	Rescuer kneels by victim's shoulders.		
		Landmark check prior to initial hand placement.		
		Proper hand position throughout.		
		Rescuer's shoulders over victim's sternum.		
		Equal compression–relaxation.		
		Compress 1 to 1 1/2 inches.		
		Keep hands on sternum during upstroke.		
		Complete chest relaxation on upstroke.		
		Say any helpful mnemonic.		
		Compression rate: 80–100/min (5 per 3–4 sec).		
4. Compression/Ventilation Cycles	Do 10 cycles of 5 compressions and 1 ventilation.	Proper compression/ventilation ratio: 5 compressions to 1 slow ventilation per cycle.		
		Observe chest rise, 1–1.5 sec/inspiration (10 cycles/60–87 sec).		
5. Reassessment†	Determine pulselessness. (If no pulse: Step 6.)‡	Feel for carotid pulse (5 sec).		
6. Continue CPR	Ventilate once.	Ventilate one time.		
		Observe chest rise; 1–1.5 sec/inspiration.		
	Resume compression/ventilation cycles	Palpate carotid pulse every few minutes.		

* If child is above age of approximately 8 years, the method for adults should be used.

† 2nd rescuer arrives to replace 1st rescuer: (a) 2nd rescuer identifies self by saying "I know CPR. Can I help?" (b) 2nd rescuer then does pulse check in Step 5 and continues with Step 6. (During practice and testing only one rescuer actually ventilates the manikin. The 2nd rescuer simulates ventilation.) (c) 1st rescuer assesses the adequacy of 2nd rescuer's CPR by observing chest rise during ventilations and by checking the pulse during chest compressions.

‡ If pulse is present, open airway and check for spontaneous breathing. (a) If breathing is present, maintain open airway and monitor breathing and pulse. (b) If breathing is absent, perform rescue breathing at 15 times/min and monitor pulse.

Instructor _____ Check: Satisfactory _____ Unsatisfactory _____

4/86

effective circulation. In such circumstances, it must be assumed that the collapse occurred more than 1 minute before the victim was discovered and the institution of basic life support procedures. In this situation, the myocardium is considered to be hypoxic, and the sequence of steps of basic life support is predicated on this fact. The *witnessed cardiac arrest* differs in that it develops in an ECG-monitored patient in the presence of the rescuer, and the steps of basic life support can be administered within 1 minute of the collapse. The sequence of management differs slightly in this situation because of the probability that the myocardium is still fairly well oxygenated at the time life support procedures are begun.

Cardiopulmonary arrest that occurs in a patient not monitored by ECG, even if the arrest is witnessed, is categorized and managed the same as is an unwitnessed cardiac arrest.

The recommended sequence of steps in the management of each of these situations is presented below. Unless the rescuer is absolutely certain that the cardiopulmonary collapse occurred within 1 minute of discovery, it must be assumed that the heart is hypoxic, and the sequence of unwitnessed cardiac arrest must be followed. Most cardiac arrests are of the unwitnessed type; however, within the dental office setting it is highly likely that office personnel will be available within 60 seconds of the collapse. Since in June 1977 the American Heart Association changed the criteria for the witnessed cardiac arrest to include only those situations in which the cardiac arrest occurs in an electrocardiographically monitored patient, the major emphasis of this section is on the unwitnessed cardiac arrest.

Cardiac Arrest in the Dental Office

Cardiac arrest (as well as any other life-threatening situation) may occur anywhere within the dental office. Medical emergencies have occurred in the waiting room, restroom, laboratory, and doctor's office, as well as in the treatment room. In all situations the victim must be placed in the supine position so that BLS may be initiated. It is possible that the victim of cardiopulmonary arrest may be seated in the dental chair at the time of collapse. The question that must then be asked is: can effective cardiopulmonary resuscitation be carried out with the victim in the dental chair? In past years, before the advent of the contoured dental chair, the answer might have been yes. However, with the

introduction of dental chairs designed for maximal comfort, it has become more difficult to adequately carry out chest compression if the victim is permitted to remain in the chair. The heart lies between two bony masses—the sternum, located anteriorly, and the spinal column, located posteriorly. With compression of the sternum toward the spinal column, intrathoracic pressure is raised, compressing the heart and blood vessels and thereby producing cardiac output. If the victim is lying on a soft object (mattress or comfortable dental chair), the spinal column flexes and the force of the compression is partially absorbed by the soft surface, thereby lessening the effectiveness of the sternal compression. When properly performed (against a hard surface), external chest compression can produce systolic blood pressure peaks of 100 torr, but the diastolic blood pressure is 0. The mean arterial blood pressure is rarely greater than 40 torr as measured in the carotid arteries. Blood flow through the carotid arteries to the cerebral circulation therefore is approximately only one quarter to one third of normal, at best. BLS performed on a soft backing proves even less effective and is therefore contraindicated.

It is usually recommended that the victim of cardiac arrest be removed from the dental chair and placed on the floor if at all possible so that BLS may be performed in a more effective manner. In many dental operatories, however, there is little or no room available on the floor on which to place the victim and still permit one or two rescuers to perform BLS. In such a situation, or if it is difficult or impossible to move a victim to the floor, BLS should be initiated with the patient in the chair. If possible, a hard object such as a solid wooden board (for example, a removable cabinet top) should be placed under the victim to support the spinal cord (Fig. 30-3). *Under no circumstances should basic life support be withheld or delayed because of the inability to move the victim to a more suitable location.*

•   •   •

In all of the following sequences, it is assumed that the patient (victim) has suffered a cardiac arrest—that is, the victim is unconscious and there is an absence of both respiration and circulation. *It is critically important for the reader to fully understand that these basic steps (ABC) are equally important in the management of ALL emergency situations—not just cardiac arrest.*

As has been demonstrated throughout this book,

one of the initial steps in the management of every emergency situation is the implementation, as needed, of the steps of basic life support. What this means is that in every situation that is considered an emergency by the doctor or any "rescuer," the steps listed below must be followed:

1. Level of consciousness assessed
2. Assistance summoned
3. Proper positioning of the victim
4. Assessment of patency of the airway (**A**) and maintenance of airway patency, if necessary
5. Assessment of spontaneous respirations (breathing, **B**) and application of artificial ventilation, if required
6. Assessment of the adequacy of circulation (**C**); if absent, activation of the emergency medical services system and application of external chest compressions

Patient response to these various steps will guide rescuers in their management. In many instances in which the victim is conscious (for example, respiratory difficulty, altered consciousness), the rescuer need only to assess A, B, and C—a process requiring only several seconds. The patient will be seen to be effectively managing A, B, and C by himself or herself, allowing the rescuer to continue to step D—definitive management.

In another situation, the rescuer may determine that the victim is unconscious. Assessment of the airway and head tilt–chin lift are required; however, assessment of B and C demonstrate adequacy of spontaneous breathing and effective pulse. The rescuer need only maintain an airway while considering the definitive management of the situation.

This must be kept in mind as the following material is read. Although A, B, and C are always assessed in every emergency situation, only those elements that are necessary for the victim's survival will be instituted clinically.

BASIC LIFE SUPPORT
Unwitnessed Cardiac Arrest

When cardiac arrest occurs in an unmonitored victim, the procedures described as follows for unwitnessed cardiac arrest must be instituted. Following the description of these steps, we will review the basic sequences for the *one-person rescue* and the *team rescue.*

The following sequence of steps should be rapidly carried out by the rescuer.

Step 1. Recognize unconsciousness. Stimulate the victim by gently shaking the shoulders and shouting. Lack of response to these sensory stimuli is a suitable criterion for establishing a diagnosis of unconsciousness (Fig. 30-4).

Many factors may be responsible for unconsciousness (Table 5-1), most of which do not lead immediately to respiratory and cardiac arrest. However, prompt management of unconsciousness from any cause follows the same format—basic life support. A differential diagnosis is reached

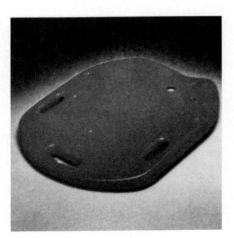

Fig. 30-3. CPR board to support victim's back and spinal cord during external chest compression.

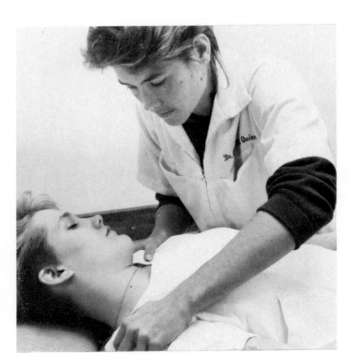

Fig. 30-4. Assess unconsciousness; shake and shout.

through the response or lack of response of the victim to each of these steps.

Step 2. Summon assistance and position patient. The rescuer will not want to treat the victim alone, therefore assistance should be called for as soon as unconsciousness is recognized. Members of the office emergency team should report to the emergency area with the drug emergency kit and a supply of oxygen and should be prepared to assist as required. This step does NOT involve activation of the emergency medical services system, just the dental office emergency team.

The patient should be placed in the supine position. The head and chest are placed parallel to the floor and the feet elevated slightly (10 degrees) to facilitate return of blood from the periphery. At this time (before determination of cardiovascular collapse), it is not yet necessary to place the victim on a hard surface. Once pulselessness is established, this procedure will be necessary.

Step 3. Assess and maintain airway. Head tilt combined with chin lift may be employed to obtain a patent airway. The rescuer places one hand on the victim's forehead, the other hand on the bony prominence of the chin (symphysis). The head is extended backward, which stretches the tissues in the neck and lifts the tongue off the posterior wall of the pharynx (Fig. 30-5). Head tilt is the single most important procedure in airway maintenance. Should head tilt be ineffective in establishing a patent airway, the jaw-thrust maneuver can be employed.

Step 4. Assess breathing and ventilate, if needed. While maintaining head tilt, the rescuer places her ear approximately 1 inch from the victim's mouth and nose so that any exhaled air may be felt and heard. The rescuer looks toward the chest of the victim to see if respiratory efforts are visible (Fig. 30-6). With cardiopulmonary arrest, respiratory efforts are absent or are so weak as to be virtually nonexistent.

Step 5. Artificial ventilation. In the absence of effective respiratory movement, artificial ventilation must immediately be started. Several techniques of artificial ventilation are discussed in Chapter 5; however, in this section only one—mouth-to-mouth ventilation—is considered. Other techniques may also be used, but it must be remembered that *no technique of artificial ventilation is effective unless a patent airway is maintained throughout the ventilatory process.* Most other devices for artificial ventilation require advanced training (advanced cardiac life support) to adequately prepare the rescuer to use them.

To perform mouth-to-mouth ventilation, head

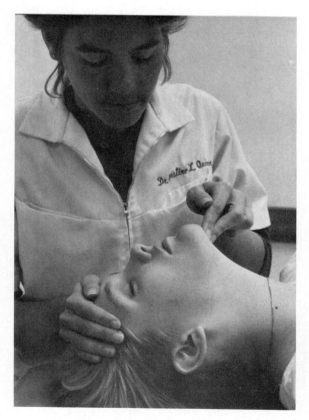

Fig. 30-5. Head tilt–chin lift.

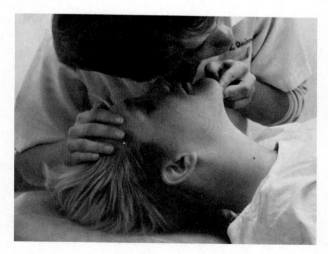

Fig. 30-6. Assess breathing: look, listen, and feel while maintaining head tilt–chin lift.

tilt must be maintained and the nose of the victim sealed (Fig. 30-7). The first ventilatory cycle is comprised of two full ventilations with adequate time (1 to 1½ seconds per breath) allowed to provide good chest expansion and decrease the possibility of gastric distention. Effective artificial ventilation is noted by the expansion of the chest of the victim. In the normal adult, the minimal volume should be 800 ml but need not exceed 1200 ml of air for adequate ventilation. Exhalation is a passive process. The rescuer removes her mouth from that of the victim, takes in a breath of fresh air, and watches the chest fall. Subsequent ventilations are performed at a rate of one every 5 seconds (12 per minute) for the adult victim. In the child, ventilations are carried out at a rate of one every 4 seconds (15 per minute), and in the infant, one every 3 seconds (20 per minute). Immediately after the first ventilatory cycle of two full breaths, the rescuer should determine the victim's cardiovascular status.

Step 6. Assess circulation. Having provided for oxygenation of the blood, the rescuer determines the presence or absence of effective circulation. A large artery must be located and carefully palpated. The femoral artery in the groin or the carotid artery in the neck are two large, central arteries. Although either may be palpated, the carotid artery is preferred. It is located in the neck region and can be reached easily without disrobing the victim. In addition, the carotid artery transports oxygenated blood to the victim's brain, which is an organ that must be perfused adequately if effective resuscitation is to be achieved.

The carotid artery is located in a groove between the trachea and the sternocleidomastoid muscle on the anterolateral aspect of the neck (Fig. 30-8). The fleshy portions of the first and second fingers should be used to feel for a pulse. Up to 10 seconds should be allowed for this procedure because the pulse, if present, may be very slow or very weak and rapid. The thumb should *never* be used to monitor pulse rate, because the thumb contains a medium-sized artery and the pulse rate recorded may be the rescuer's instead of the victim's. Unless the carotid pulse is unquestionably present, external chest compression must be initiated immediately. At this point the victim should be placed on the floor, if possible, or a hard object such as a removable table top or CPR board should be placed under the victim's back.

Step 7. Activate emergency medical system (EMS). The EMS should be activated following the check of the pulse. Many cities have a universal emergency number, 911; however, the appropriate telephone number for your locality should be

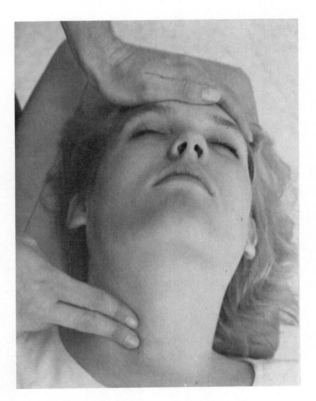

Fig. 30-8. Locate carotid artery in groove between trachea and sternocleidomastoid muscle. Head tilt must be maintained.

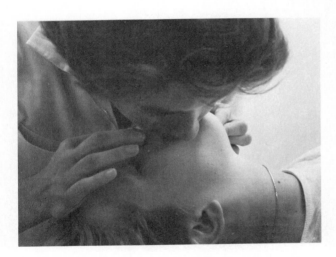

Fig. 30-7. Mouth-to-mouth ventilation.

called. Information given to the EMS dispatcher should include the following:

1. Where the emergency is (with names of cross streets if possible)
2. Number of telephone from which the call is made
3. What happened (heart attack, seizure, accident, etc.)
4. How many persons need help
5. Condition of the victim(s)
6. What aid is being given to the victim(s)
7. Any other information requested

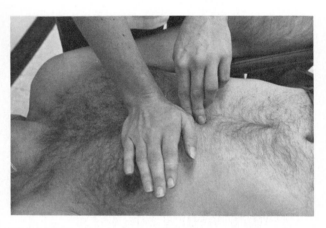

Fig. 30-9. Proper location for adult external chest compression.

To ensure that EMS personnel have no more questions, the caller should hang up last. When more than one rescuer is available, one person is sent immediately to activate the EMS. Eisenberg and others (1979) demonstrated that the shorter the time interval between collapse and the initiation of BLS and advanced cardiac life support, the greater the likelihood of survival for the victim of cardiac arrest (Table 30-1).

If only one rescuer is present, it is recommended that he continue BLS for 1 minute and then telephone for assistance as quickly as possible. Should the solo rescuer feel that there is a good chance of someone else arriving on the scene shortly, it may be decided to continue BLS until help arrives instead of making a telephone call. Should the rescuer be alone, with no telephone available, the only option is to continue BLS.

Step 8. External chest compression. External chest compression consists of the rhythmic application of pressure over the lower half of the adult sternum. The heart lies under and just to the left of the midline under the lower half of the sternum and above the spinal column. When the sternum is compressed, the intrathoracic pressure is increased; it is this increased pressure that produces cardiac output by compressing the vessels within the chest cavity and forcing blood back to and through the heart. With the release of this pressure,

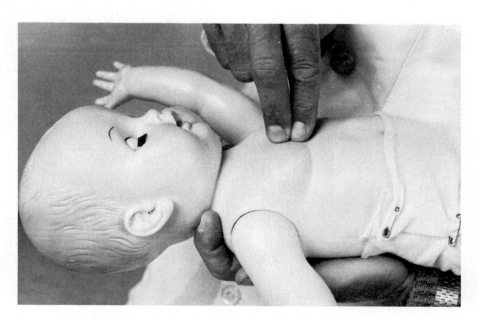

Fig. 30-10. Proper location for infant external chest compression.

blood from the periphery flows back into the heart to refill its chambers. Effective artificial ventilation and artificial circulation can provide sufficient oxygen to prevent cellular death. Two theories, the cardiac pump theory (Babbs, 1980) and the thoracic pump theory (Niemann et al., 1979), seek to explain the mechanism of blood flow during external chest compression.

Location of pressure point. To perform effective external chest compression and minimize injury to other organs (lungs, liver, heart), the rescuer's hands must be positioned properly. This area may be located by using the following maneuver (Fig. 30-9): The rescuer, located at the victim's shoulders, runs his middle finger in a superior direction along the lower border of the rib cage until the midline is reached. Directly below this midline notch (created by the convergence of the ribs) is the cartilaginous xiphoid process, which curves downward, and the liver. The rescuer's middle finger should be located in the notch, the index finger lying beside it on the lower border of the sternum. The rescuer then places the *heel* of the second hand over the midline of the sternum immediately next to the index finger. This is the proper location for external chest compression in an adult.

In the child (ages 1 to 8 years) the proper site for chest compression is located in a manner similar to that described for the adult:

1. The lower margin of the victim's rib cage is located with the rescuer's middle and index fingers.
2. The margin of the rib cage is followed with the middle finger to the notch in the midline where the right and left side ribs meet.
3. With the middle finger in this notch, the index finger is placed next to the middle finger.
4. The heel of the hand is placed next to the index finger with the long axis of the heel parallel to that of the sternum.
5. The chest is compressed with one hand to a depth of 1 to 1½ inches (2.5 to 3.8 cm) at a rate of 80 to 100 times per minute.

In the infant (under 1 year of age) the site for compression is somewhat different (Fig. 30-10). Recent evidence (Orlowski, 1984) has shown that the heart of the infant is lower in relation to external chest landmarks than was previously thought. Proper hand position for chest compression is located in the following manner:

1. An imaginary line is drawn between the nipples located over the sternum.

2. The index finger of the hand farthest from the infant's head is placed just under this intermammary line where it intersects the sternum. The area of compression is one finger's width below this intersection, at the location of the middle and ring fingers.
3. Using two or three fingers, the sternum is compressed to a depth of ½ to 1 inch (1.3 to 2.5 cm) at a rate of at least 100 compressions per minute.

Hand position. Having determined the proper location for chest compression, the rescuer must align the hands properly so that maximal effectiveness may be achieved. In the adult victim, the *heel* of the first hand is already in position on the midsternum of the victim approximately 1.5 to 2 inches (4 to 5 cm) above the xiphoid process. It is essential that only the heel of this hand be in contact with the chest wall. The heel of the second hand is next placed directly over the first hand, parallel to it (Fig. 30-11). The fingers of the two hands are then in-

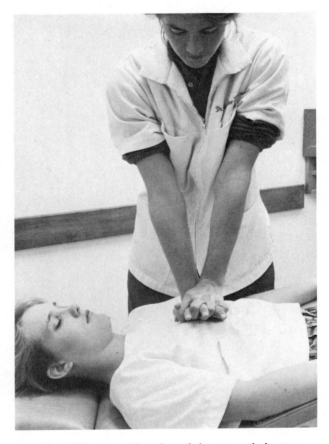

Fig. 30-11. Hand position for adult external chest compression.

terlaced, the fingers of the top hand pulling the fingers of the lower hand upward. In this manner, only the heel of the lower hand remains in contact with the victim's chest. An alternative hand position, especially useful for persons with arthritis of the hand or wrist, is to grasp the wrist of the hand on the chest with the hand that had been locating the lower end of the sternum.

These procedures are important because if the fingers of the hand contact the chest wall, the pressure exerted in chest compression will be applied over a larger area and will therefore be less effective in compressing the heart. In addition, this pressure will be exerted over the ribs, not the sternum, leading to probable rib fracture, with possible contusion and laceration of the heart and lungs.

Application of pressure. Having determined the location for chest compression and positioned the hands properly, the rescuer can begin chest com-

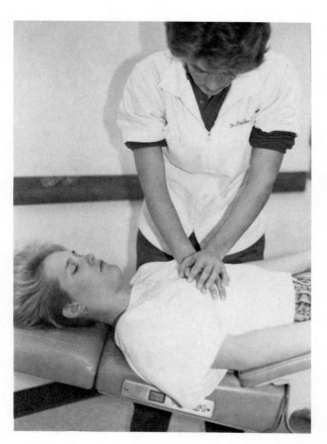

Fig. 30-12. Improper position: elbow of rescuer should be locked (straight), not bent.

pression. External chest compression (ECC) is strenuous. However, when the technique is performed properly, the trained rescuer does not become exhausted rapidly. Improperly performed external chest compression is rapidly exhausting, as well as ineffective. The following points facilitate the execution of ECC with maximal effectiveness and minimal fatigue: The shoulders of the rescuer must be located directly over the sternum of the victim, and the rescuer's arms should be locked straight (not bent) (Fig. 30-12). If the victim is lying on the floor, the rescuer must kneel beside the victim, close enough to the body that the rescuer's shoulders are directly over the victim's sternum. If the victim is in the dental chair, the rescuer stands astride the victim, and the chair is lowered so that proper positioning may be achieved (Fig. 30-13, *A*).

Improper positioning of the shoulders (at an angle to the sternum) decreases the effectiveness of chest compression and leads to the probability of complications related to costochondral separation (from stretching of ribs on one side) and fracture of ribs (from bending of ribs on the opposite side) (Fig. 30-13, *B*). Bending the elbows greatly decreases the effectiveness of chest compression and leads to rapid fatigue of the rescuer.

The rescuer then exerts pressure directly downward so that the sternum of the adult victim is depressed 1½ to 2 inches (3.8 to 5 cm). With proper shoulder and arm positioning, the rescuer allows the weight of his own body to depress the sternum of the victim. Movement of the rescuer occurs only at the hips, a gentle back-and-forth rocking motion, if the technique is properly executed. Compressions must be regular, smooth, and uninterrupted. Relaxation follows immediately and is of equal duration. The heel of the rescuer's hand must not be removed from the chest during relaxation, but pressure on the sternum should be completely released so that the sternum returns to its normal position between compressions.

The infant's chest is compressed ½ to 1 inch (1.3 to 2.5 cm) just below the intermammary line using the tips of two or three fingers, while the chest of the child is compressed 1 to 1½ inches (2.5 to 3.8 cm) using the heel of one hand (Fig. 30-14). Basic life support techniques for the adult, infant, and child are summarized in Table 30-4.

Rate of compression. The only change in rate from that recommended previously is to increase the compression rate. The rate of external chest compression should be increased to a minimum of

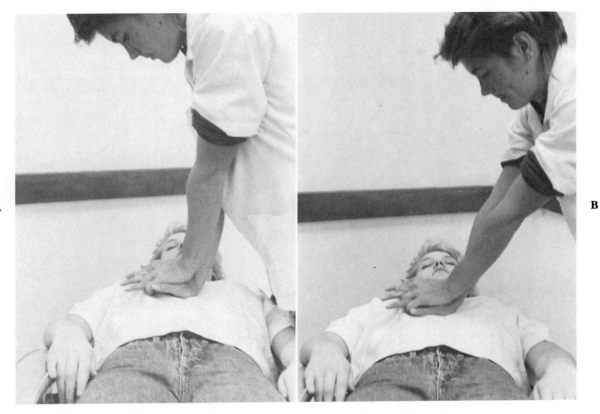

Fig. 30-13. A, Dental chair is lowered to allow rescuer to bring shoulders directly over sternum of victim. **B,** Improper positioning increases risk of injury to victim.

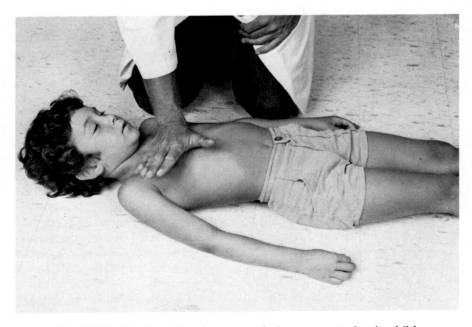

Fig. 30-14. Hand position for external chest compression in child.

Table 30-4. Summary of CPR techniques

Victim	Respirations per minute	Interval (seconds)	Ratio of compression to ventilation	Compressions				
				Rate/min	Depth (inches)	Depth (cm)	Hands	Site
Infant (<1 year of age)	20	3	5:1	100	½-1	1.3-2.5	2-3 fingers	One finger-width below intermammary line, midsternum
Child (1-8 years of age)	15	4	5:1	80-100	1-1½	2.5-3.8	1 heel	Midsternum
Adult (>8 years of age)	12	5	5:1	80-100	1½-2	3.8-5.0	2 hands	Lower half of sternum
One rescuer	8	—	15:2					
Two rescuers	12	—	5:1					

80 per minute, 100 per minute if possible. When BLS is being performed by a team of two persons, one rescuer is responsible for airway and breathing, whereas the second rescuer carries out chest compression. In this case, chest compression is performed at a rate of 80 to 100 per minute with artificial ventilation interspersed after every fifth compression. In the two-rescuer sequence, the ratio of chest compression to artificial ventilation is 5:1 with a pause of 1 to 1.5 seconds for ventilation.

When only one rescuer is available, that person is responsible for ventilation and chest compression. In the single-rescuer sequence the ratio of chest compression to artificial ventilation is 15:2. However, to compress the chest 60 times and to intersperse eight ventilations in 60 seconds, the rate of chest compressions must be faster than one per second. Fifteen chest compressions are followed by two full breaths, allowing 1 to 1.5 seconds per ventilation. Four complete cycles of 15 compressions and two ventilations should be completed in approximately 1 minute with a single rescuer. To do so effectively, it has been my experience that the 15 chest compressions should be completed in approximately 9 to 11 seconds. The remaining time permits the rescuer to move to the head, deliver two ventilations, relocate the site for chest compression, and prepare to restart chest compression.

In the infant and child, the compression to ventilation ratio is 5:1 for both single and team rescue. Compression rates are 100 per minute in infants, 80 to 100 per minute in the child. Fig. 30-2 summarizes the management of the unwitnessed cardiac arrest in the adult.

Single rescue for adults

Clinical application of the technique of basic life support for the single rescuer in a case of unwitnessed cardiac arrest is based on the techniques described earlier. When dealing with cardiac arrest and possible neurologic damage, the time element becomes critical. The chart on p. 372 presents performance criteria for one-rescuer CPR (American Heart Association).

The first steps in the sequence involve the recognition of unconsciousness, calling for assistance, and positioning the victim. The process of calling for help needs clarification: When the unconscious victim is located and the rescuer is alone, calling for help simply means yelling loudly for assistance. It does not mean leaving the victim to seek assistance, nor does it mean taking time to place a telephone call. Every second that is not spent performing BLS decreases the chance of recovery for the victim.

The rescuer is positioned so that artificial ventilation and artificial circulation may be carried out with minimal movement. The most nearly ideal position for the rescuer is astride the shoulders of the victim so that both procedures may be performed merely by bending at the waist.

Airway patency is ensured through the head tilt–chin lift or the jaw-thrust maneuver, or both, and the rescuer checks for spontaneous respiratory movement. In the absence of such movement, the rescuer ventilates the victim with two full breaths at 1 to 1.5 seconds per ventilation. Chest deflation should be noted between breaths.

With the blood of the victim now oxygenated, the

rescuer assesses the status of the circulation by palpating the carotid pulse. This important step should not be hurried; allow 5 to 10 seconds to determine pulselessness.

In the absence of effective circulation, the emergency medical services (EMS) system is activated, and external chest compression is immediately begun. The proper site for compression on the lower half of the adult sternum is located using the maneuver described earlier.

With elbows locked and shoulders directly over the sternum, the chest of the adult victim is depressed approximately 1½ to 2 inches (4 to 5 cm) at a rate of 80 to 100 compressions per minute. The rescuer should count silently or softly* to himself during this sequence and after 15 compressions immediately give two full lung inflations (1 to 1.5 seconds each), allowing complete lung deflation to occur between each breath. One complete 15:2 sequence should take approximately 15 seconds. The rescuer then immediately relocates the pressure point on the sternum and repeats the cycle of 15 compressions and two ventilations so that four complete cycles may be performed in approximately one minute. After the first four cycles and periodically thereafter, the rescuer stops to reassess the pulse and breathing of the victim.

Two-rescuer CPR for adults *(chart on p. 373)*

With two or more rescuers present to perform cardiopulmonary resuscitation, it is possible to carry out artificial ventilation and chest compressions without interruption. The new guidelines present two scenarios for two rescuers, both of which follow.

One-rescuer CPR with entry of a second rescuer. This scenario is recommended for use by persons who are not health care professionals.

When a second rescuer becomes available, he or she is sent immediately to activate the EMS system if this has not previously been done and to perform one-rescuer CPR in the event the first rescuer becomes fatigued. The following sequence is recommended:

1. Second rescuer identifies himself or herself as CPR certified and willing to help.
2. First rescuer stops CPR after two ventilations.

---

*Studies have shown that rescuers counting silently or softly can perform CPR effectively for longer durations than those counting out loud. It requires more energy expenditure to count aloud; however, when a second rescuer appears to aid, counting aloud is essential.

3. Second rescuer kneels down and checks pulse for 5 seconds.
4. If pulse is absent, second rescuer gives two breaths.
5. Then second rescuer begins external chest compression at a 15:2 ratio at a rate of 80 to 100 compressions per minute.
6. Meanwhile the first rescuer assesses the adequacy of the second rescuer's efforts.

CPR performed by two rescuers. This scenario is recommended for all health care professionals.

The use of mouth-to-mask ventilation is an acceptable alternative to mouth-to-mouth ventilation in this scenario since it is recommended that all health professionals be adequately trained to use such devices.

One person performs external chest compression while the second rescuer remains at the victim's head, maintains a patent airway, monitors the carotid pulse for adequacy of external chest compressions, and provides rescue breathing. The compression rate for two-rescuer CPR is 80 to 100 per minute with a pause of 1 to 1.5 seconds per ventilation and a compression/ventilation ratio of 5:1. When the compressor becomes fatigued, the rescuers should change position as soon as possible.

This sequence is used if one-rescuer CPR is in progress when the second rescuer arrives on the scene:

1. The most appropriate time for entrance of the second rescuer is immediately following the completion of a cycle of 15 compressions and 2 ventilations.
   a. One rescuer moves to the head of the victim, opens the airway, and checks for a pulse.
   b. The second rescuer (positioned on the opposite side of the victim (Fig. 30-15) locates the area for external chest compressions and finds the proper hand position.
2. If no pulse is present, the ventilator gives one breath and the compressor starts external chest compression at the rate of 80 to 100 per minute, counting "one-and, two-and, three-and, four-and, five."
3. After the fifth compression a pause of 1 to 1.5 seconds is allowed for ventilation.
4. The compression/ventilation ratio is 5:1.

In the event that no CPR is in progress and both professional rescuers arrive at the same time, the following sequence is followed: First, one rescuer ensures that the EMS system has been activated. If

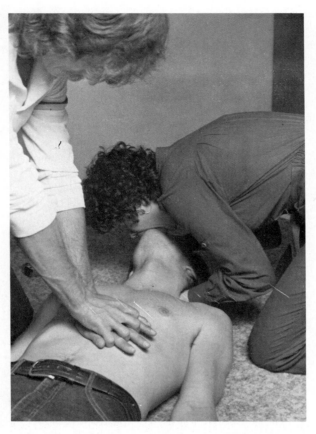

Fig. 30-15. Rescuer positions for two-person CPR.

this person must leave the area, the second rescuer initiates one-rescuer CPR. However, if both persons are available for CPR:

1. One rescuer goes to the head of the victim and
   a. Determines unresponsiveness ("shake and shout").
   b. Positions the victim.
   c. Opens the airway.
   d. Assesses breathing.
   e. If breathing is absent, says, "No breathing," and gives two ventilations.
   f. Assesses circulation.
   g. If pulse is absent, says, "No pulse."
2. The second rescuer simultaneously:
   a. Finds the location for external chest compression.
   b. Assumes the proper hand position.
   c. Initiates external chest compressions after the first rescuer states, "No pulse."

When one rescuer (usually the compressor) gets fatigued, the rescuers change position as rapidly as is possible. The sequence for change in two-rescuer

---

BASIC LIFE SUPPORT

Step 1 Recognize unconsciousness and call for help
   2 Position patient (supine)
   3 Open airway (head tilt–chin lift)
   4 Check for breathing and airway patency
      Jaw-thrust maneuver (if necessary)
      Check for breathing and airway patency (if necessary)
   5 Artificial ventilation (if necessary)
   6 Check circulation
   7 Activate EMS system
   8 External chest compression (if necessary)

CPR has been simplified in the new guidelines. The compressor calls for a switch when fatigued and completes the fifth compression. The ventilator then gives one full ventilation. Both rescuers then switch position. The original ventilator moves to the victim's chest, gets in position to administer external chest compressions, and locates the proper landmark for compressions. The original compressor moves to the victim's head, checks the carotid pulse for 5 seconds, and if it is absent says, "No pulse," and ventilates once. The new chest compressor immediately begins chest compression at the rate of 5 compressions in approximately 3 to 4 seconds. A total of 10 cycles of 5:1 should be completed in approximately 40 to 53 seconds.

The two-rescuer sequence is a more effective method of carrying out cardiopulmonary resuscitation, because it avoids interruptions in the cycle of chest compression that occur in the single-rescuer sequence. During the two-rescuer sequence it is also possible for the rescuers to change positions at any time, if desired. With the rescuers located on opposite sides of the victim, this may be readily accomplished with minimal interruption in the sequence of events. This allows the rescuers to perform BLS for longer periods of time by minimizing fatigue.

Practice, practice, and more practice is absolutely essential if the team approach to BLS is to be effective. All members of the dental office staff should be capable of working with each other in either capacity (ventilation or chest compression).

Infant resuscitation *(chart on p. 374)*

For the purposes of BLS technique, the infant is a person under 1 year of age.

Lack of responsiveness is determined by the "shake and shout" technique, as with the adult or child victim. Once unresponsiveness is determined, the rescuer will immediately call for help and place the infant in the supine (horizontal) position.

The airway is opened and assessed for patency (look, listen, and feel, as shown in Fig. 30-16) and the presence or absence of spontaneous ventilation. Three to five seconds are allowed for assessment. Two ventilations are delivered (1 to 1.5 seconds per ventilation) forcefully enough to produce chest inflation and permitting deflation between breaths. Overinflation is dangerous because it produces gastric distention, which reduces the effectiveness of subsequent ventilation and increases the risk of regurgitation. The adult rescuer's mouth can usually cover both the mouth and nose of the infant victim. If this is not possible, mouth-to-mouth or mouth-to-nose ventilation is recommended.

The pulse is next assessed. The brachial artery in the upper portion of the arm (Fig. 30-17) is palpated for 5 to 10 seconds, and if absent, the EMS system is activated and external chest compression is begun. The proper site for finger placement is midsternum one finger's width below the intermammary line (Fig. 30-10). The chest is compressed at a rate of 100 per minute (5 in 3 seconds or less) with one ventilation interspersed after every fifth compression (ratio of 5:1). The depth of compression of the infant's chest is ½ to 1 inch (1.3 to 2.5 cm), using the fleshy tips of two or three fingers held in the long axis of the sternum.

After 10 cycles (approximately 45 seconds) and periodically thereafter, the patient is reevaluated for the return of pulse and/or respiration.

Child resuscitation *(chart on p. 375)*

For the purposes of basic life support technique, the child is a person between the ages of 1 and 8 years.

Basic procedures for resuscitation of the child are similar to those previously described for the adult and infant.

The shake and shout maneuver is employed to determine lack of responsiveness, help is called for, and the patient is placed in the supine position.

The airway of the child is maintained by head tilt–chin lift and is then assessed for the presence of

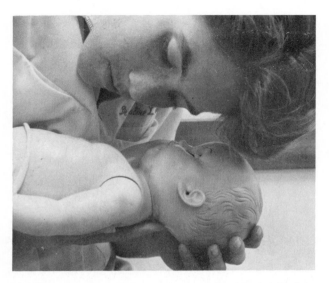

Fig. 30-16. Assess airway (look, listen, and feel) in infant victim.

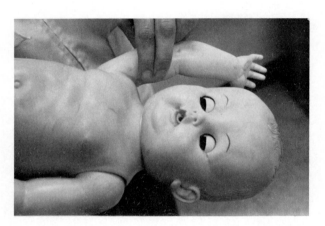

Fig. 30-17. Brachial artery in upper arm is assessed for pulse (5 to 10 seconds).

spontaneous respiratory efforts (look, listen, and feel). If absent, two full ventilations are provided.

The carotid pulse is assessed for 5 to 10 seconds, and if absent, the EMS system is activated and external chest compressions are begun. Proper hand position for the child is located by placing the middle finger into the lower border of the sternum (as in the adult) and placing the heel of one hand onto the sternum immediately superior to the index finger. The sternum is compressed 1 to 1½ inches (2.5 to 3.8 cm) at a ratio of 5 compressions to 1 ventilation, at a rate of 80 to 100 compressions per minute (5 every 3 to 4 seconds).

After 10 cycles (60 to 87 seconds) and periodically thereafter, the patient should be evaluated for the return of spontaneous pulse and/or respiration.

Monitored-Witnessed Cardiac Arrest

The monitored-witnessed cardiac arrest is one in which cardiopulmonary arrest develops in a patient who has been monitored by means of electrocardiograph and the rescuer or rescuers are able to reach the victim and begin basic life support procedures within 60 seconds of the collapse. In this sequence, the myocardium is presumed to be fairly well oxygenated because of the short period of time elapsed since the collapse. Because of this, it is possible that a small electrical stimulus delivered to the myocardium may convert ventricular tachycardia, complete AV block, or ventricular fibrillation. This stimulus may be provided by the precordial thump. As mentioned previously, most situations of cardiac arrest in the dental setting are witnessed, but few patients are monitored. Therefore the unwitnessed sequence for BLS should be employed.

Precordial thump

In the monitored-witnessed cardiac arrest, the sequence of steps in BLS is altered slightly to allow for a precordial thump to be delivered. The precordial thump, applied to the midsternum immediately following collapse, creates a small electrical stimulus that may be effective in reestablishing effective circulation in situations such as ventricular asystole caused by heart block and in reversing ventricular tachycardia or ventricular fibrillation of recent onset.

The precordial thump should be used to provide a stimulus to a potentially reactive heart. *The precordial thump is not a substitute for effective external chest compression.* In addition, only *one* precordial thump should be employed. After carrying out the precordial thump, the sequence of BLS previously described is begun; if pulse is absent, closed chest compression is immediately started.

The precordial thump is carried out as follows (Fig. 30-18): The rescuer holds a closed fist approximately 8 to 12 inches above the midpoint of the victim's sternum, with the fleshy portion of the fist facing the chest. A single, sharp, quick blow (thump) is then delivered to the sternum. If there is no immediate response (carotid pulse not present), external chest compression is started.

Evaluation of Effectiveness

It is important to evaluate the status of the victim during the administration of BLS. This evaluation determines the effectiveness of the efforts being applied and determines if the victim resumes spontaneous and effective respiratory movements and cardiac function. There are four indicators that may be observed: the color of the skin and mucous membranes, the carotid pulse, respiratory movements, and the pupils of the eye. Depending on the number of rescuers present, this monitoring may be continually or periodically carried out.

With only one rescuer present, the color of the skin and mucous membranes is the only continually observable indicator of effectiveness. With effec-

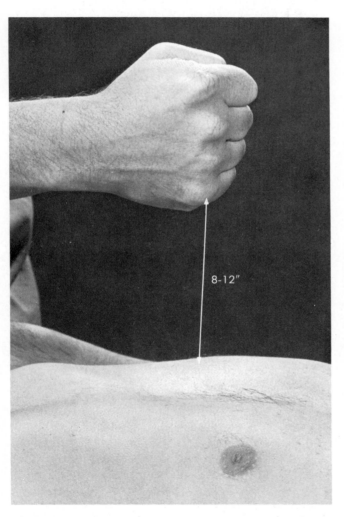

8-12″

Fig. 30-18. Precordial thump used only in monitored-witnessed cardiac arrest.

tive BLS the skin and mucous membranes should lose any cyanotic or dusky gray coloration and return to a more normal color. When performing BLS alone, it is suggested that the rescuer pause after the first minute to check for the carotid pulse (maximum 5 seconds) and observe for spontaneous respiratory movements. Subsequently the rescuer should check these indicators every 4 to 5 minutes. *Never pause for more than 5 seconds at a time, because during this time blood flow drops to zero.*

With a second rescuer present it becomes possible to monitor these important indicators with minimal interruption. The ventilation rescuer is able to monitor these indicators, as well as determine the effectiveness of external chest compression. With a finger located on the carotid artery of the victim, a pulsation should be felt with each compression. After the first minute and every 4 to 5 minutes thereafter, the sequence may be stopped (for no more than 5 seconds) to permit a determination of the effectiveness of the BLS techniques (color of skin and mucous membranes, presence or absence of spontaneous respiration, presence or absence of spontaneous cardiac rhythm, and pupillary reaction). The two-rescuer sequence described previously has a built-in delay that allows for monitoring of both respiratory and cardiac effectiveness.

Pupillary reaction to light is frequently employed as an indicator of the effectiveness of BLS. Pupils normally respond to light by constricting (narrowing). In the unconscious individual, pupils dilate. This is an indication that the brain is receiving a less than adequate supply of oxygen. If the pupils constrict when exposed to light, that is a sign that oxygenation and cerebral blood flow are adequate. Widely dilated pupils that do not react to light indicate that serious brain damage has occurred or is imminent. Pupils that are dilated but that react to light are a less ominous sign.

Pupillary response should *not* become the primary indicator of effectiveness of life support efforts. Many factors may produce variations in normal pupillary response, and for this reason it is recommended that other, more reliable factors such as skin color, respiratory movement, and cardiac activity be employed. In older persons it is not uncommon to have variations in pupillary reaction, and it is very common for alterations to occur in persons who are receiving medications (atropine and narcotic analgesics, for example).

Beginning and Termination of BLS

BLS is most effective if begun immediately after cardiac arrest has occurred. If cardiac arrest has existed for 10 minutes or more, it is highly unlikely that the victim's central nervous system will be restored to its pre–cardiac arrest status. However, individual cases are reported in the literature of effective resuscitation with little or no residual central nervous system deficit after long periods of time (1 hour and longer), usually in situations of hypothermia (submergence in cold water). Therefore it is recommended that the steps of BLS be started on all victims of cardiac arrest when any doubt exists as to the duration of the arrest. The victim should be given the benefit of the doubt when the decision must be made whether or not to start BLS.

Once cardiopulmonary resuscitation has been started, it must be continued until one of the following occurs: (1) the victim begins adequate spontaneous respiratory movement and/or adequate

---

MANAGEMENT OF CARDIAC ARREST

Unwitnessed cardiac arrest and witnessed, unmonitored cardiac arrest

Step 1 Recognize unconsciousness
  2 Position victim and call for assistance
  3 Open airway
     Head tilt–chin lift
     Check for breathing
  4 Jaw thrust maneuver (if needed)
     Assess breathing (if needed)
  5 Artificial ventilation
     Two full inflations, permitting deflation
  6 Assess circulation
     Palpate carotid pulse
  7 External chest compression
     Locate pressure point
     Hand position: heel of hand on chest (for adult)
     Application of pressure: compress sternum 1½ to 2 inches (adult)
     Rate of compression: 80-100 compressions per minute
     Single rescuer: 15 compressions, 2 ventilations
     Team rescue: 5 compressions, 1 ventilation

circulation is restored, (2) a second individual who is equally well trained in BLS is available to assist or take over the efforts of the first individual, (3) a physician arrives on the scene and assumes overall responsibility, (4) the victim is transferred to an emergency care facility that is able to continue with basic life support and/or advanced life support, or (5) the rescuer is exhausted and is physically unable to continue with resuscitation.

The last factor is not as unlikely as it might at first seem. BLS is strenuous exercise. Cases have been reported in which the rescuer has suffered cardiac arrest during the performance of BLS, with both persons subsequently dying. This factor should further motivate the doctor to see to it that all members of the dental office staff are fully trained in all BLS procedures.

Transport of Victim

The victim of cardiac arrest is ultimately transferred from the scene of the incident (that is, the dental office) to the emergency room of a hospital, where advanced life support is available (electrocardiography, defibrillation, and additional drugs to control acidosis and/or dysrhythmias). The doctor should accompany the victim in the ambulance to the hospital, assisting with BLS or overseeing its administration by other individuals (paramedics) until the victim is under the care of a physician.

Availability of Training

Training in the procedures described in this section is essential if they are to be effectively applied in life-threatening situations. Training standards have been established, and many excellent programs in BLS and advanced cardiac life support are available. It is recommended that all individuals receive certification at least annually so that a degree of proficiency may be maintained. For the location of these courses, interested individuals should contact their local dental society, dental school, American Heart Association, or American Red Cross.

BIBLIOGRAPHY

Adgey, A.A., and Partridge, J.F.: Symposium on arteriosclerotic heart disease. The prehospital phase of treatment for myocardial infarction, Geriatrics **27**:102, 1972.

Alexander, S.: Ventricular premature beats, Postgrad. Med. **60**:68, 1976.

American Heart Association: Heart facts: 1984, Dallas, 1984, American Heart Association.

American Heart Association: Instructors manual for basic life support, Dallas, 1985, American Heart Association.

American Heart Association and National Academy of Sciences, National Research Council: Standards for cardiopulmonary resuscitation (CPR) and emergency cardiac care (ECC), JAMA **227**(suppl.):833, 1974.

American Heart Association and National Academy of Sciences, National Research Council: Standards for cardiopulmonary resuscitation (CPR) and emergency cardiac care (ECC), JAMA **255**:2905, 1986.

Babbs, C.F.: New versus old theories of blood flow during CPR, Crit. Care Med. **8**:191, 1980.

Barick, B.L.: How long do you remember lifesaving CPR skills? Phy. Educ. Recreat. **3**:63, 1977.

Carveth, S.W.: Eight year experience with a stadium-based mobile coronary-care unit, Heart Lung **3**:770, 1974.

Carveth, S.W., and others: Training in advanced cardiac life support, JAMA **235**:2311, 1976.

Chiang, B.N., and others: Predisposing factors in sudden cardiac death in Tecumseh, Michigan: a prospective study, Circulation **41**:31, 1970.

Cobb, L.A., Werner, J.A., and Trobaugh, G.B.: Sudden cardiac death. I. A decade's experience with out-of-hospital resuscitation, Med. Concepts Cardiovas. Med. **49**:31, 1980.

Cobb, L.A., Werner, J.A., and Trobaugh, G.B.: Sudden cardiac death. II. Outcome of resuscitation: management and future directions, Med. Concepts Cardiovas. Med. **49**:37, 1980.

Copley, D.P., Mantle, J.A., and Rogers, W.I.: Improved outcome for pre-hospital cardiopulmonary collapse with resuscitation by bystanders, Circulation **56**:901, 1977.

Doyle, J.T.: Mechanisms and prevention of sudden death, Mod. Concepts Cardiovasc. Dis. **45**:111, 1976.

Eisenberg, M.S., Bergner, L., and Hallstrom, A.: Cardiac resuscitation in the community: importance of rapid provision and implications for program planning, JAMA **241**:1905, 1979.

Eliot, R.S.: Emotional stress and cardiac disease, JAMA **236**:2264, 1976.

Engel, G.L.: Psychologic factors in instantaneous cardiac death, editorial, N. Engl. J. Med. **294**:664, 1976.

Feinleib, M., and others: Prodromal symptoms and signs of sudden death, Circulation **52**(suppl. 3):III, 1975.

Frank, J.P., and Friedberg, D.Z.: Syncope with prolonged QT interval, Am. J. Dis. Child **130**:320, 1976.

Freeman, J.W., and Loughhead, M.G.: A coronary care ambulance controlled by radio telemetry, Med. J. Aust. **1**:132, 1975.

Friedman, G.D., Dales, L.G., and Ury, H.K.: Mortality in middle-aged smokers and nonsmokers, N. Engl. J. Med. **300**:213, 1979.

Fulton, M., Julian, D.G., and Oliver, M.F.: Sudden death and myocardial infarction, Circulation **40**(suppl. 4):IV, 1969.

Goldberg, A.H.: Cardiopulmonary arrest, N. Engl. J. Med. **290**:381, 1974.

Goldberger, E.: Treatment of cardiac emergencies, ed. 2, 1977, St. Louis, The C.V. Mosby Co.

Haerem, J.W.: Myocardial lesions in sudden, unexpected coronary death, Am. Heart J. **90**:562, 1975.

Humphries, J.O.: Treatment of non-traumatic cardiac emergencies, Postgrad. Med. **55**:159, 1974.

Inter-Society Commission for Heart Disease Resources Report: Primary prevention of the atherosclerotic diseases, Circulation **42**:3, 1972.

Jude, J.R., and Nagel, E.L.: Cardiopulmonary resuscitation 1970, Mod. Concepts Cardiovasc. Dis. **39**:133, 1970.

Kannel, W., and Gorden, T.: In The Framingham Study: an epidemiological investigation of cardiovascular disease, section 26, Shurtleff, D., editor, Washington, D.C., 1970, U.S. Government Printing Office.

Kay, C.F.: Cardiopulmonary resuscitation: a chain of many links (editorial), Ann. Intern. Med. **80:**411, 1974.

Klebba, A.J., Maurer, J.D., and Glass, E.J.: Mortality trends for leading causes of death: United States, 1950-1969. Vital and Health Statistics Series 20, Pub. No. 16, 1974, U.S. Department of Health, Education, and Welfare, Public Health Service.

Kouwenhoven, W.B., Jude, J.R., and Knickerbocker, G.G.: Closed chest cardiac massage, JAMA **173:**1064, 1960.

Kuller, L.H.: Sudden death—definition and epidemiologic considerations, Prog. Cardiovasc. Dis. **23:**1, 1980.

Kuller, L., Perper, J., and Cooper, M.: Demographic characteristics and trends in arteriosclerotic heart disease mortality: sudden death and myocardial infarction in sudden coronary death outside hospital, Proceedings, Minneapolis, 1974, AHA monograph 47, Dallas, 1975, American Heart Association.

Kushnir, B.: Primary ventricular fibrillation and resumption of work, sexual activity and driving after first acute myocardial infarction, Br. Med. J. **4:**609, 1975.

Lawrie, D.M.: Ventricular fibrillation in acute myocardial infarction, Am. Heart J. **78:**424, 1969.

Lawrie, D.M., and others: Ventricular fibrillation complicating acute myocardial infarction, Lancet **2:**523, 1968.

Loeb, H.S.: Cardiac arrest, JAMA **232:**845, 1975.

Lown, B.: Sudden cardiac death: the major challenge confronting contemporary cardiology, Am. J. Cardiol. **43:**313, 1979.

Lown, B.: Cardiovascular collapse and sudden cardiac death. In Braunwald, E., editor: Heart disease, a textbook of cardiovascular medicine, Philadelphia, 1980, W.B. Saunders Co.

Lund, I., and Skulber, A.: Cardiopulmonary resuscitation by lay people, Lancet **2:**702, 1976.

Maseri, A., and others: Coronary vasospasm as a possible cause of myocardial infarction: a conclusion derived from the study of 'preinfarction' angina, N. Engl. J. Med. **299:**1271, 1978.

McIntyre, K.M., Winslow, E.B.J., and Parker, M.R.: Sudden cardiac death. In Textbook of advanced cardiac life support, Dallas, 1983, American Heart Association.

Moss, A.J.: Prediction and prevention of sudden cardiac death, Annu. Rev. Med. **31:**1, 1980.

Myerberg, R.J., and others: A clinical, electrophysiologic, and hemodynamic profile of patients resuscitated from prehospital cardiac arrest, Am. J. Med. **68:**568, 1980.

Nagel, E.L.: Improving emergency medical care (editorial), N. Engl. J. Med. **302:**1416, 1980.

Nagel, E.L., and others: Emergency care, Circulation **51-52**(suppl. III):216, 1975.

Nalbantgil, I., Yigitbasi, O., and Kiliccioglu, B.: Sudden death with sexual activity, Am. Heart J. **91:**405, 1976.

Neimann, J.T., Garner, D., and Rosborough, J.: The mechanism of blood flow in closed chest cardiopulmonary resuscitation, Circulation **60**(suppl. 2):74, 1979.

Orlowski, J.P.: Optimal position for external cardiac massage in infants and children, Crit. Care Med. **12:**224, 1984.

Pantridge, J.F., and Geddes, J.S.: A mobile intensive care unit in the management of myocardial infarction, Lancet **2:**271, 1967.

Pozen, M.W.: Prehospital coronary care: the current case for a paramedic strategy, Am. J. Public Health **69:**13, 1979.

Rabkin, S.W., Mathewson, F.A.L., and Tate, R.B.: Chronobiology of cardiac sudden death in men, JAMA **244:**1357, 1980.

Ramirez, A., Weaver, F., and Raizner, A.: The efficacy of lay CPR instruction: an evaluation, Am. J. Public Health **67:**1093, 1977.

Renner, W.F.: Emergency medical service: the concept and coronary care, JAMA **230:**251, 1974.

Rudikoff, M.T., Freund, D., and Weisfeldt, M.D.: Mechanism of blood flow during cardiopulmonary resuscitation, Circulation **56**(suppl. 3):97, 1977.

Safer, P.: Cardiopulmonary—cerebral resuscitation including emergency airway control. In Schwartz, G.R., editor: Principles and practice of emergency medicine, Philadelphia, 1978, W.B. Saunders Co.

Salme, M.R., and others: Cardiac arrest related to anesthesia, JAMA **233:**238, 1975.

Shapter, R.K., editor: Cardiopulmonary resuscitation: basic life support, Clin. Symposia **26:**1, 1974.

Stephenson, H.E., Jr.: Cardiac arrest and resuscitation, ed. 4, St. Louis, 1974, The C.V. Mosby Co.

Thomas, C.B.: Precursors of premature disease and death, Ann. Intern. Med. **85:**653, 1976.

Thompson, R.G., Hallstrom, A.P., and Cobb, L.A.: Bystander initiated cardiopulmonary resuscitation in the management of ventricular fibrillation, Ann. Intern. Med. **90:**737, 1979.

Tomme, C.: CPR: a trend in modern dentistry, J. Am. Dent. Assoc. **95:**900, 1977.

Vaisrub, S.: Sudden death and lingering hope (editorial), JAMA **235:**1726, 1976.

Weaver, F.J., and others: Trainees' retention of cardiopulmonary resuscitation, JAMA **241:**901, 1979.

Weinblatt, E., and others: Relation of education to sudden death after myocardial infarction, N. Engl. J. Med. **299:**60, 1978.

Winslow, E.B.J.: Saving lives? (editorial), JAMA **241:**929, 1979.

QUICK-REFERENCE SECTION TO LIFE-THREATENING SITUATIONS

Section II

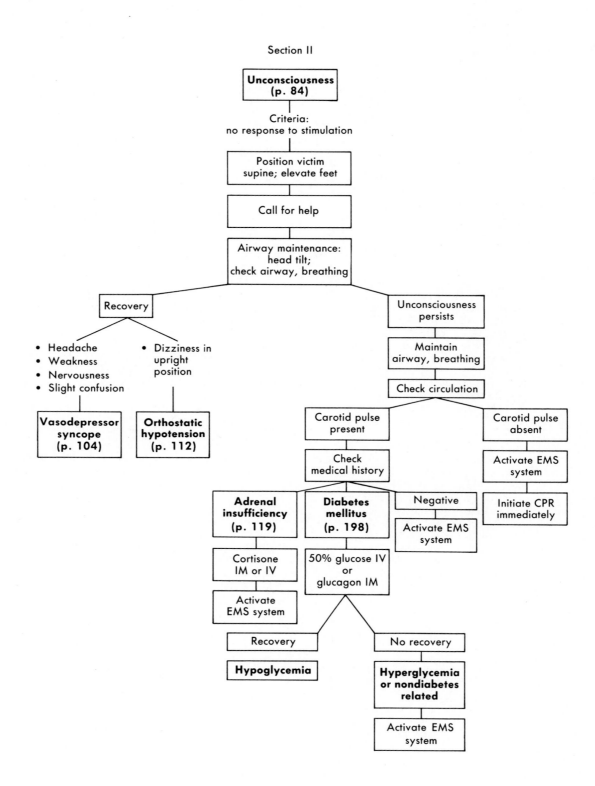

Section III

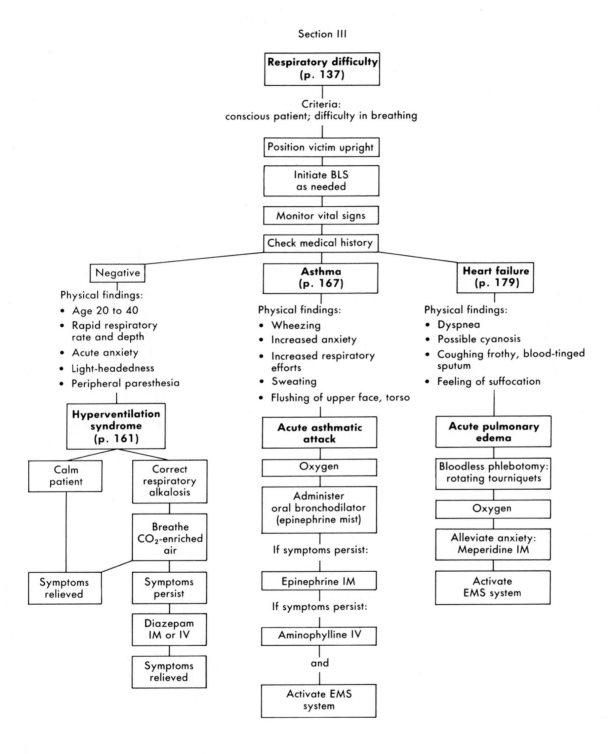

Respiratory difficulty
(p. 137)

Criteria:
conscious patient; difficulty in breathing

Position victim upright

Initiate BLS
as needed

Monitor vital signs

Check medical history

Negative

Physical findings:
- Age 20 to 40
- Rapid respiratory
  rate and depth
- Acute anxiety
- Light-headedness
- Peripheral paresthesia

Hyperventilation
syndrome
(p. 161)

Calm
patient

Correct
respiratory
alkalosis

Breathe
CO_2-enriched
air

Symptoms
relieved

Symptoms
persist

Diazepam
IM or IV

Symptoms
relieved

Asthma
(p. 167)

Physical findings:
- Wheezing
- Increased anxiety
- Increased respiratory
  efforts
- Sweating
- Flushing of upper face, torso

Acute asthmatic
attack

Oxygen

Administer
oral bronchodilator
(epinephrine mist)

If symptoms persist:

Epinephrine IM

If symptoms persist:

Aminophylline IV

and

Activate EMS
system

Heart failure
(p. 179)

Physical findings:
- Dyspnea
- Possible cyanosis
- Coughing frothy, blood-tinged
  sputum
- Feeling of suffocation

Acute pulmonary
edema

Bloodless phlebotomy:
rotating tourniquets

Oxygen

Alleviate anxiety:
Meperidine IM

Activate
EMS system

Section IV

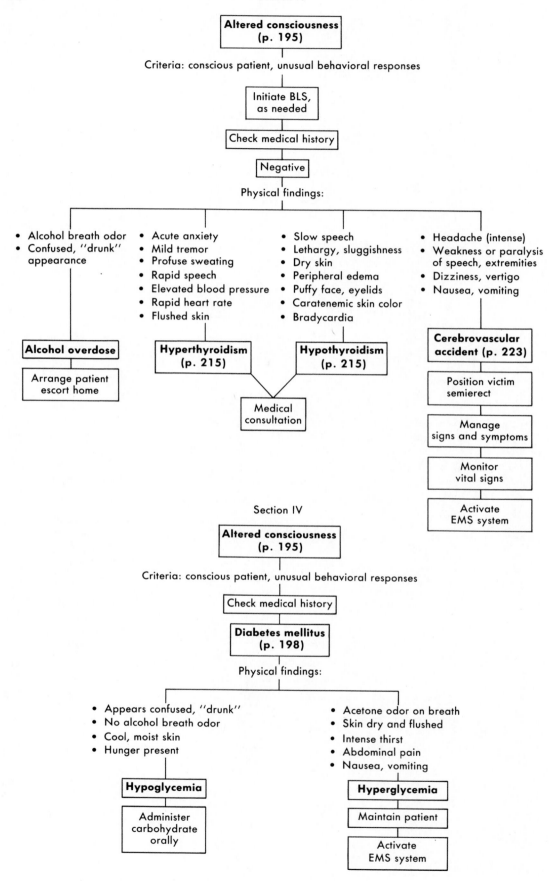

Altered consciousness (p. 195)

Criteria: conscious patient, unusual behavioral responses

Initiate BLS, as needed

Check medical history

Negative

Physical findings:

- Alcohol breath odor
- Confused, "drunk" appearance

- Acute anxiety
- Mild tremor
- Profuse sweating
- Rapid speech
- Elevated blood pressure
- Rapid heart rate
- Flushed skin

- Slow speech
- Lethargy, sluggishness
- Dry skin
- Peripheral edema
- Puffy face, eyelids
- Caratenemic skin color
- Bradycardia

- Headache (intense)
- Weakness or paralysis of speech, extremities
- Dizziness, vertigo
- Nausea, vomiting

Alcohol overdose

Arrange patient escort home

Hyperthyroidism (p. 215)

Hypothyroidism (p. 215)

Medical consultation

Cerebrovascular accident (p. 223)

Position victim semierect

Manage signs and symptoms

Monitor vital signs

Activate EMS system

Section IV

Altered consciousness (p. 195)

Criteria: conscious patient, unusual behavioral responses

Check medical history

Diabetes mellitus (p. 198)

Physical findings:

- Appears confused, "drunk"
- No alcohol breath odor
- Cool, moist skin
- Hunger present

- Acetone odor on breath
- Skin dry and flushed
- Intense thirst
- Abdominal pain
- Nausea, vomiting

Hypoglycemia

Administer carbohydrate orally

Hyperglycemia

Maintain patient

Activate EMS system

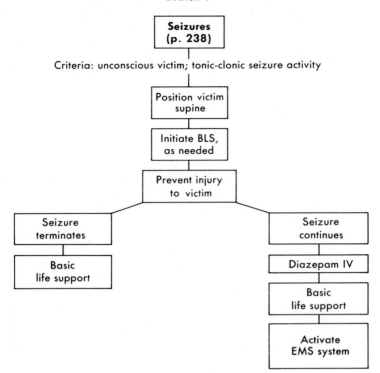

Seizures
(p. 238)

Criteria: unconscious victim; tonic-clonic seizure activity

Position victim
supine

Initiate BLS,
as needed

Prevent injury
to victim

Seizure
terminates

Basic
life support

Seizure
continues

Diazepam IV

Basic
life support

Activate
EMS system

Section VI

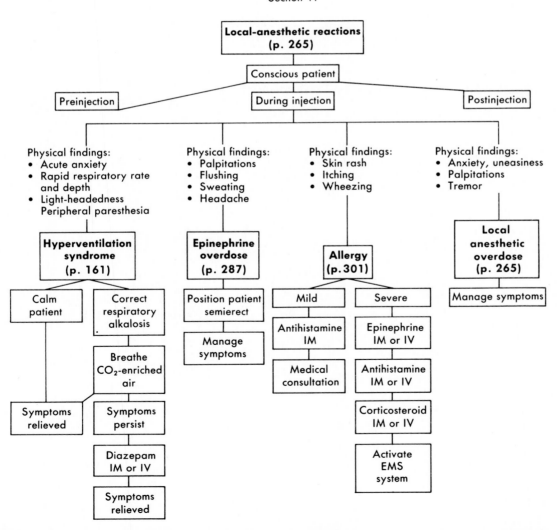

Local-anesthetic reactions
(p. 265)

Conscious patient

Preinjection

During injection

Postinjection

Physical findings:
• Acute anxiety
• Rapid respiratory rate
  and depth
• Light-headedness
  Peripheral paresthesia

Physical findings:
• Palpitations
• Flushing
• Sweating
• Headache

Physical findings:
• Skin rash
• Itching
• Wheezing

Physical findings:
• Anxiety, uneasiness
• Palpitations
• Tremor

Hyperventilation
syndrome
(p. 161)

Epinephrine
overdose
(p. 287)

Allergy
(p.301)

Local
anesthetic
overdose
(p. 265)

Calm
patient

Correct
respiratory
alkalosis

Position patient
semierect

Mild

Severe

Manage symptoms

Antihistamine
IM

Epinephrine
IM or IV

Manage
symptoms

Medical
consultation

Antihistamine
IM or IV

Breathe
CO$_2$-enriched
air

Symptoms
relieved

Symptoms
persist

Corticosteroid
IM or IV

Diazepam
IM or IV

Activate
EMS
system

Symptoms
relieved

Section VI

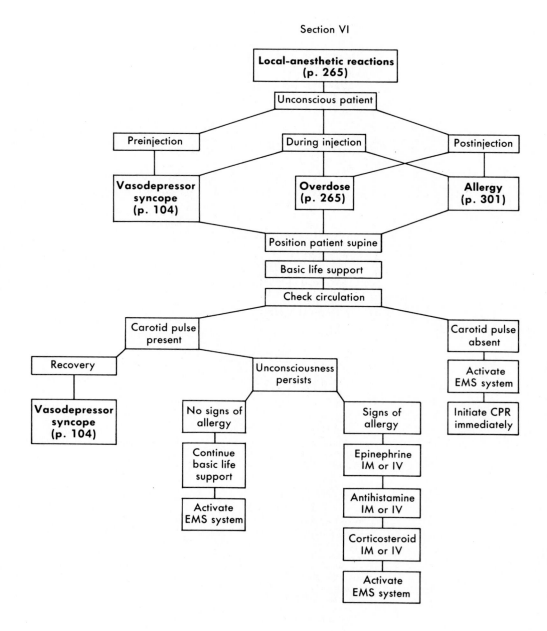

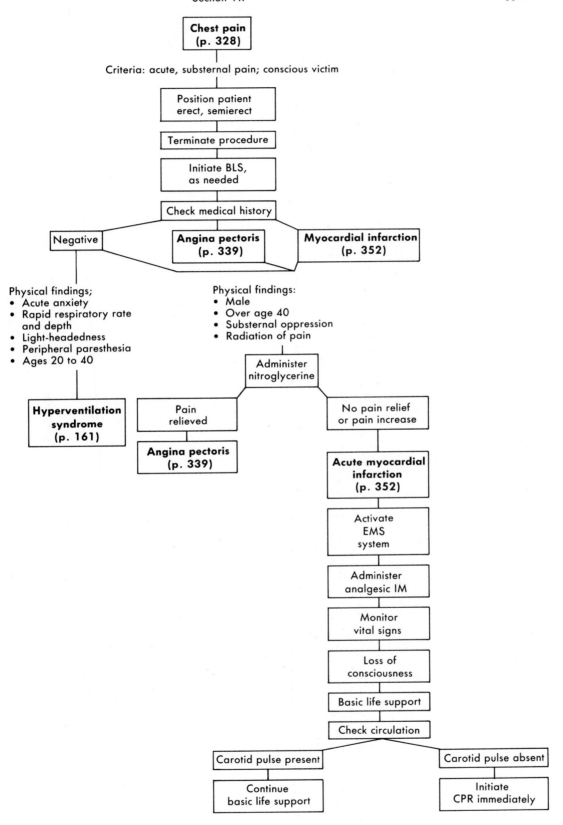

Index

Notes

Notes

Notes

Notes

Notes

Notes

Notes

Notes

Notes

Notes